Rail123

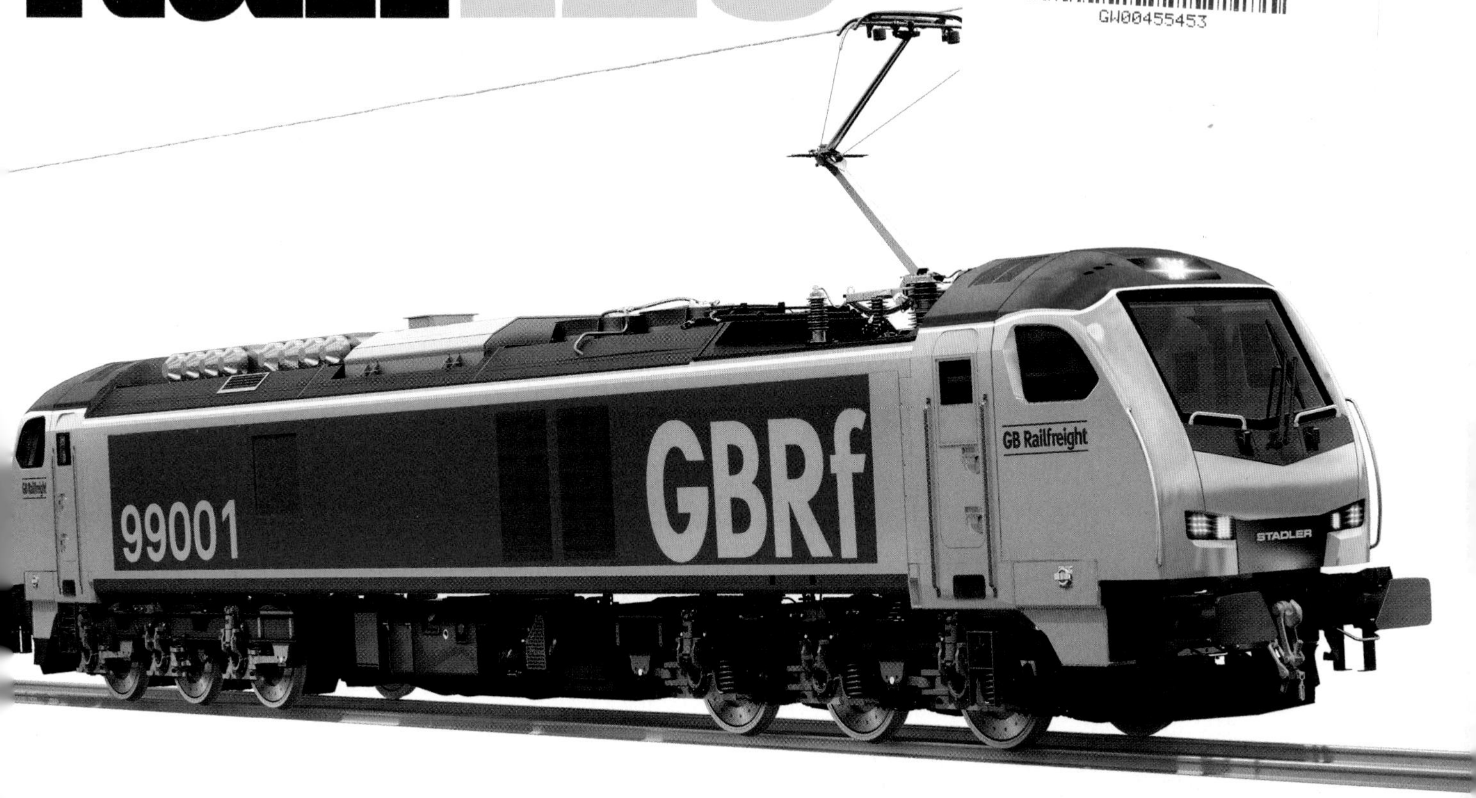

Welcome to Rail123

I am delighted to welcome readers to the 2022-2023 edition of *Rail 123*, the only annual publication produced covering all locomotives and multiple units, either in main line service, industrial use or preserved in one listing.

For many years, the main line railways and the preservation/industrial users had a very different following and thus the enthusiast publications followed the same style, but today with such a large and varied number of operators, with many 'preserved' locos and trains authorised for main line operation we considered the time was right to join all the information together in one publication. So therefore one list is provided for each class, listing main line operational, preserved, exported and industrial fleets. After considerable thought, colour coding is used to quickly identify the status of each vehicle. Full details of the colour coding used is given in the introduction section.

Since the publication of Rail 123 in summer 2021, some 8,000 changes have been recorded and advised by the rail industry, this covers withdrawn stock, new vehicles or train sets and changes to liveries, equipment and allocations. While we aim to be as up to date as possible upon publication, the rail fleets are fluid and changes are recorded most days. In the coming months we expect to see many older trains and those stored, make their final journey to the scrap yards. New trains are continuing to be delivered, with new fleets for Transport for Wales, Merseyrail and South Western Railway being handed over most months. New loco and train orders have also been placed in the 2021-2022 period, with stock for HS2 ordered from Alstom/Hitachi and new Class 93 and 99 bi-mode locomotives from Stadler.

With all these changes, the ongoing interest in railways continues, with many new enthusiasts now following the modern rail scene, this is most encouraging, after a period when interest was declining.

Rail 123 continues to give the full details of light railways and metro systems, as well as the fleets in operation on the Isle of Man and Ireland.

I hope you continue to enjoy following railways, but please keep safe while participating in your hobby.

Colin J Marsden, Editor

Editor: Colin J. Marsden
E-Mail: colin.marsden@keypublishing.com
Senior Editor Bookazines/Specials: Roger Mortimer
Publisher: Jonathan Jackson
Head of Advertising Sales: Brodie Baxter
Head of Marketing: Shaun Binnington
Head of Publishing: Finbarr O'Reilly
Group CEO: Adrian Cox

Key Publishing Ltd, PO Box 100, Stamford, Lincolnshire, PE9 1XQ.
Telephone +44 (0) 1780 755131
Fax: +44 (0)1780 757261
E-mail: enquiries@keypublishing.com
www.keypublishing.com

Printing and Origination:
Printed in Great Britain by Precision Colour Print, Telford and produced by The Railway Centre, Dawlish, Devon

ISBN: 978 1 80282 225 0

Information in Rail123 correct to 1 June 2022

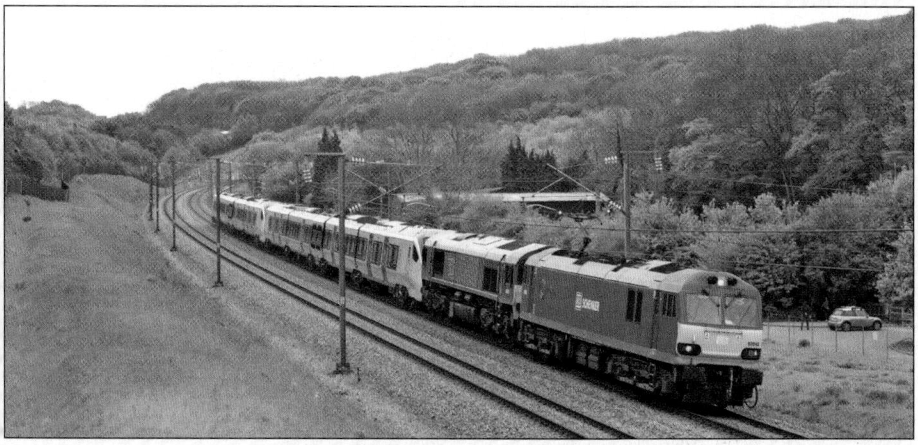

Top: *The big loco news in spring 2022 was the ordering by Beacon Rail/GBRf of 30 Class 99 Co-Co bi-mode locos. This is the artist's impression of how the class will look. The first loco is due in the UK in 2025.* **Stadler**

Left: *New trains continue to be delivered to the UK. Here a pair of Stadler 'Flirt' Class 231s Nos. 230006/005 are hauled over HS1 at Nashenden on 2 May 2022 led by Nos. 92042 and 66001.* **Jamie Squibbs**

Cover: *Freightliner Class 66/5 No. 66537 stops for a crew change at Ipswich on 18 September 2021, while powering the 08.25 Crewe Basford Hall to Felixstowe North Terminal container train. The loco sports modified two section head, marker/tail light assemblies and is viewed from the silencer end.* **CJM**

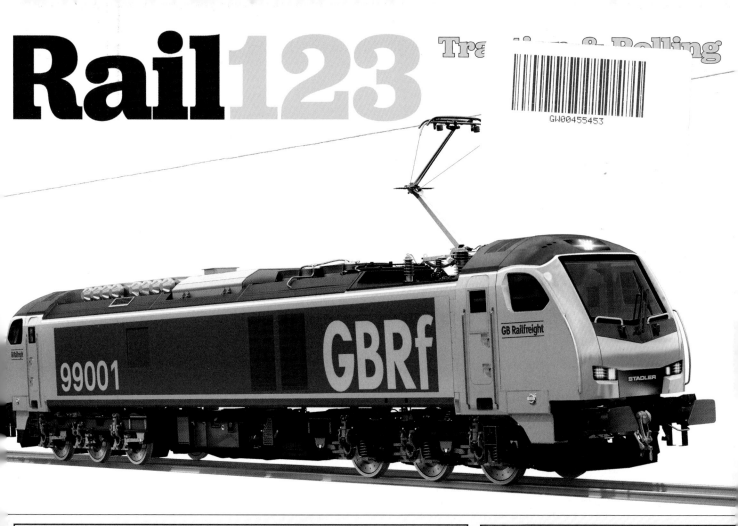

Contents

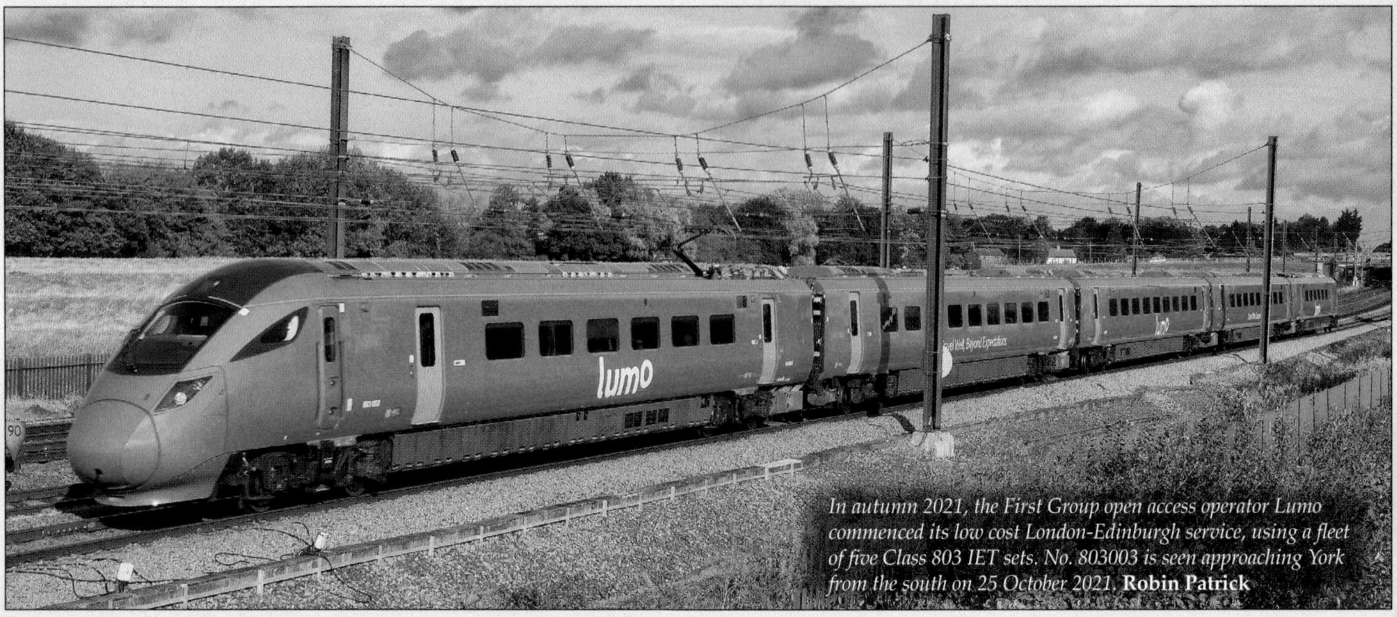

In autumn 2021, the First Group open access operator Lumo commenced its low cost London-Edinburgh service, using a fleet of five Class 803 IET sets. No. 803003 is seen approaching York from the south on 25 October 2021. **Robin Patrick**

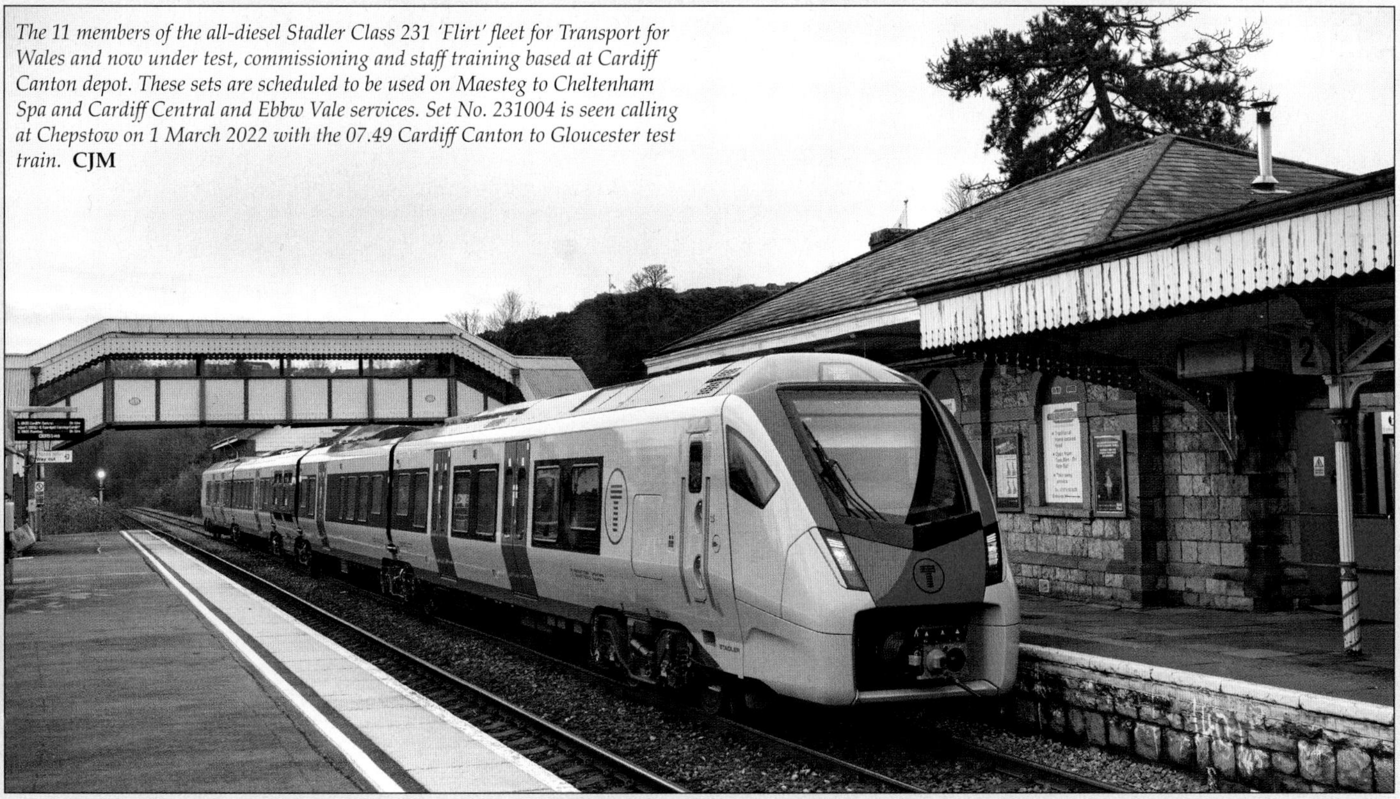

The 11 members of the all-diesel Stadler Class 231 'Flirt' fleet for Transport for Wales and now under test, commissioning and staff training based at Cardiff Canton depot. These sets are scheduled to be used on Maesteg to Cheltenham Spa and Cardiff Central and Ebbw Vale services. Set No. 231004 is seen calling at Chepstow on 1 March 2022 with the 07.49 Cardiff Canton to Gloucester test train. **CJM**

Coaching Stock

Network Rail Equipment

EuroTunnel

Metro & Light Rail

Irish Railways

Isle of Man Railways

Steam Preservation

Codes and Data

The Editor would like to thank the many railway industry staff who have assisted with information for this publication. With special thanks to Antony Christie, Nathan Williamson, Cliff Beeton and Keith Ewins, who have provided considerable help and assistance.

Operational Issues 2022

The past year, between summer 2021 and June 2022 has been a very difficult time for all UK railways, National Rail and the private sector including preservation. The Covid-19 Pandemic has continued with new mutations, seeing many travel restrictions imposed and the extension of the 'work from home' policy of the Government. This led to a considerable reduction in the number of passengers, in both the commuter and leisure markets. The downturn in passenger numbers led to a much reduced timetable introduced by all operators, with a corresponding reduction in the number of trains required. Most operators stored trains or rotated them through stored/operational status to keep fleets in a working condition.

At the end of April 2021 the railway industry, especially Great Western and LNER, was hit with a major problem, when serious cracks were identified in the aluminium frame members of Class 80x IET stock. The problem was so serious that the entire fleet was grounded for a short while, so an investigation could took place and a remedial action plan put into place. After a few weeks sets were returned to traffic, subject to a constant inspection process. The worst affected sets sidelined. It took a long time to set up a repair process, work which will get underway in spring 2022, a project likely to take several years to complete.

As detailed below in the fleet review section, new trains, especially those of the Alstom (Bombardier) 'Aventra' family have taken a very long time to be accepted, commissioned and introduced. The large number of Class 720 sets for Greater Anglia are now in service and performing well, with the entire fleet due in service this year. However, the huge fleet of Class 701 suburban replacement stock for South Western Railway are still awaited, while some 30+ sets have been delivered and used for test running, none have been accepted for service and no SWR staff training has yet commenced. These trains are now more than two years late and in early summer 2022 no planned introduction date had been announced.

Rail freight has remained buoyant, with more services and tonnage moved in the past 12 months higher than the year before. Several new flows have been won by rail and more are in the pipeline.

Traction & Rolling Stock – Locomotives

During the 2021-2022 period, several major changes have taken place in the rolling stock fleets, with some new classes introduced, older fleets withdrawn and continued delivery of new or rebuilt stock.

On a class by class basis, the **Class 08-09** shunting locos continue in mainly smaller business ownership, rather than be owned by major companies. This is a low-cost, risk-reduced option, with major hauliers not wishing to own terminal power. In places, main line locos perform shunting duties, even operating trip workings. However, in yards and terminals were shunting is required, specialist providers of such locos, such as Rail Supply Services (RSS), hold contracts to provide power at the times required. Some of the main freight operators, such as Freightliner and GB Railfreight still own a small level of shunting power.

A new class of loco entered traffic in 2021-2022 with the first of 15 **Class 18** Bo-Bo battery/hybrid locos built by Clayton of type CBD90 entering service with GB Railfreight for a trial period. The fleet is owned by Beacon Rail and will be offered on a hire basis.

The **Class 20** fleet is down to under 25 main line authorised locos, of which only around 12 are currently operational. DRS divested of the class in 2021. Several are privately owned and available for spot-hire contracts.

Just four **Class 33s** remain main line certified, working West Coast Railway, with one owned by 71A Locomotives Ltd at Swanage, this can be used for main line charter or spot hire work.

The ever popular English Electric Type 3 **Class 37** fleet still continues in front line service. Examples are operated by Colas Rail Freight, Direct Rail Services, Loco Services Ltd, Rail Operations Group, West Coast Railway, Europhoenix and UK Rail Leasing, with the fleet operating to all corners of the network. Many '37s' are in the hands of the preservation sector, with most in full running order. National Collection loco D6700 was in early 2022 leased to the Heavy Tractor Group at the Great Central Railway for a return to operation.

Class 40s, still very popular, is represented by two main line certified locos, one with Loco Services Ltd, the other with the Class 40 Preservation Society, several others are preserved.

The **HST**, or **Class 43** fleet has seen continuing changes. Three main stream operators still operate the type, Great Western, CrossCountry and Scottish Railways. These operate with power door fitted stock. Some former East Midlands '43s' operate with Data Acquisition & Testing Services (DATS) for test train use. While the former buffer-fitted power cars are now operated by European-owned Rail Adventure, operated as loco-pairs for powering new and overhauled stock in the UK and possibly main land Europe. Loco Services Ltd also operate a small HST fleet for their Midland Pullman and Staycation train sets.

The New Measurement Train continues to work with Class 43s as its prime motive power. The three regular power cars are being fitted with the latest European Rail Traffic Management System (ERTMS) and two extra ex-LNER vehicles Nos. 43290/299 were leased in 2021.

A fleet of 34 **Class 47s** were still authorised for main line operation in spring 2022, working for both passenger and freight sectors, operating for West Coast Railway, Freightliner, Loco Services Ltd, Vintage Trains, Harry Needle Railroad and GB Railfreight. A large number of Class 47s are operational in preservation.

The big **Class 50s** news in the last year has been the return to main line service of Hanson & Hall Rail / Rail Adventure No. 50008 *Thunderer* now panted in a new grey livery. GB Railfreight continue their partnership with the Class 50 Alliance, with two members working on an 'as required' basis. The Class 50 Alliance locos carry full GBRf livery.

The **Class 56** fleet remain working for Colas Rail Freight, DC Rail and GBRf. With at least 10 converted or due to be converted to Class 69s.

Three sub-class of **Class 57** still operate. Three members of the Class 57/0 sub-class are operational, two with Direct Rail Services and one with West Coast Railway. A number of the DRS locos were up for sale in early 2022. The Class 57/3 sub-class are operated by Direct Rail Services, Rail Operations Group and West Coast Railway. The DRS locos have fully operational drop-head Dellner couplings for powering Class 390s on the West Coast. The ROG locos are used to power stock transfer moves, where their drop-head auto couplers of both the Dellner and Tightlock type are used. West Coast Railway operate four Class 57/3s and one 57/6 on charter services. Great Western Railway operate four Class 57/6s on Night Riviera services between Paddington and Penzance. But in early 2022 First Group asked for expressions of interest in supply new locos for the TransPennine and Great Western routes. These are to be bi-mode electric and auxiliary power.

All but one **Class 59** are now under control of Freightliner, who use the 14 locos on Mendip aggregate duties. No. 59003 is operated by GB Railfreight, usually based in the Westbury area and used on engineering trains.

The reduced ranks of **Class 60s** remain much the same, with DB Cargo operating a fleet of 'Super-60s', refurbished a few years ago. DC Rail (Cappaga) and GB Railfreight also operate small fleets, to power heavy services, where the superior hauling power of the design can be put to good advantage. A large number of scrap examples can be found at Toton, it is unlikely that any will be returned to use, a small number are preserved.

UKs largest fleet (in terms of fleet size), the **Class 66,** continues to provide the backbone of freight power for the main operators, DB Cargo, Freghtliner, GB Railfreight, Colas Rail Freight and Direct Rail Services. The largest operator is DB-Cargo, which in addition to the UK, operates a fleet in France and Poland (although the French fleet has reduced in 2021-2022). GB Railfreight continue to expand their freight operations and have continued to seek extra locos. In 2020-2021 a number of Beacon Rail owned Class 66s which were originally delivered to Mainland Europe, have been transferred to GBRf and shipped to the UK. To meet UK operating requirements the locos have to be heavily modified, this work is done at Progress Rail in Longport and the EMD facility at Roberts Road, Doncaster. In an attempt to be more green, several examples have been modified to operate on Hydro-treated Vegetable Oil (HVO) in place of pure diesel fuel.

The 125mph **Class 67s**, which seldom if ever see post 100mph use, continue to work limited services, with many stored. Some locos have recently been modified to work with Transport for Wales Mk4 stock, with extra jumper sockets on the nose end, these have emerged in white and red TfL livery. Other locos continue to operate limited DB-C services, charter trains, the Royal Train as required and the Belmond Pullman. The two locos previously operated by Colas Rail Freight (Nos. 67023/027) have now been transferred to GB Railfreight for Caledonian Sleeper use.

The Direct Rail Services operated **Class 68** fleet of Vossloh/Stadler Type 5s, operate DRS freight services, as well as providing power for the TransPennine Express Mk5 stock, usually working on the Scarborough to Liverpool Lime Street corridor. This service has never been fully introduced due to operational problems, compounded by Covid-19. A small number of locos are leased to Chiltern Railways for Mk3 loco-hauled services, a contract due to end in autumn 2022.

Still the biggest loco news story in 2021-2022 is the conversion of **Class 69** locos, using body-shells from withdrawn Class 56s and installing EMD 710 series power units, of the same type in the Class 66. This is a major, multi-million pound project, being undertaken by Progress Rail at their Longport factory. By early summer five locos had been completed and in traffic based at Tonbridge, all carry different liveries. The driving cabs have been totally redesigned with the original desk replaced with a Class

66 style pedestal. The front ends have been redesigned, with the original horn box removed. A new AAR style jumper socket is centrally mounted, with two head/marker/tail light assemblies on each side. A high level (just below cab window height) marker light is also provided.

The General Electric-built **Class 70** fleet continues to operate with Freightliner and Colas Rail Freight, the Freightliner numbers were reduced during the peak of the Covid-19 lock down restrictions, but by summer 2022 locos are back is service.

The largest user of the dual-power **Class 73** fleet, introduced by BR Southern Region in the 1960s, is GB Railfreight. The 73/1s are operated on general freight/departmental services, while a batch of Class 73/9s are used by GBRf on Network Rail contracts. A fleet of six Class 73/9s are deployed by GBRf to power the internal Scottish legs of the Caledonian Sleeper operation and are out-based at Craigentinny. These locos have been considerably modified, with revised cabs and AAR jumper connections. Network Rail also operate a pair of heavily rebuilt 7395x locos, these are fitted with two Cummins QSK19 engines and are totally different to the GBRf rebuilds. This pair are based at the Railway Technical Centre, Derby.

In early 2021, Freightliner operated **Class 86/6s** were phased out of service, following introduction of Class 90s, inherited from Greater Anglia. The Freightliner Class 86s were stored in spring 2021, if an upturn in business materialises, some might be fully refurbished and returned to traffic. One loco has been placed on display at the Crewe Heritage Centre. Three Class 86s remain in passenger service, one with Loco Services Ltd, one with private owner Les Ross and the third with West Coast Railway.

Crewe-based Loco Services Ltd operate the sole remaining operational **Class 87**, No. 87002, previously been used by GB Railfreight on Caledonian Sleeper duties. LSL have overhauled and repainted the loco into full InterCity 'Swallow' livery and is now operated on charter services.

Direct Rail Services have a fleet of ten, high-output, bi-mode (electro-diesel) locomotives of **Class 88**, these are an electric loco with a secondary diesel engine for yard, trip or 'last mile' duties. The design is based on the Class 68, with which they can operate in multiple.

In 2020-2021, following the introduction of Stadler 'Flirt' EMUs. Of the 15 Greater Anglia **Class 90s**, 13 were taken were sold to Freightliner, bolstering their fleet and helped to replace Class 86s. DB-Cargo continue operate a fleet of Class 90s, mainly on freight/charter operations on the West Coast route, with many locos long out of service and stored.

Full introduction of IET Class 80x fleets, saw the ending of **Class 91** operations on the LNER route in 2021 during the downturn of train running due to Covid-19. However the fleet returned to front line use in June 2021 and in April/May 2022 five locos and Mk4 sets are in daily use.

The **Class 92** fleet has never been used to its full potential, designed for Channel Tunnel operations between the UK and France, the fleet saw a reduced level of work following the abandonment of overnight 'Nightstar' services. Many locos were stored and in summer 2022 only a handful are operational with DB-Cargo. Several operate with GB Railfreight, with some working freight services and others the Edinburgh/Glasgow to London legs of the Caledonian sleeper operation. A number of locos have been exported to Europe. Eight are to be refurbished by DB for domestic freight operations.

In early 2021, it was announced that Rail Operations Group, with funding from Star Capital, were to invest in up to 30 tri-mode **Class 93** locos. Based on the Class 88, the design will be a Bo-Bo with a top speed of 110mph, with an electric output of 4000kW. It will also house a Caterpillar C32 diesel, with an output of 900kW. In addition, two battery backs will be able to deliver 400kW, which can either be used to power the loco directly, or in harness with the diesel engine to give an output of 1,300kW. The first locos are now under production at the Stadler plant in Valencia, Spain, the first loco is due in the UK in the first quarter of 2023. Initially 10 locos are to be built, the remaining 20 are covered by a framework contract.

The big locomotive news in 2022 was the announcement on 30 April that GB Railfreight, through a funding package with Beacon Rail, had ordered 30 Stadler Co-Co electro-diesel locos of **Class 99** to cover business growth as well as a replacement for some Class 66s. The locos with have a 6,000kW output on electric as well as a 2,413hp (1,800kW) Cummins V12 diesel. The fleet will be built in Spain, with the first due in the UK in 2025.

Traction & Rolling Stock – Diesel Units

During 2021 we finally saw the end of 'Pacer' operations. All except a handful of Transport for Wales Class 143s were withdrawn at the end of December 2020, with the remaining sets displaced in spring 2021. However, the pacer story does not end there. A considerable number of Class 142, 143 and 144 sets have either been preserved or sold for re use in one form or another, full details are give in the fleet listings.

So far, none have returned to main line use, but this should not be ruled out.

The unique, **Class 139**, fleet of two vehicles, continues to operate on the Stourbridge Junction to Stourbridge Town 'shuttle'. The backbone of many regional services are still operated by the fleet of 1980s introduced **Class 150** design stock. Now refurbished, they operate for Northern (the largest user), Great Western and Transport for Wales. Northern operates all Class 150/0, 150/1 and 28 members of Class 150/2.

The single car **Class 153**s continue to operate, but in a much lessor form. All Northern and East Midlands sets have now been taken out of service, while the rebuilding of five vehicles for use with ScotRail to provide dedicated space for cycles and extra seating went live in summer 2021. Transport for Wales took on extra sets to allow withdrawal of 'Pacer' stock. Some of their sets do not meet the latest DDA regulations and must operate with a modified set. The unmodified vehicles have been renumbered in the 1539xx series.

The small **Class 155** fleet continue to operate for Northern, based at Neville Hill, with no plans for their replacement. On the **Class 156** front, operations remain much as in recent years, with East Midlands Railway (EMR), Northern and ScotRail running the 114 two-car sets. Some re-livery work has taken place, with EMR sets being given white, aubergine and

The former BR Southern Region flagship loco No. 73142, later 73201 Broadlands is currently operated by GB Railfreight and used for freight and departmntal duties, usually based at Tonbridge. The loco carried the BR rail blue 'heritage' livery and is seen at Tonbridge depot in January 2022. **Antony Christie**

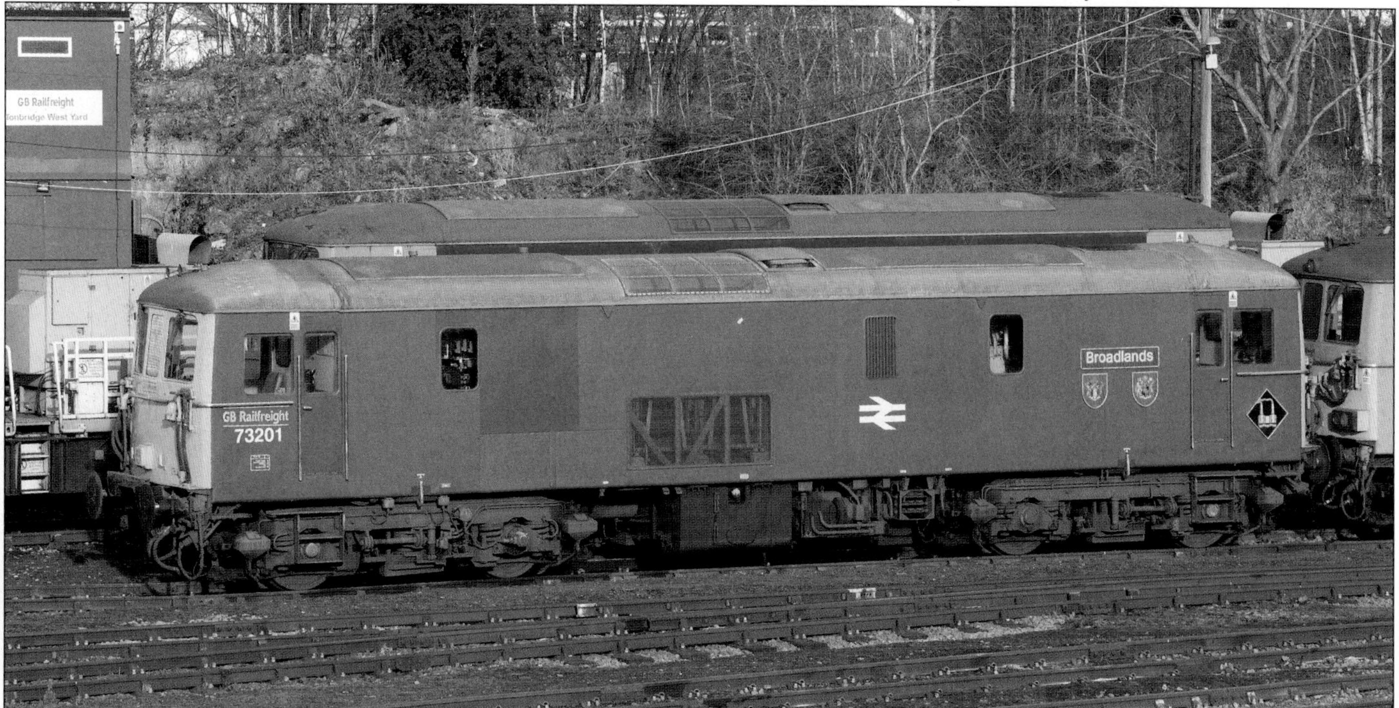

grey 'EMR-Regional' colours. Some EMR sets have been transferred to Northern over the last year.

The **Class 158s** are still regarded as some of the best second generation DMU stock, with refurbished, mainly two-car sets, working with Scottish Railways, Great Western, Northern, East Midlands Railway, Transport for Wales and South Western Railway. A small number of purpose-built three-car sets operate with Northern, with one set working on Great Western. To ease route congestion, Great Western continues to operate a small number of three-car sets formed of three driving cars. Sadly GW lost one of its two car sets No. 158763 in a serious collision and derailment at Salisbury Tunnel Junction on 31 October 2021.

The like designed **Class 159**s continue to operate with South Western Railway, these being an upgraded Class 158. Again, one set was written-off during the year after 159102 was involved in the Salisbury Tunnel Junction accident on 31 October 2021.

Built between 1990-1993 the Network SouthEast 'Networker Turbo' and 'Networker Turbo Express' **Class 165** and **Class 166** stock operate for Chiltern Railways (Class 165/0) and Great Western (Class 165/1, 166). On Great Western, Class 166s are now common on the Exeter to Barnstaple, Okehampton, Paignton and Exmouth branch services, further deployment depends on the eventual introduction of Class 769s in the London area, allowing a cascade of remaining 'Turbo' stock.

The four sub-classes of **Class 168** are the backbone of Chiltern Railways operations. Hybrid technology is now being tested with set No. 168329 having a diesel/battery system. This was introduced in early 2022.

The large fleet of **Class 170**s, formed into six sub-classes, operate for CrossCountry, Transport for Wales, Scottish Railways, East Midlands Railway, Northern and West Midlands. East Midlands Railway has recently gained sets previously used in Scotland, with their fleet set to expand further in 2022 with the transfer of some sets from West Midlands after new stock is introduced. During 2021, CrossCountry strengthened their two-car Class 170/5 fleet to three-car (Class 170/6) sets, by taking over the MS vehicles from West Midland Railways three-car units. The **Class 171**s continue to operate for GTR (Southern), no plans are on the table to replace these sets, but it has been suggested a fleet of bi-mode Class 377s could be introduced on Southern for non-electrified routes.

All four sub-classes of **Class 172** now operate on West Midlands Railway and mainly display the mauve and gold livery. The four members of non-gangwayed Class 172/1 were transferred in from Chiltern Railways in 2021 following a reduction of Chiltern services.

New stock is currently under construction for Transport for Wales to replace the two sub-classes of **Class 175** (2-car and 3-car sets). These sets will then be offered to another operator. At present, sets are still the lifeblood of longer-distance services, with the entire fleet refreshed and given the latest TfW white and red livery.

The main operator for the five-car **Class 180**s is Grand Central, with 10 sets in service. The remaining four, previously operated by First Hull Trains, are now operated on East Midlands Railway, working InterCity duties, alongside the Class 222 fleet. One Class 180 has been reduced to a four-car formation due to body corrosion. The Class 180s will continue with EMR until new Class 810 Hitachi 'Aurora' sets are introduced.

Built for TransPennine Express operation, the 51 three-car **Class 185**s operate for TPE, even after the Class 802/2 and CAF Mk5 stock was introduced. The original plan was for some sets to be phased out and returned to their lease owner, buy this was shelved and all sets will now remain with TPE.

The CAF-built **Class 195** sets, in two and three car formation were introduced in 2020, making a huge difference to Northern services, the sets are spacious, comfortable and provide a much improved regional service. Stock is finished in Northern white and blue, with the fleet based at Newton Heath depot, Manchester.

Spanish builder CAF are still assembling, in both Spain and Wales, the **Class 196** fleet, these are two-car (Class 196/0) and four-car (Class 196/1) formations and will modernise Birmingham area longer distance services. Throughout 2021 and into 2022, a handful of units were delivered to Tyseley depot, Birmingham and were placed under test, as well as taking part in staff training.

The CAF works then moved on to assembly of the **Class 197** two and three-car 'Civity' sets for Transport for Wales. The first of these sets were delivered in 2021 and should enter service in 2023-2023.

The original 'Virgin Voyager' four-car **Class 220**s and 'Virgin Super-Voyager' four/five-car **Class 221** stock, now operate with CrossCountry and Avanti West Coast. All sets are based at Central Rivers depot, near Burton-on-Trent. Announced in 2020, plans are in progress to equip one Class 220 with battery technology for dwell time and starting, thus reducing emissions. The Class 221 sets operated by Avanti West Coast, will be phased out when new Hitachi IET stock is introduced and are likely to be cascaded to CrossCountry, the first two going off-lease in June 2022.

Until the introduction of new Hitachi Class 810 'Aurora' stock, the East Midlands Railway InterCity services remain in the hands of **Class 222** stock formed in 5 and 7 car formations, these are based at Derby and owned by Eversholt leasing. These sets will need to be found a new operator when replaced by '810s'.

The conversion of former London Transport 'D' Stock into main line **Class 230** trains has continued, with five sets now delivered to Transport for Wales, in addition to the West Midlands and development trains. The TfW sets are bi-mode (diesel/battery). In November 2021, development set 230001 was shown off at the COP26 event in Glasgow operating as a pure battery train. In February 2022 it was announced that set No. 230001 reduced to a two car set, will do a years battery trial starting in summer 2022 on the West Ealing to Greenford line, using 'fast-charge' technology.

Traction & Rolling Stock – Electric Units

The 1970s introduced, 19 three-car **Class 313**/2s working for GTR Southern on the Coastway route are the oldest sets currently in regular service, no plans yet exist to replace them, this original dual power fleet are now dc only. Just one Class 313/1 remains in service with Network Rail, for ETCS development work.

The two fleets of Class 320 three-car sets, the original 22 Class 320/3 and 12 Class 320/4, converted ex Class 321 sets are allocated to Glasgow Shields Road depot and operate local services in the Glasgow area. Set No. 320305, leads a six car formation at Anniesland on 23 June 2021 with the 12.44 Airdrie to Balloch. **CJM**

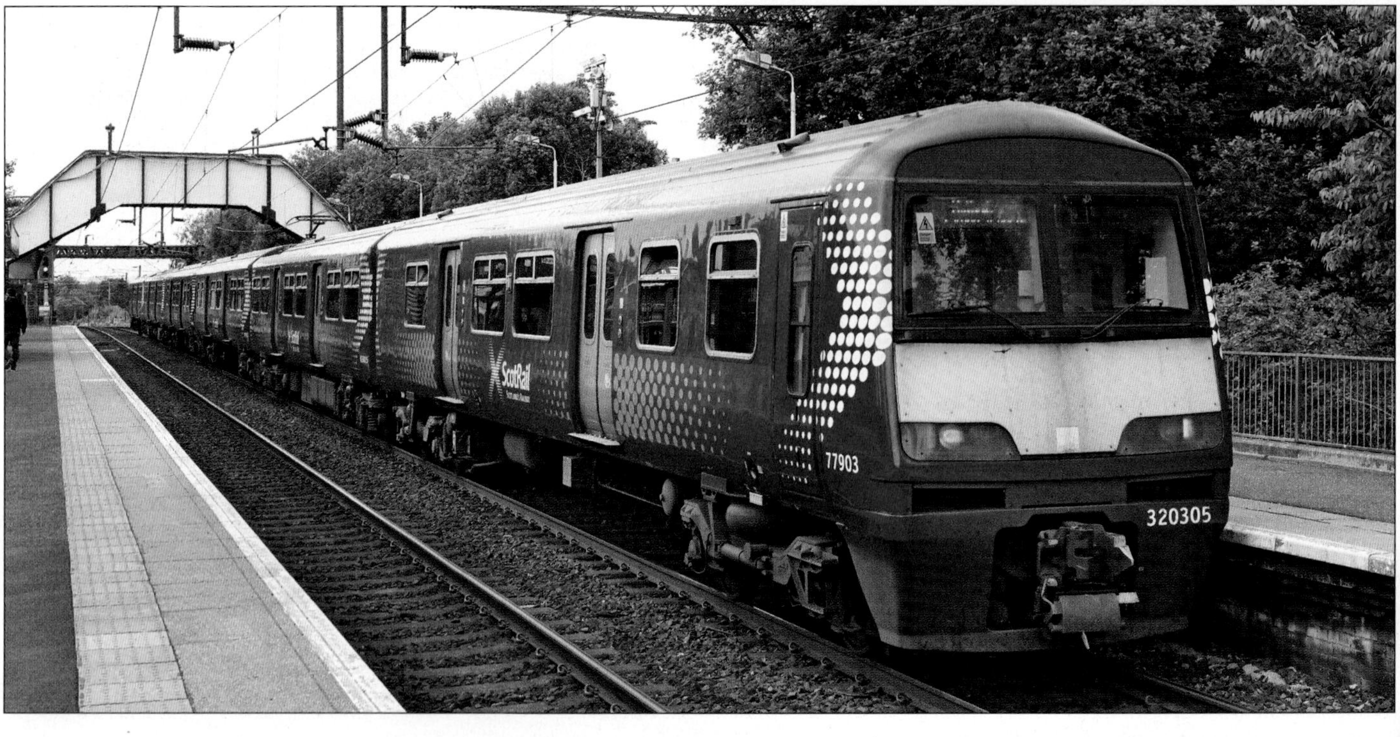

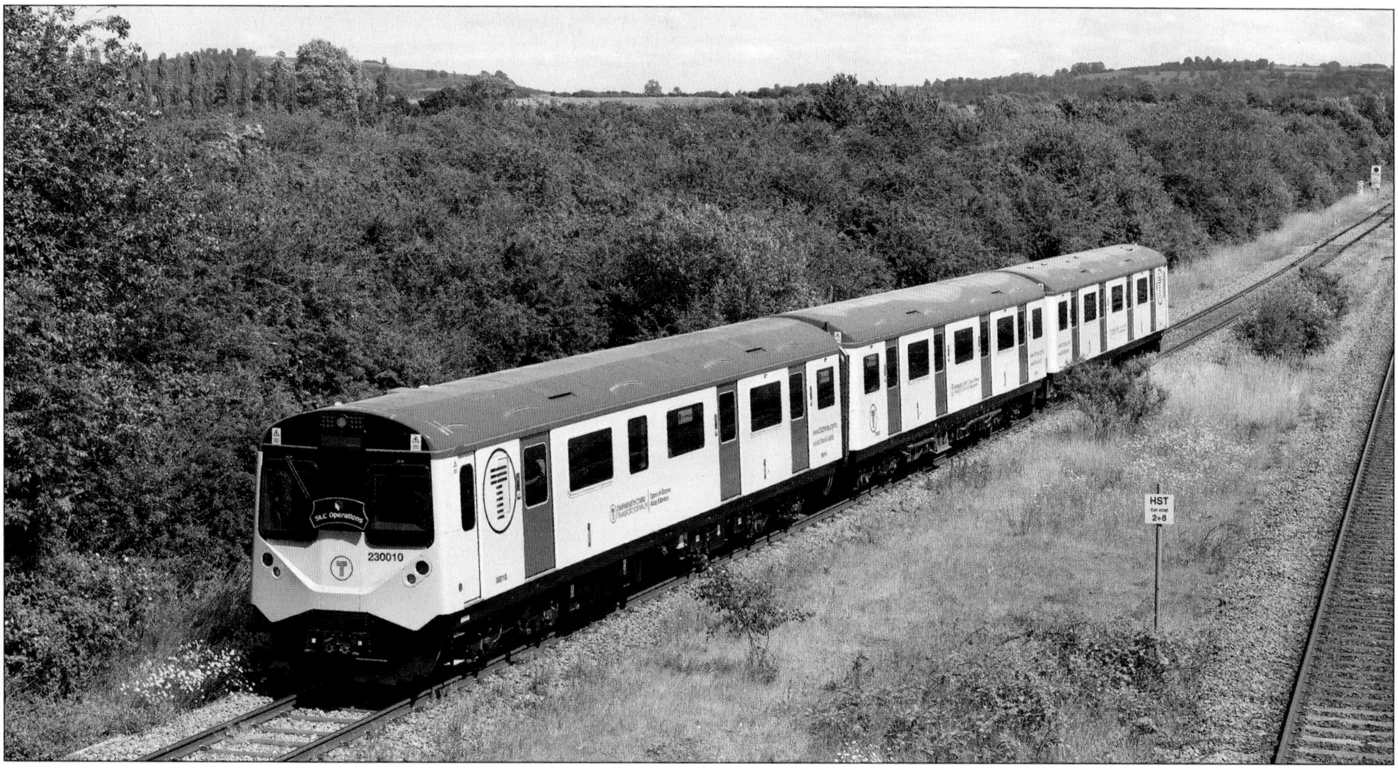

The five three-car Class 230 sets for Transport for Wales were completed by Vivarail at Long Marston in mid-2021. While testing and some training has been undertaken in the North Wales area for their introduction on the Wrexham-Bidston route, but by March 2022 none had entered service. Set No. 230010 is seen at Honeybourne during a demonstration for Rail Live 2021 on 23 June 2021. **CJM**

The handful of remaining **Class 315**s are scheduled to withdrawn from service on Liverpool Street to Shenfield by Class 345s in summer 2022.

It was planned that the remaining **Class 317**s operating on Greater Anglia, would be withdrawn in 2021, but delayed introduction of Class 720s has seen several Class 317s remain in front line service. Full deployment of 720s is scheduled for this summer which will spell the end for the '317s'.

Scottish Railways-operated **Class 318**s remain operating in the Glasgow area. The **Class 319** fleet continues to operate with Northern. Many fleet members have been converted as part of the *Porterbrook Flex* project, by installing diesel power packs under the driving cars, providing a power output to the power train line. Rail Operations Group, as part of its 'Orion' project have modified a small number of sets for parcel carrying with roller floors, those with dual power capability are reclassified as Class 768 or 769, while the electric only sets are classified as 326. Two sets has been converted as the development tool for the *Porterbrook HydroFlex* project and classified 799.

The 1990-built 22-strong **Class 320** fleet remain in use in Scotland, classified as Class 320/3 sets, these are supplemented by 12 modified Class 321s, reclassified as Class 320/4s and operate in one common pool.

Another class which should have been phased out by mid-2021 are the **Class 321**s, however, due to late delivery and commissioning of Class 720 stock on Greater Anglia, the fleet, in much reduced numbers, remain in front line service. The three Class 321/9 sets and the similar **Class 322**s were transferred from Northern to Ilford to provide extra sets meeting the PRM requirement.

New EMUs for the West Midlands Railway CrossCity will soon replace their three-car **Class 323** fleet. It is proposed, a batch of 17 will transfer to Northern, to work alongside the original Northern units, deployed on the Liverpool-Manchester-Crewe route, first sets to move in June 2023.

Currently operated by DB-Cargo, the Royal Mail owned **Class 325** sets based at Crewe, operate a small number of services over the West Coast Main Line. The fleet carries full Royal Mail red livery.

The classification **Class 326** has been allocated to the all electric version of the ROG 'Orion' light freight EMUs, but by spring 2022, sets were still carrying their previous Class 319 identities.

The **Class 331** units are the all electric version of the CAF-built Class 195, the three-car sets are based at Allerton (Liverpool) while the four-car sets are based at Neville Hill (Leeds).

Just three vehicles on the once 14 unit strong **Class 332** Heathrow Express fleet remain, all owned by Siemens and stored at their new Goole engineering facility.

The fully refurbished **Class 333** fleet, now meeting full PRM standards continue to operate on the Aire Valley routes, based at Leeds Neville Hill, a service they now share with the CAF Class 331 fleet.

Scottish Railways continues to use the 40 Alstom 'Juniper' **Class 334** sets in the Glasgow and Edinburgh area.

The 70 nine-car **Class 345** 'Aventra' units designed and built for use on the CrossRail 'Elizabeth Line', linking Reading/Heathrow in the west with Shenfield and Abbey Wood in the East, via a tunnel below central London are now entering service, following massive delays in the building and testing. All 70 sets have been built and delivered, many are now in traffic on the both the western and eastern ends of the route, and the central section between Paddington and Abbey Wood opened in May. Some sets are still stored at Old Oak Common.

The four sub-classes of **Class 350** operate with West Midlands Railway, based at Siemens Northampton depot. Each of the sub-classes have slight detail differences. The Class 350/2 fleet of 37 sets are due off-lease in 2023 following introduction of new stock. Owner Porterbrook has indicated these will be 'modernised' with battery technology, but who will operate the fleet in still unknown.

The c2c operation from Fenchurch Street to the Essex Coast is the sole operator of the **Class 357** 'Electrostar' stock. Three sub-classes now exist, the 357/3 units are designated for Metro high-occupancy operations. All sets are based at East Ham.

A class which saw major change in 2021 is the **Class 360**. The 21 four-car Class 360/0s, originally used on Greater Anglia from 2002, have now been transferred to East Midlands Railway for use on their 'EMR Connect' service from London St Pancras to Corby, where trains of up to 12 coaches operate an intense service. The fleet is based at Bedford Caldwell Road depot and in 2022 were passing through Arlington Eastleigh to be re-liveried in EMR aubergine, after entering service in branded blue. The five five-car Class 360/2 sets, displaced from the Heathrow Connect service, are now owned by Rail Operations Group and currently stored at MoD Bicester.

The 40 members of the 'Networker Express' **Class 365** fleet, have in 2021-2022 gone for scrap at either Sims Metals of Newport or Booths, Rotherham. Three vehicles have been preserved by the East Kent Railway.

The two Eurostar fleets of **Class 373** and **Class 374** saw much reduced work throughout the Corona Virus pandemic, with a very limited service operating between St Pancras and Brussels/Paris. The remaining Class 373 sets were stood down and stabled at Temple Mills, London. In February 2022 the '373' were returned to a fully operational state in preparation for a much more frequent service from spring/summer 2022.

The Electrostar **Class 375** fleet are still the main SouthEastern outer suburban and main line fleet, based at Ramsgate, they come in five sub-classes each with slight formation and detail differences. All sets carry SouthEastern blue livery.

SouthEastern 'Metro' style services from London to Dartford and other local routes are formed of **Class 376** five-car 'Electrostar' units, these are a no frills train designed for high-capacity with rapid loading/unloading reduced seats and lots of standing room. They are based at Slade Green.

Modernisation of the Southern network came in the form of various batches of **Class 377** 'Electrostar', formed in either three, four or five-car formations. All except Class 377/5 are operated by Southern, the Class 377/5s work on SouthEastern and are painted in SE blue livery. The Southern sets are painted in white and green and based at Selhurst depot. Members of the Class 377/2, 377/5 and 377/7 sub-classes are fitted with dual-voltage equipment, allowing operation from 25kV ac overhead and 750V dc third rail.

Two fleets of **Class 378** are the core traction for London Overground services. The now five-car sets, fitted with longitudinal seating are used on the busiest routes. Sets are currently in a livery transition from original London Overground white, to a more stylish black, white and blue colour, the repainting is a protracted affair, with some 75% of the fleet still in old colours after four years.

The 30 **Class 379** 'Electrostar' sets, introduced for Liverpool Street to Stansted Airport operation, displaced by Stadler Class 745s, remained with Greater Anglia to assist with longer distance services due to the late delivery of Class 720 stock. However, by January 2022 sufficient new stock was available and the Class 379s were all stood down, being stored as we closed for press.

The two modern EMU fleets of **Class 380** and **Class 385**, built by Siemens and Hitachi respectively, come in three and four-car formation operating on the core Edinburgh-Glasgow, outer suburban and local routes. All are painted in Scottish Railways blue and white.

Four sub-fleets of **Class 387** 'Electrostar' are in service with GTR, Great Western and c2c. On Great Western a batch of 12 sets (Nos. 387130-387141) are modified for use on Heathrow Express services, these have revised interiors, with extra luggage space and fitted with European Train Control System (ECTS) to enable operation over the lines into Heathrow Airport. The sets carry a special Heathrow Express livery and most are named after destination cities from around the world. The domestic GWR sets carry GWR green livery and operate Thames Valley services, all are based at Reading. The GTR units in white livery, are based at Hornsey and operate Kings Cross line services. A sub-fleet of Class 387/2s are dedicated to the Gatwick Express service and carry Gat-ex red livery. Five sets are operated by c2c, based at East Ham. However from spring 2021 these have been sub-leased to Great Western to assist with fleet shortages caused by the IET problems.

The rolling stock used on Avanti West Coast is a fleet of nine and 11-car **Class 390** 'Pendolino' sets, which in 2021-2022 were in the process of major refurbishment at the Alstom Widnes plant.

The first fleet of Hitachi trains to operate in the UK, were 29 six-car 'Javelin' **Class 395** units, introduced to work a domestic service over High Speed 1 (HS1), the units, with a top speed of 140mph (225km/h) have a basic interior, they are based at the Hitachi-operated depot in Ashford, Kent and carry SouthEastern 'high-speed' blue livery.

Introduced in 2018, a fleet of CAF-built **Class 397**s five-car stylish EMUs operate for TransPennine Express on their West Coast services from Liverpool/Manchester to Glasgow/Edinburgh. The high specification units with both first and standard class seating, were some of the first trains in the UK not to carry yellow warning ends. The sets are based in Manchester International depot.

The Sheffield 'Tram-Train' project remains in operation, using Vossloh three-section **Class 399** sets. The Government sponsored pilot project for tram-trains, sees the fleet operate between Sheffield Cathedral and Rotherham Park Gate, as well as working tram services within Sheffield city centre. The sets carry Stagecoach Super Tram blue livery.

A development of the Vossloh (now Stadler) 'Tram-Train' project is the Class 398, a fleet of 36 three car battery/electric sets for use on Cardiff Valley services. The first set is due for delivery at the end of 2022.

As part of the modernisation of South West Trains services, two major fleets of Siemens 'Desiro' units were ordered, 45 five-car express **Class 444s** and 127 four-car outer-suburban **Class 450**s. Both fleets are based at the Siemens maintenance facility at Northam, near Southampton. Delivered in 2002-2003, both class have been refurbished and currently a re-branding exercise is well advanced to apply the latest South Western Railway grey and blue colours.

The main suburban multiple unit class operated by South Western Railway continues to be the three sub-classes of **Class 455**, introduced between 1982-1985. The sets are scheduled to be replaced by Class 701 'Aventra' stock, which currently still on delivery. Once the Class 701s are commissioned, followed by a major staff training program, the SWR '455s' will be withdrawn. GTR Southern Class 455/8s were withdrawn in May 2022.

To operate alongside the Class 455s, a batch of 24 two-car **Class 456** sets were introduced in 1990, originally allocated to the SouthCentral section, later Southern were moved to South Western via refurbishment. With a massive downturn in business and the requirement for less trains, the entire Class 456 fleet were withdrawn in January 2022 and returned to their owner Porterbrook. The sets have now been moved to Long Marston for store.

At the start of privatisation in 1996, Stagecoach ordered a fleet of **Class 458** four-coach outer-suburban units. In 2013 the fleet was refurbished and strengthened to five cars by the adding of vehicles from disbanded Class 460 'Gatwick Express' units, with spare vehicles allowing extra sets to be formed. Working with South Western Railway, 28 sets are soon to be reformed as 4-car units, overhauled and deployed on main line 100mph duties from 2022-2023. Overhaul work is scheduled to be done at Alstom, Widnes.

In the days of Network SouthEast, three sub-classes of 4-car and one batch of 2-car 'Networker' units were introduced to modernise South Eastern suburban routes. Identified as **Class 465** (4-car) and **Class 466** (2-car). In 2021 the remaining Class 465/2 sets (built by Metro-Cammell) were withdrawn and are now stored awaiting disposal at Ely. The remaining Class 465s are now formed into three sub-classes all with technical differences. This stock is scheduled to be replaced in the next few years.

In November 2021 a new fleet of five two-car **Class 484** sets were introduced on the Isle of Wight, replacing the 1938 tube-stock. The Class 484s are Vivarail rebuilds of former London Underground 'D' Stock and operate from the third rail electric supply. Painted in the latest South Western Railway livery, branded Island Line, they are based at Ryde St Johns depot.

In 2021-2022 the Merseyrail electrified system was in the progress of major modernisation, with the fleets of **Class 507** and **Class 508**, 1978-1979 built three-car sets being replaced by Stadler Class 777 stock. The introduction of the new units was heavily delayed and in spring 2022 the majority of old sets were still in use with only a handful of '777s' delivered. The 507/508 fleet are unique in terms of rail vehicles, carrying a different livery on either side, silver on one and yellow on the other.

When the GTR Thameslink route was modernised, a fleet of Siemens 'Desiro City' **Class 700** units were ordered. These come in two types, 66 eight-car reduced length units and 55 12-car full length units. Based at the Siemens operated Three Bridges depot, the fleet form all Thameslink services under London on the north-south axis. The units are fitted for Automatic Train Operation (ATO), effectively working driver-less through the core tunnel section below London.

By Spring 2022, over 55 **Class 701** five and 10-car sets had been delivered to South Western Railway and were under test, none had been accepted for use. The sets, part of the Alstom (previously Bombardier) 'Aventra' family, have, in common with other like builds, been the subject of huge delays due to software and design issues. The fleet will be based at Wimbledon, with new maintenance sidings opened at Feltham. Commissioning work is undertaken from Eastleigh.

When South West Trains held the franchise for the lines radiating from Waterloo, they invested, through Angel Trains, in a fleet of 30 five-car 'Desiro-City' **Class 707** sets. As soon as the franchise changed, right at the time the '707s' were being introduced, it was announced that the fleet would not be needed, as new Class 701s would be utilised. The fleet was commissioned and introduced, but in January 2021 a start was made to transfer the fleet to SouthEastern for Metro operations in the London-Kent area, where they are now operated as the 'City-Beam' fleet.

In 2018-2020, London Overground, with funding by SMBC/Lombard, introduced a fleet of **Class 710**s, these come in three sub-classes, 710/1 - four-car 25kV ac overhead, 710/2 - four-car 25kV ac and 750V dc and 710/3 five-car dual voltage sets. These are deployed on Gospel Oak-Barking, West Anglia routes and Euston-Watford services, These are part of the Bombardier (now Alstom) 'Aventra' family and were delayed due to software issues.

In 2018, GTR had to replace its 1972-design Class 313 dual-voltage stock used on Great Northern services, this was achieved with a fleet of 25 six-car dual-voltage **Class 717** 'Desiro City' sets, similar to the Class 700s, but with end emergency gangways.

The **Class 720** five-car sets for Greater Anglia, replacing suburban and outer-suburban stock, commenced delivery in 2019, but as part of the troublesome Alston (Bombardier) 'Aventra' family, have taken a long time to enter service, with 61 of the fleet accepted by April 2022. Originally a fleet of 22 10-car and 89 five-car trains were ordered, but in late 2020 it was announced that the 22 10-car sets would be delivered as 44 five-car units. The 12 Class 720/6 sets for c2c were constructed in early 2022.

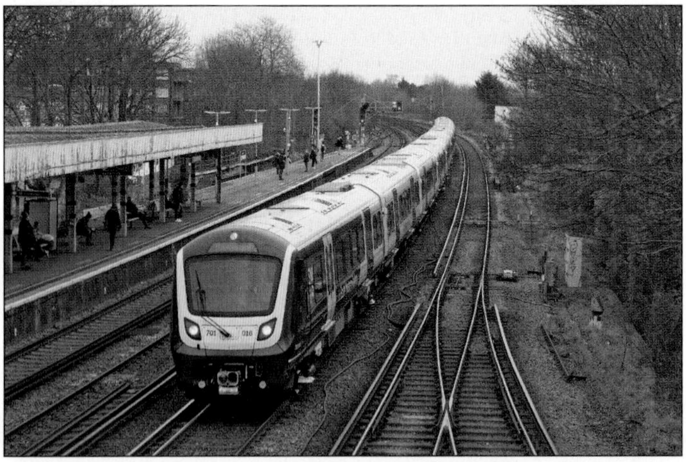

South Western Railway were facing difficult decisions in late 2021 early 2022, with the continued late or none delivery of operational Class 701 units. SWT announcing that Alstom had failed to deliver a train suitable for service, meeting the design specification. However, a number of test runs were operated and in this view at Raynes Park, set No. 701016 heads south on 26 January 2022. **Antony Christie**

As part of the total modernisation of the Greater Anglia fleet, two batches of Stadler 'Flirt' 12-car sets were introduced from 2020. The **Class 745**s are formed of six articulated pairs. The 12 Class 745/0s are InterCity sets for the London to Norwich route, while the 12 Class 745/1s are dedicated to Stansted Airport services. Both fleets are based at Norwich Crown Point.

For Greater Anglia rural services, Abellio Greater Anglia opted for a fleet of bi-mode **Class 755** three and four passenger vehicle sets, formed with an intermediate short wheelbase 'power pack' vehicle. This class is also part of the Stadler 'Flirt' platform. The sets operate as a standard electric multiple unit, but have diesel power packs for non-electrified line use.

The **Class 769** fleet of bi-mode multiple units have taken several years to build and introduce, but by early summer 2022, sets were in service. The fleet is converted from redundant Class 319s, fitted with a diesel power pack below each driving car, supplying power to the normal EMU traction package. Northern, Transport for Wales and Great Western all operate the class. The first sets to enter service were with Northern, followed by Transport for Wales with Great Western sets introduced from early summer 2022. The Great Western sets are dual voltage (25kV ac overhead and 750V dc third rail) plus diesel.

Modernisation of the Merseyrail electric system has been underway since 2020, with a fleet of 53 four-section Stadler **Class 777** EMUs slowly being delivered. Delivery has been slow, partly caused by the world pandemic, with by spring 2022 only around 25 sets in the UK. None are in service, but testing and training is ongoing. Seven sets will be fitted with traction battery equipment.

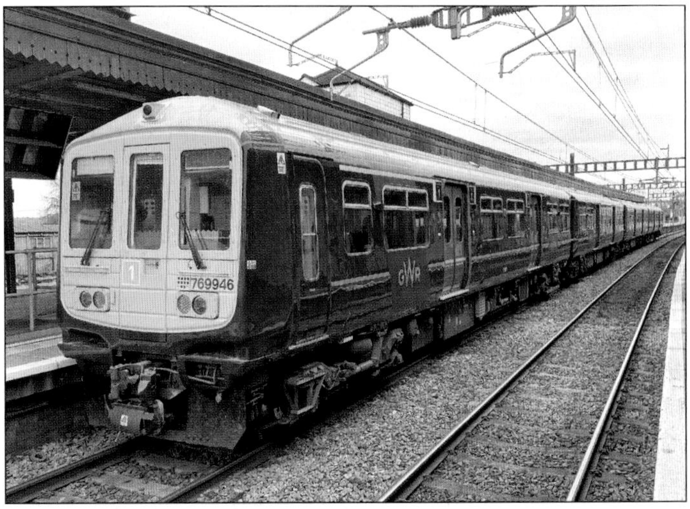

Delivery of the Class 769 four-car bi-mode units, able to operate from diesel or ac/dc electric power supply were running very late against scheduled delivery and introduction dates. During 2021-2022 a number of test runs using all three traction modes were undertaken. Here, fully finished set No. 769946 (the former 319446) is seen at Didcot with a test run on 24 November 2021. **Spencer Conquest**

InterCity Express Trains

The entire IET operation involving Great Western and LNER was thrown into chaos from 7 May 2021 when serious cracks were found in the aluminium welds on the jacking points and yaw damper brackets of Class 80x stock. As a safety measure the entire fleet was immediately grounded and most long distance trains cancelled for several days. By 13 May a limited return to service of some trains was authorised with a rigorous inspection process every day. Some sets were removed from traffic while others returned to service, this allowed a partial return of the IET timetable, but even now in spring 2022 a full IET service has not returned. Repairs to the problem which lays with Hitachi have now been agreed, but squadron repairs have yet to start. The withdrawal of sets saw some Mk4 sets return to LNER routes and on Great Western Class 387 were deployed on London-Newport, later Cardiff services, with extra units drafted in from GTR and c2c. The Hull Trains and TransPennine sets while affected were not as bad and quickly returned to traffic.

On 25 October 2021, the fleet of five **Class 803** five-car InterCity Express Trains were introduced by open access operator First East Coast, trading as Lumo, with a low-cost London King's Cross to Edinburgh service. The sets are all electric, with a battery back-up for hotel power and have standard class seating.

The 2020 announced order for IET trains to operate on Avanti West Coast consisting of 13 five-car bi-mode **Class 805**s, to replace the present 'Super Voyager' Class 221 fleet, and 10 seven-car all electric **Class 807**s to supplement the existing 'Pendolino' fleet are progressing at the Hitachi plant in Newton Aycliffe. The '807s' will operate fixed duties, as interoperability between the two fleets would not be possible, especially in terms of seat reservations.

East Midlands Railways IET fleet to replace the Class 180 and 222 stock is progressing well with a number of vehicles under assembly. EMR in partnership with Rock Rail, have ordered 33 five-car bi-mode **Class 810** sets. Based on the Hitachi AT300 design with detail differences, including four of the five vehicles being powered, with coaches that are of 24m length, two metres shorter than previous IETs. The EMR sets will be known as the 'Aurora' fleet and based in new purpose-built depot facilities at Derby.

The first tranche of rolling stock for use on the scaled-back High Speed 2 (HS2) route from London to the Midlands was announced by the Government on 9 December 2021, when 54 eight-coach 225mph (360km/h sets were ordered from a Hitachi/Alstom partnership, based on the Zefiro V300 platform.

The stock will be built at the Hitachi plant in Newton Aycliffe, with the aluminium bodies transported to Derby Litchurch Lane for fitting out. Bogies will come from a new Alstom plant at Crewe. The first train is due for completion in 2027. Each train will have four powered vehicles, have a 35 year life and be based at Washwood Heath.

LNER have issued 'expressions of interest' in providing 10 high speed trainsets, going out to the world for offers, the likely winner will be Hitachi for an upgraded AT300 product. No operator would wish to have a mixed main line high speed fleet, with 10 'different' trains roaming the network, alongside the main Class 80x fleets.

Trains On Order/Delivery 2021 - onwards

Class	Builder	Operator	Owner	Type	Number of sets/vehicles	Status
18	Clayton	Spot Hire	Beacon Rail	Bi-Mode	15	Delivery
69	Progress Rail	GB Railfreight	GB Railfreight	Co-Co	10 (+ 6 options)	In Service / Conversion
93	Stadler	Rail Operations Group	Star Capital/ROG	Bo-Bo±	30 (+ options)	Construction
99	Stadler	GB Railfreight	Beacon Rail	Co-Co±	30	Design (delivery from 2025)
196/0	CAF	West Midlands Railway	Corelink Rail	DMU	12 x 2-car (24)	Construction / Testing / Introduction
196/1	CAF	West Midlands Railway	Corelink Rail	DMU	14 x 4-car (56)	Construction / Testing / Introduction
197/0	CAF	Transport for Wales	SMBC Leasing	DMU	51 x 2-car (102)	Construction / Testing / Introduction
197/1	CAF	Transport for Wales	SMBC Leasing	DMU	26 x 3-car (78)	Construction / Testing / Introduction
230	Vivarail	Transport for Wales	Vivarail	BMU	5 x 3-car (15)	Testing / Introduction
231	Stadler	Transport for Wales	SMBC Leasing	DMU	11 x 4-car (44)	Delivery / Testing
398	Stadler	Transport for Wales	SMBC Leasing	BMU±	36 x 3-car (108)	Construction
484	Vivarail	South Western Railway	Lombard Finance	EMU	5 x 2-car (10)	In Service
701/0	Bombardier	South Western Railway	Rock Rail	EMU	60 x 10-car (600)	Delivery/Commissioning
701/5	Bombardier	South Western Railway	Rock Rail	EMU	30 x 5-car (150)	Delivery/Commissioning
720/5	Bombardier	Greater Anglia	Angel Trains	EMU	133 x 5-car (665)	Testing / In service
720/6	Bombardier	c2c	Porterbrook	EMU	6 x 10-car (60)	Testing
730/0	Bombardier	West Midlands Railway	Corelink Rail	EMU	36 x 3-car (108)	Construction / Testing
730/1	Bombardier	West Midlands Railway	Corelink Rail	EMU	29 x 5-car (145)	Construction / Testing
730/2	Bombardier	West Midlands Railway	Corelink Rail	EMU	16 x 5-car (80)	Construction / Testing
756/0	Stadler	Transport for Wales	SMBC Leasing	BMU■	7 x 3-car (21)	Construction / Delivery
756/1	Stadler	Transport for Wales	SMBC Leasing	BMU■	17 x 4-car (68)	Construction / Delivery
769/9	Wabtec	Great Western Railway	Porterbrook	BMU■	19 x 4-car (76)	Delivery / Testing / Introduction
777	Stadler	MerseyRail	Liverpool City	EMU*	53 x 4-car (212)	Delivery/Testing
803	Hitachi	First Group	Beacon Rail	EMU	5 x 5-car (25)	In Service
805	Hitachi	Avanti West Coast	Rock Rail	BMU	13 x 5-car (65)	Construction
807	Hitachi	Avanti West Coast	Rock Rail	EMU	10 x 7-car (70)	Construction
810	Hitachi	Abellio East Midlands	Rock Rail	BMU	33 x 5-car (165)	Construction / Testing
Awaited	Alstom/Hitachi	Avanti West Coast (HS2)	Awaited	EMU	54 x 8-car (432)	Design (delivery from 2027)

± Bi-mode battery / electric ■ Tri-mode battery EMU/DMU * Seven sets to have traction battery

How to use your Rail123 Traction & Rolling Stock Guide

The *Rail123 Traction & Rolling Stock Guide*, covers all locomotives, multiple units, coaches and Light Rail vehicles in the UK, Isle of Man and Ireland up to and including 1 June 2022.

The title is set out in a number of sections, covering Locomotives, Diesel Multiple Units, Electric Multiple Units, Coaches, HST stock, Fixed train formations, Network Rail infrastructure stock, EuroTunnel stock, Light Rail and Metro systems, Irish Rail, the Isle of Man railways and preserved steam.

The listings in terms of modern traction, provide one combined list for each class, containing main line certified stock, preserved vehicles, those in industrial use or exported. Each of the entries are colour coded providing immediate identification of the status of each item. This is only available in the *Rail123* annual publication, it is intended to save readers from having to refer a multiple number of publications to locate, or reference, a specific item of stock.

For items which are preserved, shown in green, the loco or vehicle number is given, followed by its last reported location. Locos or rolling stock which are in the UK but in industrial use are shown in light blue, these give where possible the National Rail (or old BR) number together with any current numeric identity, a code letter for fittings and fixtures, its livery, together with owner and latest reported location.

Locos and stock which have been exported are shown in dark orange, for these we give the former UK number with a country / location where the vehicle was exported.

Stock which is currently in service and likely to be seen in normal operation, is shown in black, with more detailed information, including current name, allocation, fittings, as well as the owner and operator.

Colour Coding Chart Examples

Operational - Black
33029 (D6547) X CS AWCA WCR WCR WCR
Preserved - Green
D2023 Kent & East Sussex Railway - 11210
Industrial - Light Blue
08484 A RSS RSS at Norwich Crown Point
Exported - Orange
07009 (D2993) Exported to Italy

Locomotives: the following information is provided, the example below is from the Class 66 section -

A	*B*	*C*	*D*	*E*	*F*	*G*	*H*
66098		A	TO	WBRT	EWS	DBC	DBC
66099		AR	TO	WBRT	EWS	DBC	DBC
66100	*Armistice 100 1918-2018*	AR	TO	WBBE	DBC	DBC	DBC

Column *A* Gives the up to date running number, with previous numbers shown in brackets.
Column *B* Shows the currently fitted nameplate. For consistency names are shown in upper and lower case, the actual style of lettering might well be different, these often use all capital letters.
Column *C* Provides a single or group of letters, this indicates the fixtures and fittings of the loco (see table below). The first letter is always the brake type.
Column *D* Shows the depot to which the locomotive is allocated, a full list of depot codes is given in a table towards the rear of the publication.
Column *E* Gives the operating pool to which the loco is allocated, a full list of pool codes is shown in the tables at the rear of the publication.
Column *F* Provides an abbreviation code for the current livery carried, again details of these can be found at the rear of the publication.
Column *G* Today, a number of different organisations and companies own locos and rolling stock, and an abbreviation for the current owner is given.
Column *H* The final column gives the present operator code, a full list is provided at the rear.

Any other notes or comments will be appended at the base of the numeric table.

Locomotive Fixture and Fitting Codes

Letters used in column C of the locomotive entries, indicate fixtures and fittings

A	Air brakes
B	Buffer fitted HST power cars
C	Combination 'swing-head' Coupling
D	Dellner Coupling
E	European Rail Traffic Management System
H	Modified for HS1 operation
K	LUL Tripcocks fitted
L	Fitted with Lickey Banker auto couplings / lights
M	Authorised for Network Rail operation
P	Slow Speed Control (SSC)
R	Radio Electronic Token Block (RETB)
S	Scharfenberg Coupling
T	Tightlock Coupling
Y	Remote Control equipped

Multiple Units: of the diesel, electric or bi-mode types, follow much of the same style, as shown in the sample below. Preserved items are shown in green, with numbers and current location provided.

A	*B*	*C*	*D*	*E*	*F*
159001	52873+58718+57873	SA	SWR	PTR	SWR
159002	52874+58719+57874	SA	SWR	PTR	SWR
159003	52875+58720+57875	SA	SWR	PTR	SWR

Column *A* Shows the current number carried, former numbers are shown in brackets.
Column *B* For multiple units the full formation is given in the operational order, with the vehicle type / formation shown in the main heading. It is not unknown for depots, enabling as many sets in traffic as possible, to cross-form units if one or more vehicles is out of service from a prolonged period. It is always worth visually checking the correct vehicles are in any given set, cross-formation is less likely with modern stock, but the Class 175s need to be watched. Computer systems have to be reset to take into account different vehicles.
Column *C* Shows the depot to which the multiple unit is allocated, a full list of depot codes is given in a table towards the rear of this publication.
Column *D* Provides an abbreviation code for the current livery, again details of these codes can be found at the rear.
Column *E* The multiple unit owner is given is this column, using a three letter code, a table of which can be found at the back.
Column *F* The final column gives the present operator code, a full list is provided at the rear of the publication.

If names are carried on multiple unit stock, these are given between columns B and C, any other specific notes will be given at the end of the tables.

Coaching Stock: Coaching stock vehicles are shown in current numerical order, with any former numbers shown in brackets, the data columns provide the following information

A	*B*	*C*	*D*	*E*	*F*	*G*	*H*
3340	FO	2f		BU	BLG	RIV	RIV
3344	FO	2f	*Scafell*	CL	PUL	LSL	LSL
3345	FO	2f		BU	BLG	RIV	RIV

Column *A* Gives the vehicle identity, with previous numbers shown in brackets, in some cases, vehicles may have been converted from stock of a different design.
Column *B* The letter code here shows the present coach type, a full list of coach types is provided in a table to the right.
Column *C* UK coaching stock vehicles are identified by a mark (Mk) number, this is shown with a suffix letter showing the variant of the design. Coaching stock mark details are documented on page 14.
Column *D* A number of passenger coaches carry names (these are mainly from the charter fleets). Names on coaching stock vehicles are usually applied in the transfer form. The listing does not indicate the case of lettering.
Column *E* In the main, coaching stock fleets are allocated to a specific depot, these are shown by the standard two letter shed code, a list of which is included in the tables section at the rear of the publication.
Column *F* Coaching stock vehicles carry a wide and diverse range of liveries, with the charter fleets these frequently change. A three letter code is used with a detail description in the tables at the rear of this publication.
Column *G* Ownership of coaching stock is again wide and varied, with in addition to the established lease companies, a number of smaller providers and charter businesses owning their own stock. The abbreviation lists are given at the rear of the publication.
Column *H* This column gives a letter code for the vehicle operator.

Departmental Stock: The listing follows much the same style as used for coaching stock, with an additional column (shown ***D***) giving a brief description of the vehicle's use.

A	*B*	*C*	*D*	*E*	*F*	*G*	*H*
975087	BSK	1	(Recovery train)	SP	NRL	NRL	NRL
975091 (34615)	BSK	1	(Test car *Mentor*)	ZA	NRL	NRL	NRL
975464 (35171)	BSK	1	(Snow train *Ptarmigan*)	SP	NRL	NRL	NRL

HST Stock: The number of HST vehicles has considerably reduced in recent years with the disposal of large numbers of Great Western, East Coast and East Midlands vehicles. However, a significant number remain in traffic, especially with Great Western and Scottish Railways. The tabular listings follow much the same style as with hauled coaching stock.

A	*B*	*C*	*D*	*E*	*F*
41182 (42278)	FO	CL	BLP	LSL	LSL
41183 (42274)	FO	CL	GWR	LSL	LSL
41185 (42313)	FO	DY	EMR	PTR	EMR

Column *A* Provides the current numeric identity, with previous numbers shown in brackets, some vehicles have carried several former identities.
Column *B* Shows the vehicle type, a list of vehicle types is given right.

Column *C* The standard two letter depot code is used for the maintenance depot where the vehicle is based.
Column *D* The present livery is shown in this column, using the standard three letter livery code.
Column *E* Unlike in the past, where the HST fleet were just owned by the rolling stock lease companies, today a number of new owners have emerged, these are detailed here.
Column *F* The current operator is shown, if the vehicle is off lease the code OLS is shown, this indicates the vehicle is currently stored and *might* return to traffic.

Vehicle Types

BCK	Brake Composite Corridor
BFK	Brake First Corridor
BSK	Brake Standard Corridor
BG	Brake Guards
BSO	Brake Standard Open
BSOT	Brake Standard Open with Micro-Buffet
BUO	Brake Unclassified Open
CK	Composite Corridor
DBSO	Driving Brake Standard Open
DSO	Driving Standard Open
DTS	Driving Trailer Standard
DVT	Driving van Trailer
FK	First Corridor
FO	First Open
FOD	First Open Disabled
GEN	Generator
GUV	General Utility Vehicle
PFK	Pullman First Kitchen
PFP	Pullman First Pantry
PSK	Pullman Standard Kitchen
PSP	Pullman Standard Pantry
RBR	Restaurant Buffet Refurbished
RFB	Restaurant First Buffet
RFM	Restaurant First Micro Buffet
RFO	Restaurant First Open
RK	Restaurant Kitchen
RLO	Restaurant Lounge Open
RMB	Restaurant Micro Buffet
RSB	Restaurant Standard Buffet
SK	Standard Corridor
SL	Sleeper Lounge
SLA	Sleeper Accessible
SLE	Sleeper either class
SLEP	Sleeper either class with Pantry
SLF	Sleeper First
SSB	Sleeper Seated Brake
TSO	Trailer Standard Open
TSOB	Trailer Standard Open Buffet
TSOD	Trailer Standard Open Disabled
TSOE	Trailer Standard Open End
TSOL	Trailer Standard Open Lavatory
TSOT	Trailer Standard Open with Micro-Buffet

HST Types

TCC	Trailer Composite Catering
TF	Trailer First
TFB	Trailer First Buffet
TGF	Trailer Guards First
TGS	Trailer Guards Standard
TRFB	Trailer Restaurant First Buffet
TS	Trailer Standard

Set Formations: While the charter train operators tend to make up train consists 'as required' for different services, the main stream operators tend to keep hauled, HST, Mk4 and Mk5 stock in semi-fixed formations. This allows a more robust method of operation ensuring vehicles 'talk' to each other, as well as providing an enhanced maintenance cycle. Vehicles can be removed from sets easily for any major issues, or extended repair. Sets are usually identified by a set number, in the example below we shown a CrossCountry HST set.

Set No.	Formation
	(DM)+TF+TBF+TS+TS+TS+TS+TGS+(DM)
XC01	41193+45001+42342+42097+42377+42374+44021

Network Rail Infrastructure and Maintenance vehicles: Today, we see a growing interest and following of the various complex machines which form the track maintenance fleet. These often unusual looking machines, mainly painted in yellow NR colours, are owned and operated by a number of companies, usually working under contract for Network Rail. Network Rail also own a significant number of vehicles. The stock are numbered in a DR series, with some now carrying their full European identities, where identified these are given in brackets after the standard number. The display of information is showed in the sample below.

A	*B*	*C*	*D*
DR77001	*Anthony Lou Phillips*	P&T AFM 2000 RT – Finishing Machine	SBR
DR77002		P&T AFM 2000 RT – Finishing Machine	SBR
DR77010 (99 70 9125 010-7)		P&T USP 6000 – Ballast Regulator	NRL

Column *A* Provides the standard number, if a full European identity is carried this is given in brackets, a large number of new machines are displaying these numbers.
Column *B* A limited number of track machines carry nameplates, these are usually of the cast type and are often of railway workers, especially those from the track maintenance departments. These are shown in this column.
Column *C* This column gives the manufacturer and type of machine. Most suppliers are shown in full but Plasser & Theurer has been shortened to P&T for reasons of space.
Column *D* This final column provides a three letter code of the vehicle owner. A list is provided at the rear.

Eurotunnel: The fleet of Eurotunnel traffic locos and rescue/engineering locos are listed and follow the standard loco format for information.

Metro and Light Rail: With an increasing interest in Light Rail and Metro systems, including London Transport (Underground) lines, a full fleet listing of all current systems in the UK and Ireland are given. The information gives the booked formation of multi-vehicle sets and tram numbers for tram systems. London Underground is broken down by line and type of stock. On this system, set numbers are not applied, but trains formations tend to remain constant for long periods.

Also included are some of the smaller 'systems' such as the Southend Pier Railway, Hythe Pier tramway and tourist attraction Seaton Tramway.

Irish Railway: The fleets operated in Northern Ireland and the Republic of Ireland are included. Northern Ireland currently operates just two fleets of diesel multiple unit stock, these are given by set and vehicle formations. NIR also operate three main line locos for engineering trains and two Class 201 locos used in the joint operation of the 'Enterprise' Belfast to Dublin service.

In the Republic of Ireland a large number of DMUs are used, plus DART metro services around Dublin, which are operated by electric units.

Dublin also operates a growing city centre tram system and these vehicles are listed by class and unit number.

Loco-hauled fleets deployed on the Belfast-Dublin and Dublin to Cork route are listed by coach number.

Isle of Man Railway: Four railway systems operate on the Isle of Man, steam services between Douglas and Port Erin, electric services between Derby Castle (Douglas) and Ramsey, electric trams between Laxey and Snaefell and a horse-drawn tramway along the sea front in Douglas. Full listings of all systems, both passenger and freight are shown.

Steam Preservation: While modern traction preservation numbers are included in the general numeric tables, preserved steam locos are quoted in numeric order as a separate group of tables, giving loco number, name (if applied), the railway 'group' from which the type came, class type, wheel arrangement and last reported location.

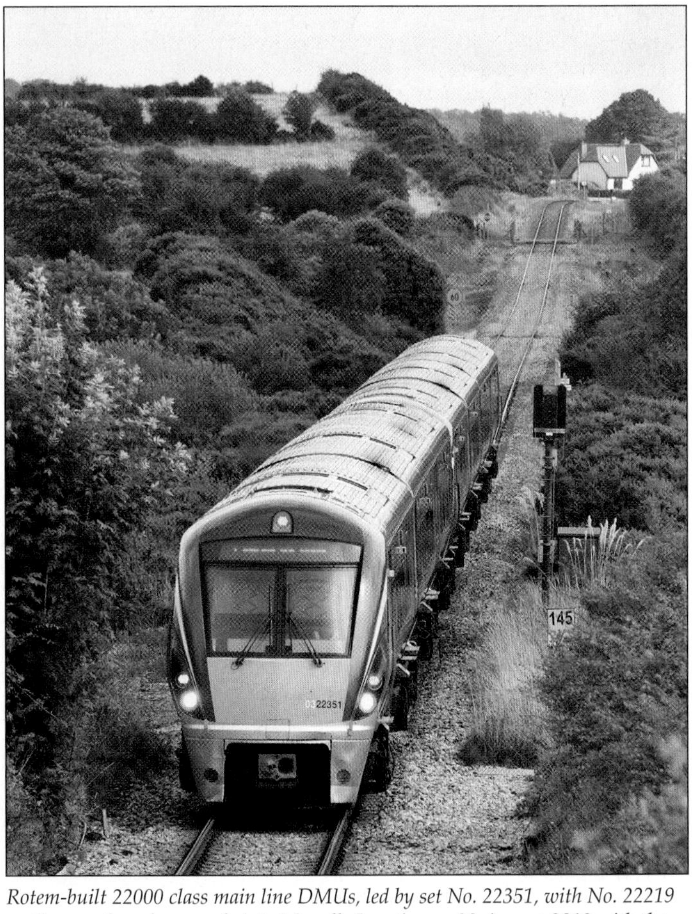

Rotem-built 22000 class main line DMUs, led by set No. 22351, with No. 22219 on the rear drop downgrade into Manulla Junction on 20 August 2019 with the, 12.45 Dublin Heuston to Westport. Much of the Irish Rail system is single line section with passing places. **CJM**

Coaching Stock Marks and Types

Mk1
The standard BR loco-hauled passenger coach built between 1951 and 1963. The design has a separate body and underframe, is usually 64ft 6in (19.66m) in length, a small number of suburban styles were constructed at 57ft (17.37m) in length. Until around 1960-1961 tungsten (bulb) lighting was used and vehicles were mounted on Mk1 bogies. In the early 1960s, some modernisation came with slightly improved interiors using fluorescent lighting. In 1961 cast style Commonwealth bogies became the standard. The Mk1 design was a mix of open and compartment vehicles, with over the years, many vehicles rebuilt with a number older coaches gaining Commonwealth or B4 bogies to improve ride.

Mk2
In 1963, the BRB unveiled a prototype of new generation passenger stock, the Mk2. This design saw semi-integral construction and was fitted with pressure heating/ventilation. The design retained older style tungsten lighting, but were mounted on a new design of B4 bogie. With some refinement from an original prototype, open and compartment vehicles of this style were built at BR Derby between 1964-1966.

The Mk2 design was furthered in 1967-1968 when a sizable fleet of Mk2a, Mk2b and Mk2c vehicles emerged from Derby. On the 2a, revised seating was fitted, aluminum was used extensively on bulkheads and doors, more modern toilets were fitted, as was fluorescent lighting and folding lime green end gangway doors. When the Mk2b emerged, this included wide wrap-around passenger doors, with no central door position. Toilets were also reduced to one per coach. By the time the Mk2c was delivered a further revised interior was used, with lower ceilings, improved decor and the use of centrally mounted ceiling fluorescent lighting. The lower ceiling panels were part of a plan to retro-fit air conditioning as this method of heating and cooling was under development. The folding end vestibule doors on this design were in red.

The most significant change in Mk2 design came with the delivery of the first Mk2d, incorporating full air conditioning, sealed double glazed passenger windows and new seats. The windows, without opening quarter lights, were of a more shallow design than on the previous Mk2s. Two further Mk2 derivatives emerged, Mk2e which incorporated smaller toilets, large end of vehicle luggage stands and bigger vestibules. The Mk2f was similar to the Mk2e but had a revised and improved air conditioning system, new style InterCity 70 seats and used an increased level of plastic and laminate for fittings and trim.

Mk3
A major step forward in coaching stock design was on the cards from the late 1960s, with a higher-speed longer vehicle being designed. This emerged as part of the original HST project, with a fleet of 75ft (23m) coaches, not only for the HST project, but also as a loco-hauled variant. Designed for 125mph (201km/h) operation and fitted with complex BT10 bogies. The design was built with first, standard and refreshment layouts and was later extended to sleeping vehicles. The coaches were of all open layout, with wrap around doors at each corner and had a streamlined skirt between the bogies. As the build progressed, a Mk3b version emerged with an improved interior, based on that of the APT. A fleet of Driving Van Trailers (DVTs) were also constructed to the Mk3 style, but with a shorter body. The HST passenger vehicles also conformed to the basic Mk3 design.

Mk4
To coincide with the modernisation and electrification of the East Coast Main Line in the late 1980s, a new design of 75ft (23m) passenger coach was developed, designated Mk4. These were vehicles designed to operate in semi-fixed formations and not as loose vehicles. The design profile would allow for tilting, but this was never installed. The open style coaches were fitted with sliding plug doors at each corner and mounted on a new design of SIG bogie, classified at BT41, allowing a maximum design speed of 140mph (225km/h), but normal speed was restricted to 125mph (201km/h). Vehicles of first, standard and refreshment design were built, together with a fleet of shorter Driving Van Trailers (DVTs).

Mk5
For two privatised operators, TransPennine and Caledonian Sleeper, Spanish builder CAF was contracted to design and build new coaching stock, designated Mk5, and are not part of the progressive designs of BR coaches. The vehicles, with a number of different layouts, first and standard class seating, cab control cars and sleeper vehicles of several styles, are based on a 72ft 10in (22.2m) body structure. They are fitted with power operated sliding plug doors at ends and mounted on CAF designed bogies.

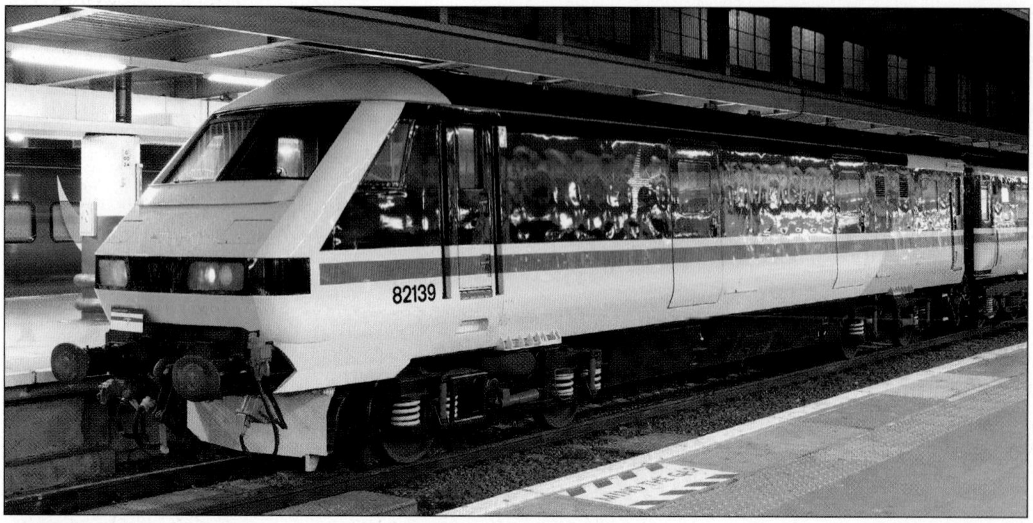

As part of the West Coast modernsation of the 1980s, a fleet of 52 Mk3b Driving Van Trailers (DVTs) were introduced from 1988. These were built on 61ft 9in (18.83m) frames. After use on West Coast, the fleet were cascaded to Greater Anglia and other routes including working with Network Rail. Some have now been preserved and two have returned to main line use with Loco Services Ltd (LSL). LSL-operated No. 82139 is seen in immaculate InterCity Swallow livery at Euston in January 2022. **Antony Christie**

The Locomotive Numbering System

Over the years, a number of different numbering systems have been used for 'modern traction' locomotives. As early examples appeared, even in the pre-grouping days, new numeric series were introduced by owners/operators for each type.

After the grouping in 1923, each of the 'Big Four' introduced different numeric series for non-steam traction, often doubling up numbers already in use on steam classes.

On the Southern Railway, early diesel shunters were numbered just 1, 2 and 3 and by the time main line electric locos emerged these were given the same numeric identification but prefixed by the loco class code 'CC'.

On the Great Western, just single numbers 1, 2 were used, while on the LNER, the company launched a new series from 6000 for electric locos and 8000 for shunting power.

The London Midland & Scottish Railway, who had by far the largest number of 'modern traction' locos, launched a new four digit series starting with a 7.

The first time any standardisation of locomotive numbering emerged was after the formation of the British Transport Commission (BTC) and Nationalisation of the railways in 1948, when a new 'Modern Traction' number series was introduced.

The range 10000-19999 was allocated to diesel or gas turbine locos, while the 20000-29999 series was allocated to electric locos. The few in traffic at the time, generally fitted around the second series, with, for example, the Southern electric locos No. CC1-CC3 renumbered to 20001-20003, and the LNER electric No. 6000 becoming No. 26000. The LMS main line prototype diesel No. 10000 just remained with its as built identity.

Detail of 1948 Numbering System

10xxx	Mainline diesel locos
11xxx	Diesel mechanical or diesel hydraulic shunters up to 299hp
12xxx	Ex-LMS shunters over 300 hp (224 kW)
13xxx	Diesel electric shunters (BTC ordered) Over 300hp
150xx	Ex-LNER shunters
151xx	Ex-GWR shunters
152xx	Ex-SR shunters
18xxx	Gas turbine locomotives
20xxx	Ex-SR electric locomotives
26xxx	Ex-LNER electric locomotives

The 1948 numbering system was satisfactory at the time, but with the rapid growth in 'modern traction' locos, and indeed multiple unit stock, a new, more robust system was required. This emerged in 1957, which became know as the '1957 Numbering System'. This prefixed all diesel locomotive numbers with a 'D' and all electric locomotives with an 'E'.

BR 1957 Numbering Basic Guide - Diesel

D1-D1999	Type 4	2000 to 2999 hp
D2000-D2999	Shunters	Below 300 hp
D3000-D4999	Shunters	300 to 799 hp
D5000-D6499	Type 2	1001 to 1499 hp
D6500-D7999	Type 3	1500 to 1999 hp
D8000-D8999	Type 1	800 to 1000 hp
D9000-D9999	Type 5	Over 3000 hp

This system was largely followed, but there were some anomalies. The Swindon-built 650hp diesel-hydraulic fleet (later Class 14) took numbers from D9500 upwards, which was outside the original plan. Also, when the original Type 2 allocated series was exceeded by extra orders, further locos received numbers from D7500 upwards.

Experimental, or trials locos tended to carry unique identities, often referring to engine builders, engine output, or the works number. The official BTC policy for trials and development locos was to use the D0xxx series.

Electric locos under the 1957 system saw different ranges used for different power types. It was planned that for AC locos the first number would be a power indication, with locos of an output between 2000-2999hp numbered in the E2000-E2999 range, while 3000-3999hp machines would be in the E3000-E3999 series.

DC locos were numbered in a different series starting E5000, with dual-power (electro-diesels) taking the E6000 range.

BR 1957 Numbering Basic Guide - Electric

E2000-E2999	AC	2000-2999hp
E3000-E3999	AC	3000-3999hp
E5000-E5999	DC	All outputs
E6000-E6999	D/DC	Electro-diesel All outputs

The 1957 numbering system worked well, but modernisation of the railways, the elimination of steam traction, compounded by the early use of computer technology, especially to loco allocation, maintenance and rostering, required a more detailed and strengthened numbering system to be introduced.

In the early 1970s, BR invested in a new computer era, the Total Operations Processing System (TOPS). This required either a five or six digit unique identity to be allocated to each loco or multiple unit, with no repetition of numbers on locos, units or coaching stock vehicles. The system used a classification-prefixed identity, where, on five digit loco numbers, the first two were the locomotive class, the third identified any sub-class, with the final two digits being an individual identity.

The TOPS based numeric system was officially introduced in 1973, and became known as the '1973 Numbering System'. However, some early re-numberings took place as far back as 1970 when a few LNER-design EM1 locos were renumbered into the 76xxx series and some AL3 and AL4 AC electric locos took on the 83xxx and 84xxx identities. The opposite occurred to the 'Western' Class 52 and 'Hymek' Class 35s which although in service until the mid-1970s did not receive TOPS numbers.

In terms of operating, the major differences of locomotives, stipulating which one could operate what type of train or service, or what equipment was fitted, led to a complex sub-class system being developed. For example, within the 500 plus Class 47 fleet, several sub-classes originally existed - 47/0 (Nos. 47001-47299) covered 'standard' locos fitted with steam-heating equipment (which might be isolated or removed), Class 47/3 (47301-47399) covered locos not fitted with any heating system, while Class 47/4 (47401-47599) covered locos fitted with electric or dual (steam/electric) train heating, 47/6, 47/9 (47601/901) covered traction development locos, Class 47/7 (47701-47717 original series) covered Scottish push-pull locos. The system was complicated and many additions and changes followed.

When allocating 'new' numbers to locos the TOPS system could not deal with a fleet starting with the number '000', such as 50000, therefore, for example, the first member of the Class 50 fleet No. D400, could not take the identity 50000 and had to be given a 'new' identity, in this case it became No. 50050. During the TOPS renumbering, a number of gaps in fleet numbering were closed up.

Under the original 1973 re-numbering policy document, issued by the BRB, the table below shows how the allocation was arranged.

BR 1973 TOPS Classification

Class 01-07	Shunters	Up to 299hp Old Nos. D2000-D2999
Class 08-14	Shunters	300-799hp Old Nos. D3000-D4999/ D9500-D9999
Class 15-20	Type 1	800-1000hp Old Nos. D8000-D8999
Class 21-32	Type 2	1001-1499hp Old Nos. D5000-D6499/ D7500-D7999
Class 33-39	Type 3	1500–1999hp Old Nos. D6500-D7499
Class 40-54	Type 4	2000-2999hp Old Nos. D1-D1999
Class 55-69	Type 5	Over 3000hp Old Nos. D9000-D9499
Class 70-79	Electric locomotives or Electro-diesel locos using direct current	
Class 80-99	Electric locomotives using alternating current	

In September 2011, the UK Rail Safety and Standards Board (RSSB), issued a revised Railway Group Standard No. GM/RT2453. This altered the use of numeric classifications to the TOPS identities. It extended the number ranges for certain types of loco to meet operating requirements and cover new classes.

The document also confirmed that British locos only operating within the UK on domestic routes, were not required to display their full 12-digit European Vehicle Number (EVN), as stipulated under UIC guidelines.

The 2011 Group Standard Revisions

Class 01-09	Diesel shunting locomotives
Class 10-79	Diesel locomotives (this authorised the 70 classification for the GE fleet)
Class 80-96	Electric locomotives
Class 73	Existing electro-diesel locomotives
Class 98	UK Heritage locomotives

The *Rail123 Traction & Rolling Stock Guide* uses the TOPS identification system, with any older 1957 series identified shown in brackets.

Multiple units now all carry a class prefixed identity, while coaching stock still uses either a three, four or five digit identity. Some multiple unit vehicles and coaches carry their full European Vehicle Number (EVN), but these are generally not shown for clarity.

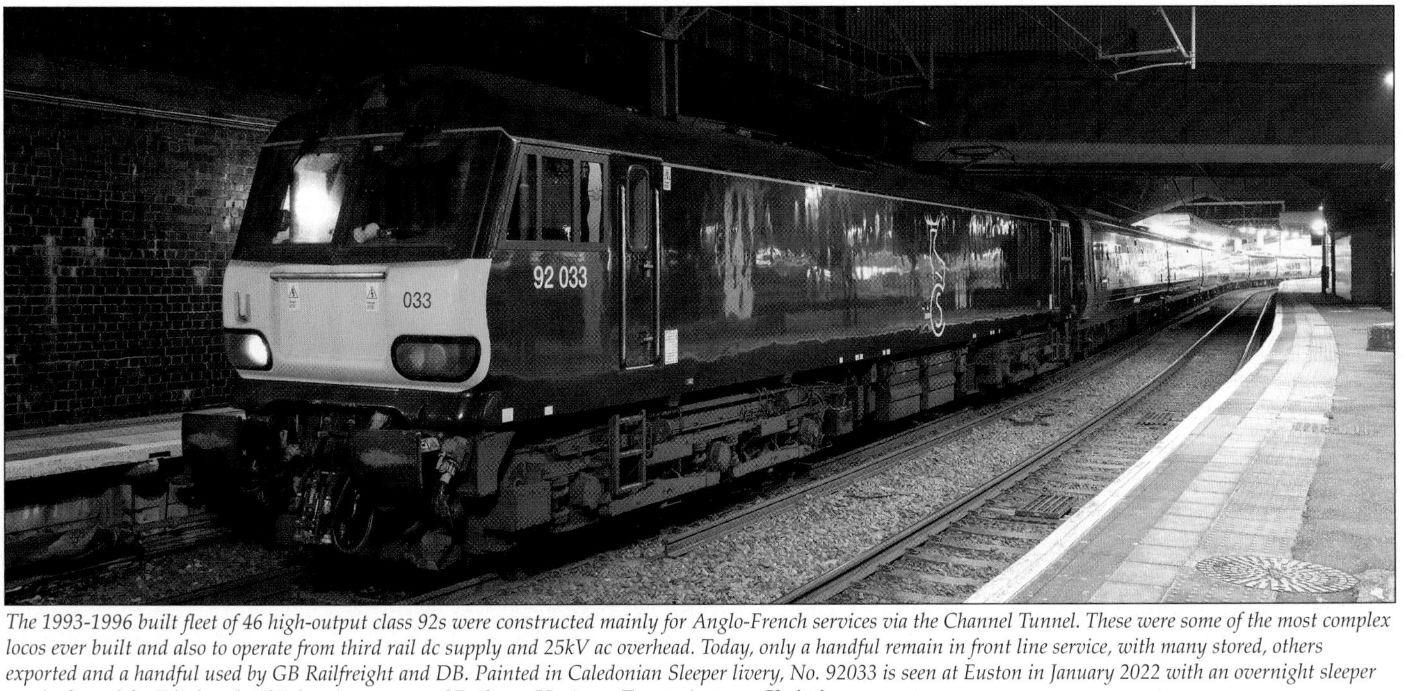

The 1993-1996 built fleet of 46 high-output class 92s were constructed mainly for Anglo-French services via the Channel Tunnel. These were some of the most complex locos ever built and also to operate from third rail dc supply and 25kV ac overhead. Today, only a handful remain in front line service, with many stored, others exported and a handful used by GB Railfreight and DB. Painted in Caledonian Sleeper livery, No. 92033 is seen at Euston in January 2022 with an overnight sleeper service bound for Edinburgh. This loco is now named Railway Heritage Trust. **Antony Christie**

Early LMS Diesel Shunting Locos
0-4-0 and 0-6-0

7050	War Department 224, 70224, 846	0-4-0DM	National Railway Museum, York
7401	(7051)	0-6-0DM	Middleton Railway
7069	War Department 18	0-6-0DE	Vale of Berkeley Railway
7103	War Department 52, 70052 Italian FS No. 700.001	0-6-0DE	Turin Ponte Mosca Station
7106	War Department 55, 70055 Italian FS No. 700.003	0-6-0DE	Rail Museum, Arezzo, Italy

NER6480 / BR26500 Class ES1
NER Bo-Bo Electric

Built: 1903
Length: 37ft 11in (11.56m)
Height: 12ft 11in (3.94m)
Width: 8ft 9in (2.67m)
Equipment: Electric 640hp (477kW)
Transmission: Electric
Tractive effort: 25,100lb (111kN)

26500 (6480) (1) National Railway Museum, Shildon

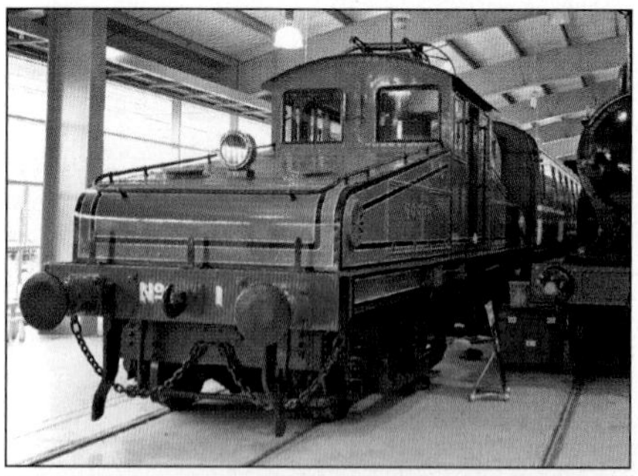

1903 vintage North Eastern Railway, later Class ES1 No. 1, BR No. 26500 on display at the National Railway Musuem, Shildon site. **Antony Christie**

18000
Brown Boveri - A1A-A1A Gas Turbine

Built: 1949
Length: 63ft 0½in (19.21m)
Height: 13ft 4in (4.06m)
Width: 9ft 2½in (2.80m)
Engine: Brown Boveri gas-turbine of 2,500hp (1,864kW)
Transmission: Electric
Tractive effort: 12,400lb (55kN)

18000 Didcot Railway Centre

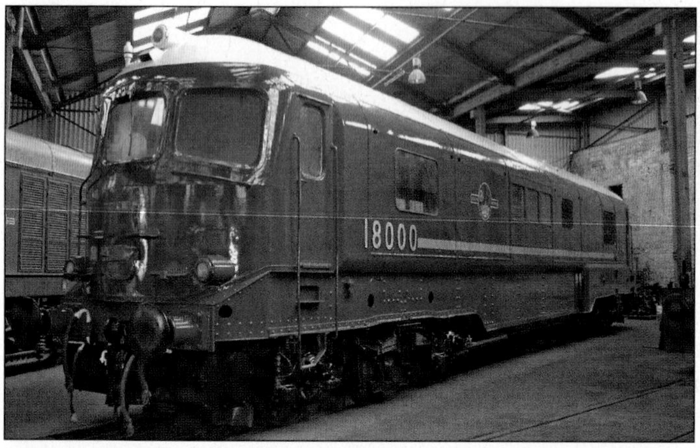

Restored to 1950s BR green, Brown-Boveri gas-turbine No. 18000 which operated on BR Western Region and was later exported to Vienna, displayed at the Mechanical Engineering Arsenal test centre. It is now preserved at Didcot Railway Centre. **Phil Barnes**

D0226
English Electric 0-6-0 Diesel-Electric

Built: 1956
Length: 31ft 8½in (9.66m)
Height: 12ft 3in (3.73m)
Width: 8ft 10in (2.69m)
Engine: English Electric 6RKT of 500hp (372.8kW)
Transmission: Electric
Tractive effort: 33,000lb (146.7kN)

D0226 (D226) Keighley & Worth Valley Railway (named *Vulcan*)

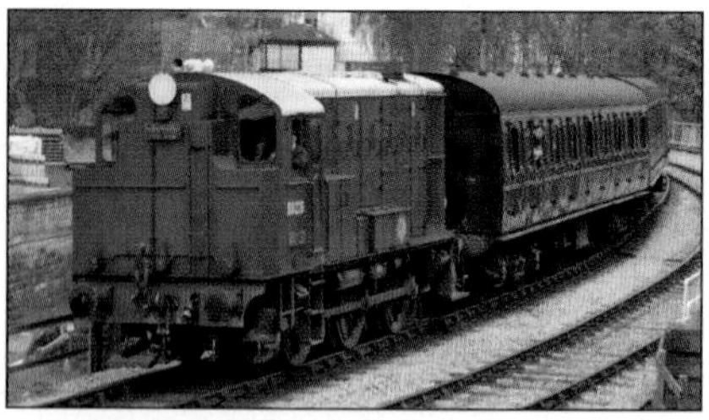

One of a pair of trial Road Switchers built by English Electric in the 1950s for trials on BR, No. D0226 is now preserved, operational at the Keighley & Worth Valley Railway. On 19 April 2022 it is seen departing Keighley, bound for Oxenhope. **Allan Clearie**

D2510 - D2519
Hudswell & Clarke 0-6-0 Diesel-Mechanical

Built: 1961
Length: 26ft 3¼in (8.00m)
Height: 12ft 0in (3.66m)
Width: 8ft 9in (2.67m)
Engine: Gardner 8L3 of 204hp (152kW)
Transmission: Mechanical
Tractive effort: 16,100lb (71.6kN)

D2511 - Keighley & Worth Valley Railway

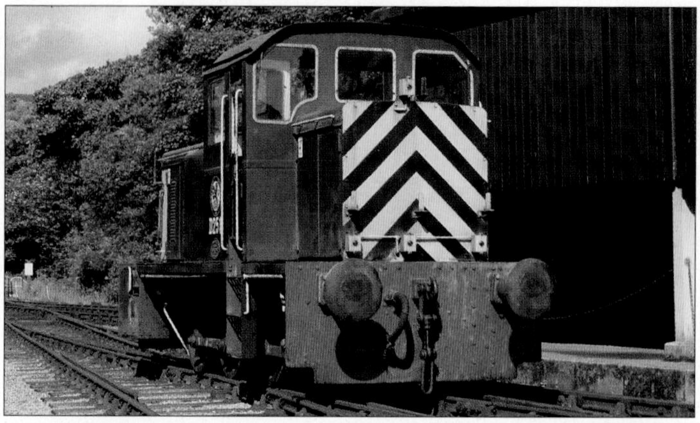

Just one example of the 10 strong Hudswell & Clarke 204hp 0-6-0 diesel mechanical fleet is preserved, No. D2511, operational at the Keighley & Worth Valley Railway. The loco is restored to 1960s green with wasp ends. **Adrian Paul**

D2708 - D2780
NBL 0-4-0 Diesel-Hydraulic

Built: 1961
Length: 24ft 5½in (7.45m)
Height: 11ft 2¾in (3.65m)
Width: 8ft 5in (2.57m)
Engine: NBL-MAN W6V of 225hp (167kW)
Transmission: Hydraulic
Tractive effort: 21,500lb (95.6kN)

D2767	-	Bo'ness & Kinneil Railway
D2774	-	Strathspey Railway

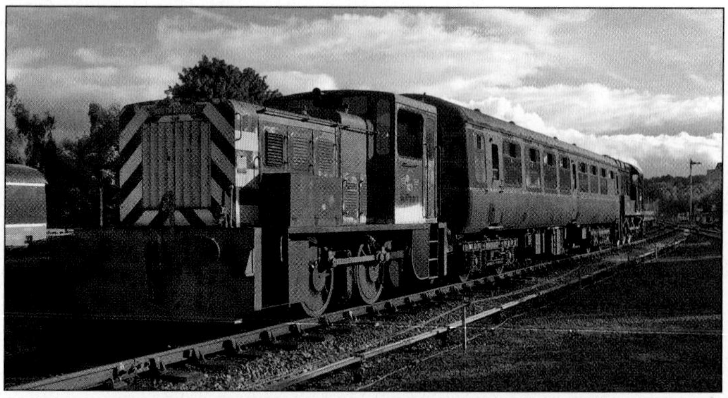

Both the preserved D2708 series NBL 0-4-0s are based in Scotland. No. D2774 is shown which is based on the Strathspey Railway. **Howard Lewsey**

Deltic - DP1
English Electric Co-Co Diesel-Electric

Built: 1955
Length: 66ft 0in (20.12m)
Height: 12ft 10½in (3.92m)
Width: 8ft 9½in (2.68m)
Engine: 2 x Napia D18-25 of 1,650hp (1,230kW)
Transmission: Electric
Tractive effort: 60,000lb (266.8kN)

DELTIC - National Railway Museum, Shildon

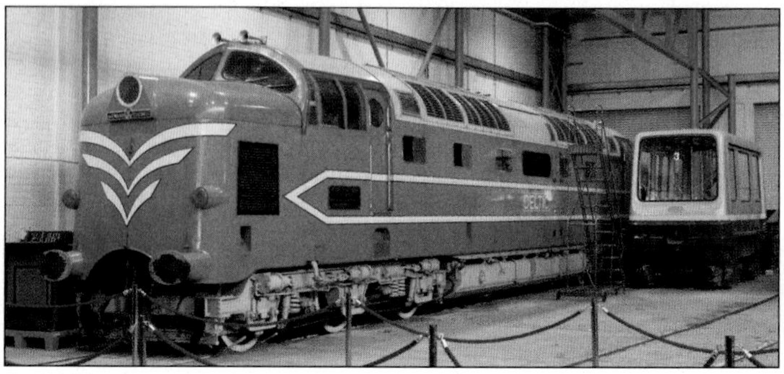

English Electric prototype 'Deltic' is preserved as part of the National Collection and is currently on display at the York site. The loco is preserved non-operational and is seen on display next to the original Birmingham Airport People Mover. **CJM**

Industrial Locomotives Class 01/5

01504 (630)		AB 0-6-0DH	Exported to Bong Mine, Liberia
01507 (425)	*Venom*	R&H 0-6-0DH	Crossley Evans Ltd, Shipley
01508 (428)		R&H 0-6-0DH	Arlington Fleet Group, Eastleigh
01509 (433)	*Lesley*	R&H 0-6-0DH	Chiltern Railways, Aylesbury
01510 (272/V320)		TH 4wDH	MoD Longtown
01511 (275/V323)		TH 4wDH	LH Group, Barton under Needwood
01512 (301/V319)	*Conductor*	TH 4wDH	DSDC Bicester
01513 (302/V318)	*Greensleeves*	TH 4wDH	DM Kineton
01514 (303/V332)		TH 4wDH	DM Longtown
01515 (304/V321)		TH 4wDH	HNRC, Barrow Hill
01520 (274/V322)		TH 4wDH	Ferrybridge WRD
01521 (278/V333)	*Flack*	TH 4wDH	DSDC Bicester
01522 (254/V272)		TH 4wDH	LH Group Barton-under-Needwood
01523 (259/V299)		TH 4wDH	Marchwood Centre
01524 (261/V301)		TH 4wDH	Ludgershall
01525 (264/V306)	*Draper*	TH 4wDH	DERA Shoeburyness
01526 (265/V307)		TH 4wDH	HNRC, Wensleydale Railway
01527 (256/V274)		TH 4wDH	MoD Glen Douglas
01528 (267/V309)		TH 4wDH	DM Kineton
01529 (268/V310)		TH 4wDH	HNRC, Wensleydale Railway
01530 (269/V311)		TH 4wDH	East Kent Railway
01531 (H4323)	*Colonel Tomline*	HUN 0-6-0DH	Peak Rail, Rowsley
01541 (260/V300)		TH 4wDH	Defence Munitions Kineton
01542 (262/V302)		TH 4wDH	Ashchurch
01543 (263/V303)		TH 4wDH	East Kent Railway
01544 (252/V270)		TH 4wDH	HNRC, Wensleydale Railway
01545 (253/V271)		TH 4wDH	HNRC, Wensleydale Railway
01546 (255/V273)		TH 4wDH	East Kent Railway
01547 (266/V308)		TH 4wDH	HNRC, Long Marston
01548 (257/V275)		TH 4wDH	MoD Ludgershall
01549 (258/V298)		TH 4wDH	MoD Marchwood
01550 (271/V324)		TH 4wDH	MoD Bicester
01551 (H016)	*Lancelot*	EE-VF 0-4-0DH	Siemens, Ardwick Depot
01552 (D3/167)		TH 0-6-0DH	HNRC, Long Marston
01553 (BR 12082)		BR Derby 0-6-0DE	Mid Hants Railway as No. 12049
01555 (D6)		HC 0-6-0DM	T J Thomson, Stcokton-on-Tees
01560 (DH25)		RR-S 4wDH	ED Murray & Son, Hartlepool
01562 (6475)	*Black Beast*	TH 0-6-0DH	Bardon Aggregates, Croft
01565 (3001)		RR-S 0-6-0DH	C F Booth, Rotherham
01567	*Elizabeth*	TH 4wDH	T J Thomson, Stockton-on-Tees
01569	*Emma*	TH 4wDH	T J Thomson, Stockton-on-Tees
01570		HB B-B DH	Hope Construction
01571 (124)	*Coral*	TH 0-6-0DH	Imerys, Bugle
01572 (5482)	*Kathryn*	RR-S 0-6-0DH	Bardon Aggregates, Croft
01573 (H006)		HUN 0-6-0DH	RMS Locotec, with Cobra Railfreight
01581 (TM4150)		TM 4wDM	York Holgate
01583 (422)		RH 0-6-0DH	Preserved Lavender Line
01585	*Scaz*	R&H 0-6-0DH	Vivarail
323-539-7	*Cheviot*	Kof II 4WDH	Northumbria Rail, at AFS

Key
HB - Hunslet Barclay, HUN - Hunslet, R&H - Ruston & Hornsby, RR-S - Rolls Royce-Sentinel, TH - Thomas Hill, TM - Trackmobile

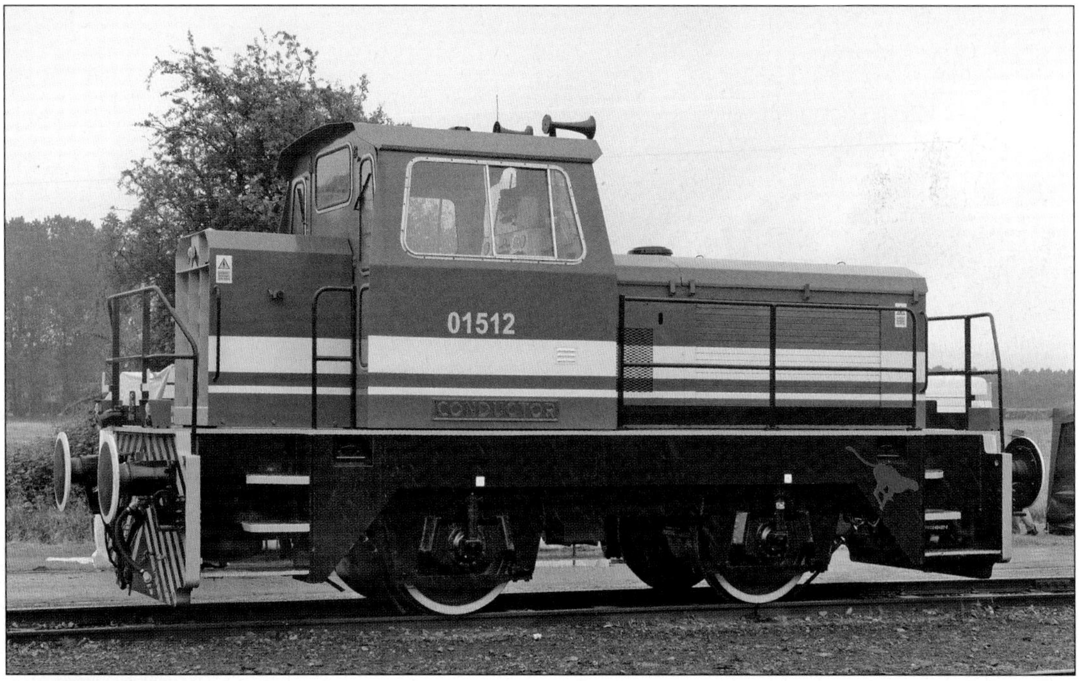

The Class 01/5 classification is reserved for Network Rail resistered industrial locomotives, these might be owned by private industry or operators such as the Ministry of Defence. They are generally not former BR-operated classes. No. 01512 Conductor is owned by the Defence, Storage and Distribution Centre (DSDC) and is currently based at Bicester. It is a Thomas Hill-built 4-wheel diesel-hydraulic. **CJM**

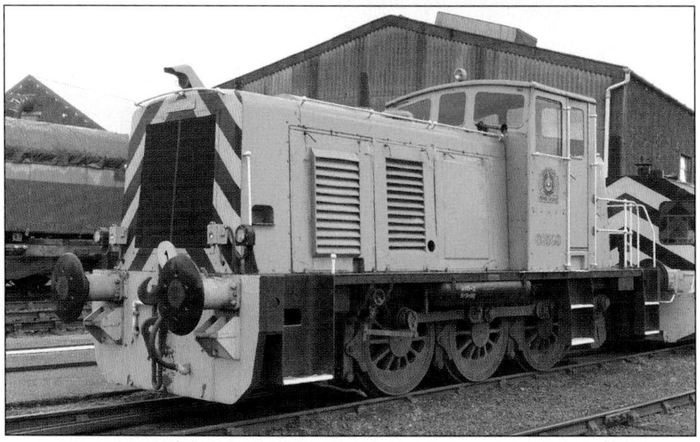

This Ruston & Hornsby 0-6-0 diesel-hydraulic, which looks very much like a BR Class 07, is used by Arlington Fleet Services, Eastleigh for works pilotage. It is painted in Arlington green and carried an Arlington Fleet Group logo on the cab side. **CJM**

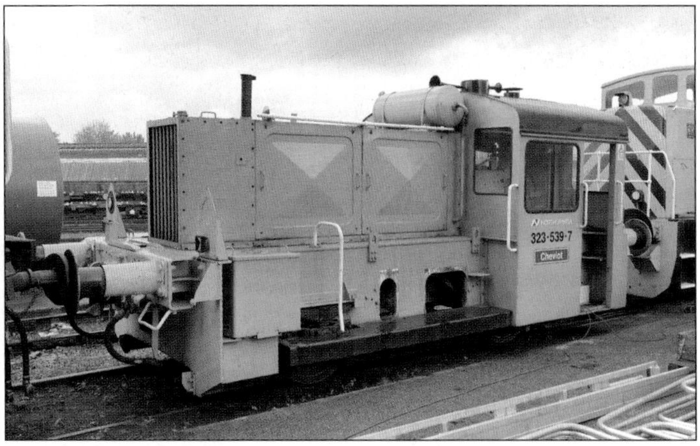

An interesting little loco at Arlington, Eastleigh, is site pilot loco No. 323 539-7. This is an import from Germany and was originally classified by DB as a Class 323, it is low-profile 0-4-0 diesel-electric, built by Kof as a DRG Kleinlokomotive of Class II. It carries Arlington Fleet Group green and carries the Northumbria Rail branding on the cab side. **CJM**

Class 01
Andrew Barclay 0-4-0 Diesel-Mechanical

Built: 1956
Length: 23ft 8in (7.21m)
Height: 11ft 10¼in (3.62m)
Width: 8ft 5in (2.57m)
Engine: Gardner 6L3 of 153hp (114kW)
Transmission: Mechanical
Tractive effort: 12,750lb (56.8kN)

D2953	11503	Peak Rail, Heritage Shunters Trust
D2956	11506	East Lancashire Railway

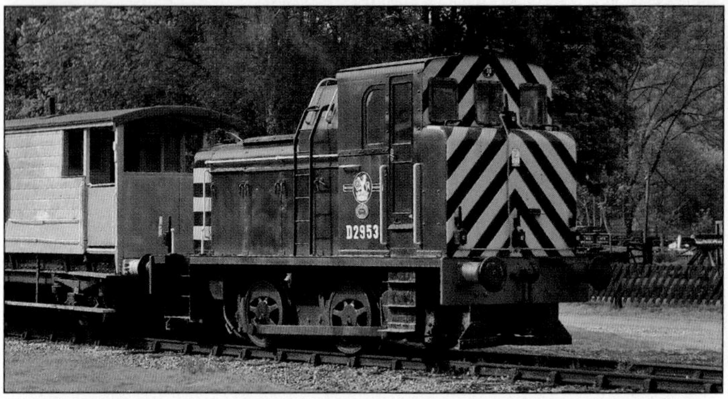

The original BR Class 01, which over the years were famous for working on the isolated Holyhead Breakwater Railway is represented by two preserved examples. No. D2953 shown, is based with the Heritage Shunters Trust at Peak Rail. **Adrian Paul**

Class 02
Yorkshire Engine Co 0-4-0 Diesel-Hydraulic

Built: 1960-61
Length: 21ft 11¾in (6.7m)
Height: 11ft 5¼in (3.49m)
Width: 8ft 6in (2.59m)
Engine: Rolls Royce C6 of 170hp (127kW)
Transmission: Hydraulic
Tractive effort: 15,000lb (66.7kN)

D2853	02003	Barrow Hill Roundhouse
D2854		Peak Rail, Heritage Shunters Trust
D2858		Midland Railway Centre
D2860		National Railway Museum
D2866		Peak Rail, Heritage Shunters Trust
D2867		Battlefield Railway
D2868		Barrow Hill Roundhouse

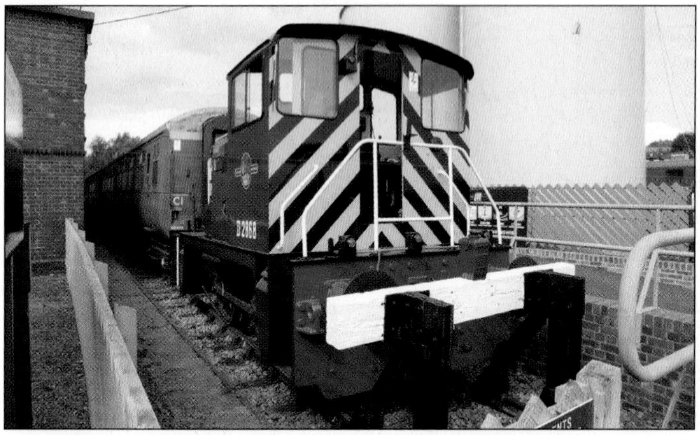

Seven of the 20 Yorkshire Engine Co built 0-4-0 diesel-hydraulic locos are preserved, these are unusual having a veranda at the cab end. No D2868 is seen at Barrow Hill, painted in 1960s BR green. **Adrian Paul**

Class 03
BR/Gardner 0-6-0 Diesel-Mechanical

Built: 1958-1962
Length: 26ft 0in (7.92m)
Height: 12ft 3½in (3.75m)
Width: 8ft 6in (2.59m)
Engine: Gardner 8L3 of 204hp (152kW)
Transmission: Mechanical
Tractive effort: 15,300lb (68kN)

03018	D2018	Mangapps Farm - as 11205					
D2019		Exported to Italy					
03020	D2020	Sonic Rail Services, Burnham - 11207					
03022	D2022	Swindon & Cricklade Railway					
D2023		Kent & East Sussex Railway - 11210					
D2024		Kent & East Sussex Railway - 11211					
03027	D2027	Peak Rail, Heritage Shunters Trust					
D2032		Exported to Italy					
D2033		Exported to Italy					
D2036		Exported to Italy					
03037	D2037	Royal Deeside Railway					
D2041		Colne Valley Railway					
D2046		Plym Valley Railway					
D2051		North Norfolk Railway					
03059	D2059	Isle of Wight Steam Railway					
03062	D2062	East Lancashire Railway					
03063	D2063	North Norfolk Railway					
03066	D2066	Barrow Hill Roundhouse					
03069	D2069	Dean Forest Railway					
03072	D2072	Lakeside & Haverthwaite Railway					
03073	D2073	Railway Age, Crewe					
03078	D2078	North Tyneside Steam Railway					
03079	D2079	Derwent Valley Light Railway					
03081	D2081	Mangapps Farm Railway Museum					
03084		X	CS	MBDL	GRN	WCR	WCR
03089	D2089	Mangapps Farm Railway Museum					
03090	D2090	National Railway Museum, Shildon					
03094	D2094	Royal Deeside Railway					
D2098		Exported to Italy					
03099	D2099	Peak Rail, Heritage Shunters Trust					
03112	D2112	Rother Valley Railway					
03113	D2113	Peak Rail, Heritage Shunters Trust					
D2117		Lakeside & Haverthwaite Railway - No. 8					
D2118		Great Central Railway, Nottingham					
03119	D2119	Epping & Ongar Railway					
03120	D2120	Fawley Hill Railway					
03128	D2128	S&D Midsomer Norton					
D2133		West Somerset Railway					
03134	D2134	Royal Deeside Railway					
D2138		Midland Railway Centre, Butterley					
D2139		Peak Rail, Heritage Shunters Trust					
03141	D2141	Pontypool & Blaenavon Railway					
03144	D2144	Wensleydale Railway					
03145	D2145	Moreton Park Rly, Moreton-on-Lugg					
D2148		Ribble Steam Railway					
03152	D2152	Swindon & Cricklade Railway					
D2153		Exported to Italy					
03158	D2158	Mangapps Farm					
03162	D2162	Llangollen Railway					
03170	D2170	Epping and Ongar Railway					
D2178		Gwili Railway					
03179	D2179	Rushden Transport Museum					
03180	D2180	Peak Rail, Rowsley					
D2182		Gloucester Warwickshire Railway					
D2184		Colne Valley Railway					
03189	D2189	Ribble Steam Railway					
D2192		Dartmouth Steam Railway					
03196		X	CS	MBDL	GRN	WCR	WCR
03197	D2197	Mangapps Farm					
D2199		Peak Rail, Heritage Shunters Trust					
03371	D2371	Dartmouth Steam Railway					
D2381		V	CS	MBDL	BLK	WCR	WCR
03399	D2399	Mangapps Farm Railway					

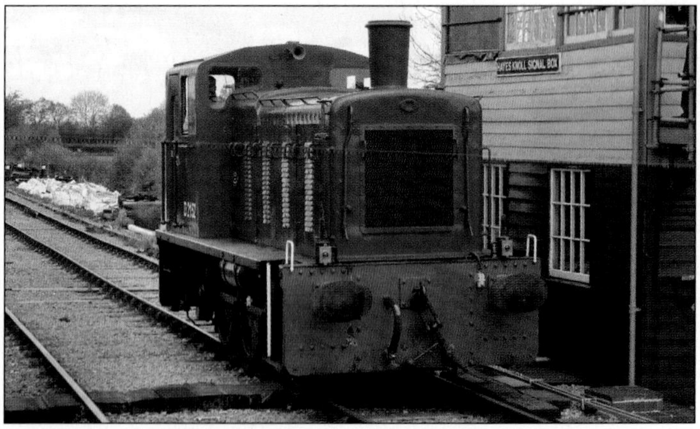

The standard design small 204hp diesel-mechanical BR shunting loco was of Class 03 and could be found operating in all corners of the network. A large number are prreserved and a handful have been exported. Preserved No. D2152 (03152) is based on the Swindon & Cricklade Railway and is seen in all-over green livery at Hayes Knoll. **Adrian Paul**

Class 04
Drewry 0-6-0 Diesel-Mechanical

Built: 1952-1961
Length: 26ft 0in (7.92m)
Height: 12ft 1⅜in (3.69m)
Width: 8ft 6in (2.59m)
Engine: Gardner 8L3 of 204hp (152kW)
Transmission: Mechanical
Tractive effort: D2200-14 - 16,850lb (74.9kN)
D2215-D2340 - 15,650lb (69.6kN)

D2203	11103	Embsay & Bolton Abbey Railway
D2205		Peak Rail, Heritage Shunters Trust
D2207	11108	North Yorkshire Moors Railway
D2216	11122	Exported to Italy
D2229	11135	Peak Rail, Heritage Shunters Trust
D2231	11150	Exported to Italy
D2245	11215	Derwent Valley Light Railway
D2246		South Devon Railway
D2271		South Devon Railway

D2272	Peak Rail, Heritage Shunters Trust
D2279	East Anglian Railway
D2280	North Norfolk Railway
D2284	Peak Rail, Heritage Shunters Trust
D2289	Peak Rail, Heritage Shunters Trust
D2295	Exported to Italy
D2298	Buckinghamshire Railway Centre
D2302	Moreton Park Rly, Moreton-on-Lugg
D2310	Battlefield Railway, Shackerstone
D2324	Peak Rail, Heritage Shunters Trust
D2325	Mangapps Farm Railway
D2334	Mid Norfolk Railway
D2337	Peak Rail, Heritage Shunters Trust

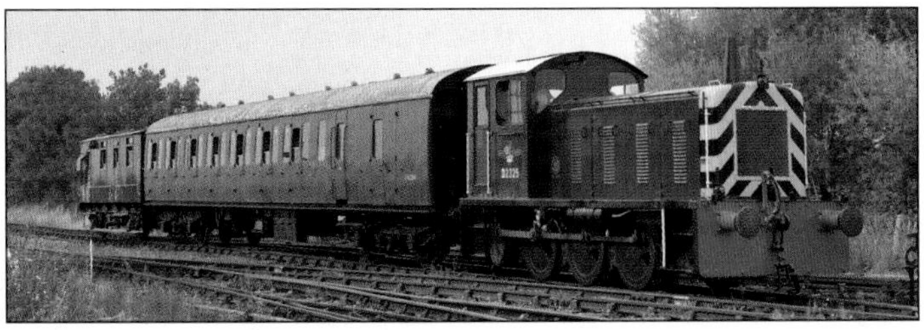

The Drewry 0-6-0 diesel-mechanical shunting locos looked very much like the BR Class 03, but had different window arrangements. Preserved at Mangapps Farm Museum, No. D2325 is seen on the railway demonstration track in summer 2021. **CJM**

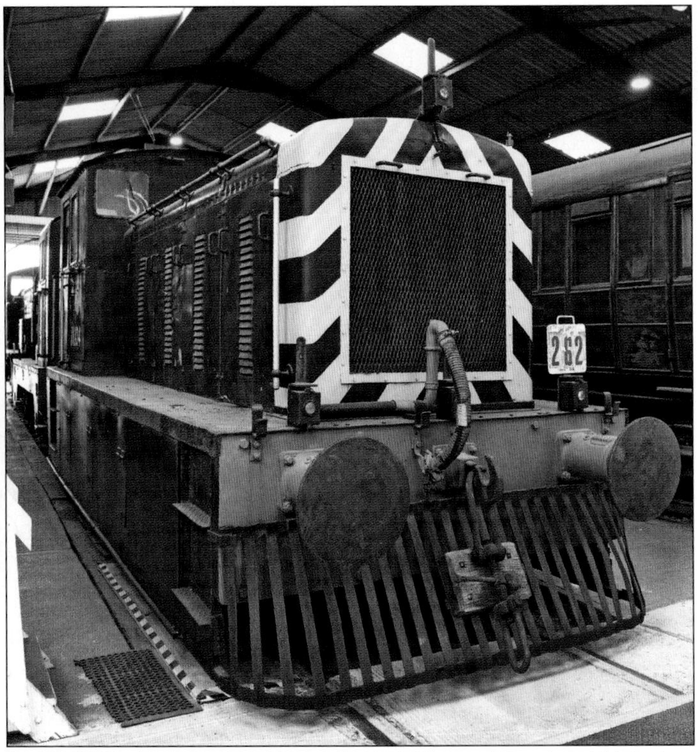

Loco No.11104 at Mangapps Farm Museum, is not what it seems, it is an industrial shunter, adapted to resemble a BR Wisbech and Upwell Tram Loco. The Number 11104 was not used in the BR Drewry series as it was carried by a departmental loco. With full front guards and side skirts the loco is seen inside the shed at Mangapps Farm. **CJM**

Class 05
Hunslet 0-6-0 Diesel-Mechanical

Built: 1955-1961
Length: 25ft 4in (7.72m)
Height: 11ft 0in (3.35m)
Width: 8ft 3in (2.51m)
Engine: Gardner 8L3 of 204hp (152kW)
Transmission: Mechanical
Tractive effort: D2550-D2573 - 14,500lb (64.9kN)
D2574-D2618 - 17,400lb (77.3kN)

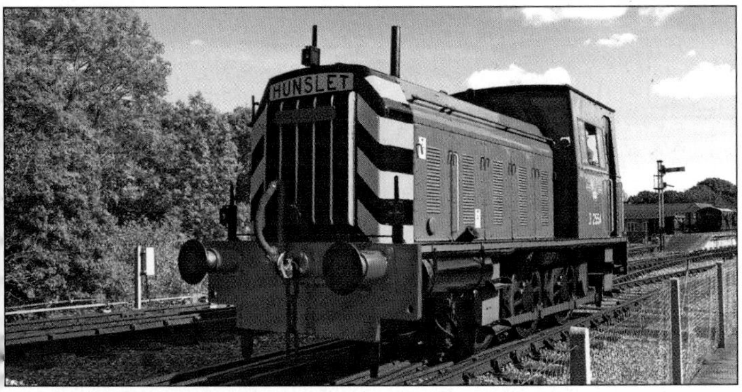

Four of the Hunslet 204hp desel-mechanical locos survive in preservation, including the only one to be renumbered into the TOPS system, 05001 (D2554) which operated in its later years on the Isle of Wight. It is shown preserved in green livery at Haven Street. **Adrian Paul**

05001	D2554	Isle of Wight Steam Railway
	D2578	Moreton Park Railway, Moreton-on-Lugg
	D2587	Peak Rail, Heritage Shunters Trust
	D2595	Ribble Steam Railway

Class 06
Andrew Barclay 0-4-0 Diesel-Mechanical

Built: 1958-1960
Length: 25ft 11in (7.90m)
Height: 11ft 10¼in (3.61m)
Width: 8ft 5in (2.57m)
Engine: Gardner 8L3 of 204hp (152kW)
Transmission: Mechanical
Tractive effort: 19,800lb (88kN)

06003	D2420	Peak Rail, Heritage Shunters Trust
-	D2432	Exported to Italy

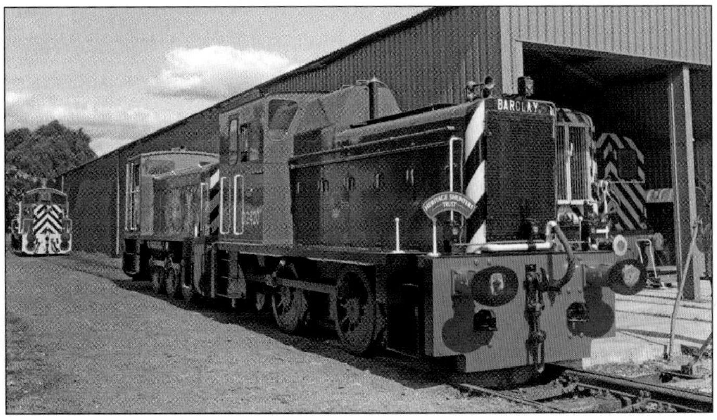

Of the 35 Barclay-built 204hp 0-4-0 locos, later of Class 06 and used exclusively in Scotland, just one is preserved. Thankfully, after departmental use at Reading signal works, No. 06003 (D2420) was saved by Peak Rail based Heritage Shunters Trust, where the loco is seen in green livery. **Adrian Paul**

Class 07
Ruston & Hornsby 0-6-0 Diesel-Electric

Built: 1962
Length: 26ft 6in (8.18m)
Height: 12ft 10in (3.92m)
Width: 8ft 6in (2.59m)
Engine: Paxman RPHL Mk3 of 275hp (205kW)
Transmission: Electric
Tractive effort: 28,800lb (128kN)

07001	D2985	Peak Rail, Heritage Shunters Trust					
07005	D2989	Great Central Railway					
07007	D2992	V	AF	MBDL	BLU	AFS	AFS
07009	D2993	Exported to Italy					
07010	D2994	Avon Valley Railway					
07011	D2995	St. Leonards Railway Engineering					
07012	D2996	HNRC Barrow Hill Roundhouse					
07013	D2997	East Lancashire Railway					

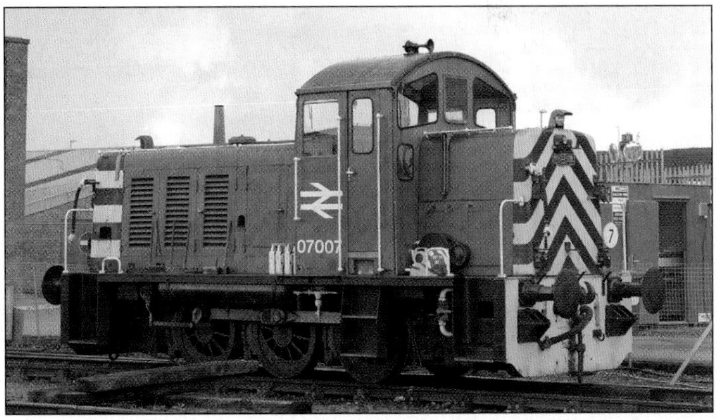

The Ruston & Hornsby 175hp diesel-electric locos, built for Southern Region use were classified 07. Six are preserved and one, No. 07007, remains operational as a works pilot at Arlington Fleet Services, Eastleigh. The loco is seen in BR blue livery. **CJM**

Class 08/09/10
BR 0-6-0 Diesel-Electric

Built: 1953-1959
Length: 29ft 3in (8.91m)
Height: 12ft 2⅝in (3.88m)
Width: 8ft 6in (2.59m)
Engine: English Electric 6K of 400hp (298kW)
Transmission: Electric
Tractive effort: 35,000lb (156kN)

-	D3000	HNRC, Worksop
-	D3002	Plym Valley Railway
-	D3014	Dartmouth Steam Railway
08011	D3018	Chinnor & Princes Risborough Railway
08012	D3019	Cambrian Heritage Railways
08015	D3022	Severn Valley Railway
08016	D3023	Heritage Shunters Trust, Peak Rail
08021	D3029	Tyseley Locomotive Works

08022	D3030	Cholsey & Wallingford Railway				
08032	D3044	Mid Hants Railway				
08046	D3059	Caledonian Railway, Brechin				
08054	D3067	Embsay & Bolton Abbey Railway				
08060	D3074	Cholsey & Wallingford Railway				
08064	D3079	National Railway Museum, Shildon				
-	D3101	Great Central Railway, Loughborough				
08102	D3167	Lincolnshire Wolds Railway				
08108	D3174	Kent & East Sussex Railway				
08114	D3180	GCR, Nottingham, on loan to Epping Ongar Railway				
08123	D3190	Cholsey & Wallingford Railway				
08133	D3201	Severn Valley Railway as No. 13201				
08164	D3232	East Lancashire Railway				
08168	D3236	Nemesis Rail, Burton-on-Trent				
-	D3261	Swindon & Cricklade Railway				
08195	D3265	Llangollen Railway as 13265				
08202	D3272	Avon Valley Railway				
08220	D3290	Nottingham Transport Centre, Ruddington				
08238	D3308	Dean Forest Railway				
08266	D3336	Keighley & Worth Valley Railway				
08288	D3358	Mid Hants Railway				
08308	D3378	Weardale Railway				
08331	D3401	Midland Railway Centre				
08359	D3429	Avon Valley Railway, loan to Bodmin & Wenford Railway				
-	D3452	Bodmin & Wenford Railway				
08375		A			RSS	RSS at Port of Boston
08377	D3462	Mid Hants Railway				
-	D3489	Spa Valley Railway				
08389		A Y	BH		HNR	EWS HNRL, Celsa Steel, Cardiff
08401		A			SPL	EMS at Hams Hall
08405		A R			EWS	RSS at Neville Hill
08410		A M			GWG	A V Dawson, Middlesborough
08411		A M			BLU	RSS at Rye Farm, Wishaw
08417		Barrow Hill Roundhouse				
08418		A	CS	MBDL	WCR	WCR WCR
08423		A			SPL	PD Ports, Middlesbrough 14/HO11
08428		A K			EWS	HNRC at Barrow Hill
08436	D3551	Swanage Railway				
08441		A			RSS	RSS at Norwich Crown Point
08442		A			ATC	Arriva Traincare, Eastleigh (S)
08443	D3558	Bo'ness & Kinneil Railway				
08444	D3559	Bodmin & Wenford Railway				
08445		A			SPL	EMS at Daventry
08447		A			SPL	Russell Group, at Hillington, Glasgow
08451		X M			ALS	Arlington, Eastleigh
08454		X M			ALS	Alstom, Widnes
08460		A			RSS	RSS at Felixstowe
08471	D3586	Severn Valley Railway				
08472		A M			WAB	EMS Hitachi, Craigentinny
08473	D3588	Dean Forest Railway (chassis only)				
08476	D3591	Swanage Railway				
08479	D3594	East Lancashire Railway				
08480		A M			RSS	RSS at Felixstowe
08483		A M	CL	LSLS	GRN	LSL LSL, Crewe Named: *Bungle*
08484		A			RSS	RSS at Norwich Crown Point
08485		A	CS	MBDL	WCR	WCR WCR, Carnforth
08490	D3605	Strathspey Railway				
08495	D3610	North Yorkshire Moors Railway				
08499		A	CF	COLO	BLU	COL COL, Cardiff
08500		X			BLU	HNRC, Worksop
08502		X			SPL	HNRC, East Kent Light Railway
08503	D3658	Barry Island Railway				
08507		Cholsey & Wallingford Railway				
08511		A			RSS	RSS at Eastleigh
08516		A			ATC	Arriva Traincare, Barton Hill
08523		X M			BLU	Weardale Railway
08525		X	NL	EMSL	EMR	EMR EMR Named: *Duncan Bedford*
08527		X			FSL	HNRC at Attero Recycling, Rossington
08528	D3690	Derwent Valley Railway				
08530		X M	FL	DFLS	FLR	PTR FLR (LH Group)
08531		X M	FL	DFLS	FLR	PTR FLR (Felixstowe)
08536		A			BLU	RSS at Rye Farm, Wishaw
08556	D3723	North Yorkshire Moors Railway				
08567		X			EWS	Arlington Fleet Services, Eastleigh
08568		X			SPL	RSS at Rye Farm, Wishaw (for sale)
08571		A M			WAB	EMS at Daventry Freight Terminal
08573		X			BLK	RMS at Weardale Railway
08575		X	FL	DHLT	FLR	PTR FLR (Nemesis Rail)
08578		X			EWS	HNRC at Worksop
08580		X M			RSS	RSS at Garston
08585		X M	FL	DHLT	FLR	PTR FLR (Southampton)
08588	H047	X			RMS	Alstom, Ilford
08590	D3757	Midland Railway Centre				
08593		X			EWS	RSS at Rye Farm, Wishaw
08596		A M Y			WAB	EMS at Hitachi, Craigentinny
08598		X			SPL	RSS at Dawsons
08600		A			SPL	A V Dawson, Middlesborough
08602	004	X			HNR	HNRC at Worksop
08604	D3771	Didcot Railway Centre				
08605		X Y			DBC	Riviera Trains at Ecclesbourne Valley Rly
08611		X M			BLU	Alstom, Wembley
08613	H064	X			RMS	PRH at Weardale Railway
08615		X M			HUN	EMS at Tata Steel, Shotton

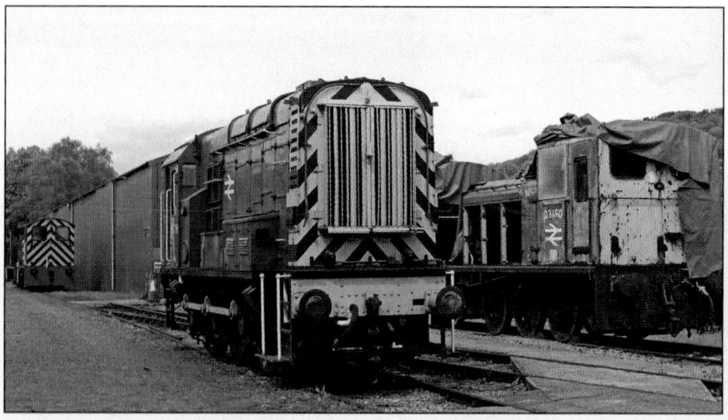

By far the largest fleet of diesel locos built for the UK was the BR standard 350hp diesel-electric 0-6-0 shunter, with almost 1,200 examples. Some remain in service, others work for industrial uses and many are preserved. Preserved No. 08016, is operated by the Heritage Shunters Trust at Peak Rail. **Adrian Paul**

08616	D3783	X	TS	EJLO	LMI	WMR WMR *Tyseley 100*
08617		X M			BLU	Alstom, Oxley
08622	H028	X			BLK	PRH at Ketton, Cement
08623		X			DBC	HNRC at Hope Cement Works
08624		X M	FL	DFLS	FLP	FLR (Trafford Pk) *Rambo Paul Ramsey*
08629	D3796	X			BLU	Progress Rail, Longport
08630	3	X Y			BLK	HNRC at Celsa Steel, Cardiff
08631		X	CL	LSLO	BLU	LSL at Weardale
08632		X Y			LOM	RSS at Loram RTC Derby
08633	D3800	Churnet Valley Railway				
08635	D3802				UOB	Hydrogen conversion at SVR
08641		X	LA	EFSH	BLU	FGP GWR Named: *Pride of Laira*
08643		X	-	-	MEN	EMS at Aggregate Industries, Merehead
08644		X M	LA	EFSH	BLU	FGP GWR Named: *Laira Diesel Depot 50 Years 1962-2012*
08645		X M	PZ	EFSH	SPL	FGP GWR Named: *St Piran*
08648		X M			BLK	RMS at Scotrail Inverness depot
08649		X			SPL	Meteor Power, VLR Centre, Dudley
08650		X			MEN	Aggregate Industries, Whatley
08652		X			RSS	Aggregate Industries, Rye Farm
08653		X			EWS	HNRC at Quinton Rail Technology
08663		A M			RSS	RSS at Port of Felixstowe
08669		A M			WAB	EMS at Wabtec
08670		A M			RSS	RSS, GBRf Bescot
08676		X			EWS	HNRC, East Kent Light Railway
08678	555	A	CS	AWCX	WCR	WCR WCR
08682		X			SPL	HNRC at Hope Cement
08683		X M			RSS	RSS at GBRf Eastleigh
08685		X			EWS	HNRC, East Kent Light Railway
08690		X	NL	EMSL	EMR	EMR EMR *David Thirkill*
08691		X M	FL	DFLS	PTR	FLR FLR (Crewe)
08694	D3861	Great Central Railway, Ruddington				
08696		A			BLU	Alstom, Wembley
08700		X			BLU	RMS at Alstom, Ilford
08701		A			SPL	HNRC at Quinton Rail Technology
08703		A			GBR	HS2 Willesden *Jermaine*
08704		X			RIV	Riviera Trains at Ecclesbourne Valley Rly
08706		Battlefield Line				
08709		X			EWS	RSS at Rye Farm, Wishaw (for sale)
08711		X C			SPL	HNRC at Nemesis Rail, Burton
08714		X			EWS	HNRC at Hope Cement Works
08721		X M			BLU	Alstom, Widnes
08724		X M			WAB	EMS at Wabtec Doncaster
08730		X			RSS	Whatley Quarry
08735		X M			ATC	Arriva Traincare, Eastleigh
08737		X	CL	LSLO	GRN	LSL LSL (Crewe)
08738		X			RSS	RSS Wishaw
08742	D3910	Barrow Hill				
08743		X			BLU	SembCorp Utilities, Wilton
08752		X Y			RSS	RSS at Wishaw
08754	H041	X M			RMS	RMS at Weardale Railway
08756		X			GRY	RMS at Weardale Railway
08757		X			GRY	GBRf, Dagenham
08762	H067	X			RMS	ERS at Yarmouth
08764		X M			BLU	Alstom at Polmadie
08765		X			HNR	HNRC at Barrow Hill
08767	D3935	North Norfolk Railway				
08769	D3937	Dean Forest Railway				
08772	D3940	North Norfolk Railway				
08773	D3941	Embsay & Bolton Abbey Railway				
08774		A			SPL	A V Dawson, Middlesborough
08780	(3948)	X	CL	LSLO	GRN	LSL LSL Named *Zippy*
08782		A Y			COR	HNRC at Barrow Hill
08783		X			EWS	EMR, Kingsbury
08784	D3952	Nottingham Heritage Railway, Ruddington				
08785		A M	FL	DFLS	GWF	RSS at Freightliner, Ipswich
08786		A			GRY	HNRC at Barrow Hill
08787		X			HAN	Hanson Quarry, Whatley
08788		X M			RMS	PRH at PD Ports, Teesport
08790		X M			BLU	Alstom, Longsight
08795	D3963	Llanelli & Mynydd Mawr Railway at Chrysalis Rail, Landore				

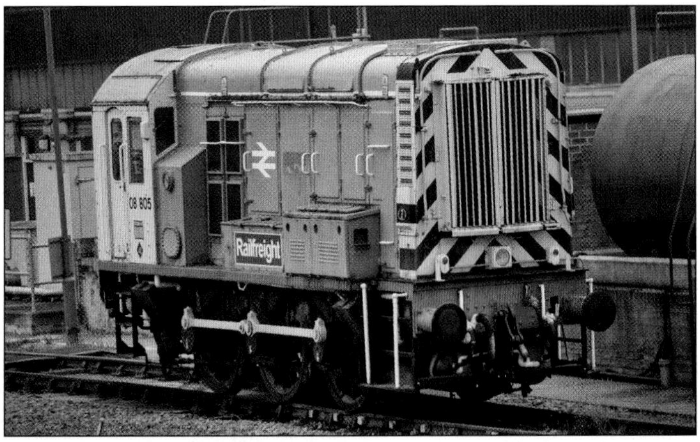

West Midlands Railway operate No. 08805 for pilotage work at its Soho depot near Birmingham, with the loco carrying former Railfreight livery. To enable attachment to Class 323 stock it carries a drop-head Tightlock coupling. **Antony Christie**

08798		X			EWS	HNRC Barrow Hill
08799	D3967)	Battlefield Line				
08802		X			EWS	HNRC at Worksop
08805		X	TS	EJLO	GRY	WMR WMR *Robin Jones 40 Years Service*
08807		A			SPL	A V Dawson, Middlesborough
08809	24	X			RMS	RMS at Hanson Cement, Ketton
08810		A			ATC	Arriva Traincare, Eastleigh
08818	4	X			GBR	HNRC at Worksop
08822		X M	PM	EFSH	ICS	FGP GWR *Dave Mills*
08823		A			HUN	EMS, Tata Steel, Shotton
08824		X C			BLK	HNRC Barrow Hill
08825	D3993	Chinnor & Princes Risborough Railway				
08830	D3998	Peak Rail, Rowsley				
08834		X			HNR	HNRC at Allerton
08836		X M	LA	EFSH	GWG	FGP GWR
08846	003	X			BLU	RSS at GBRf, March
08847		X M			COT	PRH at PD Ports, Teesport
08850	D4018	North Yorkshire Moors Railway				
08853		A M			WAB	EMS, Doncaster
08865		X			EWS	HNRC at Alstom, Barton-u-N'd
08868		X			ATC	HNRC at Arriva Traincare, Crewe
08870	H024	X			ICS	ERS, Yarmouth
08871	H074	X			COT	RMS at Wolsingham
08872		X			EWS	HNRC at EMR, Attercliffe
08874		X M			SLK	RMS at Teesport
08877		X			GRY	HNRC at Celsa Steel, Cardiff
08879		X			EWS	HNRC at Hope Cement Works
-	D4067	Great Central Railway, Loughborough				
-	D4092	Barrow Hill Roundhouse				
08881	D4095	Somerset & Dorset Railway, Midsomer Norton				
08885	H042	X			BLU	RMS at Weardale Railway
08887		A M			BLU	Alstom, Polmadie
08888	D4118	K&ESR at Avon Valley Railway for overhaul				
08891		X M			FLR	Freightliner at Barton-under-Needwood
08892		X			BLU	HNRC at Worksop
08896	D4126	Severn Valley Railway (for spares)				
08899		X	NL	EMSL	SPL	EMR EMR *Midland Counties Railway 175*
08903		X			BLU	SembCorp Utilities, Wilton
08904		X D			EWS	HNRC, Worksop
08905		X			EWS	HNRC at Hope Cement Works
08907	D4137	Great Central Railway, Loughborough				
08908		X	NL	EMSL	EMR	EMR EMR
08911	D4141	National Railway Museum				
08912		X			BLU	AV Dawson, Middledbrough
08913		X			SPL	EMR Kingsbury, pilot loco
08915	D4145	Stephenson Railway Museum				
08918		X			GRY	HNRC at Nemesis Rail, Burton
08921		X			EWS	RSS at Rye Farm, Wishaw
08922		X			GRY	RSS Rye Farm, Wishaw
08924	2	X C			GBR	HNRC at Barrow Hill
08925		X	BH	GBWM	GRN	GBR GBR at March
08927		X			GRY	RSS at GBRf Bescot
08933		X			BLU	Aggregate Industries, Whatley
08934		A	BH	GBWM	PIT	GBR GBR at March
08936		X			BLU	RMS at Hanson Cement, Ketton
08937		X			GRN	Bardon Aggregates, Dartmoor Railway
08939		X			RSS	RSS at DB Springs Branch
08943		X			HNR	HNRC at Barrow Hill
08944	D4174	East Lancashire Railway				
08947		X			BLU	Mendip Rail, LH Group
08948		A S	TI	GPSS	EPG	Eurostar, Temple Mills
08950		X	NL	EMSL	EMR	EMR EMR *David Lightfoot*
08954		X M			BLU	HNRC, Alstom, Polmadie
08956		X			GRN	London Overground, Barrow Hill
08993	D3759	Keighley & Worth Valley Railway				
08994		A			SPL	HNRC at Nemesis Rail, Burton
08995		Gwendraeth Valley Railway				
09001	D3665	Peak Rail, Rowsley				
09002		X	BH	GBWM	GRN	HNRC, Barrow Hill
09004	D3668	Swindon & Cricklade Railway				
09006		X			EWS	HNRC at Nemesis Rail, Burton
09007	D3671	X	WN	-	GRN	LOG LOG
09009		X	BH	GBWM	GRN	GBR GBR at Dean Lane
09010	D3721	South Devon Railway				
09012	D4100	Severn Valley Railway *Dick Hardy*				
09014		X			GRY	HNRC at Nemesis Rail, Burton
09015	D4103	Avon Valley Railway				
09017	D4105	National Railway Museum				
09018	D4106	Bluebell Railway				
09019	D4107	West Somerset Railway				
09022		X			BLU	Victoria Group, Port of Boston
09023		X			EWS	European Metal Reprocessing, Attercliffe
09024	D4112	East Lancashire Railway				
09025	D4113	Lavender Line				
09026	D4114	Spa Valley Railway				
09106	6	X			HNR	HNRC at Celsa Steel, Cardiff
09107	D4013	Severn Valley Railway				
09201		X			GRY	HNRC at Hope Cement Works
09204		X			ATC	Arriva Traincare, Crewe

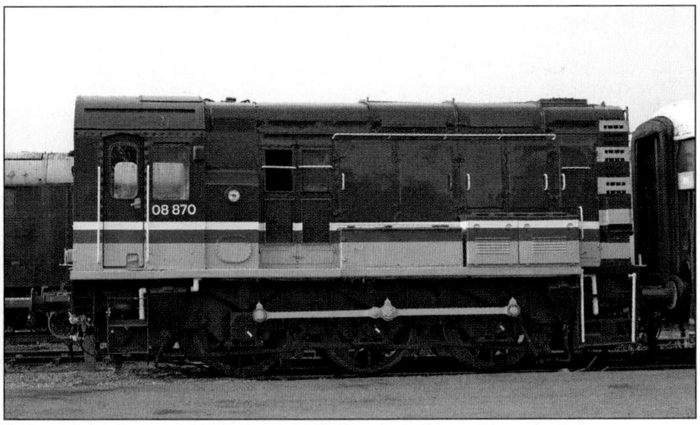

Eastern Rail Services owned No. 08870, based at Yarmouth, carries un-branded InterCity livery, with yellow side rods. This loco is fully operational, fitted with dual (air vacuum) brakes and can be made available for hire if needed. **Antony Christie**

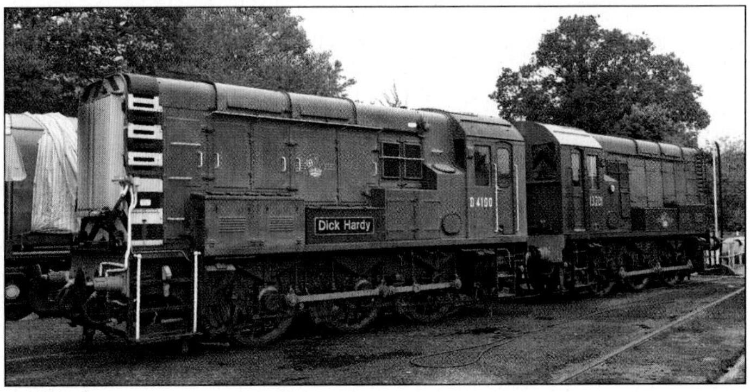

Most preserved railways have at least one standard design shunting loco on their books. Here, two of the Severn Valley Railway allocation, Nos. D4100 (09012) and 13201 (D3201 / 08133), rest on shed at Kidderminster in November 2021. No D4100 Dick Hardy, *sports high level air pipes from its former Southern Region days.* **CJM**

Class 11
LMS/BR 0-6-0 Diesel-Electric

Built: 1945-1952
Length: 29ft 1½in (8.87m)
Height: 12ft 5½in (3.80m)
Width: 8ft 7in (2.61m)
Engine: English Electric 6KT of 350hp (261kW)
Transmission: Electric
Tractive effort: 35,000lb (156kN)

12052	Caledonian Railway, Brechin
12077	Midland Railway Centre, Butterley

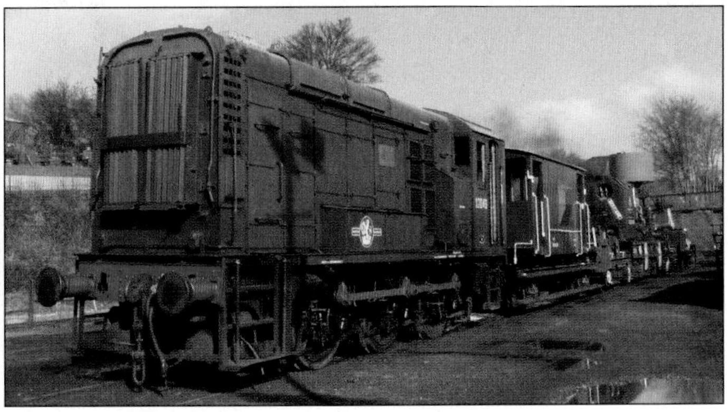

The forerunner to the BR standard shunting loco was the LMS 0-6-0, which became Class 11. Nine are preserved. This loco No. 12049, is actually No. 12082 based at the Mid-Hants Railway and carries the number of the damaged loco it replaced. **Adrian Paul**

12082	Mid Hants Railway (as 12049)
12083	Battlefield Railway
12088	Aln Valley Railway
12093	Caledonian Railway
12099	Severn Valley Railway
12131	North Norfolk Railaway
12139	North Yorkshire Moors Railway

Class 12
BR (Southern) 0-6-0 Diesel-Electric

Built: 1949
Length: 29ft 1½in (8.87m)
Height: 12ft 8¾in (3.88m)
Width: 9ft 0in (2.74m)
Engine: English Electric 6KT of 350hp (261kW)
Transmission: Electric
Tractive effort: 24,600lb (109kN)

15224	Spa Valley Line, Tunbridge Wells

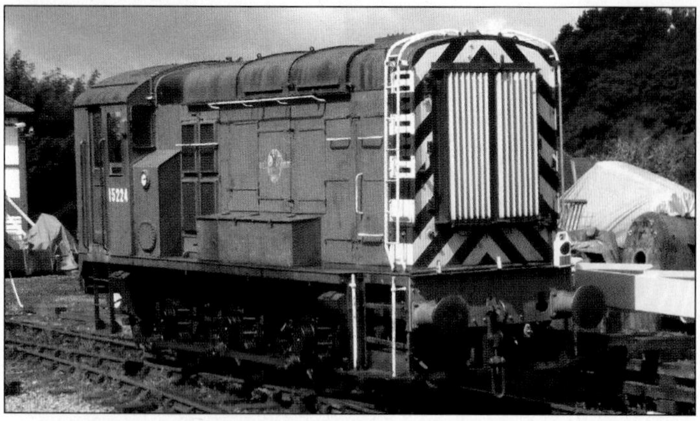

The Southern design of standard 0-6-0 shunter design is represented by just one preserved loco No. 15224, based on the Spa Valley Railway, Tunbridge Wells. The loco is seen sporting green lvery with wasp ends. **Phil Barnes**

Class 14
BR/WR 0-6-0 Diesel-Hydraulic

Built: 1964-1965
Length: 34ft 7in (10.54m)
Height: 10ft 0in (3.04m)
Width: 8ft 7½in (2.63m)
Engine: Paxman 6YJX 'Ventura' of 650hp (404kW)
Transmission: Hydraulic
Tractive effort: 30,910lb (134.4kN)

D9500	Port Elphinstone, Inverurie
D9502	East Lancashire Railway
D9504	Kent and East Sussex Railway
D9513	Embsay and Bolton Abbey Railway
D9516	Didcot Railway Centre
D9518	West Somerset Railway
D9520	Mid Norfolk Railway
D9521	Dean Forest Railway
D9523	Wensleydale Railway
D9524 (14901)	Churnet Valley Railway
D9525	Ecclesbourne Valley Railway
D9526	Kent & East Sussex Railway
D9529 (14029)	Nene Valley Railway
D9531	East Lancashire Railway
D9537	Ecclesbourne Valley Railway
D9539	Ribble Steam Railway
D9551	Severn Valley Railway
D9553	Allelys, Wishaw
D9555	Midland Railway Centre, Butterley

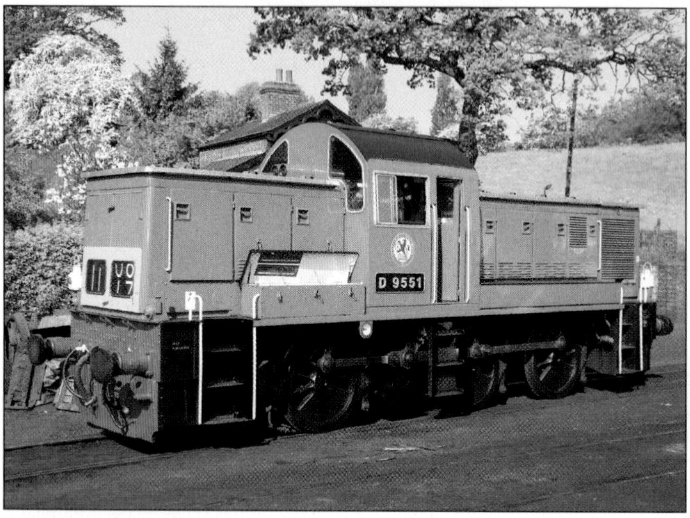

Sometimes modern traction preservation goes just a little too far, with the application o non proto-typical liveries, as is the case with Severn Valley-based Class 14 No. D9551 which sports cast number plates and golden ochre livery with a small yellow panel front end
Nathan Williamson

Class 15
Yorkshire Engine Co / BTH Type 1 Diesel-Electric

Built: 1960
Length: 42ft 0in (12.80m)
Height: 12ft 6in (3.81m)
Width: 9ft 2in (2.79m)
Engine: Paxman 16YHXL of 800hp (596.6kW)
Transmission: Electric
Tractive effort: 37,500lb (167kN)

D8233	East Lancashire Railway

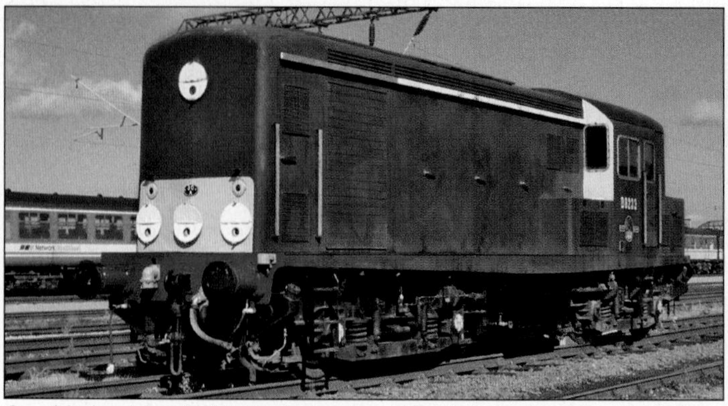

One of the few of the mid-1950s pilot scheme locos to find their way into preservation, after working in departmental use for several years, was BTH Class 15 No. D8233. It is currently under restoration at the East Lancashire Railway and is illustrated at Crewe on display in 1993. **John Stretton**

Class 17
Clayton Type 1 Diesel-Electric

Built: 1964
Length: 50ft 7in (15.42m)
Height: 12ft 8in (3.86m)
Width: 8ft 9½in (2.79m)
Engine: 2 x Paxman 6ZHXL of 450hp (671kW)
Transmission: Electric
Tractive effort: 40,000lb (178kN)

D8568	DTG at Severn Valley Railway

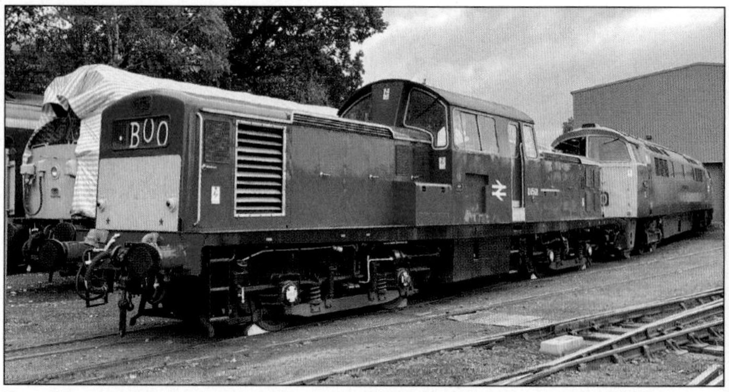

One of the gems in railway preservation is the Clayton Type 1 centre cab Class 17 No. D8568, preserved by the DTG on the Severn Valley Railway. It now sports rail blue livery with a small yellow end and is fully operational. It is shown 'on shed' at Kidderminster with 'Western' No. D1062 owned by the Western Locomotive Association. **CJM**

Class 18 (CBD90)
Clayton Equipment Co - Battery Hybrid Bo-Bo

Built: 2021-2022
Length: tba
Height: tba
Width: tba
Power: Battery Hybrid
Transmission: Electric
Tractive effort: 68,117lb (303kN)
Beacon Rail

18001	A	-	-	BLU	BEA	GBR
18002	A	-	-	BLU	BEA	BEA
18003	A	-	-	BLU	BEA	BEA
18004	A	-	-	BLU	BEA	BEA

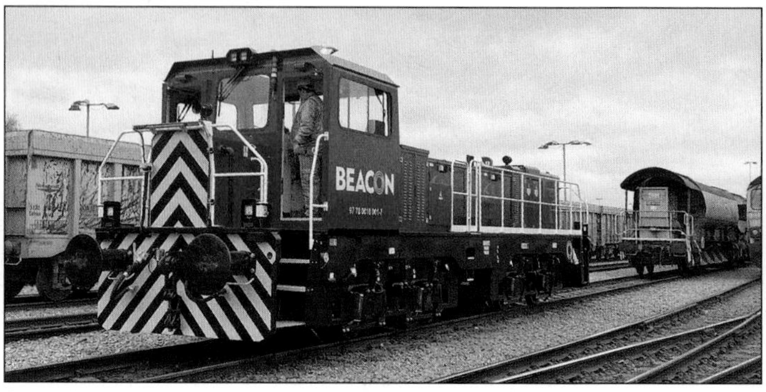

On 1 February 2022, GBRf took delivery of the first Beacon Rail Class 18 No. 18001 for a three month trial at Whitemoor Yard. The Clayton Equipment Co battery/diesel loco is classified as Clayton Equipment Hybrid+ CBD90. **GB Railfreight**

18005	A	-	-	-	BEA	BEA
18006	A	-	-	-	BEA	BEA
18007	A	-	-	-	BEA	BEA
18008	A	-	-	-	BEA	BEA
18009	A	-	-	-	BEA	BEA
18010	A	-	-	-	BEA	BEA
18011	A	-	-	-	BEA	BEA
18012	A	-	-	-	BEA	BEA
18013	A	-	-	-	BEA	BEA
18014	A	-	-	-	BEA	BEA
18015	A	-	-	-	BEA	BEA

Class 19
Lenz Labs development Bo-Bo loco

Built: 2018 from 1988 built Mk3 DVT No. 82113
Length: 61ft 9in (18.83m)
Height: 12ft 9in (3.88m)
Width: 8ft 11in (2.71m)
Engine: 2 x JCB diesel engines
Transmission: Hydraulic pump
Tractive effort: Awaited

19001	(82113)	A	SRPS, Bo'ness & Kinneil Railway

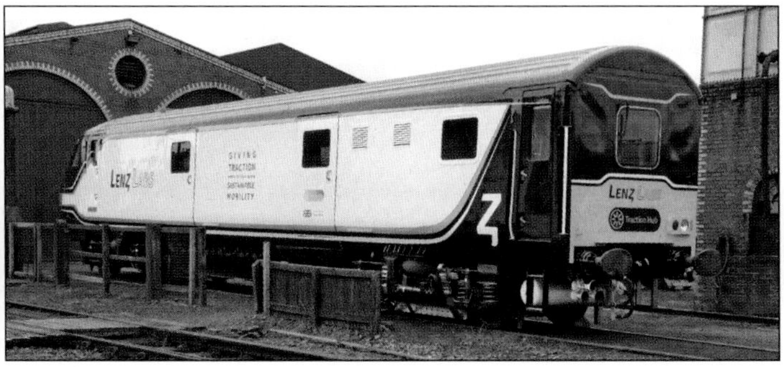

Rebuilt from former West Coast Mk3 Driving Van Trailer No. 82113, this vehicle was converted as a traction development vehicle by Edinburgh-based Damfoss. It is now operated by Lens Labs as a development vehicle for low adhesion caused by rail contamination. It uses a combination of advanced software and a 'rail hub' traction system. It is based at the Bo'ness and Kinneil Railway, north of Edinburgh. **Ian Lothian**

Class 20
English Electric Bo-Bo Diesel-Electric

Built: 1957-1968
Length: 46ft 9¼in (14.26m)
Height: 12ft 7⅝in (3.85m)
Width: 8ft 9in (2.67m)
Engine: EE8SVT Mk2 of 1000hp (746kW)
Transmission: Electric
Tractive effort: 42,000lb (187kN)

20001 (D8001)	Epping & Ongar Railway						
20007 (D8007)		X	SK	MOLO	GRN	MON	SH
20016 (D8016)	Caledonian Railway, Brechin						
20020 (D8020)	Bo'ness & Kinneil Railway, SRPS						
20031 (D8031)	Keighley & Worth Valley Railway						
20048 (D8048)	Midland Railway Centre						
20050 (D8000)	National Railway Museum						
20056 (D8056)		X	SC	HNRL	SPL	HNR	(S)
20057 (D8057)	Churnet Valley Railway						
20059 (D8059)	Mid Hants Railway						
20063 (D8063)	Battlefield Railway, Shackerstone						
20066 (D8066)		X	HC	HNRL	SPL	HNR	HOP
20069 (D8069)	HNRC at Worksop						
20081 (D8081)	Caledonian Railway, Brechin						
20087 (D8087)	HNRC at Worksop						
20088 (D8088)	Caledonian Railway, Brechin						
20096 (D8096)		X	CL	LSLO	GRN	LSL	LSL
20098 (D8098)	Great Central Railway						
20107 (D8107)	*Jocelyn Feilding 1940-2020*	X	CL	LSLO	GRN	LSL	LSL
20110 (D8110)	Battlefield Railway, Shackerstone						
20118 (D8118)	*Saltburn-by-the-Sea*	X	HC	HNRL	RFG	HNR	HOP
20121 (D8121)		X	BH	HNRL	HNR	HNR	(S)
20132 (D8132)	*Barrow Hill Depot*	X	WS	HNRL	GRY	HNR	HNR
20137 (D8137)	Gloucestershire Warwickshire Railway						
20142 (D8142)	*Sir John Betjeman*	X	SK	MOLO	GRN	MON	SH
20154 (D8154)	GCR Nottingham						
20166 (D8166)	Wensleydale Railway						
20168 (D8168)	*Sir George Earle*	X	HC	HNRL	SPL	HNR	HOP
20169 (D8169)	Private near Tebay						
20177 (D8177)	Severn Valley Railway						
20188 (D8188)	Mid Hants Railway						
20189 (D8189)		X	SK	MOLO	BLU	MON	SH
20205 (D8305)		X	SK	MOLO	BLU	C2L	SH
20214 (D8314)	Lakeside & Haverthwaite Railway						
20227 (D8327)	*Sherlock Holmes*	X	SK	MOLO	LUL	C2L	SH
20228 (D8128)	Gloucester Warwickshire Railway						
20301 (20047)		A	BH	HNRL	DRS	HNR	(S)
20302 (20084)		A	CL	LSLO	DRS	LSL	(S)
20303 (20127)		A	ZR	HNRS	DRS	HNR	(S)
20304 (20120)		A	BH	HNRL	DRS	HNR	(S)
20305 (20095)		A	CL	LSLO	DRS	LSL	(S)
20308 (20187)		A	WS	HNRS	DRS	HNR	(S)
20309 (20075)		A	WS	HNRS	DRS	HNR	(S)
20311 (20102)		A	BH	HNRL	HNR	HNR	HNR
20312 (20042)		A	WS	HNRS	DRS	HNR	(S)
20314 (20117)		A	BH	HNRL	HNR	HNR	HNR
20901 (20101)		A	WS	HNRL	GBR	HNR	HNR
20903 (20083)		A	BU	HNRS	DRS	HNR	(S)
20904 (20041)		A	BU	HNRS	DRS	HNR	(S)
20905 (20225)		A	WS	HNRL	GBR	HNR	HNR
20906 (20219)		A	HC	HNRL	SPL	HNR	HOP

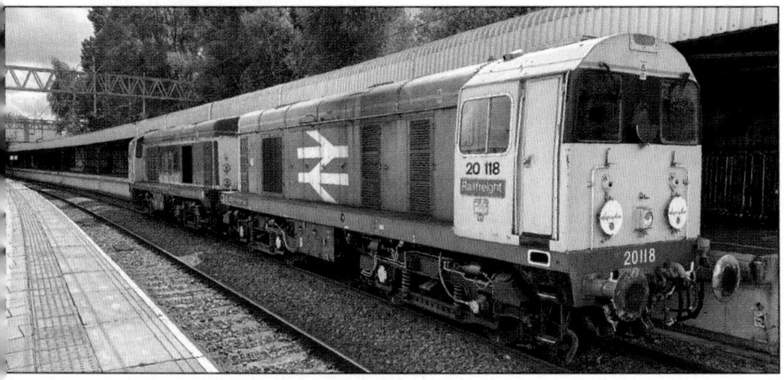

Harry Needle Railroad Company are one of the largest users of Class 20s, with some operating for industry and others on 'spot hire' basis. RAilfreight-liveried No. 20118 and ex-GBRf-liveried No. 20901 are seen at Stafford. **Spencer Conquest**

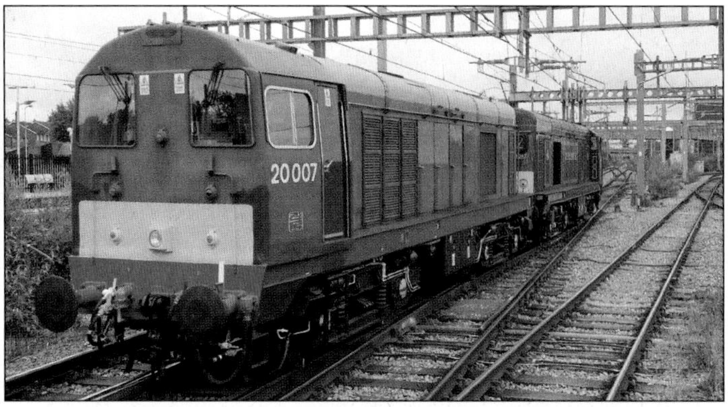

Private owner Michael Owen operates four Class 20s on 'spot hire' and are regularly seen on the main line. In this view No. 20007 in green and 20142 in London Transport livery are seen at Didcot in summer 2021. In 2021-2022 this pair carried out a number of duties with SLC Operations **Spencer Conquest**

Class 23 'Baby Deltic'
English Electric Bo-Bo Diesel-Electric

Built: 2022 (Replica, built from Class 37)
Length: 52ft 6in (16.00m)
Height: 12ft 8in (3.86m)
Width: 8ft 10¾in (2.71m)
Engine: Napier 'Deltic' T9-29 of 1,100hp (820.2kW)
Transmission: Electric
Tractive effort: 47,000lb (209kN)

D5910	Barrow Hill Roundhouse (Rebuilt from 37372 [D6859/37159]

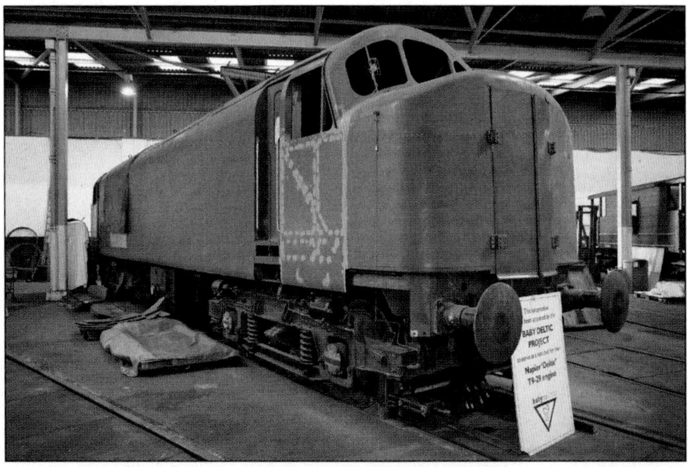

An amazing rebuild project is currently underway at Barrow Hill to build a 'new' Baby Deltic No. D5910 (the next number following the production build, from Class 37 No. 37372. This view shows the ongoing work with the cab end nearing completion. **Antony Christie**

Class 24
BR Bo-Bo Diesel-Electric

Built: 1958-1961
Length: 50ft 6in (15.39m)
Height: 12ft 8in (3.86m)
Width: 8ft 10in (2.70m)
Engine: Sulzer 6LDA28A of 1,160hp (865kW)
Transmission: Electric
Tractive effort: 40,000lb (178kN)

24032 (D5032)		North Yorkshire Moors Railway
24054 (D5054)	*Phil Southern*	East Lancashire Railway
24061 (D5061)		North Yorkshire Moors Railway
24081 (D5081)		Gloucestershire Warwickshire Railway

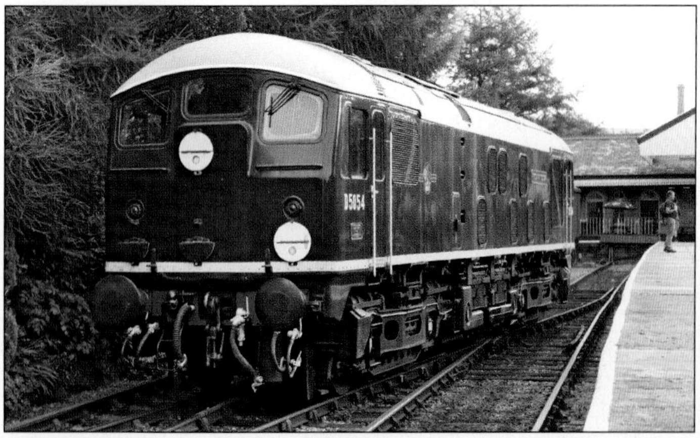

Four of the early BR Sulzer Type 2s, later Class 24 are in preservation. East Lancs Railway No. D5054 (24054) Phil Southern *is seen at Rawtenstall, from its No. 2 end displaying late 1950s all-over BR green livery.* **Adrian Paul**

Class 25
BR / Beyer Peacock Bo-Bo Diesel-Electric

Built: 1961-1966
Length: 50ft 6in (15.39m)
Height: 12ft 8in (3.86m)
Width: 9ft 1in (2.76m)
Engine: Sulzer 6LDA28B of 1,250hp (932kW)
Transmission: Electric
Tractive effort: 45,000lb (200kN)

25035 (D5185)		Great Central Railway
25057 (D5207)		HNRC Worksop, for main line use
25059 (D5209)		Keighley & Worth Valley Railway
25067 (D5217)		Nemesis Rail, Burton-on-Trent
25072 (D5222)		Caledonian Railway, Brechin
25083 (D5233)		Caledonian Railway, Brechin
25173 (D7523)		Battlefield Line, Shackerstone
25185 (D7535)		South Devon Railway
25191 (D7541)		South Devon Railway
25235 (D7585)		Bo'ness & Kinneil Railway
25244 (D7594)		Kent & East Sussex Railway
25262/25901 (D7612)		South Devon Railway
25265 (D7615)		Nemesis Rail, Burton-on-Trent
25278 (D7628)	*Sybilla*	North Yorkshire Moors Railway, Main Line
25279 (D7629)		Great Central Railway, Nottingham
25904 (D7633)		Stored - Reid Freight Services, Stoke
25309 (D7659)		Peak Rail
25313 (D7663)		HNRC for main line use
25321 (D7671)		Midland Railway Centre
25322 (D7672)		Churnet Valley Railway

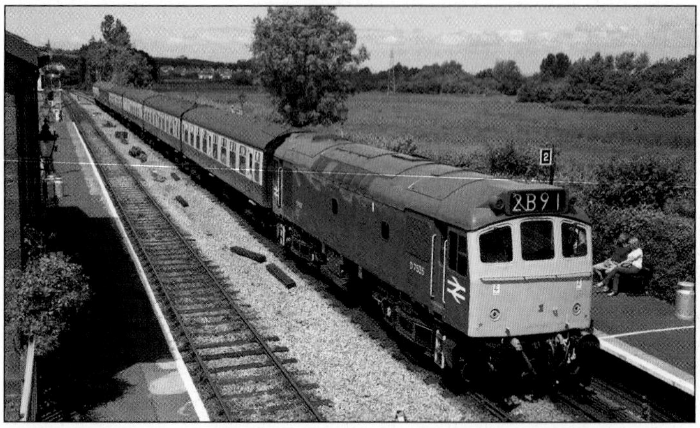

Examples of both body style of the follow-on BR Sulzer Type 2 Class 25 locos are preserved, with a total of 20 locos saved from cutting up. Rail blue liveried No. D7535 (25185) usually based on the South Devon Railway is seen at Williton while working on the West Somerset Railway. **Nathan Williamson**

Class 26
BRCW Bo-Bo Diesel-Electric

Built: 1958-1959
Length: 50ft 9in (15.47m)
Height: 12ft 8in (3.86m)
Width: 8ft 10in (2.69m)
Engine: Sulzer 6LDA28A of 1,160hp (865kW)
Transmission: Electric
Tractive effort: 42,000lb (186.8kN)

26001 (D5301)	Caledonian Railway
26002 (D5302)	Strathspey Railway
26004 (D5304)	Nemesis Rail, Burton-on-Trent
26007 (D5300)	Barrow Hill Roundhouse
26010 (D5310)	Llangollen Railway
26011 (D5311)	Nemesis Rail, Burton-on-Trent
26014 (D5314)	Caledonian Railway, Brechin
26024 (D5324)	Bo'ness & Kinneil Railway
26025 (D5325)	Strathspey Railway
26035 (D5335)	Caledonian Railway, Brechin
26038 (D5338)	Bo'ness & Kinneil Railway
26040 (D5340)	Whitrope Heritage Centre
26043 (D5343)	Gloucestershire Warwickshire Railway

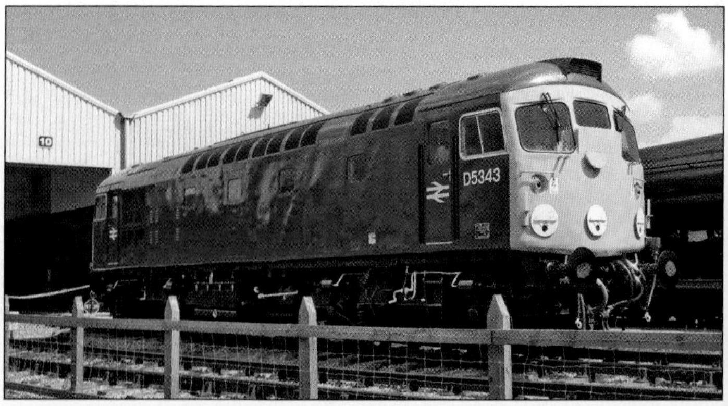

The early design of BRCW Type 2, later of Class 26 is represented by 13 preserved examples, mostly in operational condition. No. D5343 (26043) displays BR rail blue with the BR logo on the cab doors, at Toddington on the Gloucester-Warwickshire Railway. **Adrian Paul**

Class 27
BRCW Bo-Bo Diesel-Electric

Built: 1961-1962
Length: 50ft 9in (15.47m)
Height: 12ft 8in (3.86m)
Width: 8ft 10in (2.69m)
Engine: Sulzer 6LDA28B of 1,250hp (932kW)
Transmission: Electric
Tractive effort: 40,00lb (178kN)

27001 (D5347)	Bo'ness & Kinneil Railway
27005 (D5351)	Bo'ness & Kinneil Railway
27007 (D5353)	Goodman's Yard, Wishaw
27024 (D5370)	Caledonian Railway, Brechin
27050 (D5394)	Strathspey Railway
27056 (D5401)	Great Central Railway
27059 (D5410)	UKRL Leicester
27066 (D5386)	Barrow Hill Roundhouse

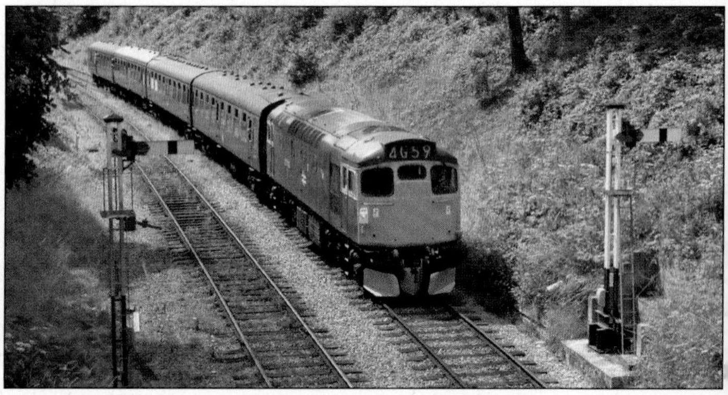

The later built BRCW Type 2 with a roof mounted headcode display, later of Class 27 has eight examples preserved. First of the class No. 27001 is seen at Groombridge on the Spa Valley Railway. **Phil Barnes**

Class 28
Metro-Vic Co-Bo Diesel-Electric

Built: 1958-1959
Length: 56ft 7½in (17.26m)
Height: 12ft 8½in (3.87m)
Width: 9ft 2½in (2.81m)
Engine: Crosssley HSTV8 of 1,200hp (895kW)
Transmission: Electric
Tractive effort: 50,000lb (224kN)

D5705	East Lancashire Railway

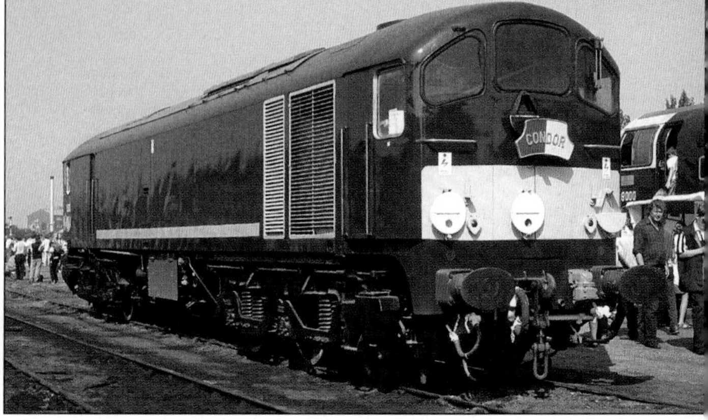

Thanks to departmental use, Co-Bo No. D5705 entered preservation and is currently under restoration at the East Lancs Railway. It is seen on display at Coalville. **Colour-Rail**

Class 31
Brush A1A-A1A Diesel-Electric

Built: 1957-1962
Length: 56ft 9in (17.30m)
Height: 12ft 7in (3.84m)
Width: 8ft 9in (2.67m)

*Engine: English Electric 12SVT of 1,470hp (1,096kW)**
Transmission: Electric
Tractive effort: 50,000lb (224kN)
** Originally Mirrlees JVS12T engine*

31018 (D5500)		National Railway Museum					
31101 (D5518)		Avon Valley Railway					
31105 (D5523)		Mangapps Farm Museum					
31106 (D5524)		X	BQ	DCRO	HAH	HAN	SH
31108 (D5526)		Midland Railway Centre					
31119 (D5537)		Embsay & Bolton Abbey Railway					
31128 (D5546)	*Charybdis*	X	BU	NRLO	BLU	NEM	SH
31130 (D5548)		Avon Valley Railway					
31162 (D5580)		Great Central Railway, Nottingham					
31163 (D5581)		Chinnor & Princes Risborough Railway					
31190 (D5613)		Plym Valley Railway					
31203 (D5627)		Pontypool & Blaenavon Railway					
31206 (D5630)		Rushden Transport Museum					
31207 (D5631)		North Norfolk Railway					
31210 (D5634)		Dean Forest Railway					
31233 (D5660)		Mangapps Farm Museum					
31235 (D5662)		Dene Forest Railway					
31255 (D5683)		Mid Norfolk Railway					
31270 (D5800)		Peak Rail, Rowsley					
31271 (D5801)		Llangollen Railway					
31285 (D5817)		Weardale Railway					
31289 (D5821)		Northampton & Lamport Railway					
31297/31463 (D5830)		Great Central Railway, Loughborough					
31327 (D5862)		Strathspey Railway					
31414 (D5814)		Midland Railway Centre					
31418 (D5522)		Midland Railway Centre					
31430 (D5695)		Spa Valley Railway					
31435 (D5600)		Embsay & Bolton Abbey Railway					
31438 (D5557)		Epping & Ongar Railway					
31452 (D5809)		ERS at Nemasis Burton					
31454 (D5654)		Stored Nemasis Burton					
31459 (D5684)		HNRC at Barrow Hill					
31461 (D5547)		Nemesis Rail, Burton-on-Trent					
31465 (D5637)		HNRC at Weardale Railway					
31466 (D5533)		Dean Forest Railway (at SVR)					
31601 (D5609)		Ecclesbourne Valley Railway					

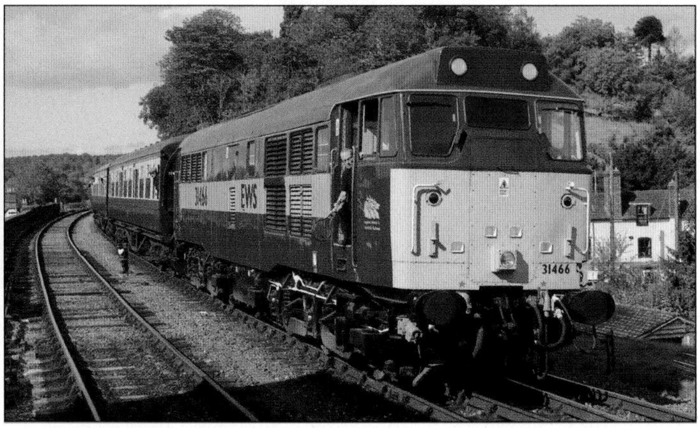

Based on the Dean Forest Railway, but recorded on the Severn Valley Railway, Class 31/4 No. 31466 displays EWS maroon and gold livery from it No. 1 end. Thirtythree Class 31s are preserved, representing all sub classes. Two remain operational on the main line and one is in industrial service. **Spencer Conquest**

Class 33
BRCW Bo-Bo Diesel-Electric

Built: 1960-1962
Length: 50ft 9in (15.47m)
Height: 12ft 8in (3.86m)
Width: 8ft 10in (2.69m) - 9ft 3in (2.81)

Engine: Sulzer 8LDA28A of 1,550hp (1,156kW)
Transmission: Electric
Tractive effort: 45,000lb (200kN)

33002 (D6501)		South Devon Railway					
33008 (D6508)		Battlefield Railway					
33012 (D6515)	*Lt Jenny Lewis RN*	X	SW	MBDL	GRN	71A	SH
33018 (D6530)		Midland Railway, Butterley					
33019 (D6534)		Nemasis Rail, Burton					
33021 (D6539)		Churnet Valley Railway					
33025 (D6543)		X	CS	AWCA	WCR	WCR	WCR
33029 (D6547)		X	CS	AWCA	WCR	WCR	WCR
33030 (D6548)		X	CS	AWCX	DRS	WCR	(S)
33035 (D6553)		Wensleydale Railway					
33046 (D6564)		East Lancashire Railway					
33048 (D6566)		West Somerset Railway					
33052 (D6570)		Bluebell Railway					
33053 (D6571)		Europhoenix, Leicester					
33057 (D6575)		West Somerset Railway					
33063 (D6583)		Spa Valley Railway					
33065 (D6585)		Spa Valley Railway					
33102 (D6513)		Churnet Valley Railway					
33103 (D6514)		Ecclesbourne Valley Railway					
33108 (D6521)		Severn Valley Railway					
33109 (D6525)		East Lancashire Railway					
33110 (D6527)		Sonic Rail, Burnham-on-Crouch					
33111 (D6528)		Swanage Railway					
33115 (D6533)		St Leonards Railway Engineering					
33116 (D6535)		NRM at Great Central Railway, Nottingham					
33117 (D6536)		East Lancashire Railway					
33201 (D6586)		Spa Valley Railway					
33202 (D6587)		Mid Norfolk Railway					
33207 (D6592)	*Jim Martin*	X	CS	AWCA	WCR	WCR	WCR
33208 (D6593)		Battlefield Railway					

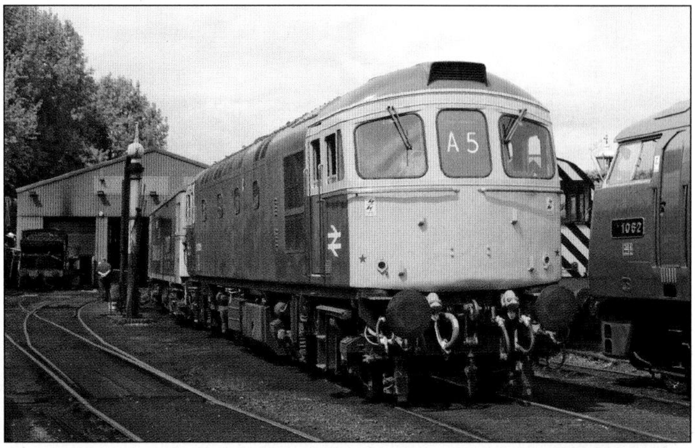

The original Southern Region-based BRCW Type 3s of Class 33 has examples of all sub-classes preserved, many in full operational condition. Class 33/0 No. 33035 is seen on shed at Bridgenorth when visiting the Severn Valley Railway, from its No. 1 end. **Adrian Paul**

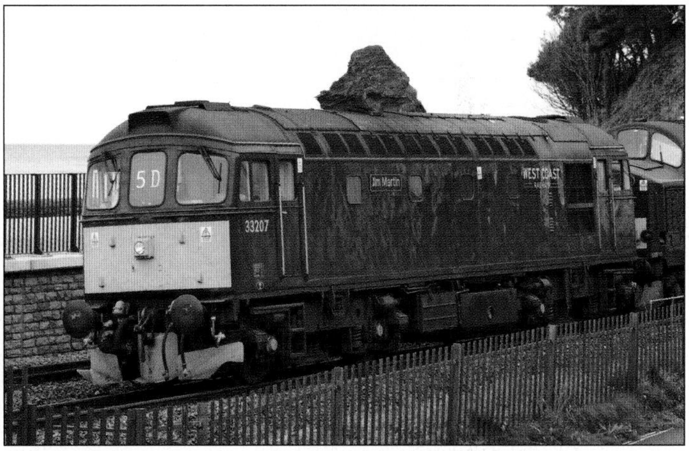

Four examples of the narrow-bodied 'Hastings' profile Class 33/2 sub-class remain, three preserved and one No. 33207 Jim Martin *operational with West Coast Railway and often used on charter or charter support services. It is frequently kept at Southall.* **CJM**

Class 35 'Hymek'
Beyer Peacock B-B Diesel-Hydraulic

Built: 1961-1964
Length: 51ft 8½in (15.76m)
Height: 12ft 10½in (3.92m)
Width: 8ft 8½in (2.65m)

Engine: Maybach MD870 of 1,700hp (1,267kW)
Transmission: Hydraulic
Tractive effort: 46,600lb (204.6kN)

D7017	D&EPG at West Somerset Railway
D7018	D&EPG at West Somerset Railway
D7029	DTG at Severn Valley Railway
D7076	East Lancashire Railway

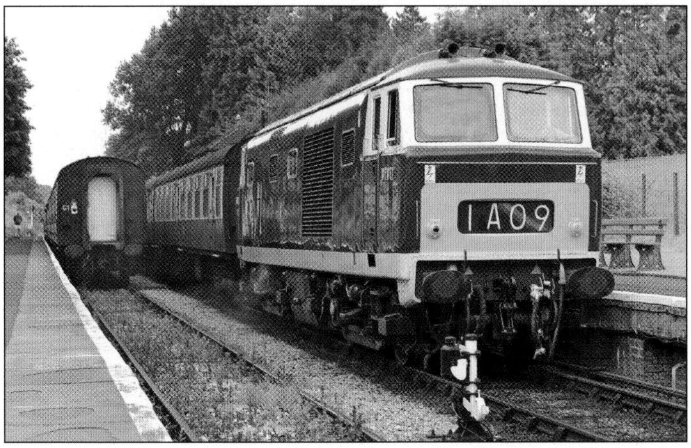

Four Beyer-Peacock 'Hymek' locos are preserved, three operational and one No. D7029 under restoration. Nos. D7017 and D7018 are owned by the D&EPG and kept on the West Somerset Railway, where No. D7017 is shown. **Adrian Paul**

Class 37
English Electric Co-Co Diesel-Electric

Built: 1960-1965
Length: 61ft 6in (18.74m)
Height: Between 12ft 9⅛in-13ft 0¼in (3.86m-3.96m)
Width: 8ft 11⅝in (2.69m)
Engine: English Electric 12CSVT of 1,750hp (1,304W)
37/9-Mirrlees MB275T of 1,800hp (1,340kW) or Ruston RK270T of 1,800hp (1,340kW)
Transmission: Electric
Tractive effort: 55,500lb (245kN)

37003 (D6703)	Private at Leicester Depot						
37009 (D6709)	Great Central Railway, Nottingham						
37023 (D6723)	Pontypool & Blaenavon Railway						
37025 (D6725)	*Inverness TMD*	X	NM	COTS	BLL	37G	COL
37029 (D6729)	Epping & Ongar Railway						
37032 (D6732)	North Norfolk Railway						
37037 (D6737)	South Devon Railway						
37038 (D6738)	(for sale 04/22)	A	KM	XSDP	DRS	DRS	DRS
37042 (D6742)	Eden Valley Railway, Warcop						
37057 (D6757)	*Barbara Arbon*	X	NM	COTS	COL	COL	COL
37059 (D6759)	(for sale 04/22)	A R	KM	XSDP	DRC	DRS	(S)
37069 (D6769)		A R	KM	XWSS	DRC	DRS	(S)
37075 (D6775)	Keighley & Worth Valley Railway						
37097 (D6797)	Caledonian Railway, Brechin						
37099 (D6799)	*Merl Evans 1947-2016*	X	NM	COTS	COL	COL	COL
37108 (D6808)	Crewe Heritage Centre						
37109 (D6809)	East Lancashire Railway						
37116 (D6816)		X	NM	COTS	COL	COL	COL
37119 (D6700)	NRM, hire to Heavy Tractor Group at Great Central Railway						
37142 (D6842)	Bodmin & Wenford Railway						
37152 (D6852)	Peak Rail, Rowsley, as 37310						
37175 (D6879)		A	NM	COTS	COL	COL	COL
37190 (D6890)	1:1 Museum, Margate						
37198 (D6898)	Head of Steam Museum, Darlington						
37207 (D6907)	VLR Centre, Dudley Hybrid Electric Power development loco						
37214 (D6914)	Bo'ness & Kenneil						
37215 (D6915)	Gloucester & Warwickshire Railway						
37216 (D6916)	Pontypool & Blaenavon Railway						
37218 (D6918)		A R	KM	XHSO	DRC	DRS	(S)
37219 (D6919)		X	NM	COTS	COL	COL	COL
37227 (D6927)	Chinnor & Princes Risborough Railway						
37240 (D6940)		X	NM	COFS	TFG	BRE	COL
37248 (D6948)	Gloucester & Warwickshire Railway						
37250 (D6950)	Wensleydale Railway						
37254 (D6954)	*Cardiff Canton*	X	NM	COTS	COL	COL	COL
37255 (D6955)	Nemesis Rail, Burton-on-Trent						
37259 (D6759)	(for sale 04/22)	A R	KM	XSDP	DRC	DRS	(S)
37261 (D6961)	Bo'ness & Kinneil Railway						
37263 (D6963)	Telford Steam Railway						
37264 (D6964)	North Yorkshire Moors Railway						
37275 (D6975)	Dartmouth Steam Railway						
37294 (D6994)	Embsay & Bolton Abbey Railway						
37308 (D6608)	Severn Valley Railway						
37372 (37159)	Barrow Hill, Baby Deltic Project - D5910						
37401 (37268)	*Mary Queen of Scots*	A R	KM	XHSO	BLL	DRS	DRS
37402 (37274)	*Stephen Middlemore 23.12.1954-6.7.2013*	A	KM	XWSS	BLL	DRS	(S)
37403 (37307)	*Isle of Mull*	X	NY	RAJV	BLL	DRS	NYM
37405 (37282)		A R	BH	HNRL	DRC	HNR	(S)
37407 (37305)	*Blackpool Tower*	X	KM	XWSS	BLL	DRS	(S)
37409 (37270)	*Lord Hinton (for sale 4/22)*	A R	KM	XSDP	BLL	DRS	DRS
37418 (37271)	*An Comunn Gaidhealach*	X	NM	COTS	BLL	PRI	COL

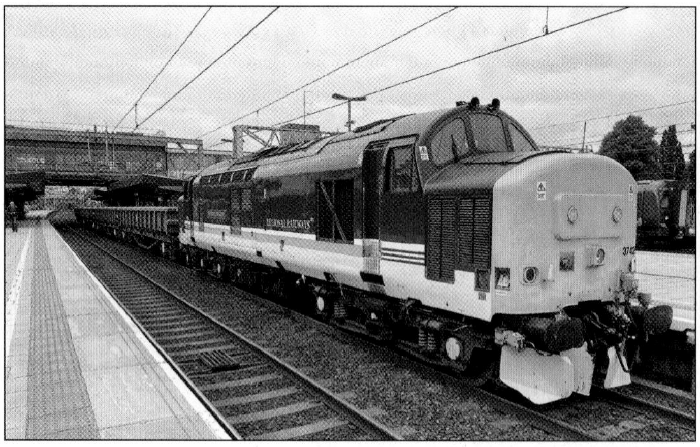

One of the most popular classes of all time, the English Electric Class 37 is still represented by a number of locos in main line service as well as a major number in preservation. Painted in Regional Railways livery with full branding, Direct Rail Services Class 37/4 No. 37425 Sir William McAlpine / Concrete Bob, *is seen passing Stafford with a southbound engineers train.* **Spencer Conquest**

37419 (37291)	*Carl Haviland 1954-2012*	A R	KM	XHSO	ICS	DRS	DRS
37421 (37267)		X	NM	COTS	BLL	COL	COL
37422 (37266)	*Victorious*	A R	KM	XHSO	DRB	DRS	DRS
37423 (37296)	*Spirit of the Lakes*	A R	KM	XWSS	BLL	DRS	(S)
37558 (37424)	*Avro Vulcan XH558*	X	KM	XHSO	BLL	DRS	DRS
37425 (37292)	*Sir Robert McAlpine / Concrete Bob*	A R	KM	XHSO	REG	DRS	DRS
37503 (D6717)	Stored at Shires Removal Group, Kinsley, Fitzwilliam						
37510 (37112)	*Orion*	A	LR	GROG	EPX	EPX	ROG
37516 (37086)	*Lord Laidon*	A	CS	AWCA	WCR	WCR	WCR
37517 (37018)		A P	CS	AWCX	WCR	WCR	(S)
37518 (37076)	*Fort William/An Gearasden*	A R	CS	AWCA	WCR	WCR	WCR
37521 (37117)		X	CL	LSLO	COL	LSL	LSL
37601 (37501)	*Perseus*	A D	LR	GROG	EPX	EPX	EPX
37602 (37502)		A R	KM	XSDP	DRC	DRS	(S)
37603 (37504)		A	WS	HNRL	DRC	HNR	(S)
37604 (37506)		A	WS	XHNC	DRC	HNR	(S)
37605 (37507)		A R	KM	HNRL	DRC	DRS	(S)
37606 (37508)		A	BU	COTS	DRC	PRI	(S)
37607 (37511)		A R	BH	COTS	BLU	HNR	COL
37608 (37512)	*Andromeda*	A R D	LR	GROG	EPX	EPX	ROG
37609 (37514)		A	WS	JNRL	DRC	HNR	(S)
37610 (37687)		A R	NM	COTS	BLU	HNR	COL
37611 (37690)	*Pegasus*	A D	LR	GROG	EPX	EPX	EPX
37612 (37691)		A	BH	COTS	BLU	HNR	COL
37667 (37151/D6851)	*Flopsie*	A R P	CL	LSLO	GRN	LSL	LSL
37668 (38257)		A E	CS	AWCA	WCR	WCR	WCR
37669 (37129)		A E	CS	AWCA	WCR	WCR	WCR
37674 (D6869)	Boat of Garten, Strathspey Railway						
37676 (37126)	*Loch Rannoch*	A	CS	AWCA	WCR	WCR	WCR
37679 (D6823)	Allelys/RSS yard Studley						
37685 (37234)	*Loch Arkaig*	A	CS	AWCA	WCR	WCR	WCR
37688 (37205)		D	CL	LSLO	TFG	LSL	LSL
37703 (37067)		X	WS	XHNC	DRS	HNR	(S)
37706 (37016)		X	CS	AWCA	WCR	WCR	WCR
37712 (37102)		A	CS	AWCX	WCR	WCR	(S)
37714 (D6724)	Great Central Rly, Loughborough						
37716 (37094)		A	KM	XHSO	DRC	DRS	DRS
37800 (37143)	*Cassiopeia*	A D	LR	GROG	EPX	EPX	ROG
37884 (37183)	*Cepheus*	A T	LR	GROG	EPX	EPX	ROG
37901 (37150)	*Mirrlees Pioneer*	A	LR	EPUK	EPX	EPX	EPX
37905 (37136)		A	LR	UKRS	GRN	URL	URL
37906 (37206)	Battlefield Railway, Shackerstone						

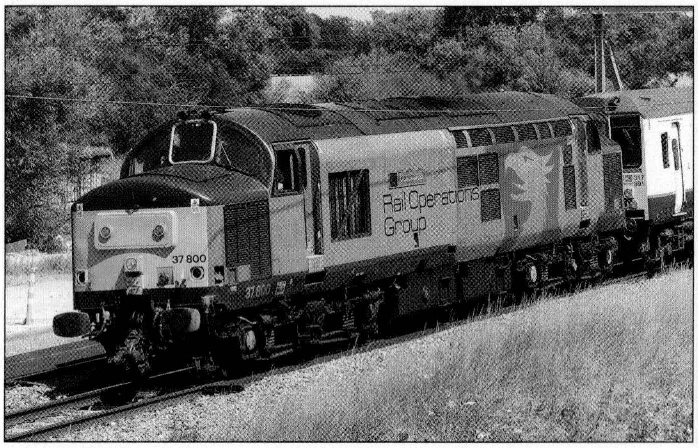

Leicester-based Europhoenix own several Class 37s , several of which are on long term hire to Rail Operations Group and fitted with drop-head Dellner or Tightlock couplings for easy coupling to multiple unit stock. Class 37/7 No. 37800 Cassiopeia is illustrated from its No. 1 end while directly coupled using its drop-head Tightlock coupling to a Class 317. **CJM**

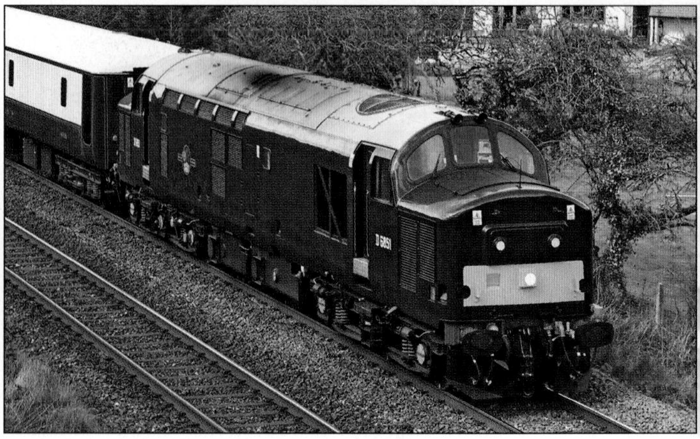

Crewe-based Loco Services Ltd (LSL) operate a small fleet of Class 37s which have been superbly restored. Displaying 1960s green livery with a small yellow warning panel end, No. D6851 (37667) is seen powering a charter train in summer 2021. The recess on the front end is where a DRS style jumper socket was previously fitted. **CJM**

Class 40
English Electric 1Co-Co1 Diesel-Electric

Built: 1958-1962
Length: 69ft 6in (21.18m)
Height: 12ft 10⅜in (3.92m)
Width: 9ft 0in (2.74m)
Engine: English Electric 16SVTMk3 of 2,000hp (1,491kW)
Transmission: Electric
Tractive effort: 52,000lb (231kN)

40012 (D212)	*Aureol*	Barrow Hill Roundhouse
40013 (D213)	*Andania*	Loco Services Limited (Main line certified - LSLO)
40106 (D306)		East Lancashire Railway

40118 (D318)	Battlefield Line
40122 (D200)	National Railway Museum, York
40135 (D335)	East Lancashire Railway
40145 (D345)	Class 40 PS at East Lancashire Railway (Main Line certified)

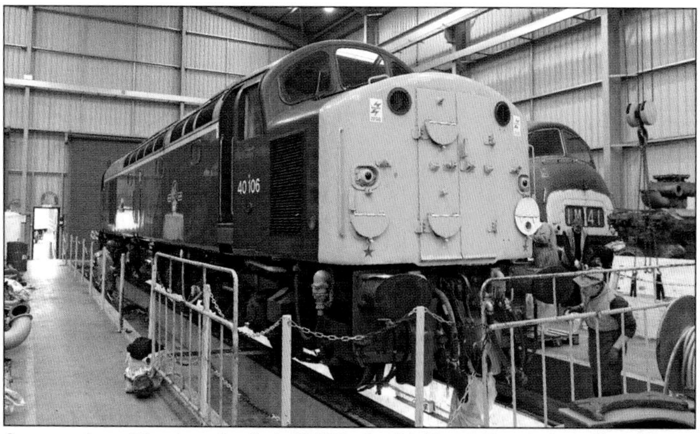

Seven members of the pioneering fleet of 2000hp English Electric Type 4s, later Class 40, are preserved, with two certified for main line operation. East Lancs Railway based No. D306 (40106) in seen inside Kidderminster depot at the Severn Valley Railway in company with 'Warship' No. D821. **CJM**

Class 41 HST Power Car (Prototype)
BREL Bo-Bo Diesel-Electric

Built: 1972
Length: 56ft 4in (17.17m)
Height: 12ft 10in (3.91m)
Width: 8ft 11in (2.72m)
Engine: Paxman 12RP200L 'Valenta' 2,250hp (1,677kW)
Transmission: Electric
Tractive effort: 17,980lb (80kN)

41001 (43000)	National Railway Museum, Shildon

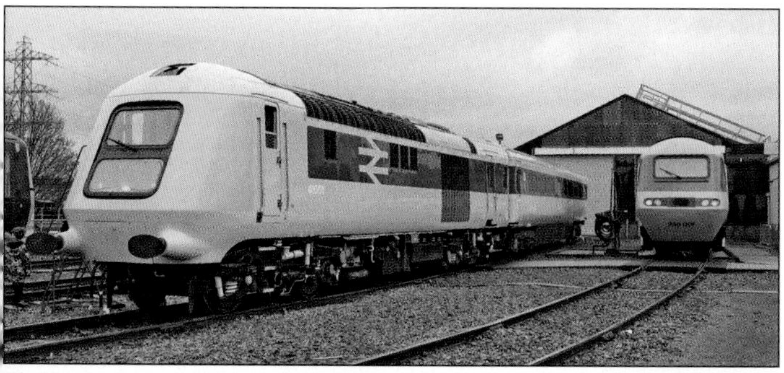

The National Railway Museum own the prototype HST power car No. 41001 (43000) which is currently on display at the Shildon Locomotion base. After development and passenger running the vehicle entered departmental service and then preservation. It is seen at Bristol St Philips Marsh posed next to pioneer production power car No. 43002. **Antony Christie**

Class 42 'Warship'
BR B-B Diesel-Hydraulic

Built: 1958-1961
Length: 60ft 0in (18.29m)
Height: 12ft 9½in (3.90m)
Width: 8ft 8½in (2.63m)
Engine: 2 x Maybach MD650 of 1,000hp (745.5kW)
Transmission: Hydraulic
Tractive effort: 52,400lb (233kN)

D821	*Greyhound*	DTG at Severn Valley Railway
D832	*Onslaught*	East Lancashire Railway

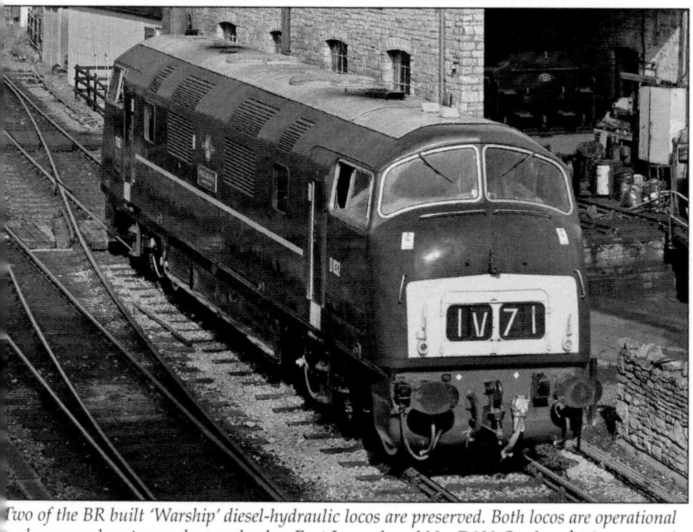

Two of the BR built 'Warship' diesel-hydraulic locos are preserved. Both locos are operational and are popular at open days and galas. East Lancs-based No. D832 Onslaught is seen on the Swanage Railway carrying BR green livery. **Adrian Paul**

Class 43 HST Power Car (Production)
BREL Bo-Bo Diesel-Electric

Built: 1976-1982
Length: 58ft 5in (17.80m)
Height: 12ft 10in (3.91m)
Width: 8ft 11in (2.72m)
Engine Original: Paxman 12RP200L 'Valenta' of 2,250hp (1,677kW)
Re-engine: Paxman 12VP185 of 2,100hp (1,565kW) or MTU 16V4000 R41R of 2,250hp (1,678lW)
Transmission: Electric
Tractive effort: 17,980lb (80kN)

43002	*Sir Kenneth Grange*	A	National Railway Museum, York				
43003		A	HA	HAPC	S7C	ANG	ASR
43004	*Caerphilly Castle*	A	LA	EFPC	GWG	ANG	GWR
43005	*St Michael's Mount*	A	LA	EFPC	GWG	ANG	GWR
43009		A	LA	EFPC	GWG	FGP	GWR
43010		A	LA	EFPC	GWG	FGP	GWR
43012		A	HA	HAPC	S7C	ANG	ASR
43013	*Mark Carne CBE*	A B	ZA	QCAR	NRL	PTR	NRL
43014	*The Railway Observer*	A B	ZA	QCAR	NRL	PTR	NRL
43015		A	HA	HAPC	S7C	ANG	ASR
43016	*Powderham Castle*	A	LA	EFPC	GWG	ANG	GWR
43017		A	EL	-	BLU	ANG	(S)
43018			Preserved Crewe Heritage Centre				
43020		A	EL	SCEL	BLU	ANG	(S)
43021		A	HA	HAPC	S7C	ANG	ASR
43022		A	LA	EFPC	GWG	FGP	GWR
43023		A	EL	SCEL	BLU	ANG	(S)
43024		A	EL	-	BLU	ANG	(S)
43025		A	EL	-	BLU	ANG	(S)
43026		A	HA	HAPC	S7C	ANG	ASR
43027		A	LA	EFPC	GWG	ANG	GWR
43028		A	HA	HAPC	S7C	ANG	ASR
43029	*Caldicot Castle*	A	LA	EFPC	GWG	ANG	GWR
43030		Angel, stored at Brodie Engineering (spares)					
43031		A	HA	HAPC	S7C	ANG	ASR
43032		A	HA	HAPC	S7C	ANG	ASR
43033		A	HA	HAPC	S7C	ANG	ASR
43034		A	HA	HAPC	S7C	ANG	ASR
43035		A	HA	HAPC	S7C	ANG	ASR
43036		A	HA	HAPC	S7C	ANG	ASR
43037		A	HA	HAPC	S7C	ANG	ASR
43040		A	LA	EFPC	GWG	ANG	GWR
43041	*St Catherine's Castle*	A	LA	EFPC	GWG	ANG	GWR
43042	*Tregenna Castle*	A	LA	EFPC	GWG	ANG	GWR
43043		A	LM	SBXL	SCE	PTR	OLS
43044		125 Group, Great Central					
43045		Northumbria Rail, Long Marston					
43046	*Geoff Drury 1930-1999 Steam Preservation and Computerised Track Recording Pioneer*	A	CL	LSLO	BLP	LSL	LSL
43047		A	CL	LSLO	BLP	LSL	LSL
43048		125 Group at Midland Railway					
43049	*Neville Hill*	A	CL	LSLO	ICS	LSL	LSL
43050		A	RJ	SBXL	SCE	PTR	(S)
43052		A	RJ	MBDL	SCE	DAS	DAS
43054		A	RJ	MBDL	SCE	DAS	DAS
43055		A	CL	LSLO	BLP	LSL	LSL
43056		Welsh Railway Trust, Gwili Railway					
43058		A	CL	LSLO	RCG	LSL	LSL
43059		A	CL	LSLO	RCG	LSL	LSL
43060		Northumbria Rail, Long Marston					
43062	*John Armitt*	A	ZA	QCAR	NRL	PTR	NRL
43064		A	LM	SBXL	SCE	PTR	(S)
43066		A	RJ	MBDL	SCE	DAS	DAS
43071		125 Heritage Ltd, Colne Valley Railway					
43073		125 Heritage Ltd, Colne Valley Railway					
43076		A	RJ	-	SCE	DAS	DAS
43078		A	LM	SBXL	BLU	PTR	(S)
43081		Preserved, Crewe Heritage Centre					
43082		125 Heritage Ltd, Colne Valley Railway					
43083		A	CL	LSLO	BLP	LSL	LSL
43086		A	LA	EFPC	GWG	PTR	(S)
43087		A	LA	EFPC	GWG	PTR	(S)
43088	*Dartmouth Castle*	A	LA	EFPC	GWG	FGP	GWR
43089		125 Group at Midland Railway					
43091		A	LA	-	GWG	PTR	(S)
43092	*Cromwell's Castle*	A	LA	EFPC	GWG	FGP	GWR

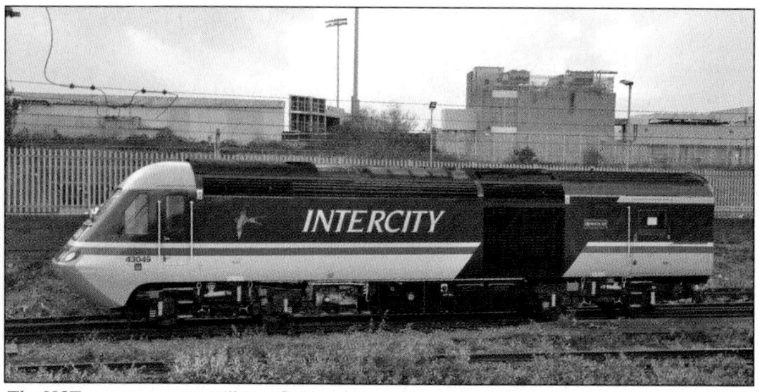

The HST power cars are still in a fluid position with many vehicles stored awaiting disposal or preservation. No. 43049 Neville Hill, restored to full InterCity Swallow livery is now operated by LSL. It is seen immaculate soon after arrival from restoration in November 2021. **Cliff Beeton**

43093	*Old Oak Common HST Depot 1976-2018*	A	LA	EFPC	SPL	FGP	GWR
43094	*St Mawes Castle*	A	LA	EFPC	GWG	FGP	GWR
43097	*Castle Drogo*	A	LA	EFPC	GWG	FGP	GWR
43098	*Walton Castle*	A	LA	EFPC	GWG	FGP	GWR
43102 (43302)	*The Journey Shrinker 148.5mph The Worlds Fastest Diesel Train*	Preserved NRM, Shildon					
43122	*Dunster Castle*	A	LA	EFPC	GWG	FGP	GWR
43124		A	HA	HAPC	S7C	ANG	ASR
43125		A	HA	HAPC	S7C	ANG	ASR
43126		A	HA	HAPC	S7C	ANG	ASR
43127		A	HA	HAPC	S7C	ANG	ASR
43128		A	HA	HAPC	S7C	ANG	ASR
43129		A	HA	HAPC	S7C*	ANG	ASR
43130		A	HA	HAPC	S7C	ANG	ASR
43131		A	HA	HAPC	S7C	ANG	ASR
43132		A	HA	HAPC	S7C	ANG	ASR
43133		A	HA	HAPC	S7C	ANG	ASR
43134	*Gordon Aikman BEM Mind Campaigner 1985-2017*	A	HA	HAPC	S7C	ANG	ASR
43135		A	HA	HAPC	S7C	ANG	ASR
43136		A	HA	HAPC	S7C	ANG	ASR
43137		A	HA	HAPC	S7C	ANG	ASR
43138		A	HA	HAPC	S7C	ANG	ASR
43139		A	HA	HAPC	S7C	ANG	ASR
43141		A	HA	HAPC	S7C	ANG	ASR
43142		A	HA	HAPC	S7C	ANG	ASR
43143		A	HA	HAPC	S7C	ANG	ASR
43144		A	HA	HAPC	S7C	ANG	ASR
43145		A	HA	HAPC	S7C*	ANG	ASR
43146		A	HA	HAPC	S7C	ANG	ASR
43147		A	HA	HAPC	S7C	ANG	ASR
43148		A	HA	HAPC	S7C	ANG	ASR
43149		A	HA	HAPC	S7C	ANG	ASR
43150		A	HA	HAPC	S7C	ANG	ASR
43151		A	HA	HAPC	S7C	ANG	ASR
43152		A	HA	HAPC	S7C	ANG	ASR
43153	*Chun Castle*	A	LA	EFPC	GWG	FGP	GWR
43154	*Compton Castle*	A	LA	EFPC	GWG	FGP	GWR
43155	*Rougemont Castle*	A	LA	EFPC	GWG	FGP	GWR
43156		A	LA	EFPC	GWG	FGP	GWR
43158	*Kingswear Castle*	A	LA	EFPC	GWG	FGP	GWR
43159		125 Group at RTC Derby					
43160	*Castle an Dinas*	A	LA	EFPC	GWG	FGP	GWR
43162	*Caerhays Castle*	A	LA	EFPC	GWG	FGP	GWR
43163		A	HA	HAPC	S7C	ANG	ASR
43164		A	HA	HAPC	S7C	ANG	ASR

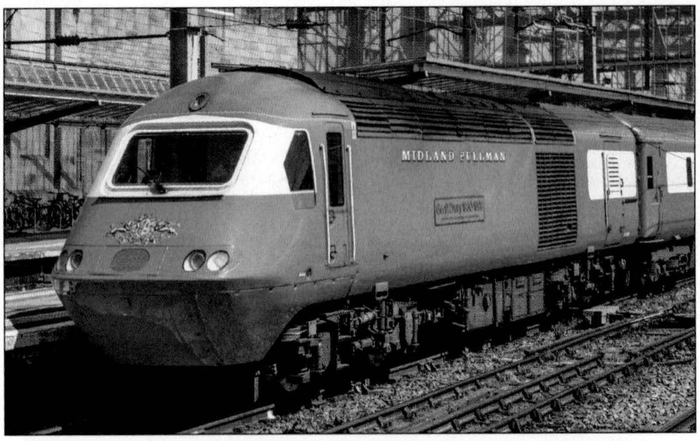

Crewe-based Loco Services Ltd operate the Midland Pullman train with three power cars and 10 trailers in Nankin blue and white livery. No. 43046 Geoff Drury 1930-1999 Steam Preservation and Computerised Track Recording Pioneer *is seen at Carlisle on 4 June 2022. Note the window in the luggage van door has been replaced by a grille, as the van now houses a generator for hotel power.* **CJM**

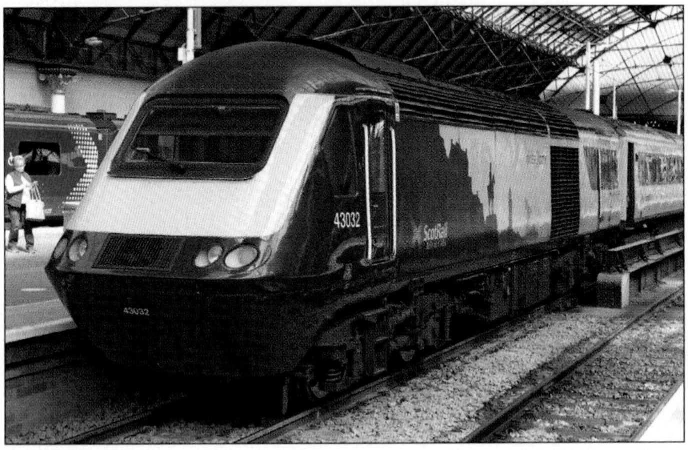

In Scotland a batch of powers are dedicated to the Inter7City (IC) services radiating north from Edinburgh and Glasgow to Inverness and Aberdeen. The Scottish power cars are all ex-Great Western vehicles and now sport a special I7C grey and blue pictogram-based scheme. No. 43032 is seen at Glasgow Queen Street. **CJM**

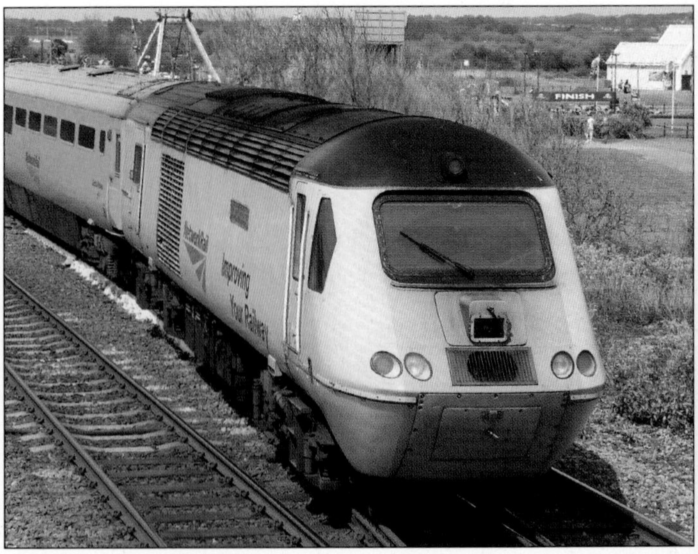

In early 2022 Network Rail were using five Class 43s to power the New Measurement Train, the three usual vehicles were undergoing an upgrade to include ETCS, so two ex-LNER power cars had been taken over to cover. Yellow-liveried No. 43062 John Armitt *is shown.* **CJM**

43165		A	EL	-	GWG	ANG	(S)
43168		A	HA	HAPC	S7C	ANG	ASR
43169		A	HA	HAPC	S7C	ANG	ASR
43170	*Chepstow Castle*	A	LA	EFPC	GWG	ANG	GWR
43171	*Raglan Castle*	A	LA	EFPC	GWG	ANG	GWR
43172	*Tiverton Castle*	A	LA	EFPC	GWG	ANG	GWR
43174		A	EL	-	GWG	ANG	(S)
43175		A	HA	HAPC	S7C	ANG	ASR
43176		A	HA	HAPC	S7C	ANG	ASR
43177		A	HA	HAPC	S7C	ANG	ASR
43179		A	HA	HAPC	S7C	ANG	ASR
43180		A	LA	-	BLU	FGP	(S)
43181		A	HA	HAPC	S7C*	ANG	ASR
43182		A	HA	HAPC	S7C	ANG	ASR
43183		A	HA	HAPC	S7C	ANG	ASR
43185		Brodie Engineering, Kilmarnock for spares					
43186	*Taunton Castle*	A	LA	EFPC	GWG	ANG	GWR
43187	*Cardiff Castle*	A	LA	EFPC	GWG	ANG	GWR
43188		A	LA	EFPC	GWG	ANG	GWR
43189	*Launceston Castle*	A	LA	EFPC	GWG	ANG	GWR
43190		A	EL	-	GWG	ANG	(S)
43191		A	EL	SCEL	GWG	ANG	(S)
43192	*Tremerton Castle*	A	LA	EFPC	GWG	ANG	GWR
43194	*Okehampton Castle*	A	LA	EFPC	GWG	FGP	GWR
43195		A	LA	EFPC	GWG	FGP	(S)
43196		A	LA	EFPC	GWG	ANG	(S)
43198	Side A: *Driver Brian Cooper 15 June 1947 - 5 October 1999* Side B: *Driver Stan Martin 25 June 1960 - 6 November 2004*	A	LA	EFPC	GWG	FGP	GWR
43206 (43006)		A	EL	-	LNE	ANG	(S)
43207 (43007)		A	LA	EHPC	AXC	ANG	AXC
43208 (43008)		A	LA	EHPC	AXC	ANG	AXC
43238 (43038)		A	EL	EMPC	LEM	ANG	(S)
43239 (43039)		A	LA	EHPC	AXC	ANG	AXC
43251 (43051)		A	ZA	COTS	COR	PTR	COL
43257 (43057)		A	ZA	COTS	COR	PTR	COL
43272 (43072)		A	ZA	COTS	COR	PTR	COL
43274 (43074)		A	ZA	COTS	COM	PTR	COL
43277 (43077)		A	ZA	COTS	COR	PTR	(S)
43285 (43085)		A	LA	EHPC	AXC	PTR	AXC
43290 (43090)		A	ZA	SBXL	LNN	PTR	NRL
43295 (43095)		A	EL	SCEL	LEM	ANG	(S)
43296 (43096)		A	WN	HHPC	LNE	HRA	(S)

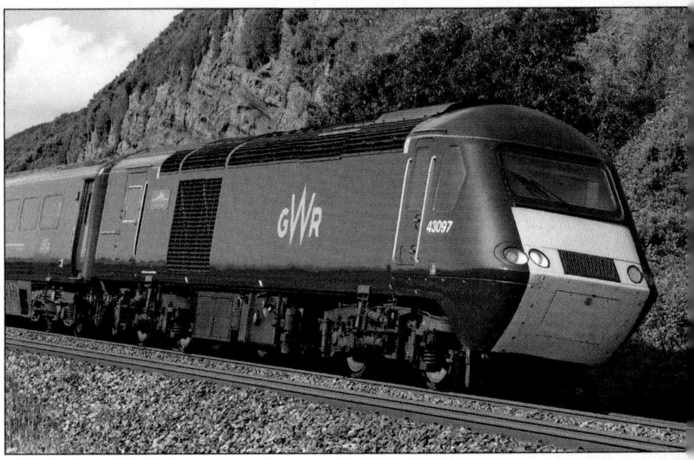

The changes of HST power car allocation after the introduction of Class 80x stock has seen Great Western retain a sizable number of power cars, allocated to Laira depot for use on 2+4 'Castle' formations, used on the Cardiff to West of England route. No. 43097 Castle Drogo *is illustrated. The naming project for the GW vehicles should be completed in 2022.* **CJM**

43299 (43099)	A	ZA	SBXL	LNN	PTR	NRL
43300 (43100)	A	NL	-	LNE	ANG	(S)
43301 (43101)	A	LA	EHPC	AXC	PTR	AXC
43303 (43103)	A	LA	EHPC	AXC	PTR	AXC
43304 (43104)	A	LA	EHPC	AXC	ANG	AXC
43305 (43105)	A	EL	SCEL	LEM	ANG	(S)
43306 (43106)	A	EL	SCEL	LEM	ANG	(S)
43307 (43107)	A	EL	SCEL	LEM	ANG	(S)
43308 (43108)	A	WN	HHPC	LNE	HRA	(S)
43309 (43109)	A	EL	SCEL	LNE	ANG	(S)
43310 (43110)	A	EL	SCEL	LEM	ANG	(S)
43311 (43111)	A	EL	SCEL	LNE	ANG	(S)
43312 (43112)	A	EL	SCEL	LNE	ANG	(S)
43314 (43114)	A	EL	SCEL	LEM	ANG	(S)
43315 (43115)	A	EL	SCEL	LNE	ANG	(S)
43316 (43116)	A	EL	SCEL	LEM	ANG	(S)
43317 (43117)	A	EL	SCEL	LEM	ANG	(S)
43318 (43118)	A	EL	SCEL	LEM	ANG	(S)
43319 (43119)	A	EL	SCEL	LEM	ANG	(S)
43320 (43120)	A	EL	SCEL	LNE	ANG	(S)
43321 (43121)	A	LA	EHPC	AXC	PTR	AXC
43357 (43157)	A	LA	EHPC	AXC	PTR	AXC
43366 (43166)	A	LA	EHPC	AXC	ANG	AXC
43367 (43167)	A	EL	SCEL	LNE	ANG	(S)
43378 (43178)	A	LA	EHPC	AXC	ANG	AXC
43384 (43184)	A	LA	EHPC	AXC	ANG	AXC

± For spares * Carries facemask

Hanson & Hall / RailAdventure
Class 43 'Power-Pairs'

43423 (43123) 92 70 0043 423-7	A B	ZG	HHPC	EMR	HRA	HRA
43465 (43065) 92 70 0043 465-8	A B	ZG	HHPC	EMR	HRA	HRA
43467 (43067) 92 70 0043 467-4	A B	ZG	HHPC	EMR	HRA	HRA
43468 (43068) 92 70 0043 468-2	A B	ZG	HHPC	HRA	HRA	HRA
43480 (43080) 92 70 0043 480-7	A B	ZG	HHPC	HRA	HRA	HRA
43484 (43084) 92 70 0043 484-9	A B	ZG	HHPC	HRA	HRA	HRA

Class 44 'Peak'
BR 1Co-Co1 Diesel-Electric

Built: 1959-1960
Length: 67ft 11in (20.7m)
Height: 12ft 10¼in (3.92m)
Width: 8ft 10½in (2.71m)
Engine: Sulzer 12LDA28A of 2,300hp (1,715kW)
Transmission: Electric
Tractive effort: 70,000lb (311kN)

44004 (D4)	*Great Gable*	Midland Railway Centre, Butterley
44008 (D8)	*Penyghent*	Peak Rail, Rowsley

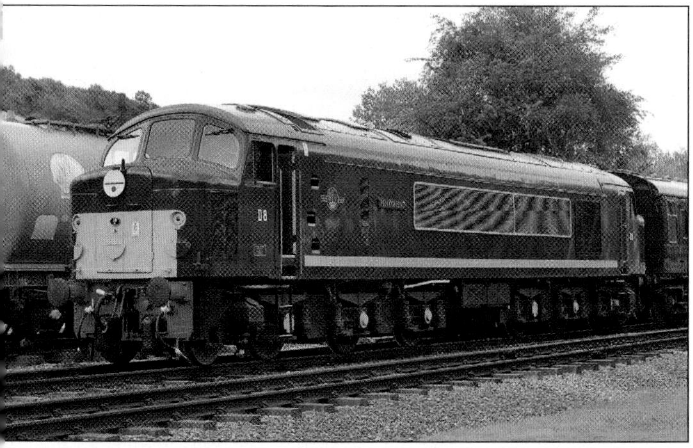

Vhen the original 10 'Peak', later Class 44s were withdrawn, two were purchased for reservation. Both are restored to a high standard, but are not certified for main line operation. Restored to 1960s green livery, No. D8 Penyghent is seen at Rowsley South with a train to Matlock. **Adrian Paul**

Class 45 'Peak'
BR 1Co-Co1 Diesel-Electric

Built: 1960-1962
Length: 67ft 11in (20.7m)
Height: 12ft 10¼in (3.92m)
Width: 8ft 10½in (2.71m)
Engine: Sulzer 12LDA28B of 2,500hp (1,864kW)
Transmission: Electric
Tractive effort: 55,000lb (244.6kN)

5015 (D14)		Battlefield, Railway (to be cut)
5041 (D53)	*Royal Tank Regiment*	Nene Valley Railway
5060 (D100)	*Sherwood Forester*	Barrow Hill Roundhouse
5105 (D86)		Barrow Hill Roundhouse
5108 (D120)		East Lancashire Railway
5112 (D61)	*Royal Army Ordnance Corps*	Nemesis Rail, Burton-on-Trent
5118 (D67)	*The Rotal Artilleryman*	LSL at Barrow Hill Roundhouse
5125 (D123)		Great Central Rly, Loughborough
5132 (D22)		Epping & Ongar Railway
5133 (D40)		Midland Railway Centre, Butterley
5135 (D99)	*3rd Carabinier*	East Lancashire Railway
5149 (D135)		Gloucester & Warwickshire Railway

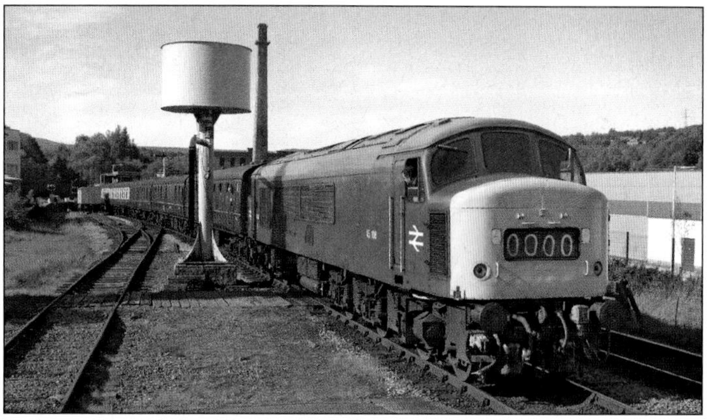

Twelve members of the first follow-on 'Peak' order, later Class 45 are preserved, carrying a variety of liveries and body styles. No. 45108 (D120) is seen in mid-1970s rail blue livery at Rawtenstall on the East Lancs Railway. **Nathan Williamson**

Class 46 'Peak'
BR 1Co-Co1 Diesel-Electric

Built: 1961-1963
Length: 67ft 11in (20.7m)
Height: 12ft 10¼in (3.92m)
Width: 8ft 10½in (2.71m)
Engine: Sulzer 12LDA28B of 2,500hp (1,864kW)
Transmission: Electric
Tractive effort: 55,000lb (244.6kN)

46010 (D147)		Great Central Railway, Nottingham
46035 (D172)		Crewe Heritage Centre
46045 (D182)	*(Ixion)*	Midland Railway Centre

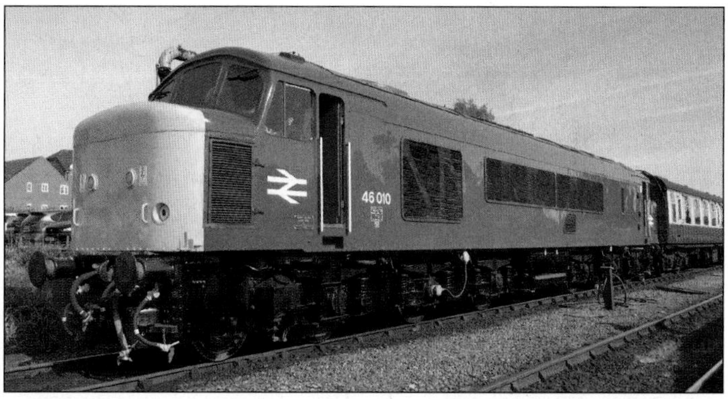

The final batch of 'Peaks' were classified as 46 and three members went into preservation. No. 46010 is shown in its final version of BR rail blue at Kidderminster on the Severn Valley Railway when attending a gala event. The loco is usually based at the Great Central Railway. **Spencer Conquest**

Class 47
BR/Brush Co-Co Diesel-Electric

Built: 1962-1965
Length: 66ft 6in (19.35m)
Height: 12ft 10⅜in (3.90m)
Width: 9ft 2in (2.79m)
Engine: Sulzer 12LDA28C of 2,580hp (1,924kW)
Transmission: Electric
Tractive effort: 60,000lb (267kN)

47004 (D1524)		Embsay & Bolton Abbey Railway					
47077 (D1661)	*North Star*	North Yorkshire Moors Railway D&EPG					
47105 (D1693)		Gloucester Warwickshire Railway					
47117 (D1705)		Great Central Rly, Loughborough					
47192 (D1842)		Ecclesbourne Valley Railway					
47194 (D1844)		X	CS	AWCX	TFG	WCR	(S)
47205 (D1855)		Northampton & Lamport Railway					
47237 (D1914)		X	CS	AWCA	WCR	WCR	WCR
47245 (D1922)	*V.E. Day 75th Anniversary*	X	CS	AWCA	WCR	WCR	WCR
47270 (D1971)		X	CS	AWCA	BLU	WCR	WCR
47292 (D1994)		Great Central Railway, Nottingham					
47306 (D1787)		Bodmin Steam Railway					
47355 (D1836)		A	CS	AWCX	BLK	WCR	(S)
47367 (D1886)		X	Mid Norfolk Railway				
47375 (D1894)		A	Exported - CRS, Hungary as 92 70 0047-375-5				
47376 (D1895)		Gloucester Warwickshire Railway					
47401 (D1500)		Midland Railway Centre					
47402 (D1501)		Peak Rail					
47417 (D1516)		Midland Railway Centre					
47449 (D1566)		Llangollen Railway					
47484 (D1662)	*Isambard Kingdom Brunel*	Rye Farm, Wishaw (Pioneer DG)					
47488 (D1713)		X	BU	MBDL	MAR	CRS	(S)
47492 (D1760)		X	CS	AWCX	RES	WCR	(S)
47501 (D1944)	*Craftsman*	X	CL	LSLO	GRN	LSL	LSL
47503 (D1946)		Colne Valley Railway					
47579 (D1778)		Mid Hants Railway					
47580 (47732)	*County of Essex*	S4G at Mid Norfolk Railway					
47593 (47790)	*Galloway Princess*	X	CL	LSLO	BLL	LSL	LSL
47596 (D1933)		Mid-Norfolk Railway					
47614 (D1733)		X	CL	LSLO	BLU	LSL	LSL

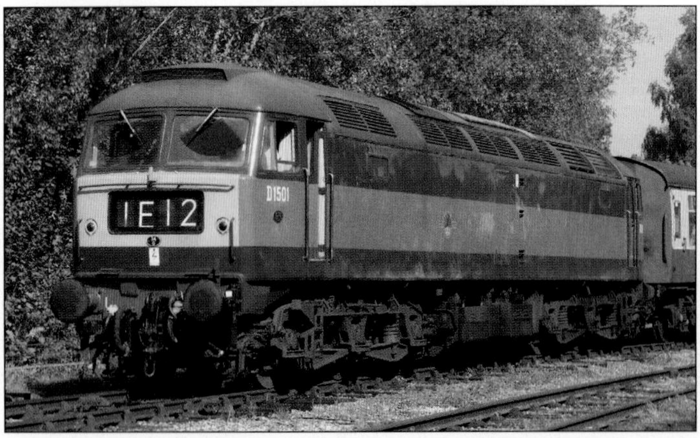

The standard BR mixed traffic loco for many years was the Brush/BR Class 47, with over 500 built in the mid 1960s. Many are still in service while a number are preserved. Preserved No. D1501 (47402) shows the original BR two-tone green livery style on the East Lancs Railway, its home base. **Adrian Paul**

47635 (D1606)		Epping & Ongar Railway					
47640 (D1921)		Nemesis Rail, Burton					
47643 (D1970)		Bo'ness & Kinneil Railway					
47701 (47493)		X	BU	MBDL	BLK	NEM	(S)
47703 (47514)		X	ZB	HNRL	BLK	HNR	WAB
47712 (47505)	*Lady Diana Spencer*	X	CL	LSLO	SCI	LSL	LSL
47714 (47511)		X	ZB	HNRL	ANG	HNR	WAB
47715 (47502)		X	WS	HNRL	NSE	HNR	HNR
47727 (47569)	*Edinburgh Castle Caisteal Dhun Eideann*	X	LR	GBDF	SCS	GBR	GBR
47739 (47594)		X D	LR	GBDF	GBB	GBR	GBR
47744 (47600)		X	BU	MBDL	EWS	NEM	(S)
47746 (47605)	*Chris Fudge 29.7.70-22.6.10*	X	CS	AWCA	WCR	WCR	WCR
47749 (47625)	*City of Truro*	X D	LR	GBDF	BLU	GBR	GBR
47760 (47562)		X	CS	AWCA	WCR	WCR	WCR
47761 (D1619)		Midland Railway Centre					
47765 (D1643)		East Lancashire Railway					
47768 (47490)		X	CS	AWCX	EWS	WCR	WCR
47769 (47491)		X	BH	HNRL	RES	HNR	HNR
47772 (47537)	*Carnforth TMD*	X	CS	AWCA	WCR	WCR	WCR
47773 (47541)		X	TM	MBDL	GRN	VTN	VTN
47776 (47578)		X	CS	AWCX	RES	WCR	(S)
47785 (D1909)		HNRC at Worksop					
47786 (47821)	*Roy Castle OBE*	X	CS	AWCA	WCR	WCR	WCR
47787 (47823)		X	CS	AWCX	WCR	WCR	(S)
47798 (D1656)	*Prince William*	National Railway Museum					
47799 (D1654)		Eden Valley Railway					
47802 (47552)		X	CS	AWCA	WCR	WCR	WCR
47804 (47792)		X	CS	AWCA	WCR	WCR	WCR
47805 (D1935)	*Roger Hosking MA 1925-2013*	X	CL	LSLO	GRN	LSL	LSL
47810 (47655)	*Crewe Diesel Depot*	X	CL	LSLO	GRN	LSL	LSL
47811 (47656)		X	CL	-	GRN	LSL	(S)
47812 (47657)		X	CS	AWCA	BLU	WCR	WCR
47813 (47658)		X	CS	AWCA	WCR	WCR	WCR
47815 (47660)	*Great Western*	X	CS	AWCA	GRN	WCR	WCR
47816 (47661)		X	CL	-	GRN	LSL	(S)
47818 (47663)		X	ZG	MBDL	BLU	AFG	(S)
47826 (47637)		X	CS	AWCA	WCR	WCR	WCR
47828 (47629)		X	CL	LSLO	ICS	D05	LSL
47830 (47649)	*Beeching's Legacy*	X	CB	DFLH	GRN	FLR	FLR
47832 (47560)		X	CS	AWCA	WCR	WCR	WCR
47841 (47622)	*The Institution of Mechanical Engineers*	One:One Railway Museum, Margate					
47843 (47623)		X	WS	HNRL	ROG	HNR	(S)
47847 (47577)		X	WS	HNRL	ROG	HNR	(S)
47848 (47632)		X	CS	AWCA	WCR	WCR	WCR
47851 (47639)		X	CS	AWCA	WCR	WCR	WCR
47854 (47674)	*Diamond Jubilee*	X	CS	AWCA	WCR	WCR	WCR

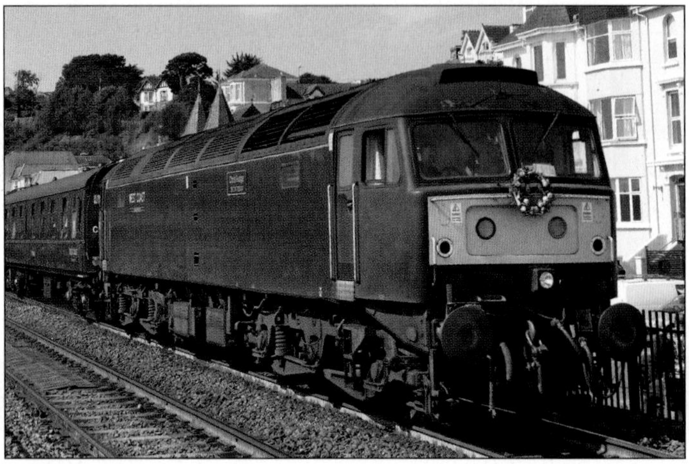

The West Coast Railway Co operate several Class 47s on charter operations. All are painted in company maroon with a small yellow warning end. No. 47746 is illustrated. This ex-Res loco was fitted with nose mounted RCH jumpers, but these are now removed. **CJM**

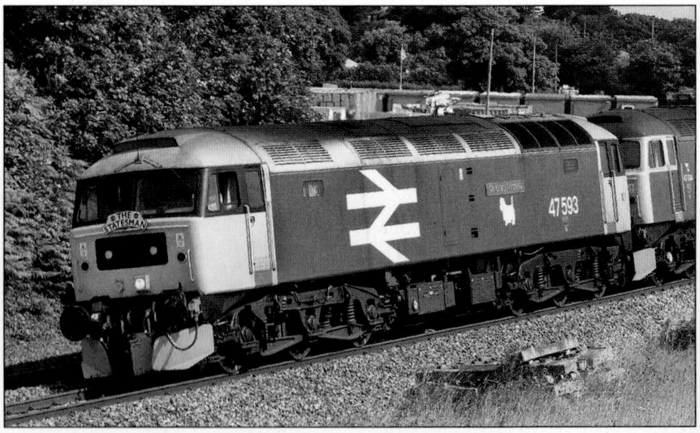

Loco services Ltd operate several wonderfully restored Class 47s, displaying a number of different livery styles. No. 47593 Galloway Princess *carried large logo blue with a 'Scottie dog' motif on the body side. Complete with yellow ploughs, the loco is seen on a charter at Dawlish Warren in July 2021.* **CJM**

Class 50
English Electric Co-Co Diesel-Electric

Built: 1967-1968
Length: 68ft 6in (20.88m)
Height: 12ft 10¾in (3.92m)
Width: 9ft 1¼in (2.77m)

Engine: EE 16SVT of 2,700hp (2,013kW)
Transmission: Electric
Tractive effort: 48,500lb (216kN)

50002 (D402)	*Supurb*	South Devon Railway					
50007 (D407)	*Hercules*	X	KR	CFOL	GBR	50A	GBR
50008 (D408)	*Thunderer*	X	LR	HVAC	GRY	HAH	HAN
50015 (D415)	*Valiant*	East Lancashire Railway					
50017 (D417)	*Royal Oak*	Great Central Railway					
50019 (D419)	*Ramillies*	Mid Norfolk Railway					
50021 (D421)	*Rodney*	Arlington Fleet Services, Eastleigh					
50026 (D426)	*Indomitable*	Arlington Fleet Services, Eastleigh §					
50027 (D427)	*Lion*	Mid Hants Railway					
50029 (D429)	*Renown*	Peak Rail, Rowsley					
50030 (D430)	*Repulse*	Peak Rail, Rowsley					
50031 (D431)	*Hood*	Severn Valley Railway					
50033 (D433)	*Glorious*	Severn Valley Railway with Class 50 Alliance					
50035 (D435)	*Ark Royal*	Severn Valley Railway					
50042 (D442)	*Triumph*	Bodmin & Wenford Railway					
50044 (D444)	*Exeter*	X	KR	CFOL	BLU	50A	50A
50049 (D449)	*Defiance*	X	KR	CFOL	GBR	50A	GBR
50050 (D400)	*Fearless*	X	NM	COFS	BLU	BOD	BOD

§ For main line certification

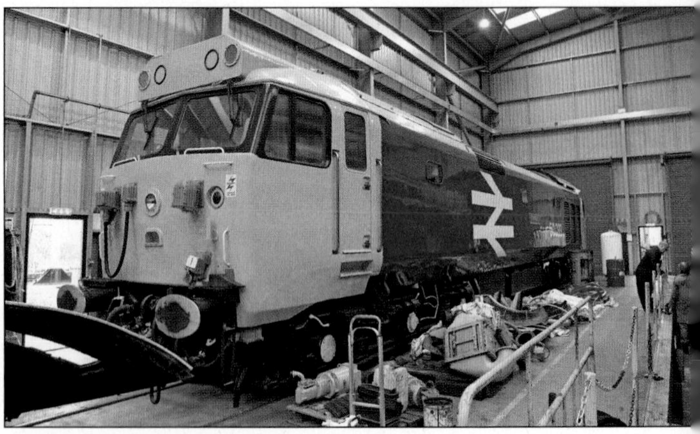

A total of 18 Class 50s were saved after withdrawal by BR, five are currently certified for main line operation. In the above view preserved No. 50033 Glorious *is seen inside the shed at Kidderminster on the Severn Valley Railway. Below No. 50008* Thunderer *is now main line certified and operated by the joint venture of Hanson & Hall and RailAdventure. The loco is see from its No.2 end at Kidderminster in November 2021. Both:* **CJM**

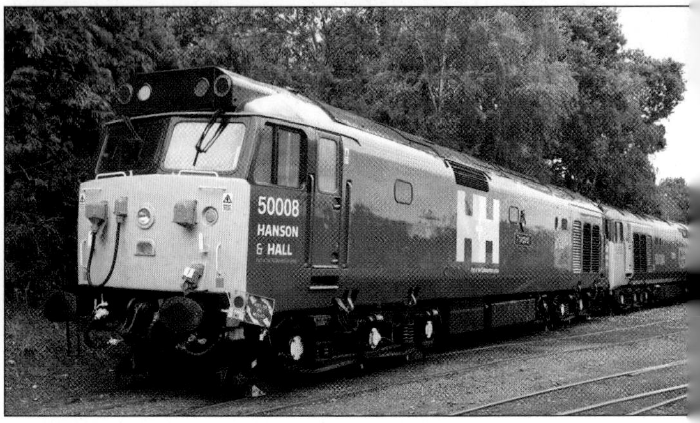

Class 52 'Western'
BR C-C Diesel-Hydraulic

Built: 1961-1964
Length: 60ft 0in (20.73m)
Height: 12ft 11¾in (3.96m)
Width: 9ft 0in (2.74m)
Engine: 2 x Maybach MD655 of 1,350hp (1,006.5kW)
Transmission: Hydraulic
Tractive effort: 70,000lb (311.3kN)

D1010	*Western Campaigner*	West Somerset Railway
D1013	*Western Ranger*	WLA at Severn Valley Railway
D1015	*Western Champion*	DTG at Severn Valley Railway
D1023	*Western Fusilier*	National Railway Museum
D1041	*Western Prince*	East Lancashire Railway
D1048	*Western Lady*	Midland Railway Centre, Butterley
D1062 (D1040)	*Western Courier*	WLA at Severn Valley Railway (As *Western Queen*)

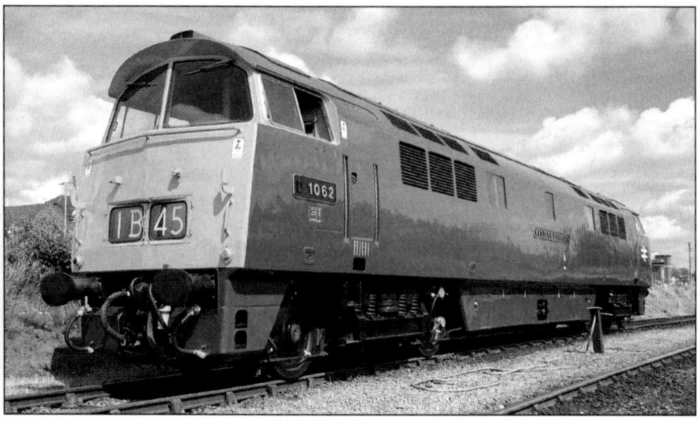

The Western Locomotive Association, based at the Severn Valley Railway have two Class 52 'Western' locos, No. D1013 which is under restoration and No. D1062 which is operational. No. D1062 Western Courier *is seen in 1970s BR rail blue.* **Roger Smith**

Class 55 'Deltic'
English Electric Co-Co Diesel-Electric

Built: 1961-1962
Length: 69ft 6in (21.18m)
Height: 12ft 11in (3.94m)
Width: 8ft 9½in (2.74m)
Engine: 2 x Napier D18.25 of 1,650hp (1,230.5kW)
Transmission: Electric
Tractive effort: 50,000lb (222kN)

55002 (D9002)	*The Kings Own Yorkshire Light Infantry*	National Railway Museum, York (ML Certified)
55009 (D9009)	*Alycidon*	DPS at Barrow Hill Roundhouse (ML Certified)
55015 (D9015)	*Tulyar*	DPS at Barrow Hill Roundhouse
55016 (D9016)	*Gordon Highlander*	1:1 Railway Museum, Margate
55019 (D9019)	*Royal Highland Fusilier*	DPS at Barrow Hill Roundhouse
55022 (D9000)	*Royal Scots Grey*	Loco Services Ltd, Crewe

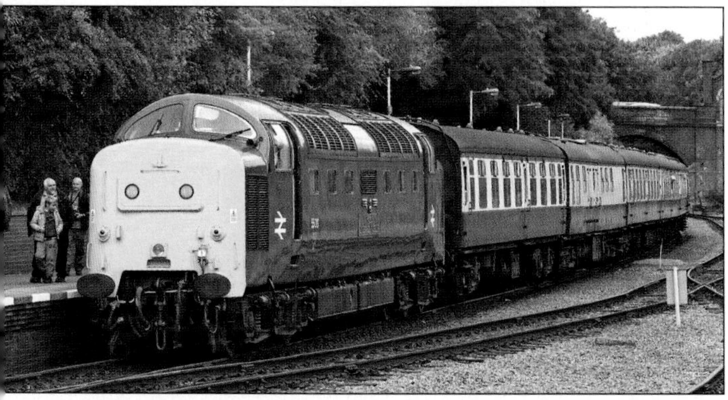

Of the fleet of 22 English Electric Type 5 'Deltic' locos, six were preserved, one in the National Collection No. 55002 (D9002). Displaying rail blue, No. 55019 Royal Highland Fusilier *is shown at Leicester North.* **Adrian Paul**

Class 56
BR/Brush Co-Co Diesel-Electric

Built: 1976-1984
Length: 63ft 6in (19.35m)
Height: 12ft 9¼in (3.89m)
Width: 9ft 2in (2.79m)
Engine: Ruston Paxman 16RK3CT of 3,250hp (2,424kW)
Transmission: Electric
Tractive effort: 61,800lb (275kN)

6006	Class 56 Group, East Lancashire Railway						
6009		A	LT	UKRS	SPL	EMD	(S)
6032		A	LT	GBGS	FER	GBR	(S)
6049	*Robin of Templecombe 1930-2013*	A	NM	COFS	COL	COL	COL
6051	*Survival*	A	NM	COFS	COL	COL	COL
6077		A	LT	UKRS	LHL	GBR	(S)
6078		A	NM	COFS	COL	COL	COL
6081		A, D	LR	GBGD	GRY	GBR	GBR
6087		A	NM	COFS	COL	BOD	GBR
6090		A	NM	COFS	COL	BOD	GBR
6091	*Driver Wayne Gaskell The Godfather*	A	LR	DCRO	DCR	DCR	DCR
56094		A	NM	COFS	COL	COL	COL
56096		A	NM	COFS	COL	BOD	COL
56097	Great Central Railway, Nottingham						
56098		A	LR	GBGD	GRY	GBR	GBR
56101		A	Exported to Hungary as 92 55 0659-001-5 - Eurogate Rail				
56103		A	LR	DCRS	DCR	DCR	(S)
56104		A	LR	UKRL	GRY	GBR	(S)
56105		A	NM	COFS	COL	BOD	COL
56106		A	LR	UKRS	FER	GBR	(S)
56113		A	NM	COFS	COL	BOD	COL
56115		A	Exported to Hungary as 92 55 0659-002-3 - Eurogate Rail				
56117		A	Exported to Hungary as 92 55 0659-003-1 - Eurogate Rail				
56301 (56045)		A	LR	UKRL	GRY	56G	SH
56302 (56124)	*PECO The Railway Modeller 2016 70 Years*	A	NM	COFS	COL	COL	COL
56303 (56125)		A	LR	HTLX	SPL	DCR	DCR
56312 (56003)		A	LR	GBGD	DCR	GBR	GBR

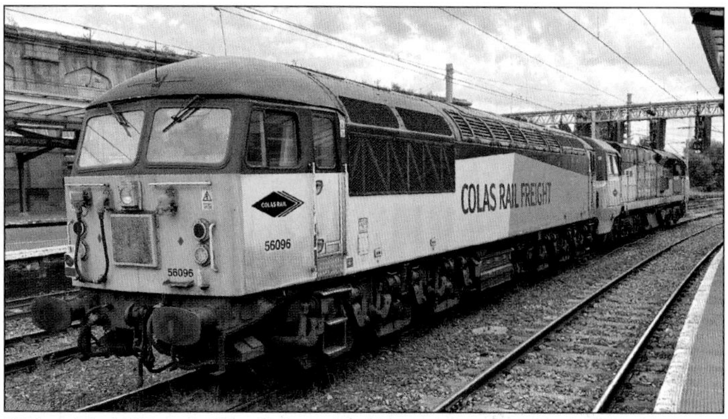

Of the original 135 strong Class 56 fleet, a handful remain operational in the UK with three exported to Hungary and now working for Eurogate Rail. Colas Rail Freight No. 56096 is shown with a Class 70 at Carlisle. **Spencer Conquest**

Class 57
Brush/BR Co-Co Diesel-Electric

Built: 1998-2004
Length: 63ft 6in (19.35m)
Height: 12ft 10⅜in (3.90m)
Width: 9ft 2in (2.79m)
Engine: 57/0 GM 645-12E3 of 2,500hp (1,860kW)
57/3, 57/5 GM 645-12F3B of 2,750hp (2,051kW)
Transmission: Electric
Tractive effort: 55,000lb (244.5kN)

57/0

57001 (47356)		A	CS	AWCA	WCR	WCR	WCR
57002 (47322)	*Rail Express*	A	KM	XHSO	DRC	DRS	DRS
57003 (47317)	(for sale 04/22)	A	KM	XSDP	DRC	DRS	DRS
57004 (47347)		A	CL	LSLO	DRC	LSL	(S)
57005 (47350)		A	CS	AWCX	WCR	WCR	(S)
57006 (47187)		A	CS	AWCA	WCR	WCR	WCR
57007 (47332)	*John Scott 12.5.45 - 22.5.12* (for sale 04/22)	A	KM	XSDP	DRC	DRS	(S)
57008 (47060)		A	CS	AWCA	DRC	WCR	WCR
57009 (47079)		A	CS	AWCA	DRC	WCR	WCR
57010 (47231)		A	CS	AWCA	DRC	WCR	WCR
57011 (47329)		A	CS	AWCA	DRC	WCR	WCR
57012 (47204)		A	CS	AWCX	DRC	WCR	(S)

57/3

57301 (47845)		AT	KM	XWSS	DRA	DRS	(S)
57302 (47827)	*Chad Varah*	AD	CL	LSLO	DRC	LSL	LSL
57303 (47705)	*Pride of Carlisle*	AT	LR	XWSS	BLU	DRS	(S)
57304 (47807)	*Pride of Cheshire*	AD	KM	XHVT	DRA	PTR	DRS
57305 (47822)		AD	LR	XHSO	ROG	DRS	DRS
57306 (47814)	*Her Majesty's Railway Inspectorate 175*	AT	KM	XHAC	DRC	DRS	DRS
57307 (47225)	Lady Penelope	AD	KM	XHVT	DRA	PTR	DRS
57308 (47846)	*Jamie Ferguson*	AD	KM	XHVT	DRA	PTR	DRS
57309 (47806)	*Pride of Crewe*	AD	KM	XHVT	DRA	PTR	DRS
57310 (47831)	*Pride of Cumbria*	AD	KM	XHSO	DRS	DRS	DRS
57311 (47817)	*Thunderbird*	AD	CL	LSLO	DRC	LSL	LSL

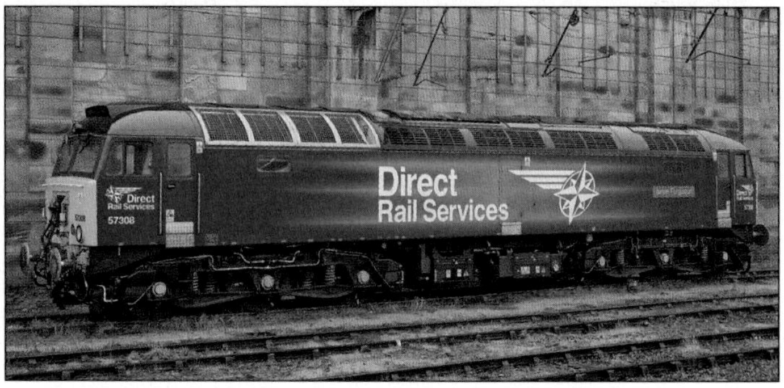

A total of 33 Class 57s were converted from Class 47s by Brush Traction, formed into three sub classes. The 16 members of Class 57/3 were originally operated by Virgin Trains as 'Thunderbird' locos, but are now operated by DRS, WCR and LSL. DRS No. 57308 Jamie Ferguson *is seen at Carlisle, note the drophead Dellner coupling.* **Antony Christie**

57312 (47330)		AD	LR	XHSO	ROG	PTR	DRS
57313 (47371)	*Scarborough Castle*	A	CS	AWCA	PUL	WCR	WCR
57314 (47372)	*Conwy Castle*	A	CS	AWCA	WCR	WCR	WCR
57315 (47234)		A	CS	AWCA	WCR	WCR	WCR
57316 (47290)	*Alnwick Castle*	A	CS	AWCA	WCR	WCR	WCR

57/6

57601 (47825)	*Windsor Castle*	A	CS	AWCA	PUL	WCR	WCR
57602 (47337)	*Restormel Castle*	A	PZ	EFOO	GWG	PTR	GWR
57603 (47349)	*Tintagel Castle*	A	PZ	EFOO	GWG	PTR	GWR
57604 (47209)	*Pendennis Castle*	A	PZ	EFOO	GWR	PTR	GWR
57605 (47206)	*Totnes Castle*	A	PZ	EFOO	GWG	PTR	GWR

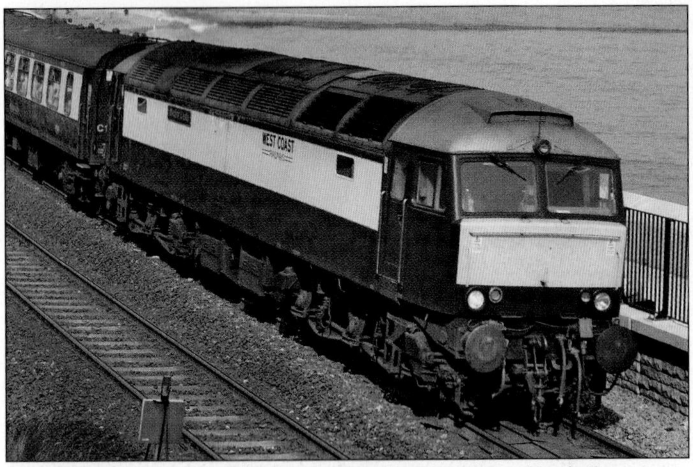

The Brush/Porterbrook Class 57/6 ETH conversion No. 57601 after working for Great Western was sold to West Coast Railway, where it now sports West Coast Pullman livery and deployed on charter services, often working 'top and tail' with a Class 47. **CJM**

Class 58
BREL Co-Co Diesel-Electric

Built: 1983-1987
Length: 62ft 9½in (19.14m)
Height: 12ft 10in (3.91m)
Width: 9ft 1in (2.77m)
Engine: Ruston Paxman 12RK3ACT of 3,300hp (2,461kW)
Transmission: Electric
Tractive effort: 61,800lb (275kN)

58001		A	ETF France
58004		A	TSO France
58005		A	ETF France
58006		A	ETF France
58007		A	TSO France
58009		A	TSO France
58010		A	TSO France
58011		A	TSO France
58012	Battlefield Line		
58013		A	ETF France
58016	UK Rail Leasing, Leicester		
58018		A	TSO France
58021		A	TSO France
58022	Ecclesbourne Valley Railway (Ivatt 10000 project)		
58023	UKRL, Leicester		
58025		A	Continental Rail, Spain
58026		A	TSO France
58027		A	Continental Rail, Spain
58032		A	ETF France
58033		A	TSO France
58034		A	TSO France
58035		A	TSO France
58036		A	ETF France
58038		A	ETF France
58039		A	ETF France
58040		A	TSO France
58041		A	Transfesa, Spain
58042		A	TSO France
58044		A	ETF France (Woippy Yard)
58046		A	TSO France
58048	Battlefield Line		
58049		A	ETF France
58050		A	Continental Rail, Spain

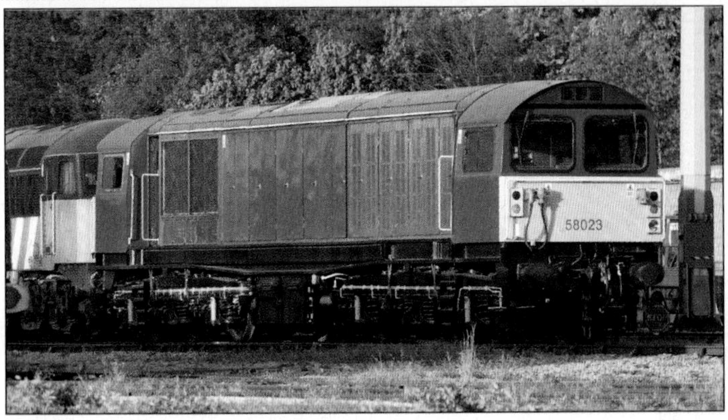

The 50 Class 58s, built as a development of the Class 56 by BREL Doncaster in 1980s, soon fell from favour. Many are currently stored in Mainland Europe, some have been broken up and four are preserved, with No. 58023 operational but not main line certified at UKRL, Leicester, which this view of the loco was recorded in Mainline Freight blue. **Antony Christie**

Class 59
General Motors/EMD Co-Co Diesel-Electric

Built: 1985-1995
Length: 70ft 0½in (21.35m)
Height: 12ft 10in (3.91m)
Width: 8ft 8¼in (2.65m)
Engine: EMD 16-645E3C of 3,000hp (2,237kW)
Transmission: Electric
Tractive effort: 122,000lb (542.6kN)

59/0

59001	*Yeoman Endeavour*	A	MD	DFHG	AGI	FLR	FLR
59002	*Alan J Day*	A	MD	DFHG	AGI	FLR	FLR
59003	*Yeoman Highlander*	A	RR	GBYH	GBN	GBR	GBR
59004	*Paul A Hammond*	A	MD	DFHG	AGI	FLR	FLR
59005	*Kenneth J Painter*	A	MD	DFHG	AGI	FLR	FLR

59/1

59101	*Village of Whatley*	A	MD	DFHG	HAN	FLR	FLR
59102	*Village of Chantry*	A	MD	DFHG	HAN	FLR	FLR
59103	*Village of Mells*	A	MD	DFHG	HAN	FLR	FLR
59104	*Village of Great Elm*	A	MD	DFHG	HAN	FLR	FLR

59/2

59201		A	MD	DFHG	RED	FLR	FLR
59202		A	MD	DFHG	GWF	FLR	FLR
59203		A	MD	DFHG	GWF	FLR	FLR
59204		A	MD	DFHG	GWF	FLR	FLR
59205		A	MD	DFHG	RED	FLR	FLR
59206	*John F. Yeoman Rail Pioneer*	A	MD	DFHG	GWF	FLR	FLR

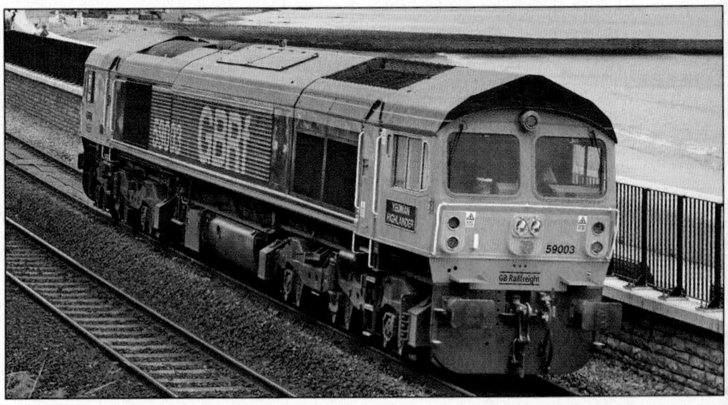

The only Class 59 not operated by Freightliner is No. 59003 Yeoman Highlander *which is owned by GB Railfreight and usually deployed in the Westbury/Eastleigh area. Carrying the latest GBRf livery and a high level marker light the loco is seen from its radiator end passing Dawlish in summer 2021 with a driver's route training run to Plymouth.* **CJM**

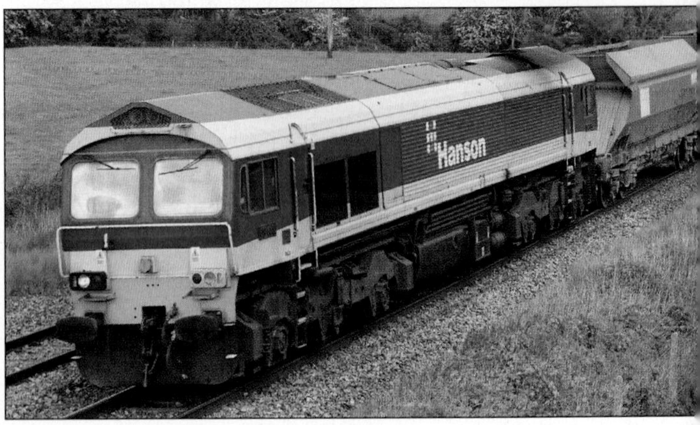

The four Class 59/1s, originally purchased by ARC Southern and then passed to Hanson Industries are now operated by Freightliner and used on their Mendip aggregate contract with members of Class 59/0 and 59/2. Carrying Hanson blue and silver colours, No. 59103 Village of Mells *powers an empty aggregate at Great Cheverell.* **CJM**

Class 60
Brush Co-Co Diesel-Electric

Built: 1989-1995
Length: 70ft 0½in (21.35m)
Height: 12ft 10in (3.91m)
Width: 8ft 8¼in (2.65m)
Engine: EMD 16-645E3C of 3,000hp (2,237kW)
Transmission: Electric
Tractive effort: 122,000lb (542.6kN)
‡ Refurbished 'Super 60'

60001‡		A	TO	WCAT	DBS	DBC	DBC
60002‡	*Graham Farish 50th Anniversary 1970-2020*	A	TO	GBTG	GBN	BEA	GBR
60003	*Freight Transport Association*	A	TO	WQCA	EWS	DBC	(S)
60004‡		A	TO	WCQA	EWS	GBR	(S)
60005		A	TO	WQCA	EWS	DBC	(S)

60007‡	*The Spirit of Tom Kendell*	A	TO	WCBT	DBS	DBC	DBC
60008	*Sir William McAlpine*	A	TO	DCRS	EWS	DCR	(S)
60009		A	TO	DCRS	EWS	DCR	(S)
60010‡		A	TO	WCBT	DBS	DBC	DBC
60011		A	TO	WCAT	DBS	DBC	DBC
60012		A	TO	WQCA	EWS	DBC	(S)
60013	*Robert Boyle*	A	TO	DCRS	GRY	DCR	(S)
60014		A	TO	WQCA	GRY	GBR	(S)
60015‡		A	TO	WCBT	DBS	DBC	DBC
60017‡		A	TO	WCBT	DBS	DBC	DBC
60018		A	TO	WQCA	EWS	GBR	(S)
60019‡	*Port of Grimsby & Immingham*	A	TO	WCAT	DBS	DBC	DBC
60020‡	*The Willows*	A	TO	WCBT	DBS	DBC	DBC
60021‡	*Penyghent*	A	TO	GBTG	GBN	BEA	GBR
60022		A	TO	DCRS	EWS	DCR	(S)
60023		A	TO	WQCA	EWS	DBC	(S)
60024‡	*Clitheroe Castle*	A	TO	WCAT	DBS	DBC	DBC
60025		A	TO	WQCA	EWS	DBC	(S)
60026‡	*Helvellyn*	A	TO	GBTG	GBB	BEA	GBR
60027		A	TO	WQCA	EWS	DBC	(S)
60028‡		A	TO	DCRO	BLU	CAP	DCR
60029‡	*Ben Nevis*	A	TO	DCRO	GRY	CAP	DCR
60030		A	TO	WQCA	EWS	DBC	(S)
60032		A	TO	WQCA	EWS	DBC	(S)
60033	*Tees Steel Express*	A	TO	WQCA	SPL	DBC	(S)
60034		A	TO	WQCA	RFE	DBC	(S)
60035		A	TO	WQCA	EWS	DBC	(S)
60036	*Gefco*	A	TO	WQCA	EWS	DBC	(S)
60037		A	TO	WQCA	EWS	DBC	(S)
60038		A	TO	DCRS	GRY	DCR	(S)
60039‡	*Dove Holes*	A	TO	WCAT	DBS	DBC	DBC
60040‡	*The Teritorial Army Centenary*	A	TO	WCAT	DBS	DBC	DBC
60043		A	TO	WQCA	EWS	DBC	(S)
60044‡	*Dowlow*	A	TO	WCAT	DBS	DBC	DBC
60045	*The Permanent Way Institution*	A	TO	WQCA	EWS	DBC	(S)
60046‡	*William Wilberforce*	A	TO	DCRO	GRY	CAP	DCR
60047‡		A	TO	GBTG	COL	BEA	GBR
60048		A	TO	WQCA	EWS	DBC	(S)
60049		A	TO	WQCA	EWS	DBC	(S)
60050	Stored at Shires Removal Group, Kinsley, Fitzwilliam						
60051		A	TO	WQCA	EWS	DBC	(S)
60052	*Glofa Twr - The last deep mine in Wales - Tower Colliery*	A	TO	WQCA	EWS	DBC	(S)
60053		A	TO	WQCA	EWS	DBC	(S)
60054‡*		A	TO	WQAA	DBC	DBC	(S)
60055‡	*Thomas Barnardo*	A	TO	DCRO	GRY	CAP	DCR
60056‡		A	TO	GBTG	COL	BEA	GBR
60057		A	TO	DCRS	RFE	DCR	(S)
60059‡	*Swinden Dalesman*	A	TO	WCBT	DBS	DBC	DBC
60060	UKRL Leicester for spares						
60061		A	TO	DCRS	GRY	DCR	(C)
60062‡	*Stainless Pioneer*	A	TO	WCAT	DBS	DBC	DBC
60063‡		A	TO	WQAA	DBS	DBC	(S)
60064		A	TO	DCRS	RFE	DCR	(S)
60065	*Spitit of Jaguar*	A	TO	WCAT	EWS	DBC	DBC
60066‡		A	TO	WCAT	ADV	DBC	DBC
60067		A	TO	WQCA	RFE	DBC	(S)
60069	*Slioch*	A	TO	WQCA	EWS	DBC	(S)
60070		A	TO	DCRS	GRY	DCR	(S)
60071	*Ribblehead Viaduct*	A	TO	WQCA	DBS	DBC	(S)
60072		A	TO	WQCA	RFE	DBC	(S)
60073		A	TO	WQCA	RFE	DBC	(S)
60074‡	*Luke*	A	TO	WCAT	SPL	DBC	DBC
60075		A	TO	DCRS	GRY	DCR	(S)
60076‡	*Dunbar*	A	TO	GBTG	COL	BEA	GBR
60077		A	TO	WQCA	RFE	DBC	(S)
60079‡		A	TO	WQBA	DBS	DBC	DBC
60080		A	TO	DCRS	GRY	DCR	(S)
60081	*Isambard Kingdom Brunel*	A	-	LSLS	GRN	LSL	S-TO
60083		A	TO	WQCA	EWS	DBC	(S)
60084		A	TO	WQCA	RFE	DBC	(S)
60085‡		A	TO	GBTG	COL	BEA	GBR
60086	Stored at Shires Removal Group, Kinsley, Fitzwilliam						
60087		A	TO	GBTG	GBR	BEA	GBR
60088		A	TO	WQCA	GRY	DBC	(S)

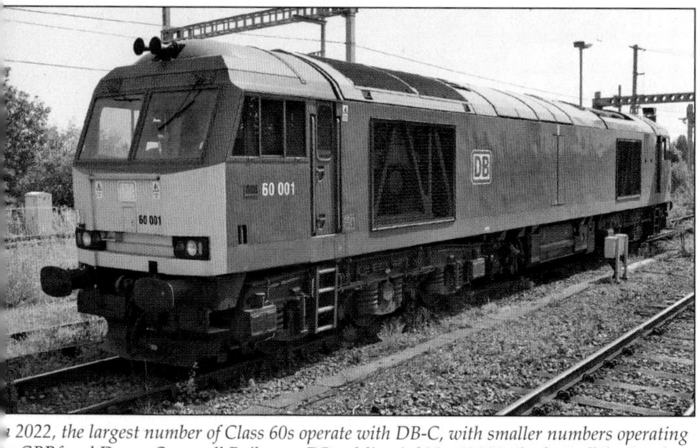

2022, the largest number of Class 60s operate with DB-C, with smaller numbers operating r GBRf and Devon Cornwall Railways. DB red-liveried No. 60001, the first off the Brush roduction line, is seen at Didcot in July 2021. **Spencer Conquest**

60090		A	TO	DCRS	RFE	DCR	(S)
60091‡	*Barry Needham*	A	TO	WQAA	DBS	DBC	(S)
60092‡		A	TO	WCBT	DBS	DBC	DBC
60093		A	TO	WQCA	EWS	DBC	(S)
60094	*Rugby Flyer*	A	TO	WQCA	EWS	DBC	DBC
60095‡		A	TO	GBTG	GBN	BEA	GBR
60096‡		A	TO	GBTG	COL	BEA	GBR
60097		A	TO	WQCA	EWS	DBC	(S)
60098		A	TO	DCRS	GRY	DCR	(S)
60099		A	TO	DRCS	TAT	DCR	(S)
60100‡	*Midland Railway - Butterley*	A	TO	WQAA	DBS	DBC	(S)
60500 (60016)		A	TO	WQCA	EWS	DBC	(S)

* HVO modified

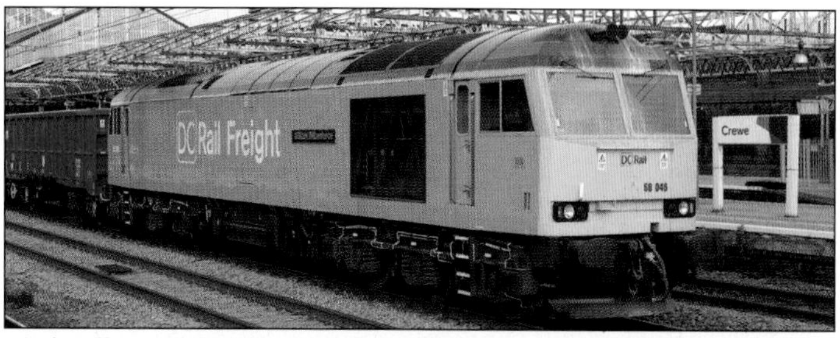

The four Class 60s operated by Devon Cornwall Railway, part of Cappagh Group mainly sport grey DC Rail Freight livery, as illustrated on No. 60046 William Wilberforce at Crewe, the exception being No. 60028 which carries Cappagh blue. **Antony Christie**

Class 66
General Motors/EMD Co-Co Diesel-Electric

Built: 1998-2020
Length: 70ft 0½in (21.35m)
Height: 12ft 10in (3.91m)
Width: 8ft 8¼in (2.65m)
Engine: EMD 12N-710 of 3,200hp (2,385kW)
Transmission: Electric
Tractive effort: 92,000-105,080lb (409-467kN)

66001		A K	TO	WBAE	DBS	DBC	DBC
66002		A	TO	WBAE	EWS	DBC	DBC
66003		A	TO	WBAE	EWS	DBC	DBC
66004		A	TO	WBAR	SPL	DBC	DBC
66005	*Maritime Intermodal One*	A	TO	WBAE	MIM	DBC	DBC
66006		A	TO	WBAR	EWS	DBC	DBC
66007		A	TO	WBAR	EWS	DBC	DBC
66009		A	TO	WBAE	DBC	DBC	DBC
66010		A	TO	WBAI	DBC	DBC	DBC
66011		A	TO	WBAE	EWS	DBC	DBC
66012		A	TO	WBAE	EWS	DBC	DBC
66013		A	TO	WBAE	EWS	DBC	DBC
66014		A	TO	WBAR	EWS	DBC	DBC
66015		A	TO	WBAE	EWS	DBC	DBC
66017		A K	TO	WBAR	DBC	DBC	DBC
66018		A	TO	WBAE	DBC	DBC	DBC
66019		A K	TO	WBAR	DBC	DBC	DBC
66020		A	TO	WBAE	DBC	DBC	DBC
66021		A	TO	WBAR	DBC	DBC	DBC
66022		A	AZ	WBEN	EWS	DBC	DB-F
66023		A	TO	WBAT	EWS	DBC	DBC
66024		A	TO	WBAE	EWS	DBC	DBC
66025		A	TO	WBAR	EWS	DBC	DBC
66026		A	TO	WBEN	EWS	DBC	DB-F
66027		A	TO	WBAE	DBC	DBC	DBC
66028		A	TO	WBAT	EWS	DBC	DBC
66029		A	TO	WGEA	EWS	DBC	DBC
66030		A	TO	WBAR	EWS	DBC	DBC
66031		A	KM	XWSS	DRA	DBC	DRS
66032		A	TO	WBAI	DBC	DBC	DBS
66033		A	AZ	WBEN	EWS	DBC	DB-F
66034		A	TO	WBAE	DBC	DBC	DBC
66035	*Resourceful*	A	TO	WBAE	DBC	DBC	DBC
66036		A	AZ	WBEN	EWS	DBC	DB-F
66037		A	TO	WQAB	EWS	DBC	(S)
66038		A	AZ	WBEN	EWS	DBC	DB-F
66039		A	TO	WBAE	EWS	DBC	DBC
66040		A	TO	WBAR	EWS	DBC	DBC
66041		A	TO	WBAR	DBC	DBC	DBC
66042		A	AZ	WBEN	EWS	DBC	DB-F
66043		A	TO	WQAB	EWS	DBC	DBC
66044		A	TO	WBAE	DBC	DBC	DBC
66045		A	AZ	WBEN	EWS	DBC	DB-F
66047	*Maritime Intermodal Two*	A	TO	WBAE	MIM	DBC	DBC
66049		A	AZ	WBEN	EWS	DBC	DB-F
66050	*EWS Energy*	A	TO	WBAE	EWS	DBC	DBC
66051	*Maritime Intermodal Four*	A	TO	WBAR	MIM	DBC	DBC
66052		A	AZ	WBEN	EWS	DBC	DB-F
66053		A	TO	WBAE	EWS	DBC	DBC
66054		A	TO	WBAR	EWS	DBC	DBC
66055	*Alan Thauvette*	A L	TO	WBLE	DBC	DBC	DBC
66056		A L	TO	WBLE	EWS	DBC	DBC
66057		A L	TO	WBAE	EWS	DBC	DBC
66059		A L	TO	WBLE	EWS	DBC	DBC
66060		A	TO	WBAR	EWS	DBC	DBC
66061		A	TO	WBAE	EWS	DBC	DBC
66062		A	AZ	WBEN	EWS	DBC	DB-F
66063		A	TO	WBAE	EWS	DBC	DBC

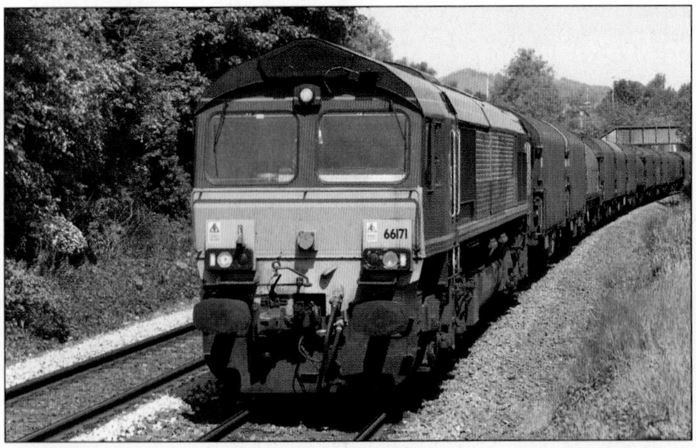

Directly after the take over of the UK main freight operations by EWS as part of privatisation, the company ordered a fleet of 250 Class 66s from General Motors, based on the Class 59, but with upgraded engine and equipment. Showing the original EWS maroon, still carried by a number of locos No. 66171 is shown, illustrating the 'swing-head coupling which was retro fitted. **CJM**

66064		A	AZ	WBEN	EWS	DBC	DB-F
66065		A	TO	WBAR	DBC	DBC	DBC
66066	*Geoff Spencer*	A	TO	WBAR	DBC	DBC	DBC
66067		A	TO	WBAR	EWS	DBC	DBC
66068		A	TO	WBAR	EWS	DBC	DBC
66069		A	TO	WBAR	DBC	DBC	DBC
66070		A	TO	WBAE	DBC	DBC	DBC
66071		A	AZ	WBEN	EWS	DBC	DB-F
66072		A	AZ	WBEN	EWS	DBC	DB-F
66073		A	TO	WBAI	DBC	DBC	DBC
66074		A	TO	WBAE	DBC	DBC	DBC
66075		A	TO	WBAE	EWS	DBC	DBC
66076		A	TO	WBAE	EWS	DBC	DBC
66077§	*Benjamin Gimbert G. C.*	A	TO	WBAR	DBC	DBC	DBC
66078		A	TO	WBAE	DBC	DBC	DBC
66079	*James Nightall GC*	A	TO	WBAR	EWS	DBC	DBC
66080		A	TO	WBAE	EWS	DBC	DBC
66082		A	TO	WBAE	DBC	DBC	DBC
66083		A	TO	WBAR	EWS	DBC	DBC
66084		A	TO	WBAR	DBC	DBC	DBC
66085§		A	TO	WBAR	DBC	DBC	DBC
66086		A	TO	WBAE	DBC	DBC	DBC
66087		A	TO	WBAE	EWS	DBC	DBC
66088		A	TO	WBAE	EWS	DBC	DBC
66089		A	TO	WBAR	EWS	DBC	DBC
66090	*Maritime Intermodal Six*	A	TO	WBAE	MIM	DBC	DBC
66091		A	KM	XHIM	DRA	DBC	DRS
66092		A	TO	WBAE	EWS	DBC	DBC
66093		A	TO	WBAE	EWS	DBC	DBC
66094		A	TO	WBAE	DBC	DBC	DBC
66095		A	TO	WBAE	EWS	DBC	DBC
66096		A	TO	WBAE	EWS	DBC	DBC
66097		A	TO	WBAE	DBS	DBC	DBC
66098		A	TO	WBAE	EWS	DBC	DBC
66099		A R	TO	WBBE	DBC	DBC	DBC
66100	*Armistice 100 1918-2018*	A R	TO	WBBE	DBC	DBC	DBC
66101		A R	TO	WBBE	DBS	DBC	DBC
66102		A R	TO	WBBE	EWS	DBC	DBC
66103		A R	TO	WBBE	EWS	DBC	DBC
66104		A R	TO	WBBT	DBC	DBC	DBC
66105		A R	TO	WBAR	DBC	DBC	DBC
66106		A R	TO	WBBE	EWS	DBC	DBC
66107		A R	TO	WBBT	DBC	DBC	DBC
66108		A R	KM	XHIM	DRA	DBC	DRS
66109	*Teesport Express*	A	TO	WBAR	SPL	DBC	DBC
66110		A R	TO	WBBE	EWS	DBC	DBC
66111		A R	TO	WBAE	EWS	DBC	DBC
66112		A R	TO	WBBE	EWS	DBC	DBC
66113		A R	TO	WBBE	DBC*	DBC	DBC
66114		A R	TO	WBBE	DBS	DBC	DBC
66115		A	TO	WBAE	DBC	DBC	DBC
66116		A	TO	WBAE	EWS	DBC	DBC
66117		A	TO	WBAE	DBC	DBC	DBC
66118		A	TO	WBAE	DBC	DBC	DBC
66119		A	TO	WBAE	EWS	DBC	DBC
66120		A	TO	WBAE	EWS	DBC	DBC
66121		A	TO	WBAE	EWS	DBC	DBC
66122		A	KM	XHIM	DRA	DBC	DRS
66123		A	AZ	WBEN	EWS	DBC	DB-F
66124		A	TO	WBAR	DBC	DBC	DBC
66125		A	TO	WBAE	DBC	DBC	DBC
66126		A	KM	XHIM	DRA	DBC	DRS
66127		A	TO	WBAT	EWS	DBC	DBC
66128		A	TO	WBAE	DBC	DBC	DBC
66129		A	TO	WBAR	EWS	DBC	DBC
66130		A	TO	WBAR	DBC	DBC	DBC
66131		A	TO	WBAE	DBC	DBC	DBC
66133		A	TO	WBAE	EWS	DBC	DBC
66134		A	TO	WBAE	DBC	DBC	DBC
66135		A	TO	WBAE	DBC	DBC	DBC
66136		A	TO	WBAE	DBC	DBC	DBC
66137		A	TO	WBAE	DBC	DBC	DBC
66138		A	TO	WQBA	EWS	DBC	DBC
66139		A	TO	WBAE	EWS	DBC	DBC
66140		A	TO	WBAE	EWS	DBC	DBC
66142	*Maritime Intermodal Three*	A	TO	WBAR	MIM	DBC	DBC
66143		A	TO	WBAE	EWS	DBC	DBC
66144		A	TO	WBAR	EWS	DBC	DBC
66145		A	TO	WQBA	EWS	DBC	DBC
66146		A	PN	WBEP	EWS	DBC	DB-P
66147		A	TO	WBAE	EWS	DBC	DBC
66148	*Maritime Intermodal Seven*	A	TO	WBAE	MIM	DBC	DBC
66149		A	TO	WBAE	DBC	DBC	DBC
66150§		A	TO	WBAE	DBC	DBC	DBC
66151		A	TO	WBAE	EWS	DBC	DBC
66152	*Derek Holmes Railway Operator*	A	TO	WBAE	DBS	DBC	DBC
66153		A	PN	WBEP	EWS	DBC	DB-P
66154		A	TO	WBAE	EWS	DBC	DBC
66155		A	TO	WBAE	EWS	DBC	DBC
66156		A	TO	WBAE	EWS	DBC	DBC
66157		A	PN	WBEP	EWS	DBC	DB-P
66158		A	TO	WBAE	EWS	DBC	DBC
66159		A	PN	WBEP	EWS	DBC	DB-P
66160		A	TO	WBAR	EWS	DBC	DBC
66161		A	TO	WBAE	EWS	DBC	DBC
66162	*Maritime Intermodal Five*	A	TO	WBAR	MIM	DBC	DBC
66163		A	PN	WBEP	DBS	DBC	DB-P
66164		A	TO	WBAE	EWS	DBC	DBC
66165		A	TO	WBAR	DBC	DBC	DBC
66166		A	PN	WBEP	EWS	DBC	DB-P
66167		A	TO	WBAE	DBC	DBC	DBC
66168		A	TO	WBAR	EWS	DBC	DBC
66169		A	TO	WBAR	EWS	DBC	DBC
66170		A	TO	WBAE	EWS	DBC	DBC
66171		A	TO	WBAR	EWS	DBC	DBC
66172	*Paul Mellene*	A	TO	WBAE	EWS	DBC	DBC
66173		A	PN	WBEP	EWS	DBC	DB-P
66174		A	TO	WBAE	EWS	DBC	DBC
66175	*Rail Riders Express*	A	TO	WBAE	DBC	DBC	DBC
66176		A	TO	WBAR	EWS	DBC	DBC
66177		A	TO	WBAE	EWS	DBC	DBC
66178		A	PN	WBEP	EWS	DBC	DB-P
66179		A	TO	WBAI	EWS	DBC	DBC
66180		A	PN	WBEP	EWS	DBC	DB-P
66181		A	TO	WBAR	EWS	DBC	DBC
66182		A	TO	WQBA	DBC	DBC	DBC
66183		A	TO	WBAE	EWS	DBC	DBC
66185	*DP World London Gateway*	A	TO	WBAE	DBS	DBC	DBC
66186		A	TO	WBAR	EWS	DBC	DBC
66187		A	TO	WBAE	EWS	DBC	DBC
66188		A	TO	WBAR	EWS	DBC	DBC
66189		A	PN	WBEP	EWS	DBC	DB-P
66190		A	TO	WBAT	EWS	DBC	DBC
66191		A	AZ	WBEN	EWS	DBC	DB-F
66192		A	TO	WBAR	DBC	DBC	DBC
66193		A	AZ	WBEN	EWS	DBC	DB-F
66194		A	TO	WBAR	EWS	DBC	DBC
66195		A	TO	WBEN	EWS	DBC	DBC
66196		A	PN	WBEP	EWS	DBC	DB-P
66197		A	TO	WBAE	DBC	DBC	DBC
66198		A	TO	WBAR	EWS	DBC	DBC
66199		A	TO	WBAE	EWS	DBC	DBC
66200		A	TO	WBAE	EWS	DBC	DBC
66201		A	AZ	WBEN	EWS	DBC	DB-F
66202		A	AZ	WBEN	EWS	DBC	DB-F
66203		A	AZ	WBEN	EWS	DBC	DB-F
66204		A	AZ	WBEN	EWS	DBC	DB-F
66205		A	TO	WBAI	DBC	DBC	DBC
66206		A	TO	WBAR	DBC	DBC	DBC
66207		A	TO	WBAE	EWS	DBC	DBC
66208		A	AZ	WBEN	EWS	DBC	DB-F
66209		A	AZ	WBEN	EWS	DBC	DB-F
66210		A	AZ	WBEN	EWS	DBC	DB-F
66211		A	AZ	WBEN	EWS	DBC	DB-F

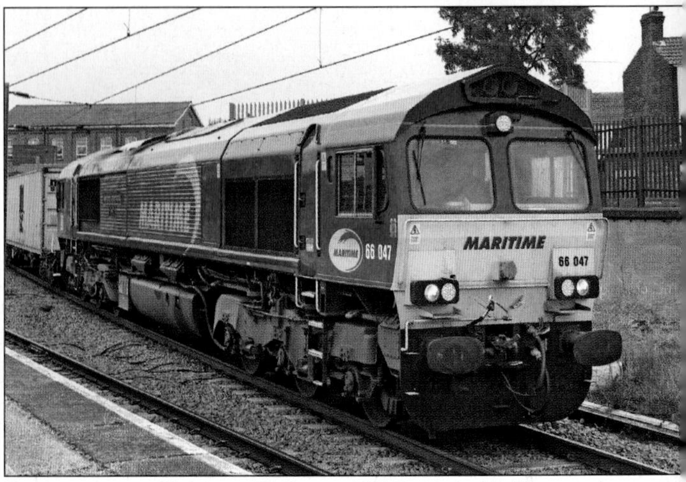

To support a partnership between DB Cargo and freight operator Maritime seven locos were repainted into Maritime blue, shown carried by No. 66047 at Doncaster on 12 October 2021. **CJM**

66212		A	AZ	WBEN	EWS	DBC	DB-F
66213		A	AZ	WBEN	EWS	DBC	DB-F
66214		A	AZ	WBEN	EWS	DBC	DB-F
66215		A	AZ	WBEN	EWS	DBC	DB-F
66216		A	AZ	WBEN	EWS	DBC	DB-F
66217		A	AZ	WBEN	EWS	DBC	DB-F
66218		A	AZ	WGEA	EWS	DBC	DB-F
66219		A	AZ	WGEA	EWS	DBC	DB-F
66220		A	PN	WBEP	DBC	DBC	DB-P
66221		A	TO	WBAR	EWS	DBC	DBC
66222		A	AZ	WBEN	EWS	DBC	DB-F
66223		A	AZ	WBEN	EWS	DBC	DB-F
66224		A	TO	WBAI	EWS	DBC	DBC
66225		A	AZ	WBEN	EWS	DBC	DB-F
66226		A	AZ	WBEN	EWS	DBC	DB-F
66227		A	PN	WBEP	EWS	DBC	DB-P
66228		A	AZ	WBEN	EWS	DBC	DB-F
66229		A	AZ	WBEN	EWS	DBC	DB-F
66230		A	TO	WQBA	DBC	DBC	(S)
66231		A	AZ	WBEN	EWS	DBC	DB-F
66232		A	AZ	WBEN	EWS	DBC	DB-F
66233		A	AZ	WBEN	EWS	DBC	DB-F
66234		A	AZ	WBEN	EWS	DBC	DB-F
66235		A	AZ	WBEN	EWS	DBC	DB-F
66236		A	AZ	WBEN	EWS	DBC	DB-F
66237		A	PN	WBEP	EWS	DBC	DB-P
66239		A	AZ	WBEN	EWS	DBC	DB-F
66240		A	AZ	WBEN	EWS	DBC	DB-F
66241		A	AZ	WBEN	EWS	DBC	DB-F
66242		A	AZ	WBEN	EWS	DBC	DB-F
66243		A	TO	WBEN	EWS	DBC	DBC
66244		A	TO	WBAI	EWS	DBC	DBC
66245		A	AZ	WBEN	EWS	DBC	DB-F
66246		A	AZ	WBEN	EWS	DBC	DB-F
66247		A	AZ	WBEN	EWS	DBC	DB-F
66248		A	PN	WBEP	DBS	DBC	DB-P
66249		A	AZ	WBEP	EWS	DBC	DB-P
66301	*Kingmoor TMD*	A	KM	XHIM	DRC	BEA	DRS
66302	*Endeavour*	A	KM	XHIM	DRA	BEA	DRS
66303	*Rail Riders 2020*	A	KM	XHIM	DRC	BEA	DRS
66304		A	KM	XHIM	DRC	BEA	DRS
66305		A	KM	XHIM	DRA	BEA	DRS
66411 as 66013FPL		A	Freightliner Poland 92 70 0066 411-4				
66412 as 66015FPL		A	Freightliner Poland 92 70 0066 412-2				
66413	*Lest We Forget*	A	LD	DFIN	GWF	AKI	FLR
66414		A	LD	DFIN	FLP	AKI	FLR
66415	*You Are Never Alone*	A	LD	DFIN	GWF	AKI	FLR
66416		A	LD	DFIN	FLP	AKI	FLR
66417 as 66014FPL		A	Freightliner Poland 92 70 0066 417-1				
66418	*Patriot*	A	LD	DFIN	FLP	AKI	FLR
66419		A	LD	DFIN	GWF	AKI	FLR
66420		A	LD	DFIN	FLP	AKI	FLR
66421	*Gresty Bridge TMD*	A	KM	XHIM	DRC	AKI	DRS
66422		A	KM	XHIM	DRC	AKI	DRS
66423		A	KM	XHIM	DRC	AKI	DRS
66424		A	KM	XHIM	DRC	AKI	DRS
66425		A	KM	XHIM	DRA	AKI	DRS
66426		A	KM	XHIM	DRA	AKI	DRS
66427		A	KM	XHIM	DRC	AKI	DRS
66428	*Carlisle Eden Mind*	A	KM	XHIM	DRA	AKI	DRS
66429		A	KM	XHIM	DRC	AKI	DRS
66430		A	KM	XHIM	DRS	AKI	DRS
66431		A	KM	XHIM	DRC	AKI	DRS
66432		A	KM	XHIM	DRC	AKI	DRS
66433		A	KM	XHIM	DRC	AKI	DRS
66434		A	KM	XHIM	DRC	AKI	DRS
66501	*Japan 2001*	A	LD	DFIM	FLR	PTR	FLR
66502	*Basford Hall Centenary 2001*	A	LD	DFIM	FLR	PTR	FLR
66503	*The Railway Magazine*	A	LD	DFIM	GWF	PTR	FLR
66504		A	LD	DFIM	FLP	PTR	FLR
66505		A	LD	DFIM	FLR	PTR	FLR
66506	*Crewe Regeneration*	A	LD	DFIM	FLR	EVL	FLR

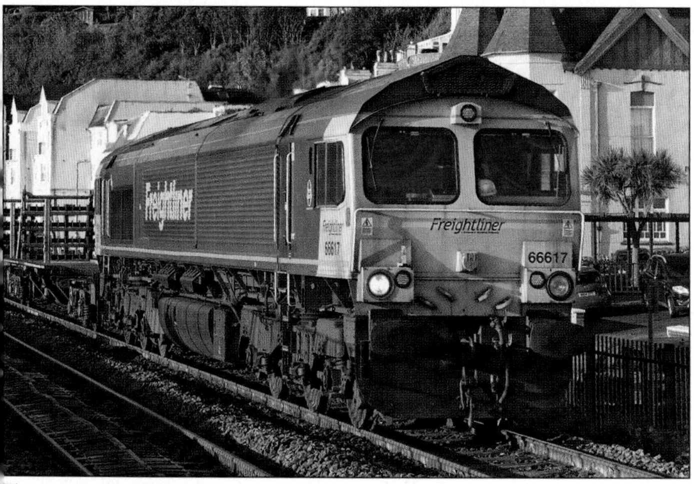

The second major UK freight operator to opt for American Class 66s was Freightliner, now part of the Genesee & Wyoming Group. High-output Class 66/6 No. 66617 is illustrated carrying Freightliner green and yellow livery. **CJM**

66507		A	LD	DFIM	FLR	EVL	FLR
66508		A	LD	DFIM	FLR	EVL	FLR
66509		A	LD	DFIM	FLR	EVL	FLR
66510		A K	LD	DFIM	FLR	EVL	FLR
66511		A	LD	DFIM	FLR	EVL	FLR
66512		A	LD	DFIM	FLR	EVL	FLR
66513		A	LD	DFIM	FLR	EVL	FLR
66514		A	LD	DFIM	FLR	EVL	FLR
66515		A	LD	DFIM	FLR	EVL	FLR
66516		A	LD	DFIM	FLR	EVL	FLR
66517		A	LD	DFIM	FLR	EVL	FLR
66518		A	LD	DFIM	FLR	EVL	FLR
66519		A	LD	DFIM	FLR	EVL	FLR
66520		A	LD	DFIM	FLR	EVL	FLR
66522		A K	LD	DFIM	FLR	EVL	FLR
66523		A	LD	DFIM	FLR	EVL	FLR
66524		A	LD	DFIM	FLR	EVL	FLR
66525		A	LD	DFIM	FLR	EVL	FLR
66526	*Driver Steve Dunn (George)*	A	LD	DFIM	FLR	PTR	FLR
66527 as 66016		A	Freightliner Poland 92 70 0066 527-7				
66528	*Madge Elliot Borders Railway Opening 2015*	A	LD	DFIM	FLP	PTR	FLR
66529		A	LD	DFIM	FLR	PTR	FLR
66530 as 66017		A	Freightliner Poland 92 70 0066 530- 1				
66531		A	LD	DFIM	FLR	PTR	FLR
66532	*P&O Nedlloyd Atlas*	A	LD	DFIM	FLR	PTR	FLR
66533	*Hanjin Express / Senator Express*	A	LD	DHLT	FLR	PTR	FLR
66534	*OOCL Express*	A	LD	DFIM	FLR	PTR	FLR
66535 as 66018		A	Freightliner Poland 92 70 0066 535-0				
66536		A	LD	DFIM	FLR	PTR	FLR
66537		A	LD	DFIM	FLR	PTR	FLR
66538		A	LD	DFIM	FLR	EVL	FLR
66539		A	LD	DFIM	FLR	EVL	FLR
66540	*Ruby*	A	LD	DFIM	FLR	EVL	FLR
66541		A	LD	DFIM	FLR	EVL	FLR
66542		A	LD	DFIM	FLR	EVL	FLR
66543		A	LD	DFIM	FLR	EVL	FLR
66544		A	LD	DFIM	FLR	PTR	FLR
66545		A	LD	DFIM	FLR	PTR	FLR
66546		A	LD	DFIM	FLR	PTR	FLR
66547		A	LD	DFIM	FLR	PTR	FLR
66548		A	LD	DFIM	FLR	PTR	FLR
66549		A	LD	DFIM	FLR	PTR	FLR
66550		A	LD	DFIM	FLR	PTR	FLR
66551		A	LD	DFIM	FLR	PTR	FLR
66552	*Maltby Raider*	A	LD	DFIM	FLR	PTR	FLR
66553		A	LD	DFIM	FLR	PTR	FLR
66554		A	LD	DFIM	FLR	EVL	FLR
66555		A	LD	DFIM	FLR	EVL	FLR
66556		A	LD	DFIM	FLR	EVL	FLR
66557		A	LD	DFIM	FLR	EVL	FLR
66558		A	LD	DFIM	FLR	EVL	FLR
66559		A	LD	DFIM	FLR	EVL	FLR
66560		A	LD	DFIM	FLR	EVL	FLR
66561		A	LD	DFIM	FLR	EVL	FLR
66562		A	LD	DFIM	FLR	EVL	FLR
66563		A	LD	DFIM	FLR	EVL	FLR
66564		A	LD	DFIM	FLR	EVL	FLR
66565		A	LD	DFIM	FLR	EVL	FLR
66566		A	LD	DFIM	FLR	EVL	FLR
66567		A	LD	DFIM	FLR	EVL	FLR
66568		A	LD	DFIM	FLR	EVL	FLR
66569		A	LD	DFIM	FLR	EVL	FLR
66570		A	LD	DFIM	FLR	EVL	FLR
66571		A	LD	DFIM	FLR	EVL	FLR
66572		A	LD	DFIM	FLR	EVL	FLR
66582 as 66009FPL		A	Freightliner Poland 92 51 3650 010-3				
66583 as 66010FPL		A	Freightliner Poland 92 51 3650 011-1				
66584 as 66011FPL		A	Freightliner Poland 92 51 3650 012-9				
66585		A	LD	DFIN	FLR	EVL	FLR
66586 as 66008FPL		A	Freightliner Poland 92 51 3650 009-5				
66587	*As One, We Can*	A	LD	DFIN	ONE	EVL	FLR
66588		A	LD	DFIN	FLR	EVL	FLR
66589		A	LD	DFIM	FLR	EVL	FLR
66590		A	LD	DFIN	FLR	EVL	FLR
66591		A	LD	DFIN	FLR	EVL	FLR
66592	*Johnson Stephens Agencies*	A	LD	DFIN	FLR	EVL	FLR
66593	*3MG Mersey Multimodal Gateway*	A	LD	DFIN	FLR	EVL	FLR
66594	*NYK Spirit of Kyoto*	A	LD	DFIN	FLR	EVL	FLR
66595 as 66595FPL		A	Freightliner Poland 92 70 0066 595-4				
66596		A	LD	DFIN	FLR	BEA	FLR
66597	*Viridor*	A	LD	DFIN	FLR	BEA	FLR
66598		A	LD	DFIN	FLR	BEA	FLR
66599±		A	LD	DFIN	FLR	BEA	FLR
66601	*The Hope Valley*	A	LD	DFHH	FLR	PTR	FLR
66602		A	LD	DFHH	GWF	PTR	FLR
66603		A	LD	DFHH	FLR	PTR	FLR
66604		A	LD	DFHH	FLR	PTR	FLR
66605		A	LD	DFHH	FLR	PTR	FLR
66606		A	LD	DFHH	FLR	PTR	FLR
66607		A	LD	DFHH	FLR	PTR	FLR
66608 as 66603FPL		A	Freightliner Poland 92 70 0066 608-5				
66609 as 66605FPL		A	Freightliner Poland 92 70 0066 609-3				
66610		A	LD	DFHH	FLR	PTR	FLR
66611 as 66604FPL		A	Freightliner Poland 92 70 0066 611-9				
66612 as 66606FPL		A	Freightliner Poland 92 70 0066 612-7				

66613		A	LD	DFHH	FLR	EVL	FLR
66614	*Poppy 2016*	A	LD	DFHH	FLR	EVL	FLR
66615		A	LD	DFHH	FLR	EVL	FLR
66616		A	LD	DFHH	FLR	EVL	FLR
66617		A	LD	DFHH	FLR	EVL	FLR
66618	*Railway Illustrated Annual Photographic Awards*	A	LD	DFHH	FLR	EVL	FLR
66619	*Derek W Johnson MBE*	A	LD	DFHH	FLR	EVL	FLR
66620		A	LD	DFHH	FLR	EVL	FLR
66621		A	LD	DFHH	FLR	EVL	FLR
66622		A	LD	DFHH	FLR	EVL	FLR
66623		A	LD	DFHH	GWF	AKI	FLR
66624 as 66002FPL		A	Freightliner Poland 92 51 3650 014-5				
66625 as 66001FPL		A	Freightliner Poland 92 51 3650 013-7				
66701		A	RR	GBBT	GBR	EVL	GBR
66702	*Blue Lightning*	A	RR	GBBT	GBN	EVL	GBR
66703	*Doncaster PSB 1981-2002*	A	RR	GBBT	GBN	EVL	GBR
66704	*Colchester Power Signal Box*	A	RR	GBBT	GBN	EVL	GBR
66705	*Golden Jubilee*	A	RR	GBBT	GBR	EVL	GBR
66706	*Nene Valley*	A	RR	GBBT	GBN	EVL	GBR
66707	*Sir Sam Fey / Great Central Railway*	A	RR	GBBT	GBN	EVL	GBR
66708	*Слава Україні Glory to Ukraine*	A	RR	GBBT	SPL	EVL	GBR
66709	*Sorrento*	A	RR	GBBT	MSC	EVL	GBR
66710	*Phil Packer BRIT*	A	RR	GBBT	GBN	EVL	GBR
66711	*Sence*	A	RR	GBBT	AGI	EVL	GBR
66712	*Peterborough Power Signalbox*	A	RR	GBBT	GBN	EVL	GBR
66713	*Forest City*	A	RR	GBBT	GBN	EVL	GBR
66714	*Cromer Lifeboat*	A	RR	GBBT	GBN	EVL	GBR
66715	*Valour*	A	RR	GBBT	GBN	EVL	GBR
66716	*Locomotive & Carriage Institution 1911-2011*	A	RR	GBBT	GBN	EVL	GBR
66717	*Good Old Boy*	A	RR	GBBT	GBN	EVL	GBR
66718	*Sir Peter Hendy CBE*	A	RR	GBLT	SPL	EVL	GBR
66719	*Metro-Land*	A	RR	GBLT	GBN	EVL	GBR
66720		A	RR	GBLT	SPL	EVL	GBR
66721	*Harry Beck*	A	RR	GBLT	SPL	EVL	GBR
66722	*Sir Edward Watkin*	A	RR	GBLT	GBN	EVL	GBR
66723	*Chinook*	A	RR	GBLT	GBN	EVL	GBR
66724	*Drax Power Station*	A	RR	GBLT	GBN	EVL	GBR
66725	*Sunderland*	A	RR	GBLT	GBN	EVL	GBR
66726	*Sheffield Wednesday*	A	RR	GBLT	GBN	EVL	GBR
66727	*Maritime One*	A	RR	GBLT	ADV	EVL	GBR
66728	*Institution of Railway Operators*	A	RR	GBLT	GBN	PTR	GBR
66729	*Derby County*	A	RR	GBLT	GBN	PTR	GBR
66730	*Whitemoor*	A	RR	GBLT	GBN	PTR	GBR
66731	*Capt. Tom Moore A True British Inspiration*	A	RR	GBLT	GNH	PTR	GBR
66732	*GBRF The First Decade 1999-2009 John Smith MD*	A	RR	GBLT	GBN	PTR	GBR
66733 (66401)	*Cambridge PSB*	A R	RR	GBFM	BLU	PTR	GBR
66734 (PB04)	*Platinum Jubilee*	A	RR	GBEB	SPL	BEA	GBR
66735 (66403)	*Peterborough United*	A	RR	GBBT	GBN	PTR	GBR
66736 (66404)	*Wolverhampton Wanderers*	A R	RR	GBFM	GBN	PTR	GBR
66737 (66405)	*Lesia*	A R	RR	GBFM	GBN	PTR	GBR
66738 (66578)	*Huddersfield Town*	A R	RR	GBBT	GBN	BEA	GBR
66739 (66579)	*Bluebell Railway*	A R	RR	GBFM	GBN	BEA	GBR
66740 (66580)	*Sarah*	A R	RR	GBFM	GBN	BEA	GBR
66741 (66581)	*Swanage Railway*	A	RR	GBBT	GBN	BEA	GBR
66742 (66406, 66841)	*Port of Immingham Centenary 1912-2012*	A	RR	GBBT	GBN	BEA	GBR
66743 (66407, 66842)		A R	RR	GBFM	ROS	BEA	GBR
66744 (66408, 66843)	*Crossrail*	A	RR	GBBT	GBN	BEA	GBR
66745 (66409, 66844)	*Modern Railways - the first 50 years*	A	RR	GBBT	GBN	BEA	GBR
66746 (66410, 66845)		A R	RR	GBFM	ROS	BEA	GBR
66747	*Made in Sheffield*	A	RR	GBEB	ADV	BEA	GBR
66748	*West Burton 50*	A	RR	GBEB	GBN	BEA	GBR
66749	*Christopher Hopcroft MBE 60 years Railway Service*	A	RR	GBEB	GBN	BEA	GBR
66750	*Bristol Panel Signal Box*	A	RR	GBEB	GBN	BEA	GBR
66751	*Inspiration Delivered Hitachi Rail Group*	A	RR	GBEB	GBN	BEA	GBR
66752	*The Hoosier State*	A	RR	GBEL	GBN	GBR	GBR
66753	*EMD Roberts Road*	A	RR	GBEL	GBN	GBR	GBR
66754	*Northampton Saints*	A	RR	GBEL	GBN	GBR	GBR
66755	*Tony Berkley OBE RFG Chairman 1997-2018*	A	RR	GBEL	GBN	GBR	GBR
66756	*The Royal Corps of Signals*	A	RR	GBEL	GBN	GBR	GBR
66757	*West Somerset Railway*	A	RR	GBEL	GBN	GBR	GBR
66758	*The Pavior*	A	RR	GBEL	GBN	GBR	GBR
66759	*Chippy*	A	RR	GBEL	GBN	GBR	GBR
66760	*David Gordon Harris*	A	RR	GBEL	GBN	GBR	GBR
66761	*Wensleydale Railway Association 25 Years 1990-2015*	A	RR	GBEL	GBN	GBR	GBR
66762		A	RR	GBEL	GBN	GBR	GBR
66763	*Severn Valley Railway*	A	RR	GBEL	GBN	GBR	GBR
66764	*Major John Poyntz Engineer & Railwayman*	A	RR	GBEL	GBN	GBR	GBR
66765		A	RR	GBEL	GBN	GBR	GBR
66766		A	RR	GBEL	GBN	GBR	GBR
66767	*Kings Cross PSB 1971-2021*	A	RR	GBEL	GBN	GBR	GBR
66768		A	RR	GBEL	GBN	GBR	GBR
66769	*LMA League Managers Association / Paul Taylor Our Inspiration*	A	RR	GBEL	SPL	GBR	GBR
66770		A	RR	GBEL	GBN	GBR	GBR
66771	*Amanda*	A	RR	GBEL	GBN	GBR	GBR
66772	*Maria*	A	RR	GBEL	GBN	GBR	GBR
66773	*Pride of GB Railfreight*	A	RR	GBNB	SPL	GBR	GBR
66774		A	RR	GBNB	GBN	GBR	GBR
66775	*HMS Argyll*	A	RR	GBNB	GBN	GBR	GBR
66776	*Joanne*	A	RR	GBNB	GBN	GBR	GBR
66777	*Annette*	A	RR	GBNB	GBN	GBR	GBR
66778	*Cambois Depot 25 Years*	A	RR	GBNB	GBN	GBR	GBR
66779	*Evening Star*	A	RR	GBEL	GRN	GBR	GBR
66780 (66008)	*The Cemex Express*	A	RR	GBOB	ADV	GBR	GBR
66781 (66016)		A	RR	GBOB	GBN	GBR	GBR
66782 (66046)		A	RR	GBOB	SPL	GBR	GBR
66783 (66058)	*The Flying Dustman*	A L	RR	GBOB	SPL	GBR	GBR
66784 (66081)		A	RR	GBOB	GBN	GBR	GBR
66785 (66132)		A	RR	GBOB	GBN	GBR	GBR
66786 (66141)		A	RR	GBOB	GBN	GBR	GBR
66787 (66184)		A	RR	GBOB	GBN	GBR	GBR
66788 (66238)	*Locomotion 15*	A	RR	GBOB	GBN	GBR	GBR
66789 (66250)	*British Rail 1948-1997*	A	RR	GBOB	SPL	GBR	GBR
66790 (T66 403)		A	RR	GBBT	GBN	BEA	GBR
66791 (T66 404)		A	RR	GBBT	BLU	BEA	GBR
66792 (T66 405)	*Collaboration*	A	RR	GBBT	GBN	BEA	GBR
66793 (29004)		A	RR	GBHH	BLU	BEA	GBR
66794 (29005)	*Steve Hannam*	A	RR	GBHH	BLU	BEA	GBR
66795 (561-05/EM05)	*Bescot LDC*	A	RR	GBHH	GBN	BEA	GBR
66796 (561-01/EM01)	*The Green Progressor*	A	RR	GBHH	SPL	BEA	GBR
66797 (513-09/ER09)		A	RR	GBEB	BLU	BEA	GBR
66798 (561-03/EM03)		A	RR	GBEB	GBN	BEA	GBR
66799 (6602/266030)		A	RR	GBEB	GBN	BEA	GBR
66846 (66573)		A	HJ	COLO	COL	BEA	COL
66847 (66574)	*Terry Baker*	A	HJ	COLO	COL	BEA	COL
66848 (66575)		A	HJ	COLO	COL	BEA	COL
66849 (66576)	*Wylam Dilly*	A	HJ	COLO	COL	BEA	COL
66850 (66577)	*David Maidment OBE*	A	HJ	COLO	COL	BEA	COL
66951		A	LD	DFIN	FLR	EVL	FLR
66952		A	LD	DFIN	FLR	EVL	FLR
66953		A	LD	DFIN	FLR	BEA	FLR
66954 as 66954FPL		A	Freightliner Poland 92 70 0066 595-4				
66955		A	LD	DFIN	FLR	BEA	FLR
66956		A	LD	DFIN	FLR	BEA	FLR
66957	*Stephenson Locomotive Society 1909-2009*	A	LD	DFIN	FLR	BEA	FLR

§ Hydro-treated Vegetable Oil (HVO) Modified ± Hydrogen demonstrator
* Carries NHS/Key Workers branding

Beacon Rail/GBRf have reserved the numbers 66351-66360 for additional Class 66s due for import from Europe in 2022-2023.

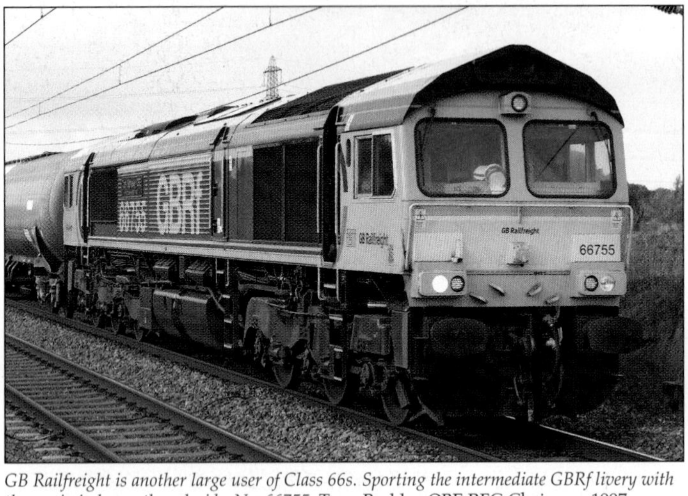

GB Railfreight is another large user of Class 66s. Sporting the intermediate GBRf livery with the semi-circles on the cab side, No. 66755 Tony Berkley OBE RFG Chairman 1997-2018 *is shown from the cooler group end. This is one of the later-built 5-door examples with reduced emissions.* **CJM**

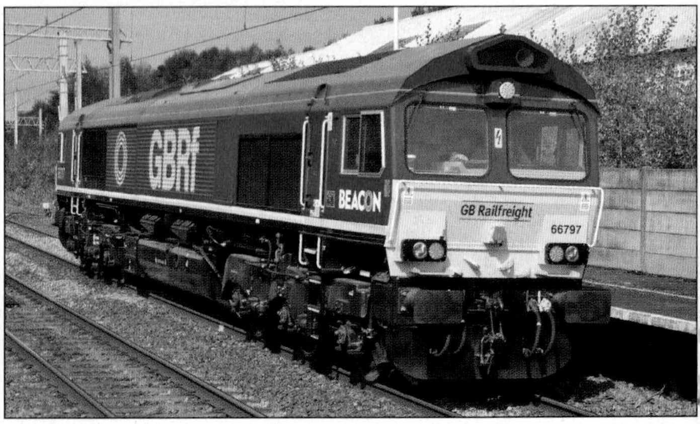

To increase the number of locos on their roster, GBRf have imported several Class 66s which previously operated in Mainland Europe, one of these is 66797. These locos can usually be identified by have brake/main reservoir pipes on either side of the coupling. This example carried its owners, Beacon Rail branding. **Cliff Beeton**

Class 67
Alstom/General Motors Bo-Bo Diesel-Electric

Built: 1999-2000
Length: 64ft 7in (19.68m)
Height: 12ft 9in (3.88m)
Width: 8ft 9in (2.66m)
Engine: EMD 12N-710G3B of 3,200hp (2,386kW)
Transmission: Electric
Tractive effort: 71,260lb (317kN)

67001		A	CE	WAAC	ATW	DBC	DBC
67002		A	CE	WAAC	ATW	DBC	DBC
67003		A	CE	WQBA	ATW	DBC	DBC
67004		A R	CE	WQAB	DBC	DBC	(S)
67005	*Queen's Messenger*	A	CE	WAAC	ROY	DBC	(S)
67006	*Royal Sovereign*	A	CE	WAAC	ROY	DBC	DBC
67007		A R	CE	WABC	EWS	DBC	DBC
67008		A	CE	WAWC	TFW	DBC	TFW
67009		A R	CE	WABC	EWS	DBC	DBC
67010		A	CE	WAWC	TFW	DBC	DBC
67011		A R	CE	WQBA	EWS	DBC	-
67012		A	CE	WAWC	TFW	DBC	DBC
67013		A	CE	WAWC	DBS	DBC	DBC
67014		A	CE	WAWC	TFW	DBC	DBC
67015		A	CE	WAWC	DBS	DBC	DBC
67016		A	CE	WAAC	EWS	DBC	DBC
67017		A	CE	WAWC	TFW	DBC	DBC
67018	*Keith Heller*	A	CE	WQBA	DBS	DBC	DBC
67019		A	CE	WQAA	EWS	DBC	-
67020		A	CE	WAWC	EWS	DBC	DBC
67021		A	CE	WAAC	PUL	DBC	DBC
67022		A	CE	WAWC	EWS	DBC	DBC
67023	*Stella*	A	EC	GBKP	COL	BEA	GBR
67024		A	CE	WAAC	PUL	DBC	DBC
67025		A	CE	WAWC	TFW	DBC	TFW
67026	*Diamond Jubilee*	A	CE	WQBA	ROJ	DBC	-
67027	*Charlotte*	A	EC	GBKP	COL	BEA	GBR
67028§		A	CE	WAAC	DBC	DBC	DBC
67029	*Royal Diamond*	A	CE	WAWC	EWE	DBC	DBC
67030		A R	CE	WQBA	EWS	DBC	(S)

§ Hydro-treated Vegetable Oil (HVO) Modified

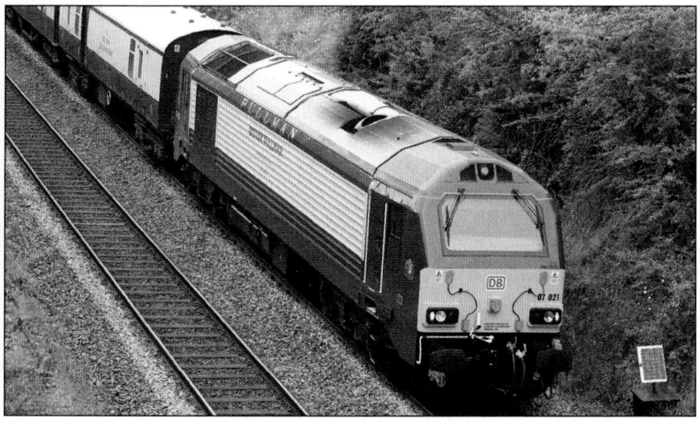

When EWS replaced its main line diesel fleet, a fleet of 30 Class 67s were ordered, with reducing traffic a number of these locos are stored. Two, Nos. 67021 and 67024 are painted in Belmond Pullman colours and are usually rostered to power the luxury land cruise train. No. 67021 is illustrated. **CJM**

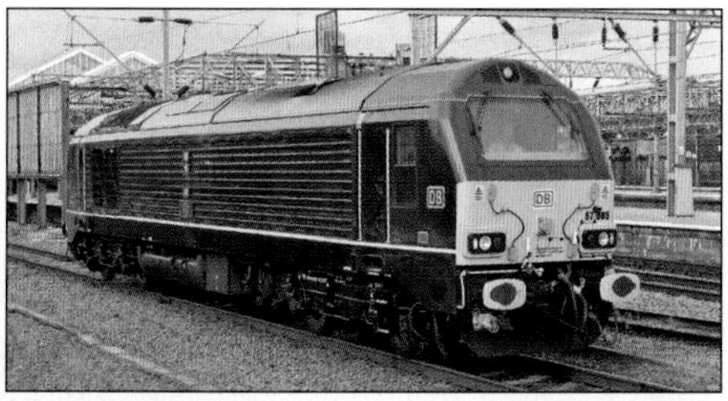

Two of the Class 67 fleet, Nos. 67005 and 67006 are maintained for use with the Royal Trains and carry Royal Claret livery, when not needed for Royal use, they operate in the general pool. No. 67005 is seen at Crewe. **Spencer Conquest**

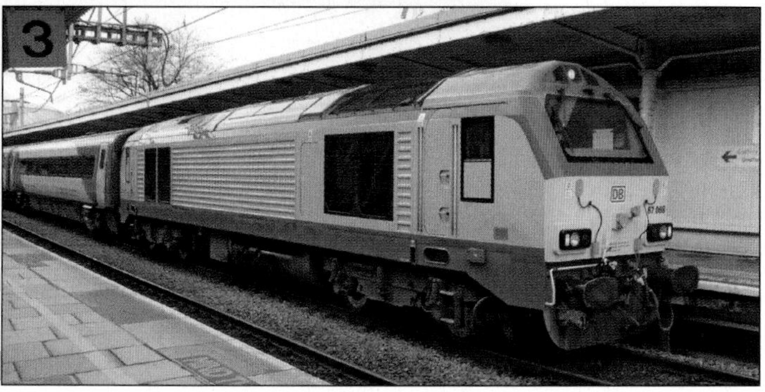

DB are contracted to supply Class 67s to power the Transport for Wales express services on the Cardiff to Holyhead corridor formed of push-pull Mk4 stock. An extra jumper socket is fitted on the end next to the AAR socket. For this work, some '67s'are repainted in TfW grey and red, but are unbranded. No. 67008 at Newport illustrates this livery. **Adrian Paul**

Class 68
Vossloh/Stadler Bo-Bo Diesel-Electric

Built: 2014-2017
Length: 67ft 3in (20.05m)
Height: 12ft 6½in (3.88m)
Width: 8ft 10in (2.69m)
Engine: Caterpillar C175-16 of 3,750hp (2,800kW)
Horsepower: Electric
Tractive effort: 31,750lb (141kN)

68001	*Evolution*	A	CR	XHVE	DRS	BEA	DRS
68002	*Intrepid*	A	CR	XHVE	DRS	BEA	DRS
68003	*Astute*	A	CR	XHVE	DRS	BEA	DRS
68004	*Rapid*	A	CR	XHVE	DRS	BEA	DRS
68005	*Defiant*	A	CR	XHVE	DRS	BEA	DRS
68006§	*Pride of the North*	A	CR	XHVE	NTS	BEA	DRS
68007	*Valiant*	A	CR	XHVE	BLU	BEA	DRS
68008	*Avenger*	A	CR	XHCS	DRS	BEA	DRS
68009	*Titan*	A	CR	XHCS	DRS	BEA	DRS
68010	*Oxford Flyer*	A	CR	XHCE	CRG	BEA	CRW
68011		A	CR	XHCE	CRG	BEA	CRW
68012		A	CR	XHCE	CRG	BEA	CRW
68013	*Peter Wreford Bush*	A	CR	XHCE	CRG	BEA	CRW
68014		A	CR	XHCE	CRG	BEA	CRW
68015	*Kev Helmer*	A	CR	XHCE	CRG	BEA	CRW
68016	*Fearless*	A	CR	XHVE	BLU	BEA	DRS
68017	*Hornet*	A	CR	XHVE	BLU	BEA	DRS
68018	*Vigilant*	A	CR	XHVE	DRS	BEA	DRS
68019	*Brutus*	A	CR	TPEX	FTN	BEA	TPE
68020	*Reliance*	A	CR	TPEX	FTN	BEA	TPE
68021	*Tireless*	A	CR	XHTP	FTN	BEA	TPE
68022	*Resolution*	A	CR	TPEX	FTN	BEA	TPE
68023	*Achilles*	A	CR	XHTP	FTN	BEA	TPE
68024	*Centaur*	A	CR	XHTP	FTN	BEA	TPE
68025	*Superb*	A	CR	XHTP	FTN	BEA	TPE
68026	*Enterprise*	A	CR	TPCF	FTN	BEA	TPE
68027	*Splendid*	A	CR	XHTP	FTN	BEA	TPE
68028	*Lord President*	A	CR	XHTP	FTN	BEA	TPE
68029	*Courageous*	A	CR	XHTP	FTN	BEA	TPE
68030	*Black Douglas*	A	CR	XHTP	FTN	BEA	TPE
68031	*Felix*	A	CR	TPEX	FTN	BEA	TPE
68032	*Destroyer*	A	CR	XHTP	FTN	BEA	TPE
68033	*The Poppy*	A	CR	XHTP	DRB	DRS	DRS
68034		A	CR	XHTP	DRB	DRS	DRS

§ § Hydro-treated Vegetable Oil (HVO) modified

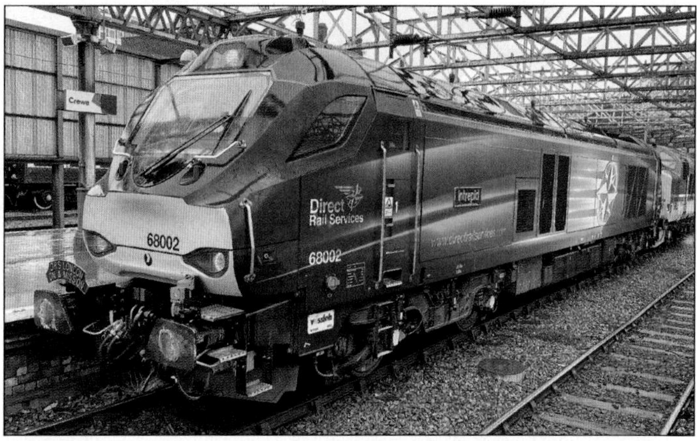

The 34 Class 68s, built by Vossloh/Stadler are leased to Direct Rail Services, a number of the fleet operate on a daily hire to TransPennine Express to work with Mk5 stock. One of the standard DRS locos, usually used for freight operations No. 68002 is seen at Crewe. These locos all have head end power for passenger train operation. **Spencer Conquest**

Class 69
Progress Rail Co-Co Diesel-Electric
Class 56 Rebuild

Built: 2020-2021
Length: 63ft 6in (19.35m)
Height: 12ft 9¼in (3.89m)
Width: 9ft 2in (2.79m)
Engine: EMD 12N-710G3B of 3,200hp (2,287kW)
Transmission: Electric
Tractive effort: 62,900lb (280kN)

69001 (56031)	*Mayflower*	A	TN	GBRG	SPL	PRO	GBR
69002 (56311)	*Bob Tiller CM&EE*	A	TN	GBRG	BLL	PRO	GBR
69003 (56018)		A	TN	GBRG	GBS	PRO	GBR
69004 (56069)		A	TN	GBRG	RTC	PRO	GBR
69005 (56007)	*Eastleigh*	A	TN	GBRG	GRN	PRO	GBR
69006 (56128)		A	TN	GBRG	?	PRO	
69007 (56037)		A	TN	GBRG	?	PRO	
69008 (56038)		A	TN	GBRG	?	PRO	
69009 (56060)		A	TN	GBRG	?	PRO	
69010 (56065)		A	TN	GBRG	?	PRO	
69011 (-)§		*Proposed for conversion*					
69012 (-)§		*Proposed for conversion*					
69013 (-)§		*Proposed for conversion*					
69014 (-)§		*Proposed for conversion*					
69015 (-)§		*Proposed for conversion*					
69016 (-)§		*Proposed for conversion*					

§ Conversion doner awaited

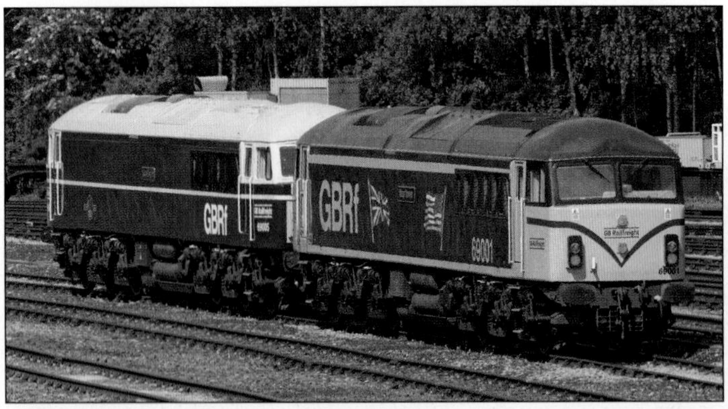

The Progress Rail/GBRf Class 69s are now entering traffic, with five locos delivered by May 2022. No. 67001 Mayflower in a joint UK/USA 'whisker' livery and No. 69005 Eastleigh in BR green colours are seen at Tonbridge on 16 May 2022. **CJM**

Class 70
General Electric Co-Co Diesel-Electric

Built: 2009-2017
Length: 71ft ½in (21.71m)
Height: 12ft 10in (3.91m)
Width: 8ft 8in (2.64m)
Engine: GE/Jenbacher V16 GEJ616 of 3,686hp (2,750kW)
Transmission: Electric
Tractive effort: 122,100lb (544kN)

70001	*PowerHaul*	A	LD	DFGI	FLP	AKI	FLR
70002		A	LD	DFGI	FLP	AKI	FLR
70003		A	LD	DFGI	FLP	AKI	FLR
70004	*The Coal Industry Society*	A	LD	DFGI	FLP	AKI	FLR
70005		A	LD	DFGI	FLP	AKI	FLR
70006		A	LD	DFGI	FLP	AKI	FLR
70007		A	LD	DFGI	FLP	AKI	FLR
70008		A	LD	DFGI	FLP	AKI	FLR
70009		A	LD	DHLT	FLP	AKI	FLR
70010		A	LD	DFGI	FLP	AKI	FLR
70011		A	LD	DFGI	FLP	AKI	FLR
70013		A	LD	DHLT	FLP	AKI	(S)
70014		A	LD	DFGI	FLP	AKI	FLR
70015		A	LD	DFGI	FLP	AKI	FLR
70016		A	LD	DFGI	FLP	AKI	FLR
70017§		A	LD	DFGI	FLP	AKI	FLR
70018		A	LD	DHLT	FLP	AKI	(S)
70019		A	LD	DHLT	FLP	AKI	(S)
70020		A	LD	DFGI	FLP	AKI	FLR
70801 (70099)		A	CF	COLO	COL	LOM	COL
70802		A	CF	COLO	COL	LOM	COL
70803		A	CF	COLO	COL	LOM	COL
70804		A	CF	COLO	COL	LOM	COL
70805		A	CF	COLO	COL	LOM	COL
70806		A	CF	COLO	COL	LOM	COL
70807		A	CF	COLO	COL	LOM	COL
70808		A	CF	COLO	COL	LOM	COL
70809		A	CF	COLO	COL	LOM	COL
70810		A	CF	COLO	COL	LOM	COL
70811		A	CF	COLO	COL	BEA	COL
70812		A	CF	COLO	COL	BEA	COL
70813		A	CF	COLO	COL	BEA	COL
70814		A	CF	COLO	COL	BEA	COL
70815		A	CF	COLO	COL	BEA	COL
70816		A	CF	COLO	COL	BEA	COL
70817		A	CF	COLO	COL	BEA	COL

§ Hydro-treated Vegetable Oil (HVO) Modified

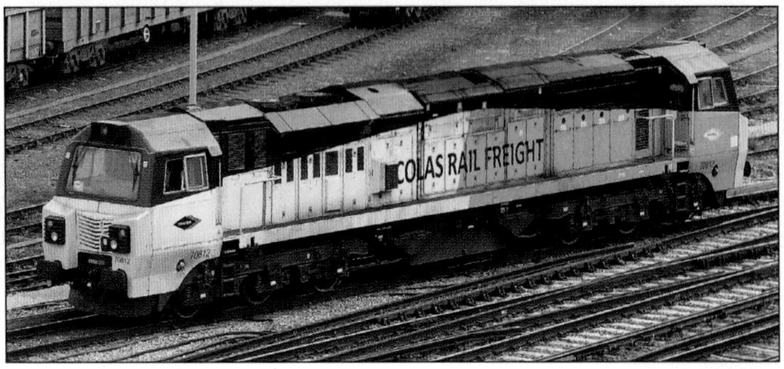

The 16 General Electric Class 70s are operated by Freightliner (70/0) and Colas Rail Freight (70/8). Colas No. 70812 is illustrated at Eastleigh, showing the cooler group end on the left. **CJM**

Class 71
BR Bo-Bo Booster-Electric

Built: 1959
Length: 50ft 7in (15.42m)
Height: 13ft 1in (3.99m)
Width: 8ft 11in (2.72m)
Power system: 750V dc third rail & overhead
Transmission: Electric
Tractive effort: 43,000lb (191.2kN)

71001 (E5001) National Railway Museum, Shildon

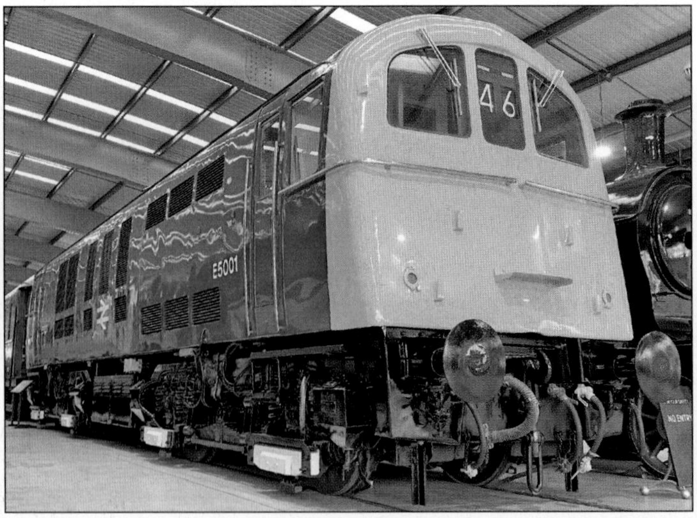

Recently restored to late 1960s BR rail blue, No. E5001 is currently on display at the NRM Locomotion exhibition in Shildon. **Spencer Conquest**

Class 73
BR/English Electric Bo-Bo Electro-Diesel

Built: 1965-1967
Length: 52ft 6in (16.00m)
Height: 12ft 5⅜in (3.79m)
Width: 8ft 8in (2.64m)
Engine: 73/1, 73/2 EE4SRKT of 600hp (447kW)
73/95 2x Cummins QSK19 of 750hp (559kW)
73/96 MTU 8V 4000R43L of 1,600hp (1,193kW)
Transmission: Electric
Tractive effort: max 40,000lb (179kN)

73001 (E6001)		Loco Services Ltd, Crewe					
73002 (E6002)		Loco Services Ltd, Eastleigh					
73003 (E6003)		Restoration at Eastleigh					
73101(S)		X	ZG	GBZZ	PUL	GBR	(S)
73107	*Tracy*	X	SE	GBED	GBN	GBR	GBR
73109	*Battle of Britain 80th Anniversary*	X	SE	GBED	GBN	GBR	GBR
73110		X	ZG	GBSD	BLU	GBR	(S)
73114 (E6020)		Battlefield Railway, Shackerstone					
73118 (E6024)		Barry Island Railway					
73119	*Borough of Eastleigh*	X	SE	GBED	GBN	GBR	GBR
73128	*O.V.S. Bulleid C.B.E.*	X	SE	GBED	GBN	GBR	GBR
73129 (E6036)		Cambrian Railway, Oswestry					
73130 (E6037)		MoD Bicester					
73133		X	ZG	MBED	GRN	TTS	TTS
73134		X	WS	GBZZ	ICS	GBR	(S)
73136	*Mhairi*	X	SE	GBED	GBB	GBR	GBR
73138		Peak Rail					
73139		X	ZA	GBZZ	NSE	GBR	(S)
73140 (E6047)		Spa Valley Railway					
73141	*Charlotte*	X	SE	GBED	GBB	GBR	GBR
73201 (73142)	*Broadlands*	X	SE	GBED	BLU	GBR	GBR
73202 (73137)	*Graham Stenning*	X	SL	MBED	SOU	PTR	GTR
73210 (E6022)		Ecclesbourne Valley Railway					
73212 (73102)	*Fiona*	X	SE	GBED	GBB	GBR	GBR
73213 (73112)	*Rhodalyn*	X	SE	GBED	GBB	GBR	GBR
73235 (73125)		X	BM	HYWD	SPL	PTR	SWR
73951 (73104)	*Malcolm Brinded*	A	ZA	QADD	NRL	NRL	NRL
73952 (73211)	*Janis Kong*	A	ZA	QADD	NRL	NRL	NRL
73961 (73209)	Alison	A	SE	GBNR	GBN	GBR	GBR
73962 (73204)	*Dick Mabbutt*	A	SE	GBNR	GBB	GBR	GBR
73963 (73206)	*Janice*	A	SE	GBNR	GBB	GBR	GBR
73964 (73205)	*Jeanette*	A	SE	GBNR	GBB	GBR	GBR
73965 (73208)	*Des O'Brian*	A	SE	GBNR	GBB	GBR	GBR
73966 (73005)		A	EC	GBCS	SCS	GBR	SCS
73967 (73006)		A	EC	GBCS	SCS	GBR	SCS
73968 (73117)		A	EC	GBCS	SCS	GBR	SCS
73969 (73105)		A	EC	GBCS	SCS	GBR	SCS
73970 (73103)		A	EC	GBCS	SCS	GBR	SCS
73971 (73207)		A	EC	GBCS	SCS	GBR	SCS

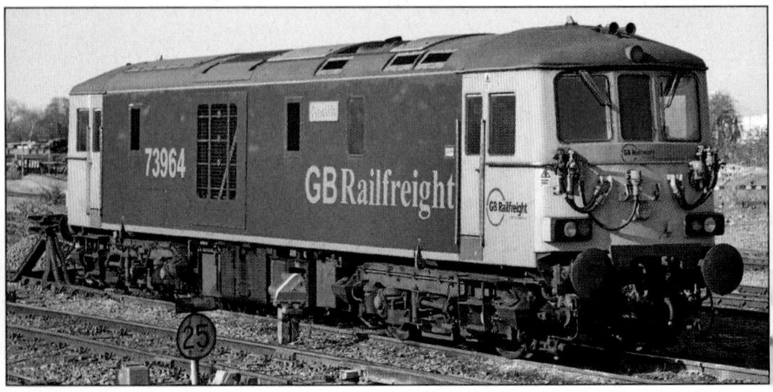

The original Southern Region dual-power Class 73s are still front line traction for GBRf, many examples are also preserved. Refurbished and re-engineered No. 73964, used for freight and departmental operations is seen. Note the triangulation marker light arrangement and the additional AAR style front end jumper socket. **Mark V. Pike**

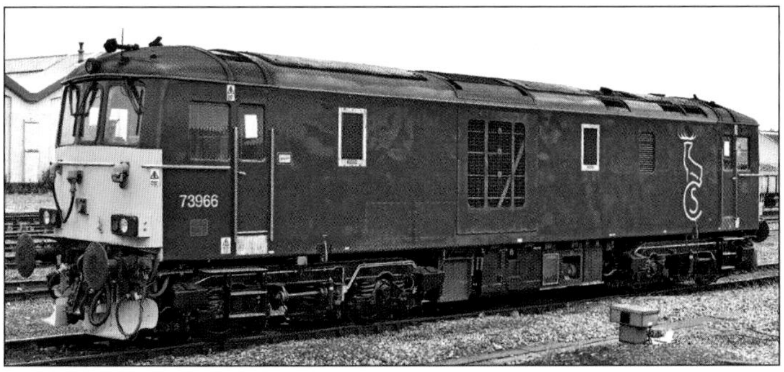

The six Class 73/0s refurbished for GBRf and deployed on Caledonian Sleeper operations were refurbished slightly different, losing their high level air pipes and Pullman rubbing plant and fitted with a drop-head Dellner coupling. No. 73966 is shown stabled at Eastleigh. **Mark V. Pike**

Class 76
LNER/BR Bo-Bo Electric

Built: 1941-1953	*Power system: 1,500V dc overhead*
Length: 50ft 4in (15.34m)	*Transmission: Electric*
Height: 13ft 0in (3.96m)	*Tractive effort: 45,000lb (200.1kN)*
Width: 9ft 0in (2.74m)	

76020 (E26020)	National Railway Museum, York

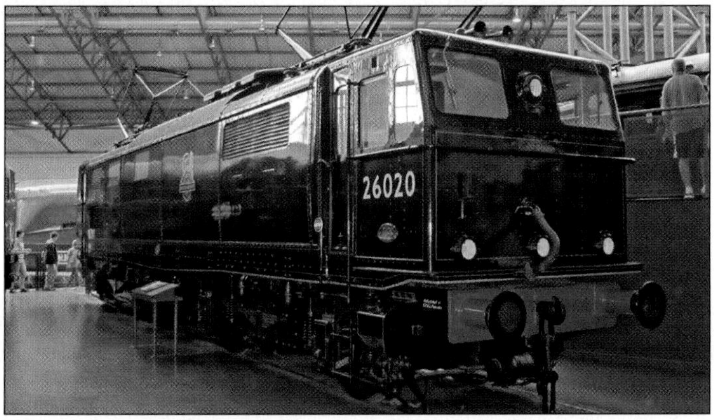

After withdrawal, Woodhead electric Class 76 No. 76020 was claimed for the National Collection. It was cosmetically refurbished at BREL Doncaster Works and sports 1950s BR black livery. It is currently on display at York museum. **Derek Holmes**

Class 77
BR Co-Co Electric

Built: 1953-1954	*Power system: 1,500V dc overhead*
Length: 59ft 0in (17.98m)	*Transmission: Electric*
Height: 13ft 0in (3.96m)	*Tractive effort: 45,000lb (200.1kN)*
Width: 8ft 10in (2.69m)	

E27000	*Electra*	Midland Railway Centre
E27001	*Ariadne*	Museum of Science & Ind, Manchester
E27003	*Diana*	Dutch National Railway Museum, Utracht

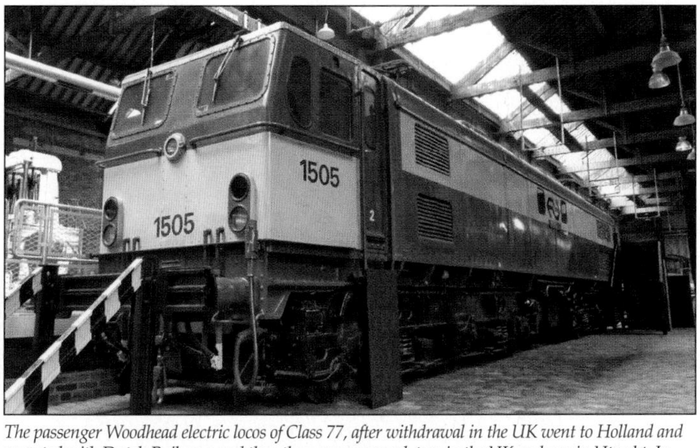

The passenger Woodhead electric locos of Class 77, after withdrawal in the UK went to Holland and operated with Dutch Railways and thus three are preserved, two in the UK and one in Utrecht. In Dutch Railways livery No 1505 (E27001) is seen at MSI, Manchester. **Phil Barnes**

Class 81
BRCW Bo-Bo Electric

Built: 1959-1964	*Power system: 25,000V ac overhead*
Length: 56ft 6in (17.98m)	*Transmission: Electric*
Height: 13ft 0½in (3.97m)	*Tractive effort: 50,000lb (222.4kN)*
Width: 8ft 8½in (2.65m)	

81002 (E3003)	AC Loco Group Barrow Hill Roundhouse

Just one Class 81 is preserved, No. 81002, the original E3003. This is in the care of the AC Locomotive Group and usually kept at Barrow Hill Roundhouse, where this view was taken showing it under restoration. **P Booth**

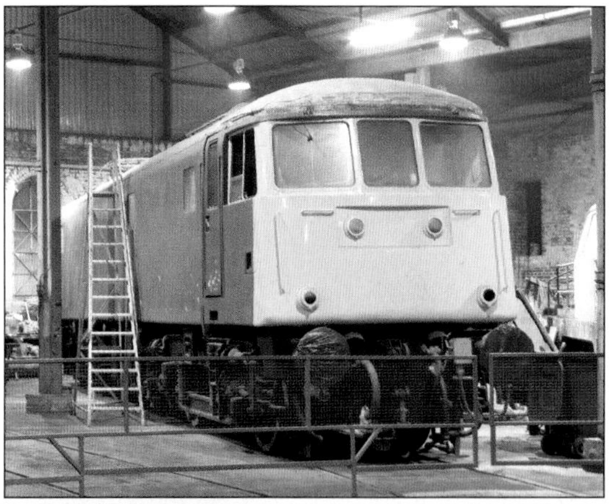

Class 82
Beyer Peacock Bo-Bo Electric

Built: 1960-1961	*Power system: 25,000V ac overhead*
Length: 56ft 0in (17.07m)	*Transmission: Electric*
Height: 13ft 0½in (3.97m)	*Tractive effort: 50,000lb (222.4kN)*
Width: 8ft 9in (2.67m)	

82008 (E3054)	AC Loco Group Barrow Hill Roundhouse

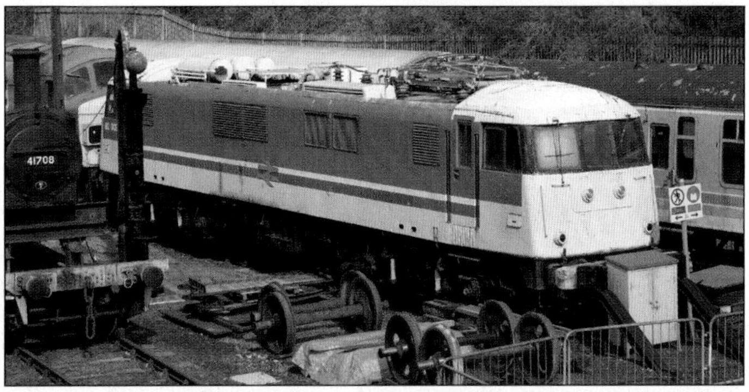

After withdrawal Beyer Peacock Class 82 No. 82008, the original No. E3054 was saved for preservation and is currently based with the AC Loco Group at Barrow Hill. The loco is seen, in need of some cosmetic attention in April 2022. **Antony Christie**

Class 83
EE Bo-Bo Electric

Built: 1960-1962	*Power system: 25,000V ac overhead*
Length: 52ft 6in (16m)	*Transmission: Electric*
Height: 13ft 0½in (3.97m)	*Tractive effort: 38,000lb (169kN)*
Width: 8ft 8½in (2.65m)	

83012 (E3054)	AC Loco Group Barrow Hill Roundhouse

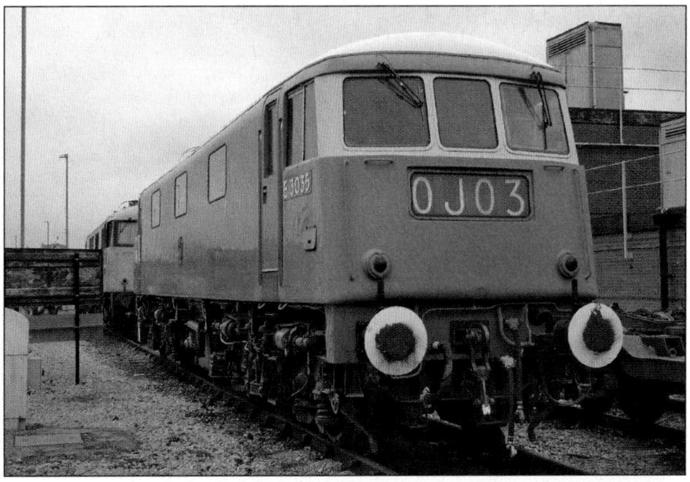

The sole preserved Class 83 No. 83012 (E3054) is restored to early electric blue livery, with a white cab roof and window surrounds. It is usually based at Barrow Hill. **Nathan Williamson**

Class 84
NBL Bo-Bo Electric

Built: 1960-1961	*Power system: 25,000V ac overhead*
Length: 53ft 6in (16.31m)	*Transmission: Electric*
Height: 13ft 0½in (3.97m)	*Tractive effort: 50,000lb (222.4kN)*
Width: 8ft 8¼in (2.65m)	

84001 (E3036)	NRM, at Barrow Hill Roundhouse

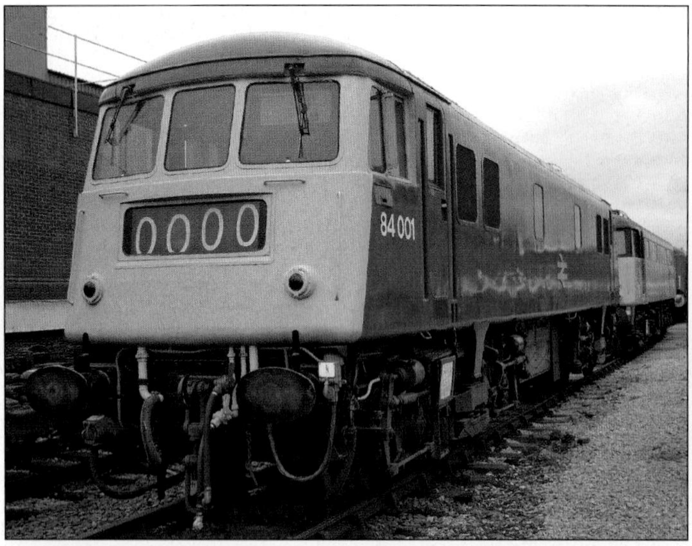

One example of the North British Loco Co AC electric class AL4 (84) is preserved by the National Railway Museum and is currently on loan to the AC Loco Group Barrow Hill Roundhouse. **Nathan Williamson**

Class 85
BR Bo-Bo Electric

Built: 1961-1964
Length: 56ft 6in (17.22m)
Height: 13ft 0½in (3.97m)
Width: 8ft 8¼in (2.65m)
Power system: 25,000V ac overhead
Transmission: Electric
Tractive effort: 50,000lb (222.4kN)

85101 (85006 / E3061)	AC Loco Group Barrow Hill Roundhouse

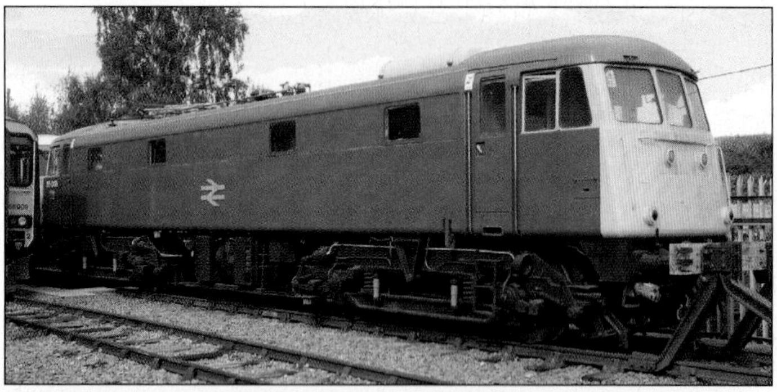

One member of the AL5, Class 85 design is preserved, No. 85006, which again is looked after by the AC Loco Group and kept at Barrow Hill Roundhouse. It currently sports BR rail blue with yellow ends, and is seen on shed in 2021. **Adrian Paul**

Class 86
BR/English Electric Bo-Bo Electric

Built: 1961-1964
Length: 56ft 6in (17.22m)
Height: 13ft 0½in (3.97m)
Width: 8ft 8¼in (2.65m)
Power system: 25,000V ac overhead
Transmission: Electric
Tractive effort: 50,000lb (222.4kN)

86101	Sir William A Stanier FRS	X	CL	LSLO	ICS	LSL	LSL
86213		A	Bulmarket, Bulgaria - 91 52 00 87703-2 (85002)				
86215		A	Eurogate Rail, Hungary - 91 55 0450-005-8				
86217		A	Eurogate Rail, Hungary - 91 55 0450-006-6				
86218		A	Eurogate Rail, Hungary - 91 55 0450-004-1				
86228		A	Eurogate Rail, Hungary - 91 55 0450-007-4				
86231		A	Bulmarket, Bulgaria - 91 52 00 85005-4				
86232		A	Eurogate Rail, Hungary - 91 55 0450-003-3				
86233		A	Bulmarket, Bulgaria - stored				
86234		A	Bulmarket, Bulgaria - 91 52 00 85006-2				
86235		A	Bulmarket, Bulgaria - 91 52 00 87704-0				
86242		A	Eurogate Rail, Hungary - 91 55 0450-008-2				
86248		A	Eurogate Rail, Hungary -91 55 0450-001-7				
86250		A	Eurogate Rail, Hungary -91 55 0450-002-5				
86259	*Les Ross/Peter Pan*	X	RU	MBEL	BLU	PPL	PPL
86401	*Mons Meg*	X	CS	AWCA	SCS	WCR	WCR
86424		A	Eurogate Rail, Hungary - 91 55 0450-009-0				
86604 (86404)		A	CB	DHLT	FLR	FLR	(S)
86605 (86405)		A	CB	DHLT	FLR	FLR	(S)
86607 (86407)		A	CB	DHLT	FLR	FLR	(S)
86608 (86501)		A	CB	DHLT	FLR	FLR	(S)
86609 (86409)		A	CB	DHLT	FLR	FLR	(S)
86610 (86410)		A	CB	DHLT	FLR	FLR	(S)
86612 (86412)		A	CB	DHLT	FLR	FLR	(S)
86613 (86413)		A	CB	DHLT	FLR	FLR	(S)
86614 (86414)		A	CB	DHLT	FLR	FLR	(S)
86622 (86422)		Crewe Heritage Centre					
86627 (86427)		A	CB	DHLT	FLR	FLR	(S)
86628 (86428)		A	CB	DHLT	FLR	FLR	(S)
86632 (86432)		A	CB	DHLT	FLR	FLR	(S)
86637 (86437)		A	CB	DHLT	FLP	FLR	(S)
86638 (86438)		A	CB	DHLT	FLR	FLR	(S)
86639 (86439)		A	CB	DHLT	FLR	FLR	(S)
86701 (86205)		A	Bulmarket, Bulgaria - 91 52 00 85001-3				
86702 (86260)		A	Bulmarket, Bulgaria - 91 52 00 85002-1				

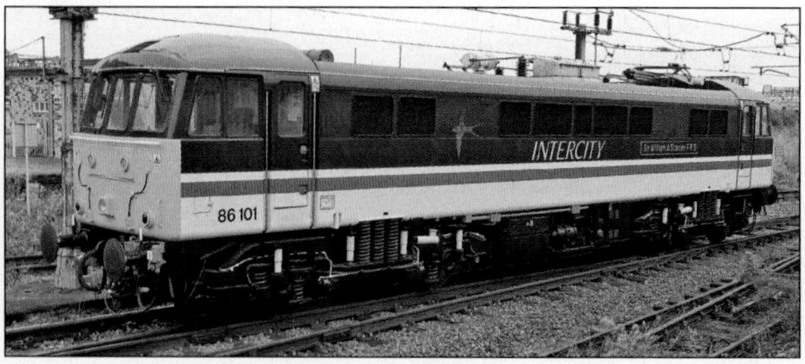

With the Freightliner Class 86s now long term stored, only three Class 86s are main line certified with three private operators and used to power charter and railtour trains. Loco Services Ltd at Crewe operate Class 86/1 No. 86101 which is seen in immaculate full InterCity Swallow livery at Crewe. **Spencer Conquest**

Class 87
BREL Bo-Bo Electric

Built: 1973-1974
Length: 58ft 6in (17.83m)
Height: 13ft 1¼in (3.97m)
Width: 8ft 8¼in (2.65m)
Power system: 25,000V ac overhead
Transmission: Electric
Tractive effort: 58,000lb (258kN)

87001	*Royal Scot*	National Railway Museum					
87002	*Royal Sovereign*	A	CL	LSLO	ICS	LSL	LSL
87003		A	BZK Bulgaria - 91 52 00 87003-0				
87004		A	BZK Bulgaria - 91 52 00 87004-8				
87006		A	BZK Bulgaria - 91 52 00 87006-3				
87007		A	BZK Bulgaria - 91 52 00 87007-1				
87008		A	BZK Bulgaria - 91 52 00 87008-9				
87009		A	Bulmarket Bulgaria - 91 52 00 87009-4				
87010		A	BZK Bulgaria - 91 52 00 87010-5				
87012		A	BZK Bulgaria - 91 52 00 87012-1				
87013		A	BZK Bulgaria - 91 52 00 87013-9				
87014		A	BZK Bulgaria - 91 52 00 87014-7				
87017		A	Bulmarket Bulgaria - 91 52 00 87017-7				
87019		A	BZK Bulgaria - 91 52 00 87019-6				
87020		A	BZK Bulgaria - 91 52 00 87020-4				
87022		A	BZK Bulgaria - 91 52 00 87022-0				
87023		A	Bulmarket Bulgaria - 91 52 00 87023-5				
87025		A	Bulmarket Bulgaria - 91 52 00 87025-0				
87026		A	BZK Bulgaria - 91 52 00 87026-1				
87028		A	BZK Bulgaria - 91 52 00 87028-8				
87029		A	BZK Bulgaria - 91 52 00 87029-2				
87033		A	BZK Bulgaria - 91 52 00 87033-7				
87034		A	BZK Bulgaria - 91 52 00 87034-5				
87035	*Robert Burnes*	A	Crewe Heritage Centre				

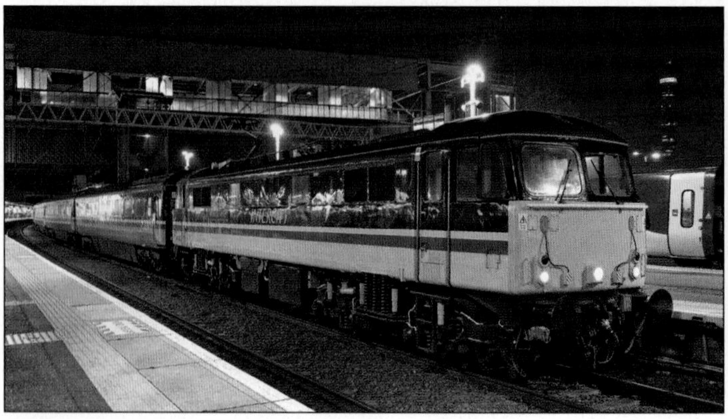

One Class 87, No. 87002 is certified for main line operation, working with LSL. It is used to power the InterCity charter set, complete with a Mk3 DVT at the remote end. The loco is seen at Euston in January 2022. **Antony Christie**

Class 88
Stadler Bo-Bo Bi-Mode

Built: 2017
Length: 67ft 3in (20.5m)
Height: 12ft 6½in (3.82m)
Width: 8ft 10in (2.69m)
Power system: 25,000V ac overhead or Caterpillar C27 engine of 950hp (708kW)
Transmission: Electric
Tractive effort: 71,260lb (317kN)

88001	*Revolution*	A	KM	XHVE	DRA	BEA	DRS
88002	*Prometheus*	A	KM	XHVE	DRA	BEA	DRS
88003	*Genesis*	A	KM	XHVE	DRA	BEA	DRS
88004	*Pandora*	A	KM	XHVE	DRA	BEA	DRS
88005	*Minerva*	A	KM	XHVE	DRA	BEA	DRS
88006	*Juno*	A	KM	XHVE	DRA	BEA	DRS

88007	*Electra*	A	KM	XHVE	DRA	BEA	DRS
88008	*Ariadne*	A	KM	XHVE	DRA	BEA	DRS
88009	*Diana*	A	KM	XHVE	DRA	BEA	DRS
88010	*Aurora*	A	KM	XHVE	DRA	BEA	DRS

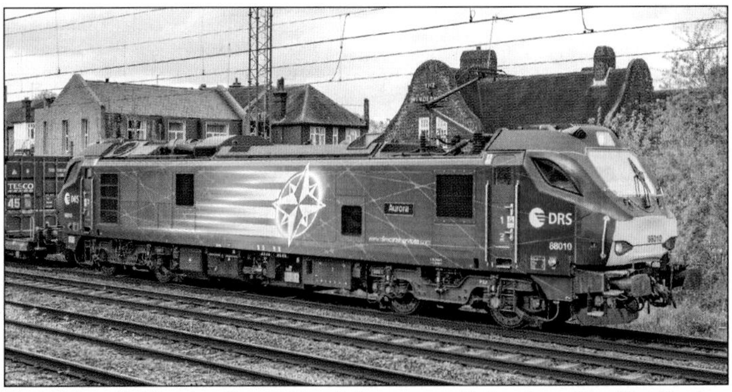

The 10 Direct Rail Services Class 88 bi-mode locos are usually found operating West Coast freight operations, and occasionally flask traffic in the Carlisle-Sellafield area. No. 88010 Aurora is illustrated, displaying the latest DRS livery/branding. **Antony Christie**

Class 89
Brush Co-Co Electric

Built: 1987
Length: 64ft 11in (19.79m)
Height: 13ft 0½in (3.97m)
Width: 8ft 11½in (2.73m)
Power system: 25,000V ac overhead
Transmission: Electric
Tractive effort: 46,100lb (205kN)

89001	*Avocet*	A	CL	LSLO	ICS	ACL	LSL

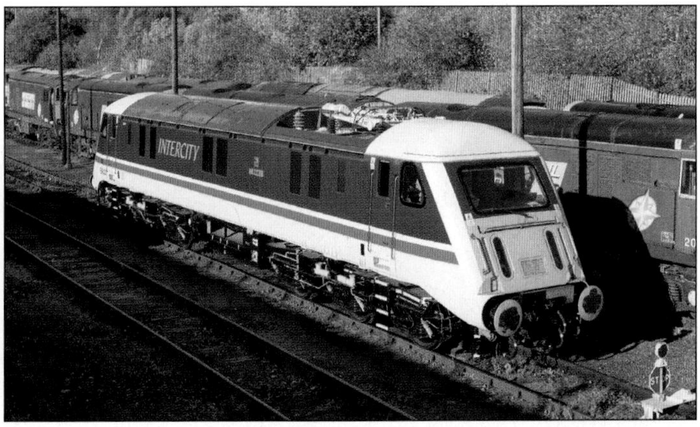

With the Cass 89 now under the control of Loco Services Ltd at Crewe and the announcement that it will return to the main line for charter train use, we look forward to soon seeing with futuristic looking loco back in service. It is shown at Barrow Hill. **Steve Donald**

Class 90
BREL Bo-Bo Electric

Built: 1987-1990
Length: 61ft 6in (18.74m)
Height: 13ft 0¼in (3.97m)
Width: 9ft 0in (2.74m)
Power system: 25,000V ac overhead
Transmission: Electric
Tractive effort: 58,000lb (258kN)

90001	*Royal Scot*	A	CL	LSLO	ICS	LSL	LSL
90002	*Wolf of Badenoch*	A	CL	LSLO	ICS	LSL	LSL
90003		A	CB	DFLC	GWF	FLR	FLR
90004		A	CB	DFLC	GWF	FLR	FLR
90005		A	CB	DFLC	GWF	FLR	FLR
90006	*Roger Ford / Modern Railways Magazine*	A	CB	DFLC	GWF	FLR	FLR
90007		A	CB	DFLC	GWF	FLR	FLR
90008		A	CB	DFLC	GWF	FLR	FLR
90009		A	CB	DFLC	GWF	FLR	FLR
90010		A	CB	DFLC	GWF	FLR	FLR
90011		A	CB	DFLC	GWF	FLR	FLR
90012		A	CB	DFLC	GWF	FLR	FLR
90013		A	CB	DFLC	GWF	FLR	FLR
90014	*Over the Rainbow*	A	CB	DFLC	GWF	FLR	FLR
90015		A	CB	DFLC	GWF	FLR	FLR
90016		A	CB	DFLC	FLR	FLR	FLR
90017		A	CE	WQCA	EWS	DBC	(S)
90018	*The Pride of Bellshill*	A	CE	WQAB	DBS	DBC	(S)
90019	*Multimodal*	A	CE	WEDC	DBC	DBC	(S)
90020		A	CE	WEDC	BLK	DBC	(S)
90021 (90221)	*Donald Malcolm*	A	CE	WEAC	SPL	DBC	DBC
90022 (90222)	*Freightconnection*	A	CE	WQCA	RFE	DBC	(S)
90023 (90223)		A	CE	WQCA	EWS	DBC	(S)
90024 (90224)		A	CE	WEAC	SPL	DBC	(S)
90025 (90225)		A	CE	WQCA	RFD	DBC	(S)
90026		A	CE	WEDC	BLK	DBC	(S)
90027 (90227)	*Allerton T&RS Depot*	A	CE	WQCA	RFD	DBC	(S)
90028	*Sir William McAlpine*	A	CE	WEDC	DBC	DBC	DBC
90029		A	CE	WEDC	BLK	DBC	(S)
90030 (90130)		A	CE	WQCA	EWS	DBC	(S)
90031 (90131)	*The Railway Children Partnership Working For Street Children Worldwide*	A	CE	WQCA	EWS	DBC	(S)
90032 (90132)		A	CE	WQCA	EWS	DBC	(S)
90033 (90233)		A	CE	WQCA	RFE	DBC	(S)
90034 (90134)		A	CE	WEDC	DRB	DBC	(S)
90035 (90135)		A	CE	WEAC	DBC	DBC	(S)
90036 (90136)	*Driver Jack Mills*	A	CE	WEDC	DBS	DBC	(S)
90037 (90137)	*Christine*	A	CE	WEAC	SPL	DBC	DBC
90038 (90238)		A	CE	WQCA	RFE	DBC	(S)
90039 (90239)	*The Chartered Institute of Logistics & Transport*	A	CE	WEDC	SPL	DBC	DBC
90040 (90140)		A	CE	WQAB	DBS	DBC	(S)
90041		A	CB	DFLC	FLR	FLR	FLR
90042		A	CB	DFLC	FLP	FLR	FLR
90043		A	CB	DFLC	FLP	FLR	FLR
90044		A	CB	DFLC	GWF	FLR	FLR
90045		A	CB	DFLC	FLP	FLR	FLR
90046		A	CB	DFLC	FLR	FLR	FLR
90047		A	CB	DFLC	GWF	FLR	FLR
90048		A	CB	DFLC	GWF	FLR	FLR
90049		A	CB	DFLC	FLP	FLR	FLR
90050 (90150)		A	CB	DHLT	FLG	FLR	(S)

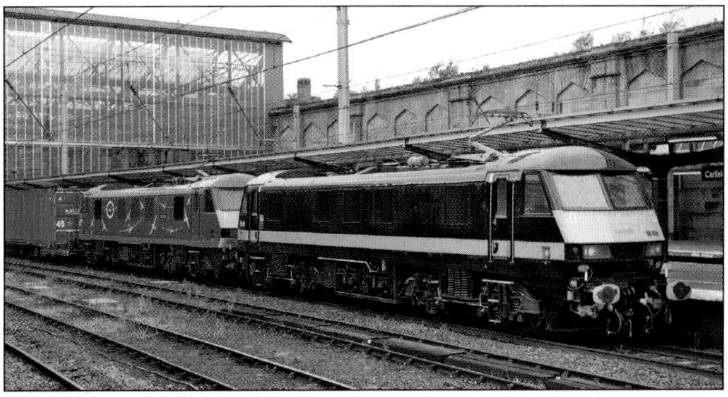

A large number of the DB operated Class 90s are long out of service and stored at Crewe, a handful still operate main line services, mainly over the West Coast route. Black-liveried No. 90020 and 90037 in red with glider images and the legend 'Hans-Georg Werner Thank You & Good Luck' honouring the retiring DB Chief Executive Officer are seen at Carlisle. **Antony Christie**

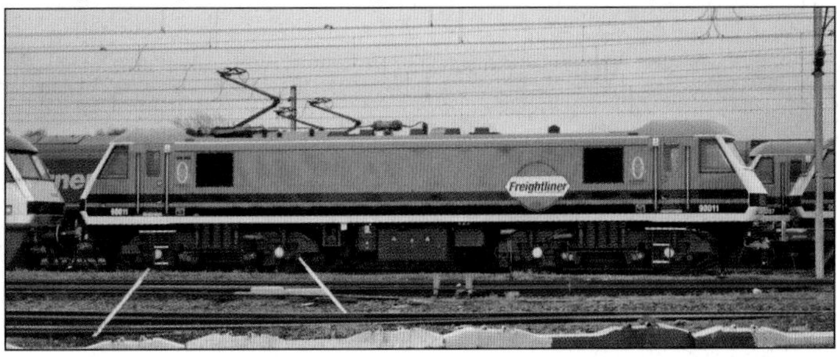

All of the recently arrived ex-Greater Anglia Class 90 fleet are now in Freightliner orange livery and many have lost their previous cast nameplates. No. 90011 is seen at Crewe, the home base for the Freightliner '90' fleet. **Cliff Beeton**

Class 91
BREL Bo-Bo Electric

Built: 1988-1991
Length: 63ft 8in (19.40m)
Height: 12ft 4in (3.76m)
Width: 9ft 0in (2.74m)
Power system: 25,000V ac overhead
Transmission: Electric
Tractive effort: 43,000lb (190kN)

91101 (91001)	*Flying Scotsman*	A	NL	IECA	SPL	EVL	LNR
91105 (91005)		A	NL	IECA	LNR	EVL	LNR
91106 (91006)		A	NL	IECA	LNR	EVL	LNR
91107 (91007)	*Skyfall*	A	NL	IECA	LNR	EVL	LNR
91109 (91009)	*Sir Bobby Robson*	A	NL	IECA	LNR	EVL	LNR
91110 (91010)	*Battle of Britain Memorial Flight* (for preservation at NRM, York)	A	NL	IECA	SPL	EVL	LNR
91111 (91011)	*For the Fallen*	A	NL	IECA	SPL	EVL	LNR
91112 (91012)		A	DR	SAXL	LNR	EVL	(S)
91114 (91014)	*Durham Cathedral*	A	NL	IECA	LNR	EVL	LNR
91115 (91015)	*Blaydon Races*	A	DR	SAXL	LNR	EVL	(S)
91116 (91016)		A	DR	SAXL	LNR	EVL	(S)
91117 (91017)		A	BH	EPEX	EPX	EPX	(S)
91118 (91018)	*The Fusiliers*	A	DR	SAXL	LNR	EVL	(S)
91119 (91019)	*Bounds Green InterCity Depot 1977-2017*	A	NL	IECA	ICS	EVL	LNR
91120 (91020)		A	BH	EPEX	EPX	EPX	(S)
91121 (91021)		A	DR	-	LNR	EVL	(S)
91122 (91022)		A	CY	EROG	LNR	EVL	(S)
91124 (91024)		A	NL	IECA	LNR	EVL	LNR
91125 (91025)		A	DR	SAXL	LNR	EVL	(S)
91127 (91027)		A	NL	IECA	LNR	EVL	LNR
91128 (91028)	*InterCity 50*	A	CY	EROG	LNR	EVL	(S)
91130 (91030)	*Lord Mayor of Newcastle*	A	NL	IECA	LNR	EVL	LNR
91131 (91031)	Scheduled for preservation by by SRPS at Bo'ness						

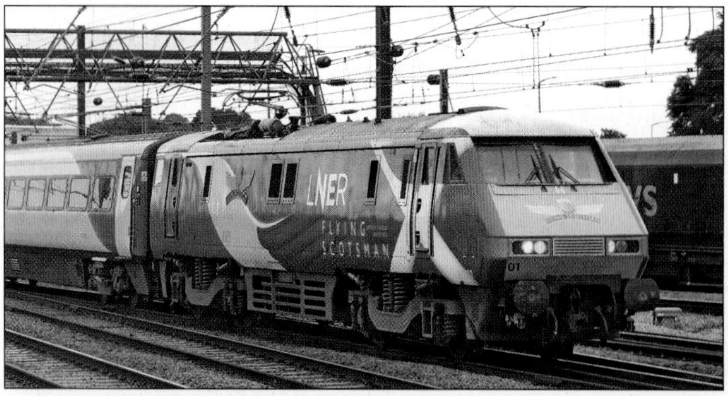

Even with a full compliment of Class 80x trains, LNER still require around three Class 91/Mk4 formations each day, mainly operating King's Cross-Leeds/York services. No. 91101 in Flying Scotsman colours is shown arriving at Doncaster heading to Leeds in October 2021. **CJM**

Class 92
BR/Brush Co-Co Dual Voltage Electric

Built: 1993-1995
Length: 70ft 1in (21.36m)
Height: 13ft 0in (3.96m)
Width: 8ft 8in (2.64m)
Power system: 25,000V ac overhead, 75V dc third rail
Transmission: Electric
Tractive effort: 90,000lb (400kN)

92001	*Mircea Eliade*	A	Locotech, Russia 91 53 0472 002-1				
92002	*Lucian Blaga*	A	Locotech, 91 53 0472 003-9, stored Hungary				
92003		A	DB Romania 91 53 0472 xxx-x				
92004	*Jane Austen*	A	CE	WQCA	RFE	DBC	(S)
92005		A	Locotech, 91 53 0472 005-4, stored Hungary				
92006		AD	WB	GBSL	SCS	GBR	GBR
92007	*Schubert*	A	CE	WQBA	RFE	DBC	(S)
92008	*Jules Verne*	A	CE	WQCA	RFE	DBC	(S)
92009	*Marco Polo*	AH	CE	WQCA	DBS	DBC	(S)
92010		ADH	WB	GBST	SCS	GBR	GBR
92011	*Handel*	AH	CE	WFBC	RFE	DBC	DBC
92012	*Mihai Eminescu*	A	Locotech, 91 53 0472 001-3, stored Hungary				
92013	*Puccini*	A	CE	WQBA	RFE	DBC	(S)
92014		AD	WB	GBSL	SCS	GBR	SCS
92015		AH	CE	WFBC	DBS	DBC	DBC
92016		AH	CE	WQCA	DBS	DBC	(S)
92017	*Bart the Engine*	A	CE	WQCA	SPL	DBC	(S)
92018		ADH	WB	GBST	SCS	GBR	SCS
92019	*Wagner*	AH	CE	WFBC	RFE	DBC	DBC
92020	*Billy Stirling*	AD	WB	GBSL	GBN	GBR	GBR
92021		A	WS	GBSD	EPG	GBR	(S)
92022		A	DB, Bulgaria 91 52 1688 022-1				
92023		ADH	WB	GBSL	SCS	GBR	SCS
92024	*Marin Preda*	A	Locotech, 91 53 0472 004-7, stored Hungary				
92025		A	DB, Bulgaria 91 52 1688 025-1				
92026		A	DB, Romania 91 53 0472 026-x				
92027		A	DB, Bulgaria 91 70 1688 027-1				
92028		AD	WB	GBST	GBN	GBR	SCS
92029	*Dante*	A	CE	WQAB	RFE	DBC	(S)
92030		A	DB, Bulgaria 91 52 1688 030-1				
92031		AH	CE	WQBA	DBS	DBC	(S)
92032	*IMechE Railway Division*	ADH	WB	GBCT	GBN	GBR	GBR
92033	*Railway Heritage Trust*	AD	WB	GBSL	SCS	GBR	SCS
92034	*Kipling*	A	DB, Bulgaria 91 52 1688 034-3				
92035	*Mendelssohn*	A	CE	WQCA	RFE	DBC	(S)
92036	*Bertolt Brecht*	AH	CE	WFBC	RFE	DBC	DBC
92037	*Sullivan*	A	CE	WQCA	RFE	DBC	(S)
92038		A	WB	GBST	SCS	GBR	SCS
92039	*Eugen Ionescu*	A	DB, Romania 91 53 0472 006-2				
92040	*Goethe*	A	WS	GBSD	EPG	GBR	(S)
92041	*Vaughan Williams*	AH	CE	WFBC	RFE	DBC	DBC
92042		AH	CE	WFBC	DBS	DBC	DBC
92043		ADH	WB	GBST	GBN	GBR	GBR
92044	*Couperin*	AH	WB	GBCT	SCS	GBR	GBR
92045	*Chaucer*	A	WS	GBSD	EPG	GBR	(S)
92046	*Sweelinck*	A	WS	GBSD	EPG	GBR	(S)

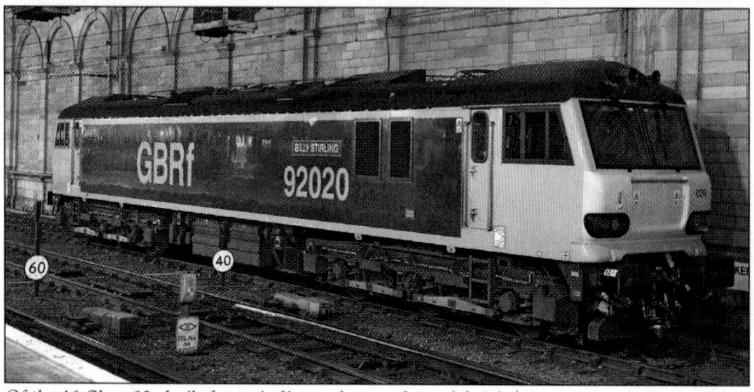

Of the 46 Class 92s built for main line and cross-channel freight/passenger operations only a handful remain in service, mainly with GB Railfreight. In full GBRf blue and orange livery, No. 92020 Billy Stirling is seen at Edinburgh Waverley on 11 November 2021 awaiting to take over the London bound Caledonian Sleeper service. **CJM**

Class 97/3 (former 37)
English Electric Co-Co Diesel-Electric

Built: 1960-1965
Length: 61ft 6in (18.74m)
Height: Between 12ft 9⅛in-13ft 0¼in (3.86m-3.96m)
Width: 8ft 11⅝in (2.69m)
Engine: English Electric 12CSVT of 1,750hp (1,304W)
Transmission: Electric
Tractive effort: 55,500lb (245kN)

97301 (37100)		AE	ZA	QETS	NRL	NRL	NRL
97302 (37170)	*Rheilffyrdd Ffestiniog Ffestiniog & Welsh Highland Railways*	AE	ZA	QETS	NRL	NRL	NRL
97303 (37178)	*Dave Berry*	AE	ZA	QETS	NRL	NRL	NRL
97304 (37217)	*John Tiley*	AE	ZA	QETS	NRL	NRL	NRL

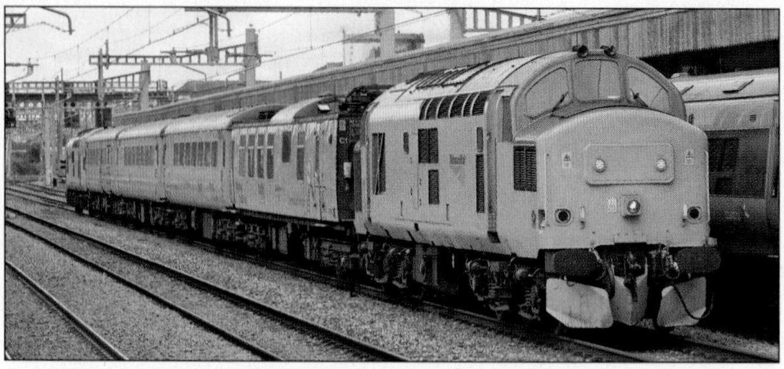
Four Class 97/3s are operated by Network Rail for test train and Cambrian Coast work and classified in the departmental series as 973xx. The fleet sport full Network Rail branded yellow livery and are based at the RC Derby. No. 97303 is seen leading a test train at Cardiff in July 2021. This loco was subsequently named Dave Berry. **Spencer Conquest**

Class 97/6 (PWM shunters)
Ruston & Hornsby 0-6-0 Diesel-Electric

Built: 1953-1959
Length: 28ft 8½in (7.53m)
Height: Between 11ft (3.35m)
Width: 8ft 6in (2.59m)
Engine: English Electric Ruston 6VPHL of 165hp
Transmission: Electric
Tractive effort: 17,000ib (76kN)

97650 (PWM650)	Peak Rail
97651 (PWM651)	Swindon & Cricklade Railway
97654 (PWM654)	Peak Rail

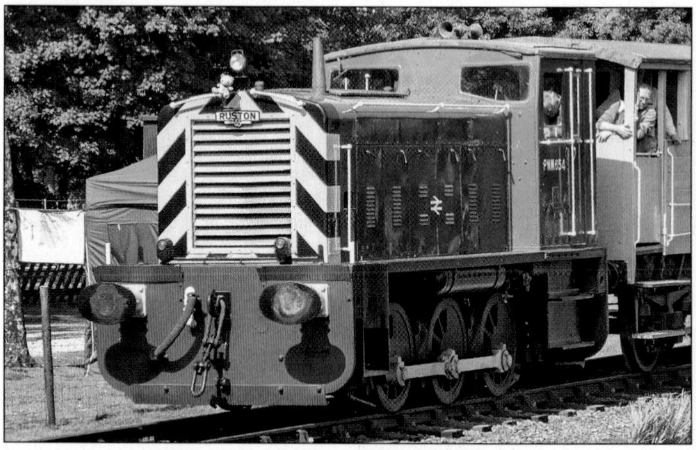

Now preserved by the Heritage Shunters Trust at Peak Rail, Ruston & Hornsby 0-6-0 No. PWM65, later Class 97/6 No. 97654 is seen at Peak Rail, painted in 1970s BR rail blue carrying its Permanent Way Machinery (PWM) number **John Stretton**

Class Di8 Mak
Mak Bo-Bo Diesel-Electric

Built: 1996-1997
Length: 57ft 1in (17.4m)
Height: 14ft 4½in (4.38m)
Width: 9ft 10in (3.00m)
Engine: Caterpillar 3516 DI-TA of 2,110hp (1,570kW)
Transmission: Electric

801 (8.701)	Operational
802 (8.702)	Operational
803 (8.703)	Out of use, awaiting parts
804 (8.704)	Operational
808 (8.708)	Operational
812 (8.712)	Withdrawn, spares donor
816 (8.716)	Out of use, awaiting parts
817 (8.717)	Operational
818 (8.718)	Withdraw, spares donor
819 (8.719)	Out of use, awaiting parts
820 (8.720)	Withdrawn, spares donor

GB Railfreight provide heavy-duty shunting locos for British Steel, Scunthorpe, with a fleet of 11 Class Di8 Bo-Bo diesel-electrics. In yellow/red livery No. 8.704 (804) is shown. **Richard Tuplin**

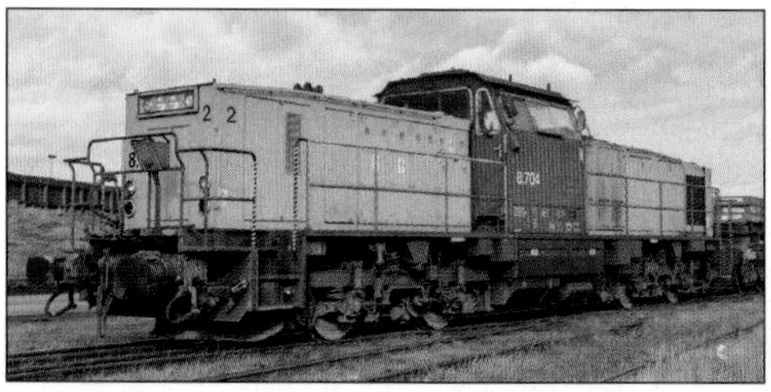

At a Glance - UK Main Line Locomotives 2022-2023

Class	No. Range	Builder	Type	Output	Introduced	Operator
03	03018-03399	BR	0-6-0DM	204hp (152kW)	1958	WCR, industry
07	07001-07013	Ruston & Hornsby	0-6-0DE	275hp (205kW)	1962	AFS, industry
08	08001-09204	BR	0-6-0DE	400hp (298kW)	1953	AFS, COL, EMR, FLR, GBR, GWR, HNR, LOG, LSL, WCR, WMR
18	18001-18015	Clayton	Bo-Bo	558hp (416kW)	2021	Beacon Rail, GBR
19	19001	Damfoss	Bo-Bo		2018	Damfoss
20	20001-20906	English Electric	Bo-Bo	1,000hp (746kW)	1957	189, C2L, EEP, HNR, LSL
33	33012-33207	Birmingham RCW	Bo-Bo	1,500hp (1,156kW)	1960	71A, WCR
37	37025-37905	English Electric	Co-Co	1,750hp (1,304kW)	1960	COL, DRS, EPX, LSL, ROG, URL, WCR
43	43003-43484	BR	Bo-Bo	2,250hp (1,677kW)	1976	ASR, AXC, COL, DAS, EMR, GWR, LSL, NRL
47	47194-47854	BR/Brush	Co-Co	2,580hp (1,924kW)	1962	GBR, HNR, LSL, ROG, S4G, VIN, WAB, WCR
50	50007-50050	English Electric	Co-Co	2,700hp (2,013kW)	1967	50A, BOD, GBR, HAN
56	56007-56312	BR/Brush	Co-Co	3,250hp (2,424kW)	1976	BOD, COL, DCR, GBR
57/0	57001-57012	Brush/BR	Co-Co	2,500hp (1,860kW)	1998	DRS, WCR
57/3	57301-57316	Brush/BR	Co-Co	2,750hp (2,051kW)	2002	DRS, ROG, WCR
57/6	57601-57605	Brush/BR	Co-Co	2,750hp (2,051kW)	2001	WCR, GWR
59	59001-59206	GM/EMD	Co-Co	3,000hp (2,237kW)	1985	GBR, FLR
60	60001-60500	Brush	Co-Co	3,000hp (2,237kW)	1985	DBC, DCR, GBR
66	66001-66957	GM/EMD	Co-Co	3,200hp (2,385kW)	1998	COL, DBC, DRS, FLR, GBR
67	67001-67030	GM/Alstom	Bo-Bo	3,200hp (2,385kW)	1999	GBR, DBC, TFW
68	68001-68034	Vossloh/Stadler	Bo-Bo	3,750hp (2,800kW	2014	CRW, DRS, TPE
69	69001-69106	Progress Rail	Co-Co	3,200hp (2,385kW)	2021	GBR
70	70001-70817	General Electric	Co-Co	3,686hp (2,750kW)	2009	COL, FLR
73/1,2	73101-73235	English Electric	Bo-Bo	Electric 1,600hp (1,193kW) Diesel 600hp (447kW)	1966	GBR, NRL, SWR, TTS, GTR
73/95	73951-73952	RVEL	Bo-Bo	Elrctric 1,328hp (990kW) Diesel 1,500hp (1,120kW)	2014	NRL
73/96	73961-73971	Brush	Bo-Bo	Electric 1,600hp (1,195kW) Diesel 1,600hp (1,193kW)	2014	GBR, NRL, SCS
86	86101-86639	BR	Bo-Bo	5,000hp (3,728kW)	1966	LSL, PRI, WCR
87	87002	BREL	Bo-Bo	5,000hp (3,728kW)	1973	LSL
88	88001-88010	Stadler	Bo-Bo	Eletric 5,360hp (4,000kW) Diesel 940hp (708kW)	2016	DRS
90	90001-90049	BREL	Bo-Bo	5,000hp (3,728kW)	1987	DBC, FLR, LSL
91	91101-91131	BREL	Bo-Bo	6,300hp (4,700kW)	1988	LNE, ROG, EPX
92	92001-92046	Brush	Co-Co	6,760hp (5,040kW)	1993	DBC, GBR
97	97301-97304	English Electric	Co-Co	1,750hp (1,304kW)	1960	NRL
Di8	801-820	Mak	Bo-Bo	2,110hp (1,570kW)	1996	GBR

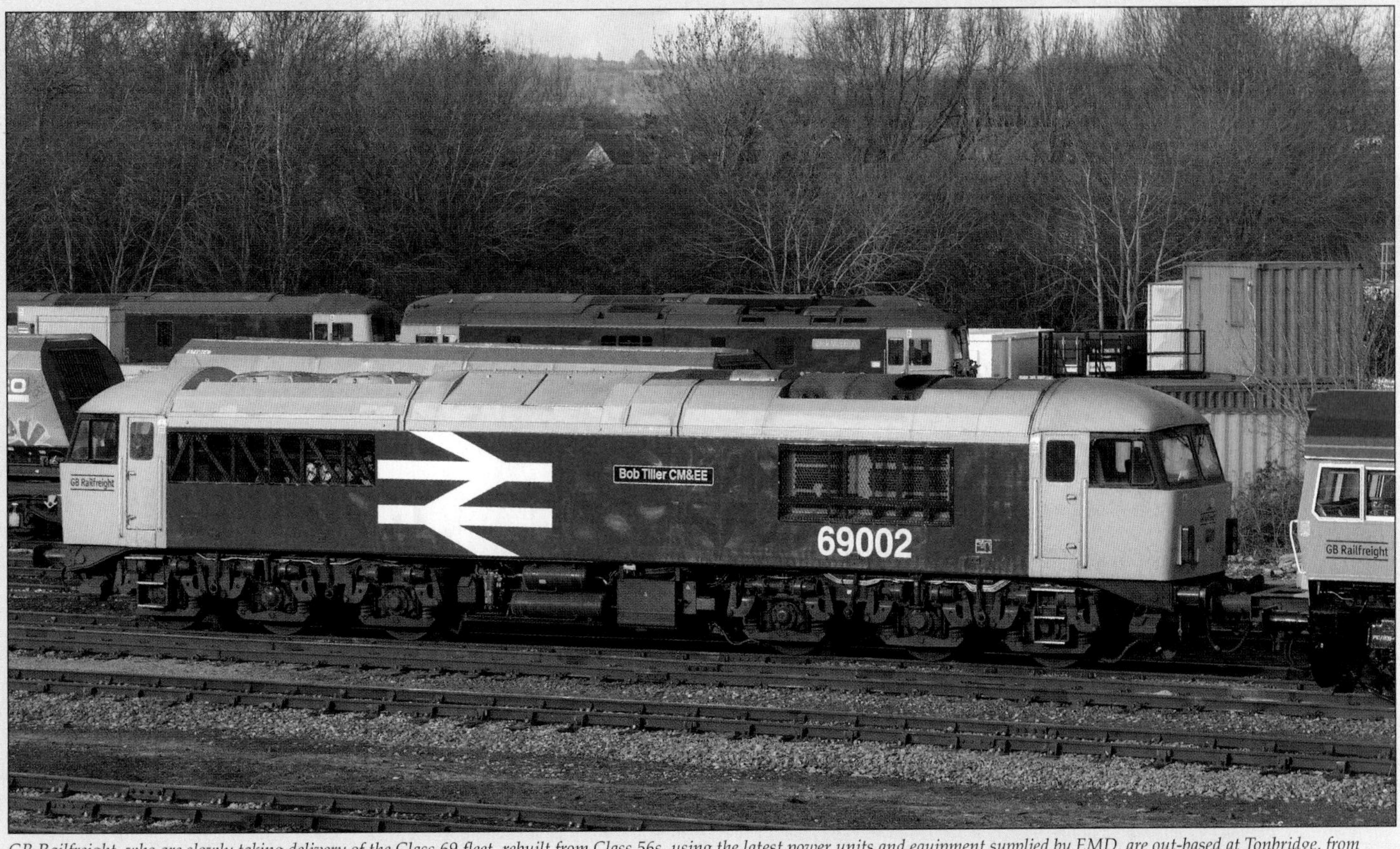

GB Railfreight, who are slowly taking delivery of the Class 69 fleet, rebuilt from Class 56s, using the latest power units and equipment supplied by EMD, are out-based at Tonbridge, from were they operated limited services on Network Rail flows and freight duties, frequently involving the Gypsum flow from Mountfield. In immaculate large logo blue with wrap around yellow end livery, No. 69002 Bob Tiller CM&EE *is seen at Tonbridge on 27 January 2022.* **Antony Christie**

Diesel Multiple Units

Non TOPS Classes

GWR 4	National Railway Museum
GWR 20	Kent & East Sussex Railway
GWR 22	Didcot Railway Centre
APT-E	National Railway Museum
LEV1	National Railway Museum at Wensleydale
LEV3	Downpatrick & County Down Railway
RB002	Riverstone Old Corn Railway, USA
RB004	Waverley Route Heritage Centre

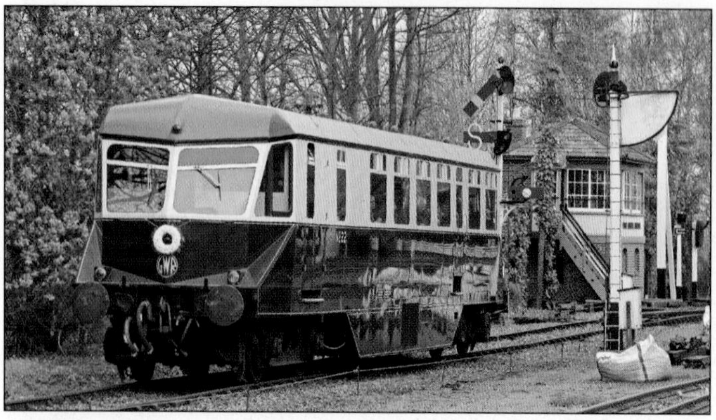

Great Western Railway design double ended railcar No. W22 is preserved at the Didcot Railway Centre, where this image was captured. **Martyn Tattam**

First Generation DMMU

50015	114	Midland Railway Centre
50019	114	Midland Railway Centre
50160	101	North Yorkshire Moors Railway
50164	101	North Yorkshire Moors Railway
50170	101	Ecclesbourne Valley Railway
50193	101	Great Central Railway
50203	101	Great Central Railway
50204	101	North Yorkshire Moors Railway
50222	101	Barry Island Railway
50253	101	Ecclesbourne Valley Railway
50256	101	Wensleydale Railway
50266	101	Great Centrtal Railway
50321	101	Great Central Railway
50338	101	Barry Island Railway
50413	103	Helston Railway
50416	109	Llangollen Railway
50437	104	Llangollen Railway
50447	104	Llangollen Railway
50454	104	Llangollen Railway
50455	104	East Lancashire Railway
50479	104	East Lancashire Railway
50494	104	East Lancashire Railway
50517	104	East Lancashire Railway
50528	104	Llangollen Railway
50531	104	Telford Steam Railway
50599	108	Ecclesbourne Valley Railway
50619	108	Dean Forest Railway
50628	108	Keith & Dufftown Railway
50632	108	Dean Forest Railway
50645	108	Great Central Railway North
50746	111	Wensleydale Railway
50926	108	Great Central Railway North
50928	108	Keighley & Worth Valley Railway
50933	108	Severn Valley Railway
50971	108	Kent & East Sussex Railway
50980	108	Weardale Railway
51017	126	Bo'ness & Kinneil Railway
51043	126	Bo'ness & Kinneil Railway
51073	119	Ecclesbourne Valley Railway
51074	119	Swindon & Cricklade Railway
51104	119	Swindon & Cricklade Railway
51118	100	Midland Railway Centre
51131	116	Battlefield Line
51138	116	Great Central Railway North
51151	116	Great Central Railway North
51187	101	Cambrian Railway
51188	101	NRM at Ecclesbourne Valley Railway
51189	101	Keighley & Worth Valley Railway
51192	101	National Railway Museum at NNR
51205	101	Cambrian Railway
51210	101	Wensleydale Railway
51213	101	East Anglian Railway Museum
51226	101	Mid Norfolk Railway
51228	101	Mid Norfolk Railway
51317	118	Arlington Eastleigh
51321	118	Battlefield Line
51339	117	Colne Valley Railway
51342	117	Epping & Ongar Railway
51347	117	Gwili Railway
51351	117	Pontypool & Blaenavon Railway
51352	117	South Devon Railway
51353	117	Wensleydale Railway
51354	117	West Somerset Railway
51356	117	Swanage Railway
51360	117	Gloucestershire Warwickshire Railway
51363	117	Gloucestershire Warwickshire Railway
51365	117	Plym Valley Railway
51367	117	Strathspey Railway
51370	117	Mid Norfolk Railway
51371	117	North Somerset Rly at Eastleigh
51372	117	Gloucestershire Warwickshire Railway
51375	117	Chinnor and Princes Risborough Rly
51376	117	South Devon Railway
51381	117	Mangapps Farm Museum
51382	117	Colne Valley Railway
51384	117	Epping and Ongar Railway
51388	117	Swanage Railway (main line certified)
51392	117	Swanage Railway
51396	117	Great Central Railway
51397	117	Pontypool & Blaenavon Railway
51400	117	Wensleydale Railway
51401	117	Gwili Railway
51402	117	Strathspey Railway
51405	117	Gloucestershire Warwickshire Railway
51407	117	Plym Valley Railway
51412	117	Mid Norfolk Railway
51413	117	North Somerset Rly at Eastleigh
51427	101	Great Central Railway
51434	101	Mid Norfolk Railway
51485	105	East Lancashire Railway
51499	101	Mid Norfolk Railway
51503	101	Mid Norfolk Railway
51505	101	Ecclesbourne Valley Railway
51511	101	North Yokshire Moors Railway
51512	101	Cambrian Railway
51562	108	National Railway Museum
51565	108	Keighley & Worth Valley Railway
51566	108	Dean Forest Railway
51567	108	Ecclesbourne Valley Railway
51568	108	Keith & Dufftown Railway
51571	108	Kent & East Sussex Railway
51572	108	Wensleydale Railway
51591	127	Midland Railway Centre
51610	127	Midland Railway Centre
51616	127	Helston Railway
51618	127	Llangollen Railway
51622	127	Helston Railway at Vincent Eng, Henstridge, Somerset
51625	127	Midland Railway Centre
51655	115	Rosyth Dockyard
51663	115	West Somerset Railway (frame only)
51669	115	Midland Railway, Butterley
51803	101	Keighley & Worth Valley Railway
51813	110	East Lancashire Railway
51842	110	East Lancashire Railway
51849	115	Midland Railway, Butterley
51859	115	West Somerset Railway
51880	115	West Somerset Railway
51886	115	Birmingham Railway Museum
51887	115	West Somerset Railway
51899	115	Buckingham Railway Centre
51907	108	Llangollen Railway
51909	108	East Somerset Railway
51914	108	Dean Forest Railway
51919	108	Garw Valley Railway
51922	108	National Railway Museum
51933	108	Swanage Railway
51937	108	Poulton & Wyre Railway
51941	108	Severn Valley Railway

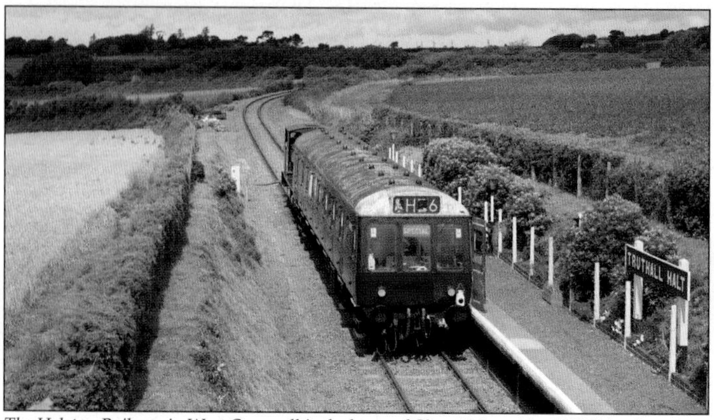

The Helston Railway in West Cornwall is the home of Class 127 car No. M51616, where it is restored in non-authentic maroon livery. It is seen on the railway at Truthall Halt on 22 August 2021. **Antony Christie**

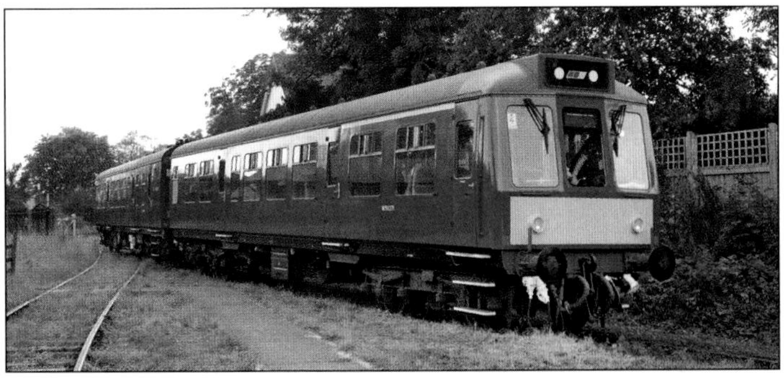

Painted in BR rail blue with a small yellow warning end, Class 108 Driving Trailer Composite No. M56271 is seen coupled to vehicle M51909 at the East Somerset Railway, Cranmore in September 2021. **Antony Christie**

51942	108	Mid Norfolk Railway
51947	108	East Somerset Railway
51950	108	Telford Steam Railway
51990	107	Strathspey Railway
51993	107	Tanat Valley Railway (for sale 09/21)
52005	107	Tanat Valley Railway (for sale 09/21)
52006	107	Avon Valley Railway
52008	107	Strathspey Railway
52012	107	Tanat Valley Railway (for sale 09/21)
52025	107	Avon Valley Railway
52029	107	Fife Heritage Railway, Leven
52030	107	Strathspey Railway
52031	107	Tanat Valley Railway (for sale 09/21)
52044	108	Dean Forest Railway
52048	108	Garw Valley Railway
52053	108	Keith & Dufftown Railway
52054	108	Weardale Railway
52062	108	Telford Steam Railway
52064	108	Severn Valley Railway
52071	110	Lakeside & Haverthwaite Railway
52077	110	Lakeside & Haverthwaite Railway
54223	108	Llangollen Railway
54270	108	Mid Norfolk Railway
54504	108	Swanage Railway
55000	122	South Devon Railway
55001	122	East Lancashire Railway
55003	122	Gloucestershire Warwickshire Railway
55005	122	Battlefield Line
55006	122	Ecclesbourne Valley Railway
55009	122	Great Central Railway
55012	122	Weardale Railway
55019	122	Llanelli & Mynydd Mawr Railway
55020	121	Bodmin & Wenford Railway
55022	121	LNWR Heritage Centre, Crewe
55023	121	Chinnor & Princes Risborough Railway
55024	121	Chinnor & Princes Risborough Railway
55025	121	Honeybourne Airfield
55027	121	Ecclesbourne Valley Railway
55028	121	Swanage Railway
55029	121	Rushden Transport Museum
55031	121	Eccclesbourne Valley Railway
55032	121	Wensleydale Railway
55033	121	Colne Valley Railway
55034	121	Locomotive Services, Crewe
56006	114	Midland Railway Centre
56015	114	Midland Railway Centre
56055	101	Cambrian Railway
56057	101	Strathspey Railway
56062	101	North Norfolk Railway
56097	100	Midland Railway Centre
56121	105	East Lancashire Railway
56160	103	Bodfari, Denbigh (private)
56169	103	Helston Railway
56171	109	Llangollen Railway
56182	104	North Norfolk Railway
56207	108	BSC Scunthorpe
56208	108	Severn Valley Railway
56224	108	Keith & Dufftown Railway
56271	108	East Somerset Railway
56274	108	Wensleydale Railway
56279	108	Lavendar Line (for sale 09/21)
56287	121	Epping & Ongar Railway
56289	121	East Lancashire Railway
56301	100	Mid Norfolk Railway
56342	101	Great Central Railway
56343	101	Wensleydale Railway
56347	101	Mid Norfolk Railway
56352	101	NRM at Ecclesbourne Valley Railway
56356	101	Barry Island Railway
56358	101	East Anglian Railway Museum
56408	101	Lavender Line
56456	105	Llangollen Railway
56484	108	Poulton & Wyre Railway
56490	108	Llangollen Railway
56491	108	Keith & Dufftown Railway
56492	108	Dean Forest Railway
56495	108	Kirklees Light Railway
59003	116	Dartmouth Steam Railway
59004	116	Dartmouth Steam Railway
59117	110	Mid Norfolk Railway
59137	104	East Lancashire Railway
59228	104	East Lancashire Railway
59245	108	BSC Scunthorpe
59250	108	Severn Valley Railway
59276	120	Great Central Railway
59303	101	Ecclesbourne Valley Railway
59387	108	Dean Forest Railway
59404	126	Bo'ness & Kinneil Railway
59444	116	Chasewater Railway
59486	117	Swanage Railway (main line certified)
59488	117	Dartmouth Steam Railway
59492	117	Swanage Railway
59493	117	South Devon Railway
59494	117	Dartmouth Steam Railway
59500	117	Wensleydale Railway (static)
59501	117	Great Central Railway North
59503	117	Dartmouth Steam Railway
59505	117	Gloucestershire Warwickshire Railway
59506	117	Great Central Railway
59507	117	Dartmouth Steam Railway
59508	117	Gwili Railway
59509	117	Wensleydale Railway
59510	117	Gloucestershire Warwickshire Railway
59511	117	Strathspey Railway
59513	117	Dartmouth Steam Railway
59514	117	Swindon & Cricklade Railway
59515	117	Yeovil Railway Centre
59517	117	Dartmouth Steam Railway
59520	117	Dartmoor Railway
59521	117	Helston Railway
59522	117	Nottingham Transport Heritage Trust
59539	101	North Yorkshire Moors Railway
59575	111	Great Central Railway
59603	127	Chasewater Railway
59609	127	Midland Railway Centre
59659	115	Midland Railway Centre
59664	115	Talybont-on-Usk
59678	115	West Somerset Railway
59701	110	East Lancashire Railway
59719	115	Mid Hants Railway
59740	115	South Devon Railway
59761	115	Buckinghamshire Railway Centre
59791	107	Tanat Valley Railway (for sale 09/21)
79018	-	Ecclesbourne Valley Railway
79443	-	Bo'ness & Kinneil Railway
79612	-	Ecclesbourne Valley Railway
79900	-	Ecclesbourne Valley Railway
79960	-	Ribble Steam Railway
79962	-	Keighley & Worth Valley Railway
79963	-	East Anglian Railway
79964	-	Keighley & Worth Valley Railway
79976	-	Nemesis Rail, Burton
79978	-	Swindon & Cricklade Railway
79998	-	Royal Deeside Railway (Battery electric)
79999	-	Royal Deeside Railway (Battery electric)
977020	-	Downpatrik Steam Railway
998900	-	Middleton Railway
999507	-	Lavender Line

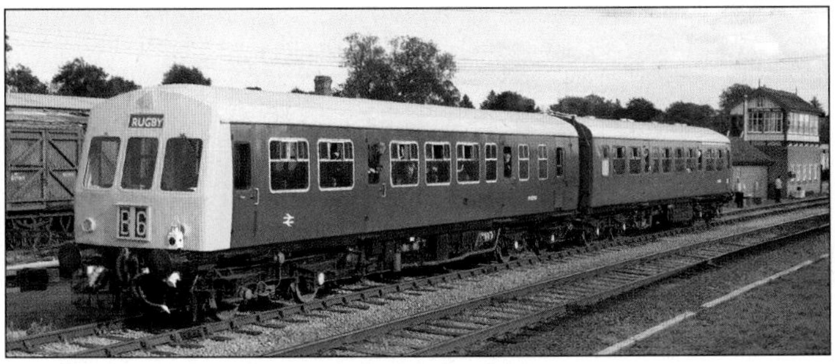

Restored to perfect 1970s BR rail blue with full wrap around yellow end and aluminum frames to the passenger windows, a Class 101 two-car with DMSB 50203 nearest the camera is seen at Swithland on the Great Central Railway. **Nathan Williamson**

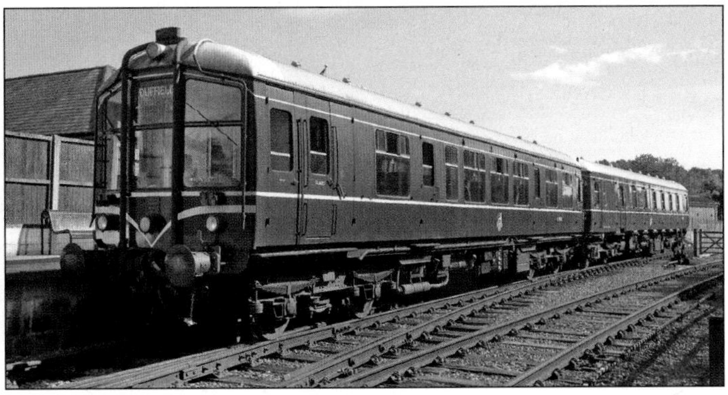

Only a handful of first generation DMMU vehicles are preserved. 'Bubble' car No. M79900 is preserved at the Ecclesbourne Valley Railway in 1950s green. After passenger service this vehicle became Derby RTC test car 975010 Iris *before preservation.* **Nathan Williamson**

Second Generation Diesel Units

TOPS Classes

Class 139
Parry People Mover 4-wheel vehicle

Built: 2007-2008
Length: 28ft 6in (8.7m)
Height: 12ft 3in (3.77m)
Width: 7ft 10in (2.4m)
Engine: Ford MVH-420 of 86hp (64kW)
Transmission: Hydrostatic

	Formation: DMS				
139001	39001	SJ	WMR	PMO	WMT
139002	39002	SJ	WMR	PMO	WMT

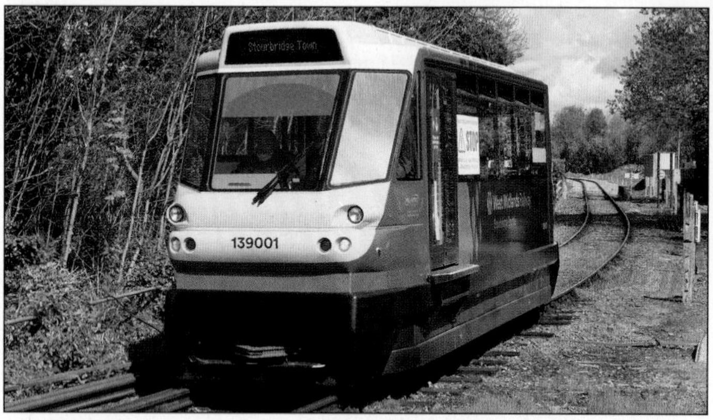

A pair of Parry People Mover cars are used on the West Midlands Railway Stourbridge Junction to Stourbridge Town 'shuttle'. Based in a small shed at Stourbridge Junction, one vehicle operates at a time. They carry mauve and gold WMR livery. No. 139001 is seen at Stourbridge Junction. **CJM**

Class 140
BR / Leyland Railbus 4-wheel Railbus

Built: 1981
Vehicle length: 57ft 5½in (15.98m)
Height: 11ft 5¾in (3.53m)
Width: 8ft 0½in (2.45m)
Engine: 1 x Leyland TL11 per car
Horsepower: 200hp (149kW) per car
Transmission: Mechanical

	Formation: DMS+DMSL	
140001	55500+55501	Keith & Dufftown Railway

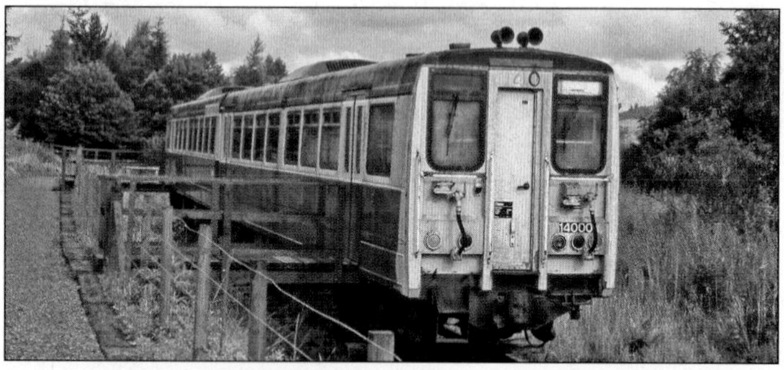

The early prototype for the Railbus concept was built by Leyland and BR at the RTC, Derby before entering test and limited passenger service. After a period of store, it entered preservation and is at the Keith & Dufftown Railway, Scotland. **Colour-Rail**

Class 141
BREL / Leyland Railbus 4-wheel Railbus

Built: 1985
Vehicle length: 50ft ¼in (15.45m)
Height: 12ft 8¾in (3.88m)
Width: 8ft 2½in (2.50m)
Engine: 1 x Leyland TL11 per car
Horsepower: 205hp (153kW) per car
Transmission: Mechanical

	Formation: DMS+DMSL		
141001	141102	55502+55522	Exported to Iran 2000
141004	141105	55505+55525	Exported to Iran 2001
141005	141106	55506+55526	Exported to Holland
141006	141107	55507+55527	Exported to Iran 2000
141007	141108	55508+55528	Loco Services, Margate
141008	141109	55509+55529	Exported to Iran 2000
141010	141111	55511+55531	Exported to Iran 2000
141011	141112	55512+55532	Exported to Holland
141012	141113	55513+55533	Midland Railway Centre
141013	141114	55514+55534	Exported to Iran 2000
141014	141115	55515+55535	Exported to Iran 2000
141015	141116	55516+55536	Exported to Iran 2001
141016	141117	55517+55537	Exported to Iran 2000
141017	141118	55518+55538	Exported to Iran 2001
141018	141119	55519+55539	Exported to Iran 2000
141019	141120	55520+55540	Exported to Iran 2000

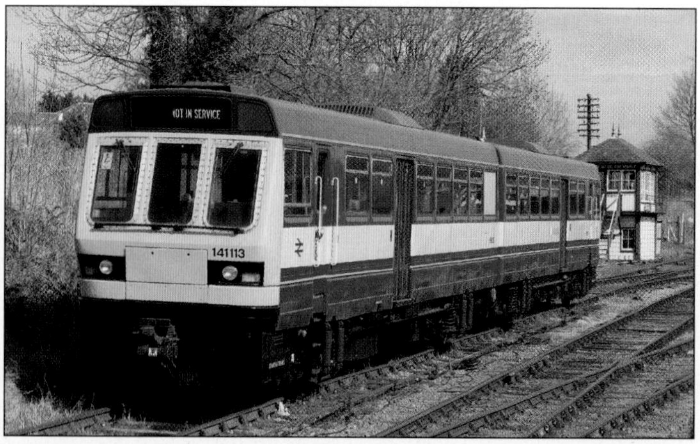

The first production Railbus sets, classified 141, did not remain in traffic with BR for many years, most were exported to Iran in 2000-2001. Thankfully two are preserved and available for use. No. 141113, the original No. 141012 is based at the Midland Railway Centre, where this view was recorded in April 2022. **Antony Christie**

Class 142
BREL / Leyland Railbus 4-wheel Railbus

Built: 1985-1987
Vehicle length: 50ft 0½in (15.55m)
Height: 12ft 8in (3.86m)
Width: 9ft 2¼in (2.80m)
Engine: 1 x Cummins LTA10R per car
Horsepower: 225hp (165kW) per car
Transmission: Mechanical

	Formation: DMS+DMSL	
142001	55542+55592	National Railway Museum, Shildon
142003	55544+55594	LSL, for dsplay at 1:1 Museum, Margate
142004	55545+55595	Telford Steam Railway
142006	55547+55597	Llanelli & Mynydd Mawr Railway
142007	55548+55598	LSL, stored AFS Eastleigh
142011	55552+55602	Midland Railway Centre
142013	55554+55604	Midland Railway Centre
142014	55555+55605	Arlington Fleet Services, Eastleigh
142017	55558+55608	East Kent Railway
142018	55559+55609	Wensleydale Railway
142019	55560+55610	Waverley Route Heritage Centre, Whiterope
142020	55561+55611	Waverley Route Heritage Centre, Whiterope
142023	55564+55614	Plym Valley Railway
142027	55568+55618	Chasewater Railway (spares)
142028	55569+55619	Wensleydale Railway
142029	55570+55620	Chasewater Railway
142030	55571+55621	Chasewater Railway
142033	55574+55624	South Wales Police Development, Bridgend
142035	55576+55626	Wensleydale Railway
142036	55577+55627	East Kent Railway
142038	55579+55629	Mid Norfolk Railway
142041	55582+55632	Wensleydale Railway
142043	55584+55634	Sussex Fire Training School, Kingstanding
142045	55586+55636	Kirk Merrington School, Spennymoor
142047	55588+55638	Stored Gascoigne Wood
142055	55705+55751	Pacer Group at Foxfield Railway
142056	55706+55752	Arlington Fleet Services, Eastleigh
142058	55708+55754	Telford Steam Railway
142060	55710+55756	Wensleydale Railway
142061	55711+55757	Mid-Norfolk Railway
142078	55728+55768	Wensleydale Railway
142084	55734+55780	Rushden, Higham & Wellingborough Railway
142087	55737+55783	Wensleydale Railway
142089	55739+55785	Arlington Fleet Services, Eastleigh
142090	55740+55786	Wensleydale Railway
142091	55741+55787	Rushden, Higham & Wellingborough Railway
142094	55744+55790	Embsay & Boton Abbey

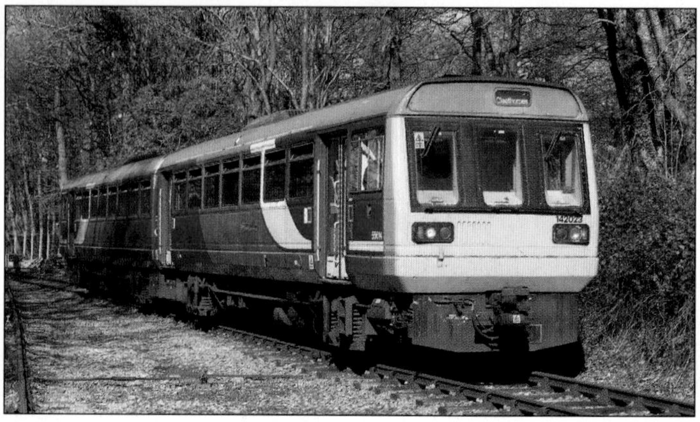

Often despised by enthusiasts and passenger it is amazing that 30 Class 142s are preserved, with seven in industrial use and two still awaiting disposal. However these two-car light weight sets are ideal for preservation sites and a good design for all year operation when the cost of running locomotives (steam or diesel) is prohibitive. No. 142023 is seen in Northern colours at the Plym Valley Railway. **Dan Phillips**

Class 143
Walter Alexander / Andrew Barclay 4-wheel Railbus

Built: 1985-1986
Vehicle length: 51ft 0½in (15.55m)
Height: 12ft 2¾in (3.73m)
Width: 8ft 10½in (2.70m)
Engine: 1 x Cummins LTA10R per car
Horsepower: 225hp (165kW) per car
Transmission: Mechanical

Formation: DMS+DMSL

143601	55642+55667	Tanat Valley Railway
143602	55651+55668	Nene Valley Railway
143603	55658+55689	Vale of Berkeley Railway, stored RSS, Wishaw
143606	55647+55672	Llanelli & Mynydd Mawr Railway
143607	55648+55673	Llanelli & Mynydd Mawr Railway
143608	55649+55674	Wensleydale Railway (to be delivered)
143612	55653+55678	Llanelli & Mynydd Mawr Rly, for Vale of Berkeley Rly
143616	55657+55682	Tanat Valley Railway
143617	55644+55683	Stored GWR at Bristol St Philips Marsh
143618	55659+55684	Plym Valley Railway
143619	55660+55685	Stored GWR at Bristol St Philips Marsh
143622	55663+55688	Llanelli Goods Shed Trust
143623	55664+55689	Wensleydale Railway
143625	55666+55691	Keighley & Worth Valley Railway (spares)

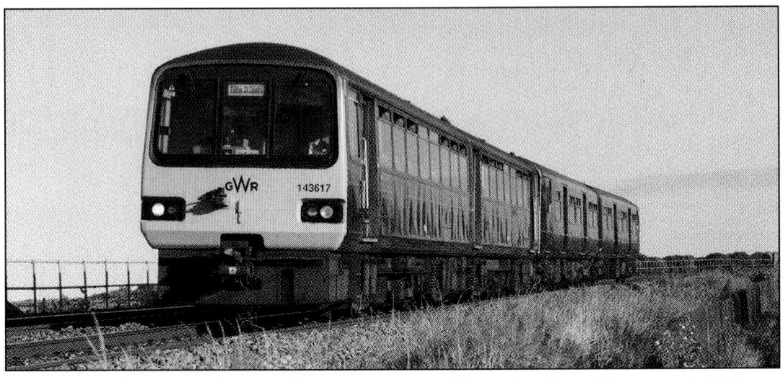

As with the Class 142s, when the Class 143s were withdrawn by Great Western and TfW many entered preservation. Currently, two sets Nos. 143617 and 143619 are still on the books of Great Western stored at St Philips Marsh, Bristol. In happier days No. 143617 is seen working with a Class 150 at Cockwood with a Paignton-Exeter service. **CJM**

Class 144
Walter Alexander / BREL 4-wheel Railbus

Built: 1986-1987
Vehicle length: 50ft 2in (15.29m)
Height: 12ft 2¾in (3.73m)
Width: 8ft 10½in (2.70m)
Engine: 1 x Cummins LTA10R per car
Horsepower: 225hp (165kW) per car
Transmission: Mechanical

Formation: DMS+DMSL or DMS+MS+DMSL

144001	55801	Airdale General Hospital
	55824	Platform 1 Charity, Huddersfield station
144002	55802+55825	Dayles School, Blyth, classroom
144003	55803+55826	Great Central Railway (Ruddington)
144004	55804+55827	Aln Valley Railway
144005	55805+55828	Loram, Derby RTC
144006	55806+55829	Cambrian Railway, Oswestry
144007	55807+55830	Cambrian Railway, Oswestry
144008	55831	Corby & District Model Railway
	55808	Fagley Primary School, Bradford
144009	55809+55832	Greater Manchester Fire & Rescue at ELR
144010	55810+55833	East Lancs Railway
144011	55811+55834	Keighley & Worth Valley Railway
144012	55812+55835	Network Rail, stored Long Marston
144013	55813+55836	Telford Steam Railway
144014	55814+55850+55837	Vintage Trains, Tyseley
144016	55816+55852+55839	Aln Valley Railway
144017	55817+55853+55840	Woodhead Her Gp at Appleby/Frodingham
144018	55818+55854+55841	Mid Norfolk Railway
144019	55819+55855+55842	Vintage Trains, Tyseley
144020	55820+55856+55843	Wensleydale Railway
144022	55822+55858+55845	Keith & Dufftown Railway
144023	55823+55846	Vintage Trains, Tyseley

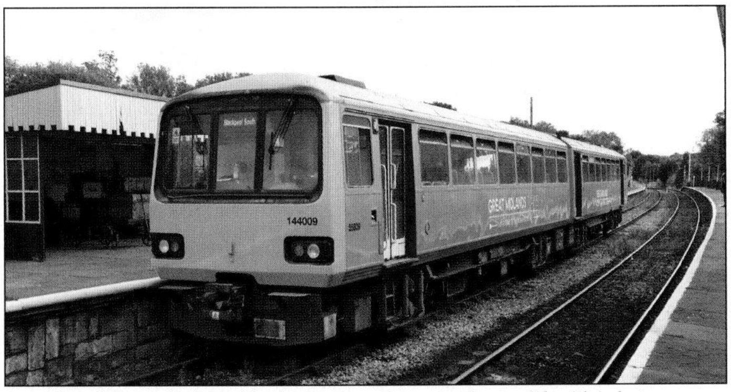

A number of Class 144s have either been preserved or entered a new life with industry or providing accommodation for schools or hospitals. In a fictional livery of Great Midlands Trains, set No. 144009 is seen at the East Lancs Railway. **Adrian Paul**

Class 150/0
BREL 3-car 'Sprinter'

Built: 1984, (1985-86 - 150003-006)
Vehicle length: 65ft 9¾in (20.06m)
Height: 12ft 4½in (3.77m)
Width: 9ft 3¼in (2.82m)
*Engine: 1 x Cummins NT855R4 per car**
Horsepower: 285hp (213kW) per car
Transmission: Hydraulic
**150003-006 - 1 x Cummins NT855R5 per car*

Formation: DMSL+MS+DMS

150001	55200+55400+55300	NH	NNR	ANG	NOR
150002	55201+55401+55301	NH	NNR	ANG	NOR

Formation: DMSL+DMS+DMS

150003	52116+57209+57116	NH	NNR	ANG	NOR
150004	52112+57212+57112	NH	NNR	ANG	NOR
150005	52117+52223+57117	NH	NNR	ANG	NOR
150006	52147+57223+57147	NH	NNR	ANG	NOR

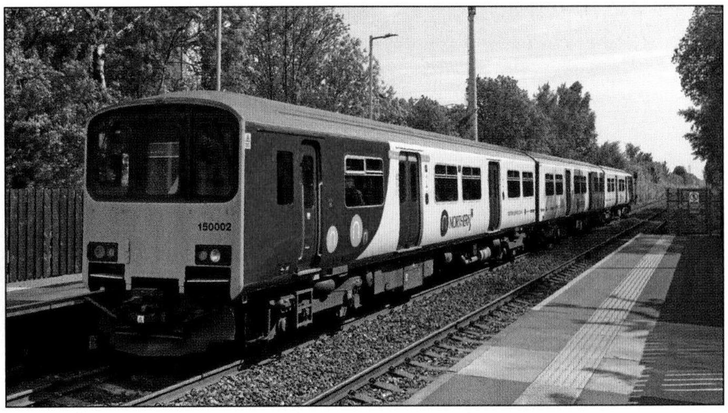

Two three-car Class 150/0s as built and four 150/1s with a Class 150/2 intermediate vehicle operate for Northern, based at Newton Heath. One of the original three-car sets No. 150002 is shown. The original two sets, 150001, 150002 were the prototype units for the entire 'Sprinter' fleets. **CJM**

Class 150/1
BREL 2-car 'Sprinter'

Built: 1985-1986
Vehicle length: 65ft 9¾in (20.06m)
Height: 12ft 4½in (3.77m)
Width: 9ft 3¼in (2.82m)
Engine: 1 x Cummins NT855R5 per car
Horsepower: 285hp (213kW) per car
Transmission: Hydraulic

Formation: DMSL+DMS

150101	52101+57101	NH	NNR	ANG	NOR
150102	52102+57102	NH	NNR	ANG	NOR
150103	52103+57103	NH	NNR	ANG	NOR
150104	52104+57104	NH	NNR	ANG	NOR
150105	52105+57105	NH	NNR	ANG	NOR
150106	52106+57106	NH	NNR	ANG	NOR
150107	52107+57107	NH	NNR	ANG	NOR
150108	52108+57108	NH	NNR	ANG	NOR
150109	52109+57109	NH	NNR	ANG	NOR
150110	52110+57110	NH	NNR	ANG	NOR
150111	52111+57111	NH	NNR	ANG	NOR
150113	52113+57113	NH	NNR	ANG	NOR
150114	52114+57114	NH	NNR	ANG	NOR
150115	52115+57115	NH	NNR	ANG	NOR
150118	52118+57118	NH	NNR	ANG	NOR
150119	52119+57119	NH	NNR	ANG	NOR
150120	52120+57120	NH	NNR	ANG	NOR
150121	52121+57121	NH	NNR	ANG	NOR
150122	52122+57122	NH	NNR	ANG	NOR
150123	52123+57123	NH	NNR	ANG	NOR
150124	52124+57124	NH	NNR	ANG	NOR
150125	52125+57125	NH	NNR	ANG	NOR
150126	52126+57126	NH	NNR	ANG	NOR
150127	52127+57127	NH	NNR	ANG	NOR
150128	52128+57128	NH	NNR	ANG	NOR
150129	52129+57129	NH	NNR	ANG	NOR
150130	52130+57130	NH	NNR	ANG	NOR
150131	52131+57131	NH	NNR	ANG	NOR
150132	52132+57132	NH	NNR	ANG	NOR
150133	52133+57133	NH	NNR	ANG	NOR
150134	52134+57134	NH	NNR	ANG	NOR
150135	52135+57135	NH	NNR	ANG	NOR
150136	52136+57136	NH	NNR	ANG	NOR
150137	52137+57137	NH	NNR	ANG	NOR
150138	52138+57138	NH	NNR	ANG	NOR
150139	52139+57139	NH	NNR	ANG	NOR
150140	52140+57140	NH	NNR	ANG	NOR
150141	52141+57141	NH	NNR	ANG	NOR
150142	52142+57142	NH	NNR	ANG	NOR
150143	52143+57143	NH	NNR	ANG	NOR
150144	52144+57144	NH	NNR	ANG	NOR
150145	52145+57145	NH	NNR	ANG	NOR
150146	52146+57146	NH	NNR	ANG	NOR
150148	52148+57148	NH	NNR	ANG	NOR
150149	52149+57149	NH	NNR	ANG	NOR
150150	52150+57150	NH	NNR	ANG	NOR

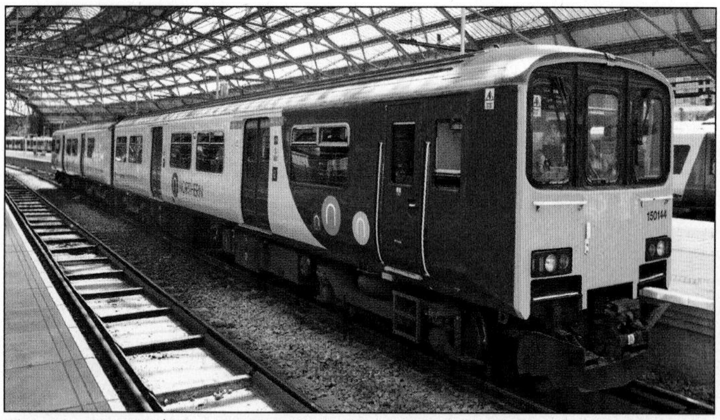

The entire Class 150/1 fleet operate with Northern, based at Manchester Newton Heath and be found throughout the Northern operating area. All sets are refurbished to meet PRM requirements and all sport the Northern white livery. Set No. 150144 is seen at Liverpool Lime Street in summer 2021. **CJM**

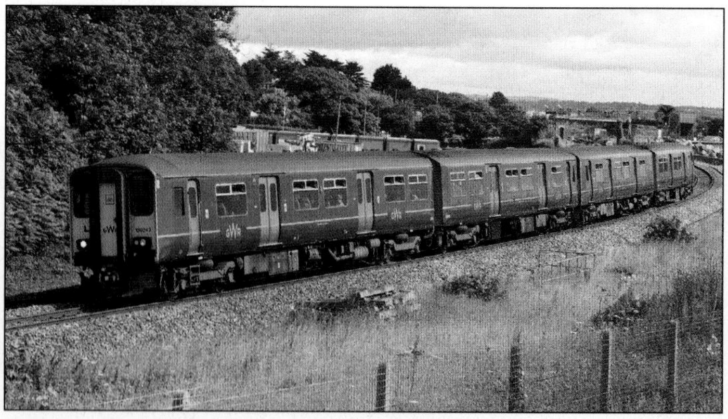

The Great Western Railway-operated Class 150s are based at the enlarged and modernised Exeter depot, located adjacent to Exeter St Davids station. The fleet operate Exeter-Paignton, Penzance, Exmouth, Barnstaple and Oxehampton duties as well as Cornish branch lines. Set No. 150243 is shown in full GWR green and light grey livery. **CJM**

Class 150/2
BREL 2-car 'Sprinter'

Built: 1986-1987
Vehicle length: 65ft 9¾in (20.06m)
Height: 12ft 4½in (3.77m)
Width: 9ft 3¼in (2.82m)
Engine: 1 x Cummins NT855R5 per car
Horsepower: 285hp (213kW) per car
Transmission: Hydraulic

	Formation: DMSL+DMS					
150201	52201+57201		NL	NNR	ANG	NOR
150202	52202+57202		EX	GWG	ANG	GWR
150203	52203+57203		NL	NNR	ANG	NOR
150204	52204+57204		NL	NNR	ANG	NOR
150205	52205+57205		NL	NNR	ANG	NOR
150206	52206+57206		NL	NNR	ANG	NOR
150207	52207+57207		EX	GWG	ANG	GWR
150208	52208+57208		CV	ATT	PTR	TFW
150210	52210+57210		NH	NNR	ANG	NOR
150211	52211+57211		NL	NNR	ANG	NOR
150213	52213+57213		CV	ATT	PTR	TFW
150214	52214+57214		NL	NNR	ANG	NOR
150215	52215+57215		NL	NNR	ANG	NOR
150216	52216+57216		EX	GWG	ANG	GWR
150217	52217+57217		CV	TFW	PTR	TFW
150218	52218+57218		NL	NNR	ANG	NOR
150219	52219+57219		EX	FGB	PTR	GWR
150220	52220+57220		NL	NNR	ANG	NOR
150221	52221+57221		EX	GWG	PTR	GWR
150222	52222+57222		NL	NNR	ANG	NOR
150224	52224+57224		NH	NNR	ANG	NOR
150225	52225+57225		NH	NNR	ANG	NOR
150226	52226+57226		NH	NNR	ANG	NOR
150227	52227+57227		CV	TFW	PTR	TFW
150228	52228+57228		NL	NNR	PTR	NOR
150229	52229+57229		CV	ATT	PTR	TFW
150230	52230+57230		CV	ATT	PTR	TFW
150231	52231+57231		CV	ATT	PTR	TFW
150232	52232+57232		EX	GWG	PTR	GWR
150233	52233+57233	*Peter West OBE*	EX	GWG	PTR	GWR
150234	52234+57234		EX	GWG	PTR	GWR
150235	52235+57235		CV	TFW	PTR	TFW
150236	52236+57236		CV	TFW	PTR	TFW
150237	52237+57237		CV	TFW	PTR	TFW
150238	52238+57238		EX	FGB	PTR	GWR
150239	52239+57239		EX	GWG	PTR	GWR
150240	52240+57240		CV	TFW	PTR	TFW
150241	52241+57241		CV	TFW	PTR	TFW
150242	52242+57242		CV	TFW	PTR	TFW
150243	52243+57243		EX	GWG	PTR	GWR
150244	52244+57244		EX	GWG	PTR	GWR
150245	52245+57245		CV	TFW	PTR	TFW
150246	52246+57246		EX	GWG	PTR	GWR
150247	52247+57247		EX	GWG	PTR	GWR
150248	52248+57248		EX	GWG	PTR	GWR
150249	52249+57249		EX	GWG	PTR	GWR
150250	52250+57250		CV	ATT	PTR	TFW
150251	52251+57251		CV	TFW	PTR	TFW
150252	52252+57252		CV	ATT	PTR	TFW
150253	52253+57253		CV	TFW	PTR	TFW
150254	52254+57254		CV	TFW	PTR	TFW
150255	52213+57255		CV	TFW	PTR	TFW
150256	52256+57256		CV	TFW	PTR	TFW
150257	52257+57257		CV	TFW	PTR	TFW
150258	52258+57258		CV	ATT	PTR	TFW
150259	52259+57259		CV	TFW	PTR	TFW
150260	52260+57260		CV	ATT	PTR	TFW
150261	52261+57261		EX	GWG	PTR	GWR
150262	52262+57262		CV	ATT	PTR	TFW
150263	52263+57263		EX	GWG	PTR	GWR
150264	52264+57264		CV	ATT	PTR	TFW
150265	52265+57265		EX	GWG	PTR	GWR
150266	52266+57266		EX	GWG	PTR	GWR
150267	52267+57267		CV	TFW	PTR	TFW
150268	52268+57268		NL	NNR	PTR	NOR
150269	52269+57269		NH	NNR	PTR	NOR
150270	52270+57270		NL	NNR	PTR	NOR
150271	52271+57271		NL	NNR	PTR	NOR
150272	52272+57272		NL	NNR	PTR	NOR
150273	52273+57273		NL	NNR	PTR	NOR
150274	52274+57274		NL	NNR	PTR	NOR
150275	52275+57275		NL	NNR	PTR	NOR
150276	52276+57276		NL	NNR	PTR	NOR
150277	52277+57277		NL	NNR	PTR	NOR
150278	52278+57278		CV	TFW	TFW	TFW
150279	52279+57279		CV	ATT	PTR	TFW
150280	52280+57280		CV	ATT	PTR	TFW
150281	52281+57281		CV	ATT	PTR	TFW
150282	52282+57282		CV	TFW	PTR	TFW
150283	52283+57283		CV	TFW	PTR	TFW
150284	52284+57284		CV	TFW	PTR	TFW
150285	52285+57285		CV	ATT	PTR	TFW

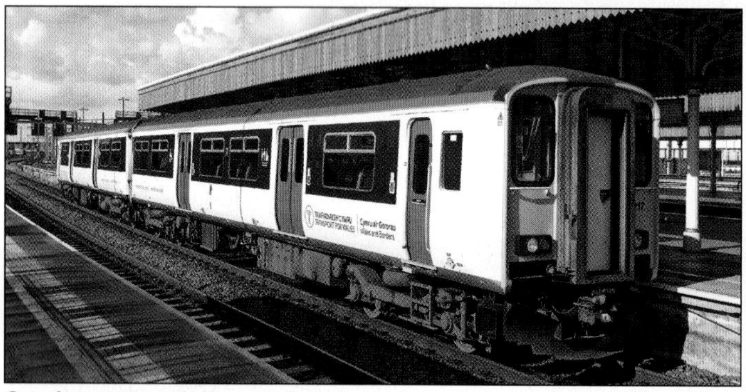

Over the past 18 months Transport for Wales has progressively upgraded their Class 150/2 fleet, even though they will soon be replaced. Sets now sport the light grey livery, red doors and black window band. Set 150217 is illustrated at Cardiff on a valley line service. **CJM**

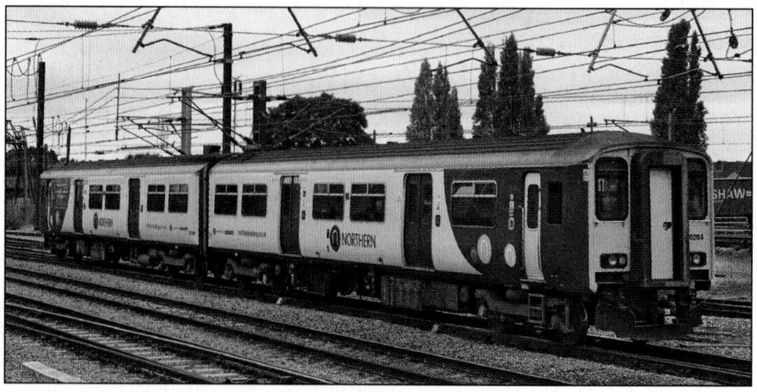

The Northern Class 150/2 allocation is split between Leeds Neville Hill and Manchester Newton Heath depots, with Neville Hill having the larger allocation. All sport Northern white and blue livery. Set No. 150204 is illustrated departing from Doncaster on a Sheffield duty. **CJM**

Class 153
Leyland / Hunslet Barclay One-car 'Super Sprinter'

Built: 1991-1992 (as 155 1987-1988)
Vehicle length: 76ft 5in (23.29m)
Height: 12ft 3⅜in (3.75m)
Width: 8ft 10in (2.69m)
Engine: 1 x Cummins NT855R5 per car
Horsepower: 285hp (213kW) per car
Transmission: Hydraulic

	Formation: DMSL				
153301	52301	EL	NOR	ANG	OLS
153303	52303	CV	TFW	TFW	TFW
153304	52304	EL	NOR	ANG	OLS
153305	52305	CK	ASB	ANG	ASR

153906§	52306		CV	TFW	PTR	TFW
153307	52307		CV	NOR	ANG	*
153308	52308		EL	EMR	ANG	OLS
153909§	52309		CV	TFW	PTR	TFW
155910§	52310		CV	TFW	PTR	TFW
153311	52311		LM	EMR	PTR	NRL
153312	52312		CV	TFW	TFW	TFW
153913§	52313		CV	TFW	PTR	TFW
153914§	52314		CV	TFW	PTR	TFW
153315	52315		EL	NOR	ANG	OLS
153316	52316	*John 'Longitude' Harrison Inventor of the Marine Chronometer*	HT	NOR	PTR	OLS
153317	52317		EL	NOR	ANG	OLS
153918§	52318		CV	EMR	TFW	TFW
153319	52319		EL	EMR	ANG	OLS
153320	52320		CV	TFW	PTR	TFW
153921§	52321		CV	TFW	PTR	TFW
153922§	52322		CV	TFW	PTR	TFW
153323	52323		CV	TFW	PTR	TFW
153324	52324		LM	NOR	PTR	OLS
153325	52325		CV	TFW	PTR	TFW
153926§	52326		CV	TFW	PTR	TFW
153327	52327		CV	TFW	TFW	TFW
153328	52328		CV	NOR	ANG	*
153329	52329		CV	TFW	ANG	TFW
153330	52330		LM	NOR	PTR	OLS
153331	52331		CV	NOR	ANG	*
153332	52332		LM	NOR	ANG	OLS
153333	52333		CV	TFW	PTR	TFW
153334	52334		LM	LMI	PTR	OLS
153935§	52335		CV	TFW	PTR	TFW
153351	57351		EL	NOR	ANG	OLS
153352	57352		CV	NOR	ANG	*
153353	57353		CV	TFW	TFW	TFW
153354	57354		LM	LMI	PTR	OLS
153355	57355		EL	EMR	ANG	OLS
153356	57356		LM	LMI	PTR	OLS
153357	57357		EL	EMR	ANG	OLS
153358	57358		LM	NOR	PTR	OLS
153359	57359		LM	NOR	PTR	OLS
153360	57360		LM	NOR	PTR	OLS
153361	57361		CV	TFW	ANG	TFW
153362	57362		CV	TFW	ANG	TFW
153363	57363		LM	NOR	PTR	OLS
153365	57365		LM	LMI	PTR	OLS
153367	57367		CV	TFW	PTR	TFW
153968§	57368		CV	EMR	TFW	TFW
153369	57369		CV	TFW	ANG	TFW
153370	57370		CK	ASB	ANG	ASR
153371	57371		LM	LMI	PTR	TFW
153972§	57372		CV	EMR	TFW	TFW
153373	57373		CK	ASB	ANG	ASR
153374	57374		CF	EMR	ANG	TFW
153375	57375		LM	LMI	PTR	OLS
153376	57376		ZA	EMR	PTR	NRL
153377	57377		CK	ASB	ANG	ASR
153378	57378		EL	NOR	ANG	OLS
153379	57379		LM	EMR	PTR	OLS
153380	57380		CK	ASB	ANG	ASR
153381	57381		LM	EMR	PTR	OLS
153982§	57382		CV	EMR	TFW	TFW
153383	57383	*Ecclesbourne Valley Railway 150 Years*	LM	EMR	PTR	OLS
153384	57384		LM	EMR	PTR	OLS
153385	57385		ZA	EMR	PTR	NRL

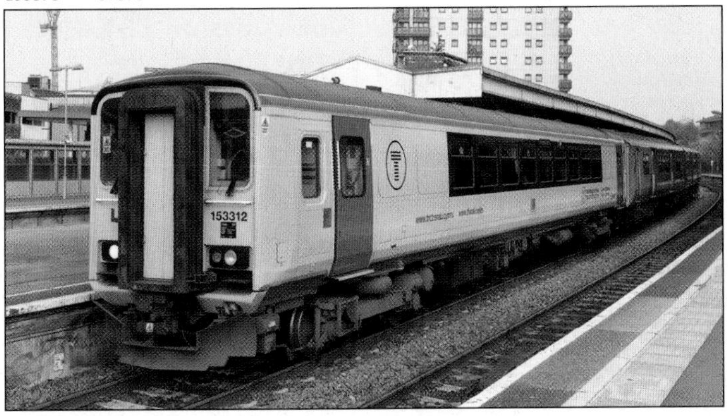

Over the last year the number of working Class 153s has considerably reduced with both Northern and East Midlands Railway taking the class out of use A number of the Transport for Wales sets have received an upgrade to meet PRM requirements and have been repainted in the latest light grey, orange and black livery, as shown on No. 153312. **CJM**

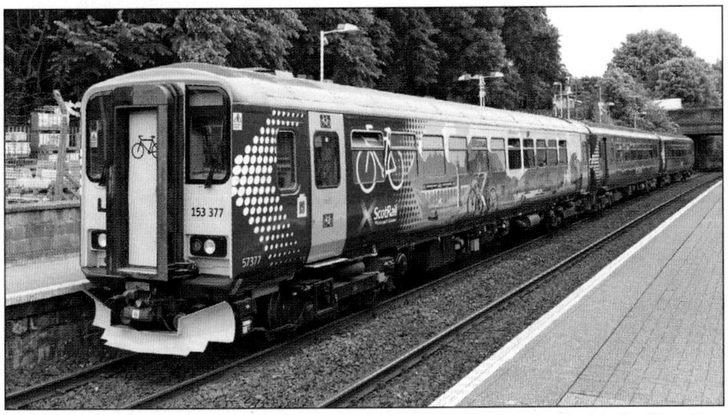

In Scotland, five Class 153s have been overhauled by Brodie Engineering for 'Active Travel' services between Glasgow and Oban, Fort William and Mallaig route. Internally the vehicles have been rebuilt to provide space for sports equipment with seating retained at one end. St No. 153377 is shown. Note the front end handrails have been removed. **CJM**

§ Renumbered from 1533xx as non-PRM compliant
NRL sets Video Inspection Units (VIU)
* For conversion to 'Active Travel' vehicles for TfW

With a large number of off-lease Class 153s, Network Rail took over three ex East Midlands examples for adaptation to Video Inspection Units (VIUs). Some external modifications have been carried out with nose end cameras and recording equipment and some windows have been replaced by ventilation grilles. No. 153376 is seen stabled at Manningtree. **Jamie Dyke**

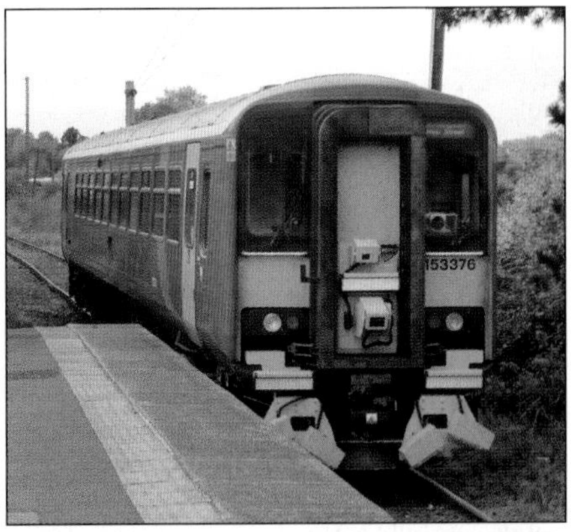

Class 155
Leyland 2-car 'Super Sprinter'

Built: 1987-1988
Vehicle length: 76ft 5in (23.29m)
Height: 12ft 3¾in (3.75m)
Width: 8ft 10in (2.69m)
Engine: 1 x Cummins NT855R5 per car
Horsepower: 285hp (213kW) per car
Transmission: Hydraulic

	Formation: DMSL+DMS				
155341	52341+57341	NL	NNR	PTR	NOR
155342	52342+57342	NL	NNR	PTR	NOR
155343	52343+57343	NL	NNR	PTR	NOR
155344	52344+57344	NL	NNR	PTR	NOR
155345	52345+57345	NL	NNR	PTR	NOR
155346	52346+57346	NL	NNR	PTR	NOR
155347	52347+57347	NL	NNR	PTR	NOR

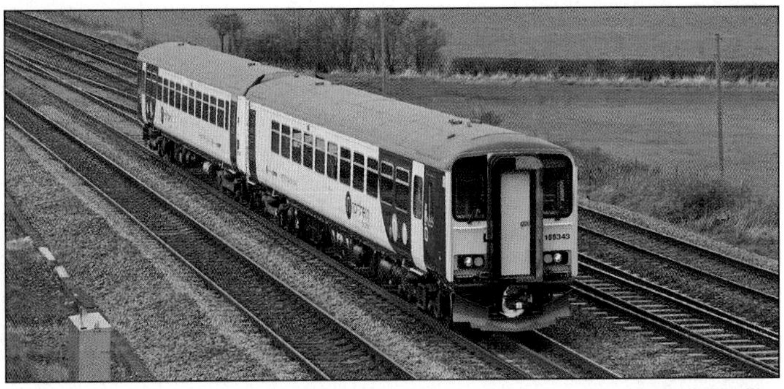

Northern operate five two-car Class 155 Leyland 'Super Sprinter' sets based at Leeds Neville Hill. Refurbished and now carrying the Northern white livery, No. 155342 is seen near York. The units are usually deployed on Leeds to Hull and Scarborough routes. **Adrian Paul**

Class 156
Metro-Cammell 2-car 'Super Sprinter'

Built: 1987-1989
Vehicle length: 75ft 6in (23.03m)
Height: 12ft 6in (3.81m)
Width: 8ft 11in (2.73m)
Engine: 1 x Cummins NT855R5 per car
Horsepower: 285hp (213kW) per car
Transmission: Hydraulic

	Formation: DMSL+DMS				
156401	52401+57401	NH	EMR	PTR	NOR
156402	52402+57402	NH	NOR	PTR	NOR
156403	52403+57403	NM	EMR	PTR	EMR
156404	52404+57404	NM	EMR	PTR	EMR
156405	52405+57405	NM	EMI	PTR	EMR
156406	52406+57406	NM	EMI	PTR	EMR
156907	(156407) 52407+57407	BH	EMI	PTR	OLS
156408	52408+57408	NM	EMR	PTR	EMR
156409	(156909) 52409+57409	DY	EMI	PTR	OLS
156410	52410+57410	NM	EMR	PTR	EMR
156411	52411+57411	NM	EMR	PTR	EMR
156412	52412+57412	NH	NOR	PTR	NOR
156413	52413+57413	NM	EMR	PTR	EMR
156414	52414+57414	NM	BLU	PTR	EMR
156415	52415+57415	NH	EMR	PTR	NOR
156916	(156416) 52416+57416	BH	EMI	PTR	OLS

156917	(156417) 52417+57417	DY	EMI	PTR	OLS
156918	(156418) 52418+57418	BH	EMI	PTR	OLS
156919	(156419) 52419+57419	DY	EMI	PTR	OLS
156420	52420+57420	NH	NNR	PTR	NOR
156421	52421+57421	HT	NNR	PTR	NOR
156422	52422+57422	DY	NNE	PTR	EMR
156423	52423+57423	NH	NNR	PTR	NOR
156424	52424+57424	NH	NNR	PTR	NOR
156425	52425+57425	NH	NNR	PTR	NOR
156426	52426+57426	NH	NNR	PTR	NOR
156427	52427+57427	NH	NNR	PTR	NOR
156428	52428+57428	NH	NNR	PTR	NOR
156429	52429+57429	NH	NNR	PTR	NOR
156430	52430+57430	CK	SCR	ANG	ASR
156431	52431+57431	CK	SCR	ANG	ASR
156432	52432+57432	CK	SCR	ANG	ASR
156433	52433+57433	CK	SCR	ANG	ASR
156434	52434+57434	CK	SCR	ANG	ASR
156435	52435+57435	CK	SCR	ANG	ASR
156436	52436+57436	CK	SCR	ANG	ASR
156437	52437+57437	CK	SCR	ANG	ASR
156438	52438+57438	HT	NNR	ANG	NOR
156439	52439+57439	CK	SCR	ANG	ASR
156440	52440+57440	HT	NNR	PTR	NOR
156441	52441+57441	NH	NNR	PTR	NOR
156442	52442+57442	CK	SCR	ANG	ASR
156443	52443+57443	HT	NNR	ANG	NOR
156444	52444+57444	HT	NNR	ANG	NOR
156445	52445+57445	CK	SCR	ANG	ASR
156446	52446+57446	CK	SCR	ANG	ASR
156447	52447+57447	HT	NNR	ANG	NOR
156448	52448+57448	HT	NNR	ANG	NOR
156449	52449+57449	HT	NNR	ANG	NOR
156450	52450+57450	CK	SCR	ANG	ASR
156451	52451+57451	HT	NNR	ANG	NOR
156452	52452+57452	NH	NNR	PTR	NOR
156453	52453+57453	CK	SCR	ANG	ASR
156454	52454+57454	HT	NNR	ANG	NOR
156455	52455+57455	NH	NNR	PTR	NOR
156456	52456+57456	CK	SCR	ANG	ASR
156457	52457+57457	CK	SCR	ANG	ASR
156458	52458+57458	CK	SCR	ANG	ASR
156459	52459+57459	NH	NNR	PTR	NOR
156460	52460+57460	NH	NNR	PTR	NOR
156461	52461+57461	NH	NNR	PTR	NOR
156462	52462+57462	CK	SCR	ANG	ASR
156463	52463+57463	HT	NOR	ANG	NOR
156464	52464+57464	NH	NNR	PTR	NOR
156465	52465+57465	HT	NNR	ANG	NOR
156466	52466+57466	NH	NNR	PTR	NOR
156467	52467+57467	CK	SCR	ANG	ASR
156468	52468+57468	HT	NNR	ANG	NOR
156469	52469+57469	HT	NNR	ANG	NOR
156470	52470+57470	NM	EMR	PTR	EMR
156471	52471+57471	HT	NNR	ANG	NOR
156472	52472+57472	HT	NNR	ANG	NOR
156473	52473+57473	NM	EMR	PTR	EMR
156474	52474+57474	CK	SCR	ANG	ASR
156475	52475+57475	HT	NNR	ANG	NOR
156476	52476+57476	CK	SCR	ANG	ASR
156477	52477+57477	CK	SCR	ANG	ASR
156478	52478+57478	CK	SCR	BRO	ASR
156479	52479+57479	HT	NNR	ANG	NOR
156480	52480+57480	HT	SPL	ANG	NOR
156481	52481+57481	HT	NNR	ANG	NOR
156482	52482+57482	HT	NNR	ANG	NOR
156483	52483+57483	HT	NNR	ANG	NOR
156484	52484+57484	HT	NNR	ANG	NOR
156485	52485+57485	HT	NNR	ANG	NOR
156486	52486+57486	HT	NNR	ANG	NOR
156487	52487+57487	HT	NNR	ANG	NOR
156488	52488+57488	HT	NNR	ANG	NOR
156489	52489+57489	HT	NNR	ANG	NOR

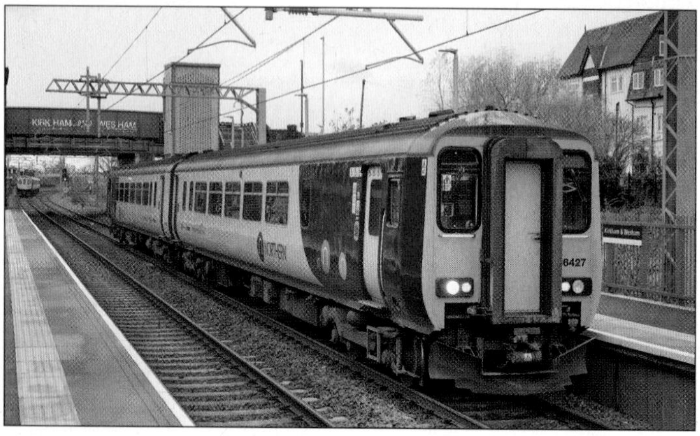

A fleet of 114 two-car Class 156 'Super Sprinter' sets were built by Metro-Cammell. Today these are allocated to East Midlands Railway, Northern and Scottish Railways. Painted in Northern white and blue, set No. 156427 is seen calling at Kirkham and Wesham in December 2021. **Antony Christie**

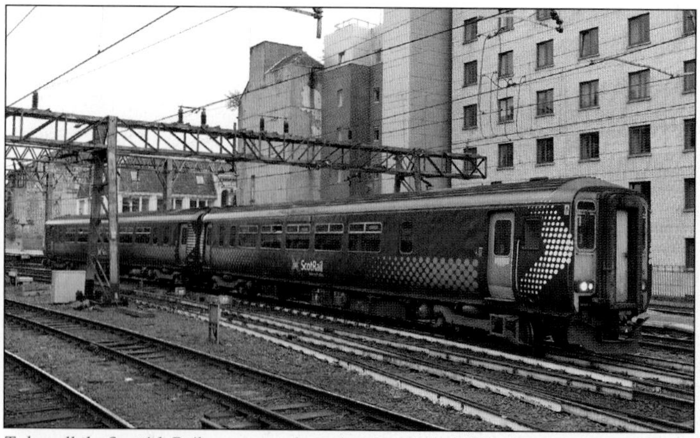

Today, all the Scottish Railway operated sets, based at Corkerhill depot are painted in the Scottish Railway blue and white Saltire livery, with contrasting mid-grey passenger doors. Set No. 156505 is seen at Glasgow Central. **CJM**

156490	52490+57490	HT	NNR	ANG	NOR
156491	52491+57491	HT	NNR	ANG	NOR
156492	52492+57492	CK	SCR	ANG	ASR
156493	52493+57493	CK	SCR	ANG	ASR
156494	52494+57494	CK	SCR	ANG	ASR
156495	52495+57495	CK	SCR	ANG	ASR
156496	52496+57496	HT	NNR	ANG	NOR
156497	52497+57497	NM	EMR	PTR	EMR
156498	52498+57498	NM	EMR	PTR	EMR
156499	52499+57499	CK	SRB	ANG	ASR
156500	52500+57500	CK	SCR	ANG	ASR
156501	52501+57501	CK	SCR	ANG	ASR
156502	52502+57502	CK	SCR	ANG	ASR
156503	52503+57503	CK	SCR	ANG	ASR
156504	52504+57504	CK	SCR	ANG	ASR
156505	52505+57505	CK	SCR	ANG	ASR
156506	52506+57506	CK	SCR	ANG	ASR
156507	52507+57507	CK	SCR	ANG	ASR
156508	52508+57508	CK	SCR	ANG	ASR
156509	52509+57509	CK	SCR	ANG	ASR
156510	52510+57510	CK	SCR	ANG	ASR
156511	52511+57511	CK	SCR	ANG	ASR
156512	52512+57512	CK	SCR	ANG	ASR
156513	52513+57513	CK	SCR	ANG	ASR
156514	52514+57514	CK	SCR	ANG	ASR

Class 158
BREL 2 or 3-car 'Express'

Built: 1990-1992
Vehicle length: 76ft 1¾in (23.20m)
Height: 12ft 6in (3.81m)
Width: 9ft 3¼in (2.82m)

Engine: 1 x Cummins NT855R5 per car
Horsepower: 350hp (260kW) per car§
Transmission: Hydraulic
§ 158863-872 engine set to 400hp (300kW)

Formation: DMSL(A)+DMSL(B) or DMSL+DMCL or DMSL+MS+DMSL

158701	52701+57701	IS	SCR	PTR	ASR
158702	52702+57702	IS	SCR	PTR	ASR
158703	52703+57703	IS	SCR	PTR	ASR
158704	52704+57704	IS	SCR	PTR	ASR
158705	52705+57705	IS	SCR	PTR	ASR
158706	52706+57706	IS	SCR	PTR	ASR
158707	52707+57707	IS	SCR	PTR	ASR
158708	52708+57708	IS	SCR	PTR	ASR
158709	52709+57709	IS	SCR	PTR	ASR
158710	52710+57710	IS	SCR	PTR	ASR
158711	52711+57711	IS	SCR	PTR	ASR
158712	52712+57712	IS	SCR	PTR	ASR
158713	52713+57713	IS	SCR	PTR	ASR
158714	52714+57714	IS	SCR	PTR	ASR
158715	52715+57715	IS	SCR	PTR	ASR
158716	52716+57716	IS	SCR	PTR	ASR
158717	52717+57717	IS	SCR	PTR	ASR
158718	52718+57718	IS	SCR	PTR	ASR
158719	52719+57719	IS	SCR	PTR	ASR
158720	52720+57720	IS	SCR	PTR	ASR
158721	52721+57721	IS	SCR	PTR	ASR
158722	52722+57722	IS	SCR	PTR	ASR
158723	52723+57723	IS	SCR	PTR	ASR
158724	52724+57724	IS	SCR	PTR	ASR
158725	52725+57725	IS	SCR	PTR	ASR
158726	52726+57726	CK	SCR	PTR	ASR
158727	52727+57727	IS	SCR	PTR	ASR
158728	52728+57728	IS	SCR	PTR	ASR
158729	52729+57729	CK	SCR	PTR	ASR
158730	52730+57730	CK	SCR	PTR	ASR
158731	52731+57731	CK	SCR	PTR	ASR
158732	52732+57732	CK	SCR	PTR	ASR
158733	52733+57733	CK	SCR	PTR	ASR
158734	52734+57734	CK	SCR	PTR	ASR
158735	52735+57735	CK	SCR	PTR	ASR
158736	52736+57736	CK	SCR	PTR	ASR
158737	52737+57737	CK	SCR	PTR	ASR
158738	52738+57738	CK	SCR	PTR	ASR

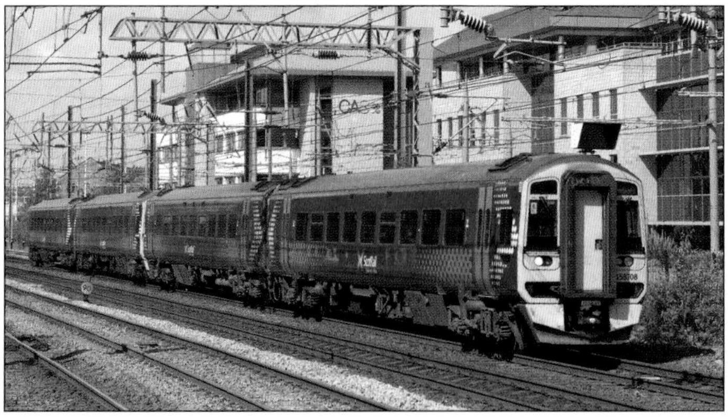

One of the most numerous modern DMU types is the Class 158 'Express' unit, first introduced in 1990 for use in Scotland. Set No. 158708 in Scottish Railways livery is illustrated approaching Edinburgh Haymarket in June 2021. The Scottish sets sport a slightly revised front end and plough style. **CJM**

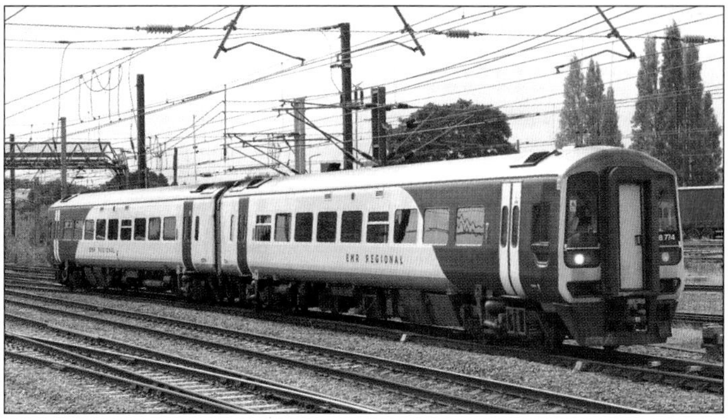

For longer distance East Midlands Railway Regional services a fleet of Class 158 two-car sets are based at Nottingham Eastcroft. These are progressively appearing in EMR purple and white livery with EMR Regional branding. Set No. 158774 is seen at Doncaster with a service from Lincoln. **CJM**

158739	52739+57739	CK	SCR	PTR	ASR
158740	52740+57740	CK	SCR	PTR	ASR
158741	52741+57741	CK	SCR	PTR	ASR
158745	52745+57745	PM	GWR	PTR	GWR
158747	52747+57747	PM	GWR	PTR	GWR
158749	52749+57749	PM	GWG	PTR	GWR
158750	52750+57750	PM	GWG	PTR	GWR
158752	52752+58716+57752	NL	NNR	PTR	NOR
158753	52753+58710+57753	NL	NNR	PTR	NOR
158754	52754+58708+57754	NL	NNR	PTR	NOR
158755	52755+58702+57755	NL	NNR	PTR	NOR
158756	52756+58712+57756	NL	NNR	PTR	NOR
158757	52757+58706+57757	NL	NNR	PTR	NOR
158758	52758+58714+57758	NL	NNR	PTR	NOR
158759	52759+58713+57759	NL	NNR	PTR	NOR
158760	52760+57760	PM	GWG	PTR	GWR
158762	52762+57762	PM	GWG	PTR	GWR
158763(S)	52763+57763	LM	GWG	PTR	-
158765	52765+57765	PM	GWG	PTR	GWR
158766	52766+57766	PM	GWG	PTR	GWR
158767	52767+57767	PM	GWG	PTR	GWR
158769	52769+57769	PM	GWG	PTR	GWR
158770	52770+57770	NM	SCE	PTR	EMR
158773	52773+57773	NM	EMI	PTR	EMR
158774	52774+57774	NM	EMI	PTR	EMR
158777	52777+57777	NM	SCE	PTR	EMR
158780	52780+57780	NM	SCE	ANG	EMR
158782	52782+57782	NL	NNR	ANG	NOR
158783	52783+57783	NM	SCE	ANG	EMR
158784	52784+57784	NL	NNR	ANG	NOR
158785	52785+57785	NM	SCE	ANG	EMR
158786	52786+57786	NL	NNR	ANG	NOR
158787	52787+57787	NL	NNR	ANG	NOR
158788	52788+57788	NM	SCE	ANG	EMR
158789	52789+57789	NL	NNR	ANG	NOR
158790	52790+57790	NL	NNR	ANG	NOR
158791	52791+57791	NL	NNR	ANG	NOR
158792	52792+57792	HT	NNR	ANG	NOR
158793	52793+57793	NL	NNR	ANG	NOR
158794	52794+57794	NL	NNR	ANG	NOR
158795	52795+57795	NL	NNR	ANG	NOR
158796	52796+57796	NL	NNR	ANG	NOR
158797	52797+57797	NL	NNR	ANG	NOR
158798	52798+58715+57798	PM	GWG	PTR	GWR
158799	52799+57799	NM	SCE	PTR	EMR
158806	52806+57806	NM	SCE	PTR	EMR
158810	52810+57810	NM	SCE	PTR	EMR
158812	52812+57812	NM	SCE	PTR	EMR
158813	52813+57813	NM	SCE	PTR	EMR
158815	52815+57815	HT	NNR	ANG	NOR
158816	52816+57816	HT	NNR	ANG	NOR
158817	52817+57817	HT	NNR	ANG	NOR
158818	52818+57818	MN	TFW	ANG	TFW
158819	52819+57819	MN	TFW	ANG	TFW
158820	52820+57820	MN	TFW	ANG	TFW
158821	52821+57821	MN	TFW	ANG	TFW
158822	52822+57822	MN	TFW	ANG	TFW
158823	52823+57823	MN	TFW	ANG	TFW
158824	52824+57824	MN	TFW	ANG	TFW
158825	52825+57825	MN	TFW	ANG	TFW
158826	52826+57826	MN	TFW	ANG	TFW
158827	52827+57827	MN	TFW	ANG	TFW
158828	52828+57828	MN	TFW	ANG	TFW
158829	52829+57829	MN	TFW	ANG	TFW
158830	52830+57830	MN	TFW	ANG	TFW
158831	52831+57831	MN	TFW	ANG	TFW
158832	52832+57832	MN	TFW	ANG	TFW
158833	52833+57833	MN	TFW	ANG	TFW
158834	52834+57834	MN	TFW	ANG	TFW
158835	52835+57835	MN	TFW	ANG	TFW
158836	52836+57836	MN	TFW	ANG	TFW
158837	52837+57837	MN	TFW	ANG	TFW
158838	52838+57838	MN	TFW	ANG	TFW
158839	52839+57839	MN	TFW	ANG	TFW
158840	52840+57840	MN	TFW	ANG	TFW
158841	52841+57841	MN	TFW	ANG	TFW
158842	52842+57842	HT	NNR	ANG	NOR
158843	52843+57843	HT	NNR	ANG	NOR
158844	52844+57844	HT	NNR	ANG	NOR
158845	52845+57845	HT	NNR	ANG	NOR
158846	52846+57846	NM	SCE	ANG	EMR
158847	52847+57847	NM	SCE	ANG	EMR
158848	52848+57848	HT	NNR	ANG	NOR
158849	52849+57849	HT	NNR	ANG	NOR
158850	52850+57850	HT	NNR	ANG	NOR
158851	52851+57851	HT	NNR	ANG	NOR
158852	52852+57852	NM	SCE	ANG	EMR
158853	52853+57853	HT	NNR	ANG	NOR
158854	52854+57854	NM	SCE	ANG	EMR
158855	52855+57855	HT	NNR	ANG	NOR
158856	52856+57856	NM	SCE	ANG	EMR
158857	52857+57857	NM	SCE	ANG	EMR
158858	52858+57858	NM	SCE	ANG	EMR
158859	52859+57859	HT	NNR	ANG	NOR
158860	52860+57860	HT	NNR	ANG	NOR
158861	52861+57861	HT	NNR	ANG	NOR
158862	52862+57862	NM	SCE	ANG	EMR
158863	52863+57863	NM	SCE	ANG	EMR
158864	52864+57864	NM	SCE	ANG	EMR
158865	52865+57865	NM	SCE	ANG	EMR
158866	52866+57866	NM	SCE	ANG	EMR
158867	52867+57867	NL	NNR	ANG	NOR
158868	52868+57868	NL	NNR	ANG	NOR
158869	52869+57869	NL	NNR	ANG	NOR
158870	52870+57870	NL	NNR	ANG	NOR
158871	52871+57871	NL	NNR	ANG	NOR
158872	52872+57872	NL	NNR	ANG	NOR
158880 (158737)	52737+57737	SA	SWN	PTR	SWR
158881 (158742)	52742+57742	SA	SWN	PTR	SWR
158882 (158743)	52743+57743	SA	SWN	PTR	SWR
158883 (158744)	52744+57744	SA	SWN	PTR	SWR
158884 (158772)	52772+57772	SA	SWN	PTR	SWR
158885 (158775)	52775+57775	SA	SWN	PTR	SWR
158886 (158779)	52779+57779	SA	SWN	PTR	SWR
158887 (158781)	52781+57781	SA	SWR	PTR	SWR
158888 (158802)	52802+57802	SA	SWR	PTR	SWR
158889 (158808)	52808+57808	NM	EMR	PTR	EMR
158890 (158814)	52814+57814	SA	SWR	PTR	SWR
158901	52901+57901	NL	NNR	EVL	NOR
158902	52902+57902	NL	NNR	EVL	NOR
158903	52903+57903	NL	NNR	EVL	NOR
158904	52904+57904	NL	NNR	EVL	NOR
158905	52905+57905	NL	NNR	EVL	NOR

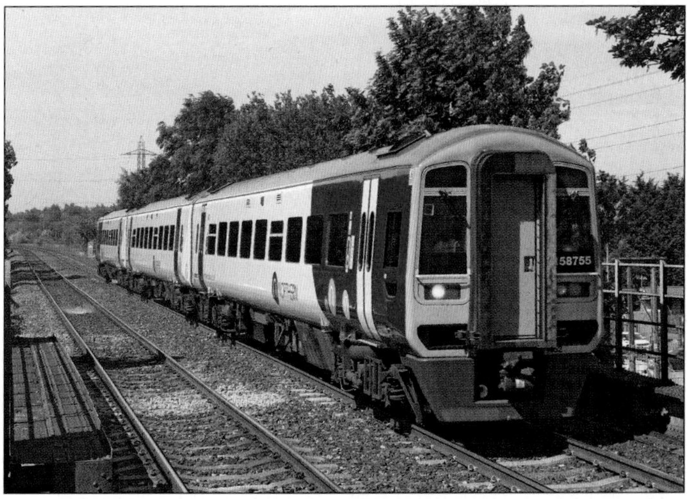

Northern operate a fleet of two and fixed three-car sets, with an intermediate Motor Standard. Sets are based at both Leeds Neville Hill and Newcastle Heaton depots and sport the standard Northern white livery. Three-car set No. 158755 is shown. **CJM**

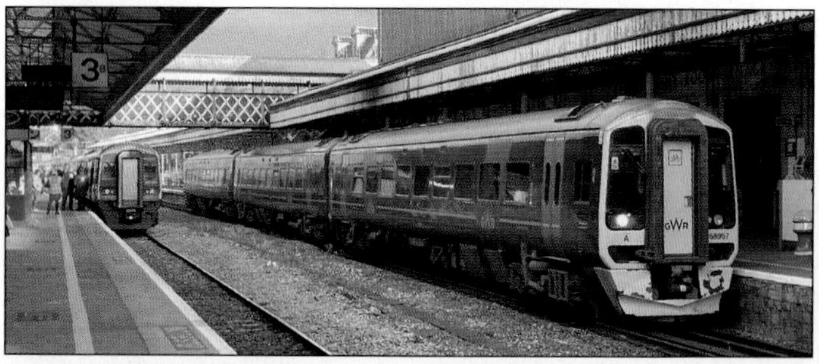

Great Western operate a fleet of two and three-car Class 158s. All but one of the three-car sets are formed of three driving cars, one fixed three-car set is also on the roster. The three-car sets are based a St Philips Marsh and the two-car sets at Exeter. No. 158957 is shown. **CJM**

158906	52906+57906	NL	NNR	EVL	NOR
158907	52907+57907	NL	NNR	EVL	NOR
158908	52908+57908	NL	NNR	EVL	NOR
158909	52909+57909	NL	NNR	EVL	NOR
158910	52910+57910	NL	NNR	EVL	NOR
158950 (158761/751)	57751+52761+57761	EX	GWG	PTR	GWR
158951 (158764/751)	52751+52764+57764	EX	GWG	PTR	GWR
158956 (158748/768)	57748+52768+57768	EX	GWG	PTR	GWR
158957 (158748/771)	52748+52771+57771	EX	GWG	PTR	GWR
158958 (158746/776)	57746+52776+57776	EX	GWG	PTR	GWR
158959 (158746/778)	52746+52778+57778	EX	GWG	PTR	GWR

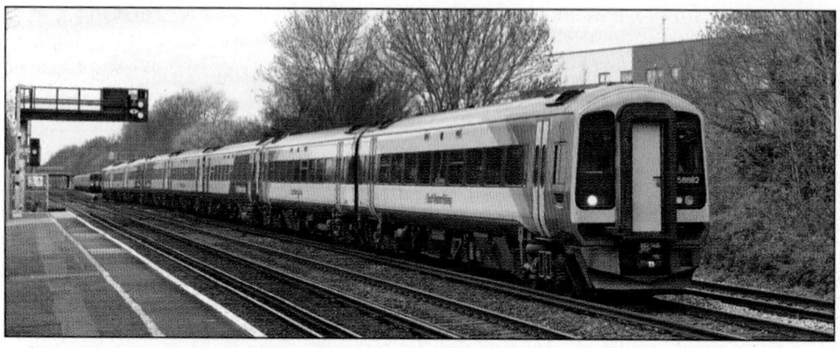

Salisbury depot of South Western Railway is home to 11 two-car sets Nos 158880-158890, used to strengthen Class 159 formed services and work non-electrified routes. Painted in the old Stagecoach-style livery with SWR branding, No. 158992 passes Raynes Park. **CJM**

Class 159
BREL 3-car 'Express'

Built: 159/0 - 1992-1993, 159/1 2006
Vehicle length: 76ft 1¾in (23.20m)
Height: 12ft 6in (3.81m)
Width: 9ft 3¼in (2.82m)
Engine: 1 x Cummins NT855R5 per car
Horsepower: 159/0 - 400hp (300kW)
159/1 - 350hp (260kW) per car
Transmission: Hydraulic

159/0 Formation: DMCL+MSL+DMSL

159001	52873+58718+57873	SA	SWR	PTR	SWR
159002	52874+58719+57874	SA	SWR	PTR	SWR
159003	52875+58720+57875	SA	SWR	PTR	SWR
159004	52876+58721+57876	SA	SWR	PTR	SWR
159005	52877+58722+57877	SA	SWR	PTR	SWR
159006	52878+58723+57878	SA	SWR	PTR	SWR
159007	52879+58724+57879	SA	SWR	PTR	SWR
159008	52880+58725+57880	SA	SWR	PTR	SWR
159009	52881+58726+57881	SA	SWR	PTR	SWR
159010	52882+58727+57882	SA	SWR	PTR	SWR
159011	52883+58728+57883	SA	SWR	PTR	SWR
159012	52884+58729+57884	SA	SWR	PTR	SWR
159013	52885+58730+57885	SA	SWR	PTR	SWR
159014	52886+58731+57886	SA	SWR	PTR	SWR
159015	52887+58732+57887	SA	SWR	PTR	SWR
159016	52888+58733+57888	SA	SWR	PTR	SWR
159017	52889+58734+57889	SA	SWR	PTR	SWR
159018	52890+58735+57890	SA	SWR	PTR	SWR
159019	52891+58736+57891	SA	SWR	PTR	SWR
159020	52892+58737+57892	SA	SWR	PTR	SWR
159021	52893+58738+57893	SA	SWR	PTR	SWR
159022	52894+58739+57894	SA	SWR	PTR	SWR

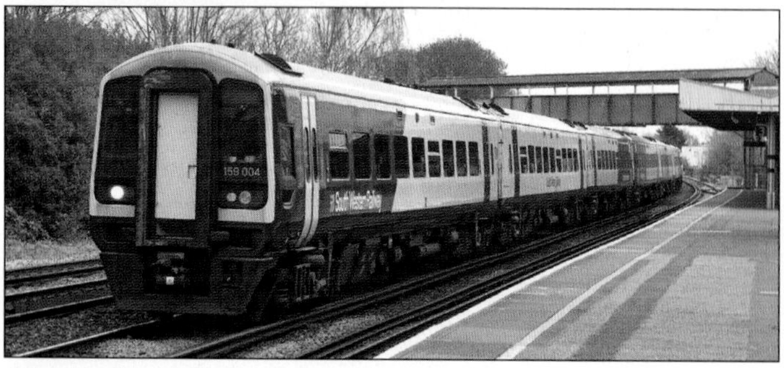

A fleet of 22 three-car Class 159/0s are based at Salisbury for use on the Waterloo-Exeter route, all members carry the new South Western Railway grey and blue livery with lemon ends. Set No. 159004 heads west at Raynes Park in May 2021. **CJM**

159/1 Formation: DMCL+MSL+DMSL

159101 (158800)	52800+58717+57800	SA	SWN	PTR	SWR
159102 (158803)(S)	52803+58703+57803	LM	SWN	PTR	-
159103 (158804)	52804+58704+57804	SA	SWN	PTR	SWR
159104 (158805)	52805+58705+57805	SA	SWN	PTR	SWR
159105 (158807)	52807+58707+57807	SA	SWN	PTR	SWR
159106 (158809)	52809+58709+57809	SA	SWN	PTR	SWR
159107 (158811)	52811+58711+57811	SA	SWN	PTR	SWR
159108 (158801)	52801+58701+57801	SA	SWN	PTR	SWR

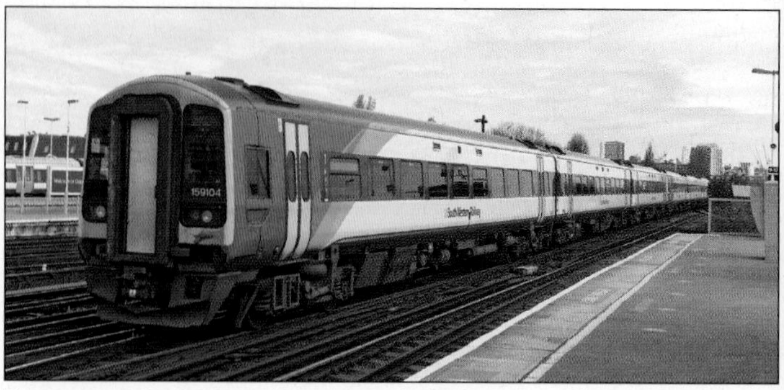

The seven operational Class 159/1s, operating alongside the Class 159/0s carry the older Stagecoach based swirl livery with South Western Railway branding. Set No. 159102 was seriously damaged in a collision and derailment at Salisbury Tunnel Junction on 31 October 2021 and is stored at Long Marston and is unlikely to be repaired. No. 159104 is seen at Clapham Junction. **CJM**

Class 165
BREL 2 and 3-car 'Networker Turbo'

Built: 1990-1993
Vehicle length: Driving - 75ft 2½in (22.92m)
Intermediate - 74ft 6½in (22.72m
Height: 12ft 5¼in (3.79m)
Width: 9ft 2½in (2.81m)
Engine: 1 x Perkins 2006THW per car
Horsepower: 350hp (260kW)
Transmission: Hydraulic

165/0 Formation: DMSL+DMS or DMSL+MS+DMS Trip-Cock fitted

165001	58801+58834	AL	CRW	ANG	CRW
165002	58802+58835	AL	CRW	ANG	CRW
165003	58803+58836	AL	CRW	ANG	CRW
165004§	58804+58837	AL	CRW	ANG	CRW
165005	58805+58838	AL	CRW	ANG	CRW
165006	58806+58839	AL	CRW	ANG	CRW
165007	58807+58840	AL	CRW	ANG	CRW
165008	58808+58841	AL	CRW	ANG	CRW
165009	58809+58842	AL	CRW	ANG	CRW
165010	58810+58843	AL	CRW	ANG	CRW
165011	58811+58844	AL	CRW	ANG	CRW
165012	58812+58845	AL	CRW	ANG	CRW
165013	58813+58846	AL	CRW	ANG	CRW
165014	58814+58847	AL	CRW	ANG	CRW
165015	58815+58848	AL	CRW	ANG	CRW
165016	58816+58849	AL	CRW	ANG	CRW
165017	58817+58850	AL	CRW	ANG	CRW
165018	58818+58851	AL	CRW	ANG	CRW
165019	58819+58852	AL	CRW	ANG	CRW
165020	58820+58853	AL	CRW	ANG	CRW
165021	58821+58854	AL	CRW	ANG	CRW
165022	58822+58855	AL	CRW	ANG	CRW
165023	58873+58867	AL	CRW	ANG	CRW
165024	58874+58868	AL	CRW	ANG	CRW
165025	58875+58869	AL	CRW	ANG	CRW
165026	58876+58870	AL	CRW	ANG	CRW
165027	58877+58871	AL	CRW	ANG	CRW
165028	58878+58872	AL	CRW	ANG	CRW
165029	58823+55404+58856	AL	CRW	ANG	CRW
165030	58824+55405+58857	AL	CRW	ANG	CRW
165031	58825+55406+58858	AL	CRW	ANG	CRW
165032	58826+55407+58859	AL	CRW	ANG	CRW
165033	58827+55408+58860	AL	CRW	ANG	CRW
165034	58828+55409+58861	AL	CRW	ANG	CRW
165035	58829+55410+58862	AL	CRW	ANG	CRW
165036	58830+55411+58863	AL	CRW	ANG	CRW
165037	58831+55412+58864	AL	CRW	ANG	CRW
165038	58832+55413+58865	AL	CRW	ANG	CRW
165039	58833+55414+58866	AL	CRW	ANG	CRW

§ 165004 fitted with Magtec HyDrive battery / diesel system

165/1 Formation: DMSL+MS+DMS or DMSL+DMS

165101	58953+55415+58916	PM	GWG	ANG	GWR
165102	58954+55416+58917	RG	GWG	ANG	GWR
165103	58955+55417+58918	RG	GWG	ANG	GWR
165104	58956+55418+58919	RG	GWG	ANG	GWR
165105	58957+55419+58920	RG	GWG	ANG	GWR
165106	58958+55420+58921	RG	GWG	ANG	GWR
165107	58959+55421+58922	RG	GWG	ANG	GWR
165108	58960+55422+58923	RG	GWG	ANG	GWR
165109	58961+55423+58924	RG	GWG	ANG	GWR
165110	58962+55424+58925	RG	GWG	ANG	GWR
165111	58963+55425+58926	RG	GWG	ANG	GWR
165112	58964+55426+58927	PM	GWG	ANG	GWR
165113	58965+55427+58928	RG	GWG	ANG	GWR
165114	58966+55428+58929	RG	GWG	ANG	GWR

165116	58968+55430+58931	RG	GWG	ANG	GWR
165117	58969+55431+58932	RG	GWG	ANG	GWR
165118	58879+58933	RG	GWG	ANG	GWR
165119	58880+58934	RG	GWG	ANG	GWR
165120	58881+58935	RG	GWG	ANG	GWR
165121	58882+58936	RG	GWG	ANG	GWR
165122	58883+58937	RG	GWG	ANG	GWR
165123	58884+58938	RG	GWG	ANG	GWR
165124	58885+58939	RG	GWG	ANG	GWR
165125	58886+58940	RG	GWG	ANG	GWR
165126	58887+58941	RG	GWG	ANG	GWR
165127	58888+58942	RG	GWG	ANG	GWR
165128	58889+58943	PM	GWG	ANG	GWR
165129	58890+58944	PM	GWG	ANG	GWR
165130	58891+58945	PM	GWG	ANG	GWR
165131	58892+58946	RG	GWG	ANG	GWR
165132	58893+58947	PM	GWG	ANG	GWR
165133	58894+58948	PM	GWG	ANG	GWR
165134	58895+58949	PM	GWG	ANG	GWR
165135	58896+58950	PM	GWG	ANG	GWR
165136	58897+58951	PM	GWG	ANG	GWR
165137	58898+58952	PM	GWG	ANG	GWR

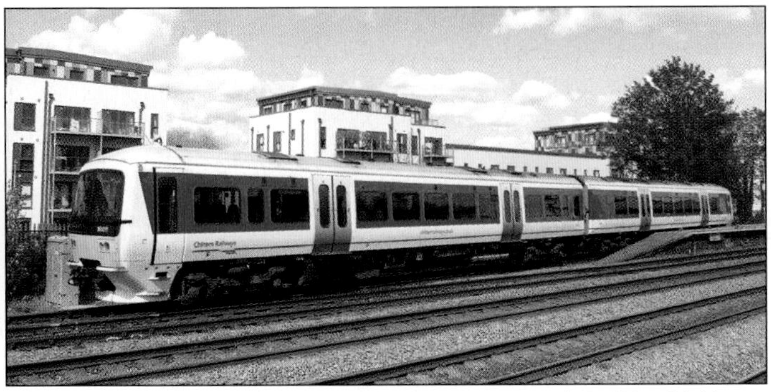

Chiltern Railways Class 159 fleet of two and three-car sets are now air conditioned (with no opening windows) and have a smooth front. Sets based at Aylesbury carry white and blue local livery, No. 165011 departs from Leamington Spa. **CJM**

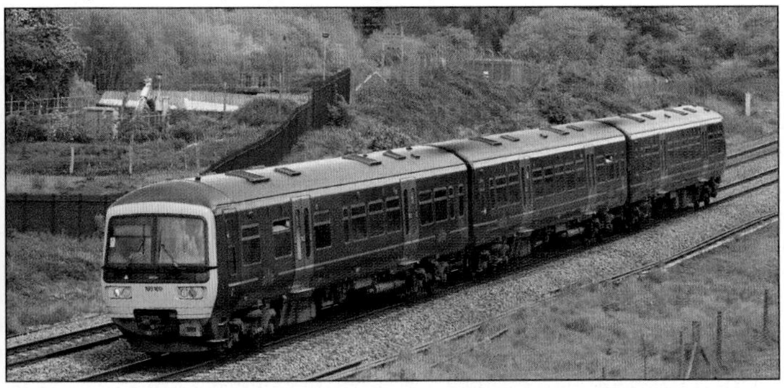

Great Western Railway-operated two and three-car Class 165s still sport opening top windows and the earlier style front end. The fleet based at Reading/St Philips Marsh operate in the Thames Valley, Avon and Exeter areas. Three-car set No. 165109 is recorded passing Hungerford on a Reading to Bedwyn service. **CJM**

Class 166
BREL 3-car 'Networker Turbo Express'

Built: 1992-1993
Vehicle length: Driving - 75ft 2½in (22.92m)
Intermediate - 74ft 6½in (22.72m
Height: 12ft 5¼in (3.79m)
Width: 9ft 2½in (2.81m)
Engine: 1 x Perkins 2006THW per car
Horsepower: 350hp (260kW)
Transmission: Hydraulic

Formation: DMSL+MS+DMS

166201	58101+58601+58122		PM	FGB	ANG	GWR
166202	58102+58602+58123		PM	FGB	ANG	GWR
166203	58103+58603+58124		PM	FGB	ANG	GWR
166204	58104+58604+58125	*Norman Topsom MBE*	PM	GWG	ANG	GWR
166205	58105+58605+58126		PM	GWG	ANG	GWR
166206	58106+58606+58127		PM	GWG	ANG	GWR
166207	58107+58607+58128		PM	FGB	ANG	GWR
166208	58108+58608+58129		PM	GWG	ANG	GWR
166209	58109+58609+58130		PM	FGB	ANG	GWR
166210	58110+58610+58131		PM	GWG	ANG	GWR
166211	58111+58611+58132		PM	FGB	ANG	GWR
166212	58112+58612+58133		PM	GWG	ANG	GWR
166213	58113+58613+58134		PM	GWG	ANG	GWR
166214	58114+58614+58135		PM	GWG	ANG	GWR
166215	58115+58615+58136		PM	FGB	ANG	GWR
166216	58116+58616+58137		PM	GWG	ANG	GWR
166217	58117+58617+58138		PM	GWG	ANG	GWR
166218	58118+58618+58139		PM	GWG	ANG	GWR
166219	58119+58619+58140		PM	GWG	ANG	GWR
166220	58120+58620+58141	*Roger Watkins - The GWR Master Train Planner*	PM	GWG	ANG	GWR
166221	58121+58621+58142	*Reading Train Care Depot*	PM	FGB	ANG	GWR

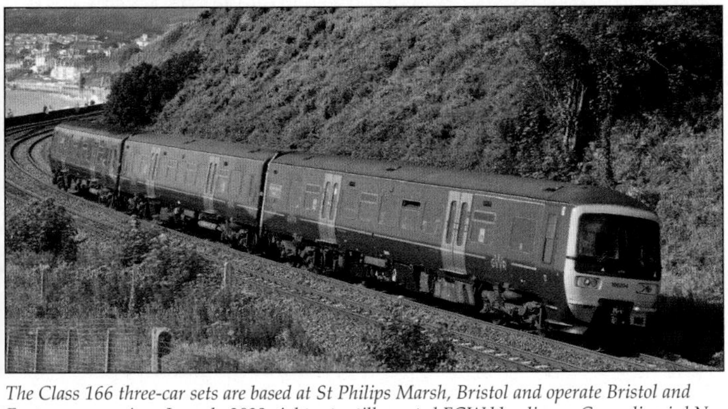

The Class 166 three-car sets are based at St Philips Marsh, Bristol and operate Bristol and Exeter area services. In early 2022 eight sets still sported FGW blue livery. Green-liveried No. 166204 Norman Topsom MBE *is seen approaching Dawlish Warren.* **CJM**

Class 168
BREL 3 and 4-car 'Clubman'

Built: 1997-2006
Vehicle length: Driving - 75ft 2½in (22.92m)
Intermediate - 74ft 6½in (22.72m
Height: 12ft 5¼in (3.79m)
Width: 9ft 2½in (2.81m)
Engine: 1 x Perkins 2006THW per car
Horsepower: 350hp (260kW)
Transmission: Hydraulic

168/0 Formation: DMSL+MS+MS+DM Trip-Cock fitted

168001	58151+58651+58451+58251	AL	CRG	PTR	CRW
168002	58152+58652+58452+58252	AL	CRG	PTR	CRW
168003	58153+58653+58453+58253	AL	CRG	PTR	CRW
168004	58154+58654+58454+58254	AL	CRG	PTR	CRW
168005	58155+58655+58455+58255	AL	CRG	PTR	CRW

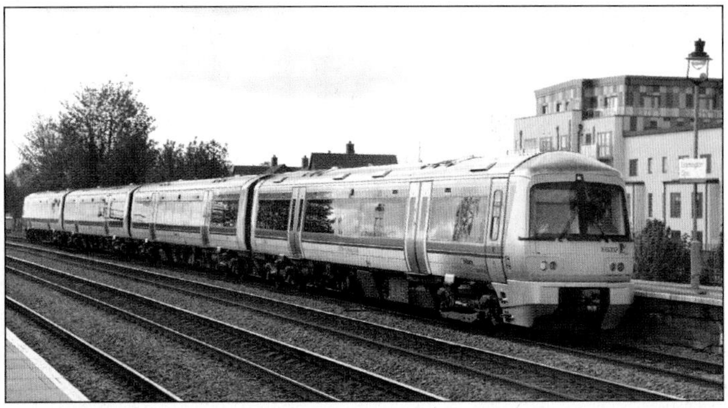

Chiltern Railways operate the original five of the 'Turbostar' DMUs, known as Clubman sets These have a different body profile to the later standard 'Turbostar' design. Set No. 168002 is seen arriving at Leamington Spa with a Birmingham to Marylebone service in May 2021. All Chiltern Class 168s are fitted with trip cocks. **CJM**

168/1 Formation: DMSL+MS+MS+DMS or DMSL+MS(L)+DMS Trip-Cock fitted

168106	58156+58756+58456+58256	AL	CRG	PTR	CRW
168107	58157+58457+58757+58257	AL	CRG	PTR	CRW
168108	58158+58458+58258	AL	CRG	PTR	CRW
168109	58159+58459+58259	AL	CRG	PTR	CRW
168110	58160+58460+58260	AL	CRG	PTR	CRW
168111	58161+58461+58261	AL	CRG	EVL	CRW
168112	58162+58462+58262	AL	CRG	EVL	CRW
168113	58163+58463+58263	AL	CRG	EVL	CRW

168/2 Formation: DMSL+MS+MS+DMS or DMSL+MS(L)+DMS Trip-Cock fitted

168214	58164+58464+58264	AL	CRG	PTR	CRW
168215	58165+58465+58365+58265	AL	CRG	PTR	CRW
168216	58166+58466+58366+58266	AL	CRG	PTR	CRW
168217	58167+58467+58367+58267	AL	CRG	PTR	CRW
168218	58168+58468+58268	AL	CRG	PTR	CRW
168219	58169+58469+58269	AL	CRG	PTR	CRW

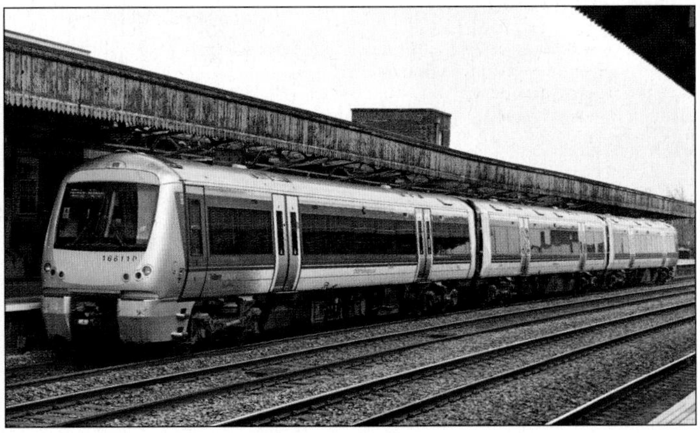

Members of Class 168/1, 168/2 and 168/3 have the standard Turbostar body style, as shown on set No. 168110 at Leamington Spa. Sets come in a mix of two, three and four-car formations. **CJM**

168/3	Formation: DMSL+DMSL Trip-Cock fitted					
168321	(170301)	50301+79301	AL	CRG	PTR	CRW
168322	(170302)	50302+79302	AL	CRG	PTR	CRW
168323	(170303)	50303+79303	AL	CRG	PTR	CRW
168324	(170304)	50304+79304	AL	CRG	PTR	CRW
168325	(170305)	50305+79305	AL	CRG	PTR	CRW
168326	(170306)	50306+79306	AL	CRG	PTR	CRW
168327	(170307)	50307+79307	AL	CRG	PTR	CRW
168328	(170308)	50308+79308	AL	CRG	PTR	CRW
168329	(170309, 170399)	50399+79399	AL	SPL	PTR	CRW

168329 fitted with HybridFLEX diesel/battery system

§ 58461 was originally 58661, 58462 was originally 58662, 58463 was originally 58663

* Carries NHS/Key Workers branding

Class 170

AdTranz/Bombardier 2 and 3-car 'Turbostar'

Built: 1998-2005
Vehicle length: 76ft 6in (23.62m)
Height: 12ft 4½in (3.77m)
Width: 8ft 10in (2.69m)
Engine: 1 x MTU 6R 183TD 13H per car
Horsepower: 422hp (315kW)
Transmission: Hydraulic

170/1	Formation: DMSL+MS+DMCL or DMSL+DMCL				
170101	50101+55101+79101	TS	AXC	PTR	AXC
170102	50102+55102+79102	TS	AXC	PTR	AXC
170103	50103+55103+79103	TS	AXC	PTR	AXC
170104	50104+55104+79104	TS	AXC	PTR	AXC
170105	50105+55105+79105	TS	AXC	PTR	AXC
170106	50106+55106+79106	TS	AXC	PTR	AXC
170107	50107+55107+79107	TS	AXC	PTR	AXC
170108	50108+55108+79108	TS	AXC	PTR	AXC
170109	50109+55109+79109	TS	AXC	PTR	AXC
170110	50110+55110+79110	TS	AXC	PTR	AXC
170111	50111+79111	TS	AXC	PTR	AXC
170112	50112+79112	TS	AXC	PTR	AXC
170113	50113+79113	TS	AXC	PTR	AXC
170114	50114+79114	TS	AXC	PTR	AXC
170115	50115+79115	TS	AXC	PTR	AXC
170116	50116+79116	TS	AXC	PTR	AXC
170117	50117+79117	TS	AXC	PTR	AXC

170/2	Formation: DMSL+MS+DMSL or DMSL+DMSL				
170201	50201+56201+79201	CV	TFW	PTR	TFW
170202	50202+56202+79202	CV	TFW	PTR	TFW
170203	50203+56203+79203	CV	TFW	PTR	TFW
170204	50204+56204+79204	CV	TFW	PTR	TFW
170205	50205+56205+79205	CV	TFW	PTR	TFW
170206	50206+56206+79206	CV	TFW	PTR	TFW
170207	50207+56207+79207	CV	TFW	PTR	TFW
170208	50208+56208+79208	CV	TFW	PTR	TFW
170270	50270+79270	CV	TFW	PTR	TFW
170271	50271+79271	CV	TFW	PTR	TFW
170272	50272+79272	CV	TFW	PTR	TFW
170273	50273+79273	NM	EMP	PTR	EMR

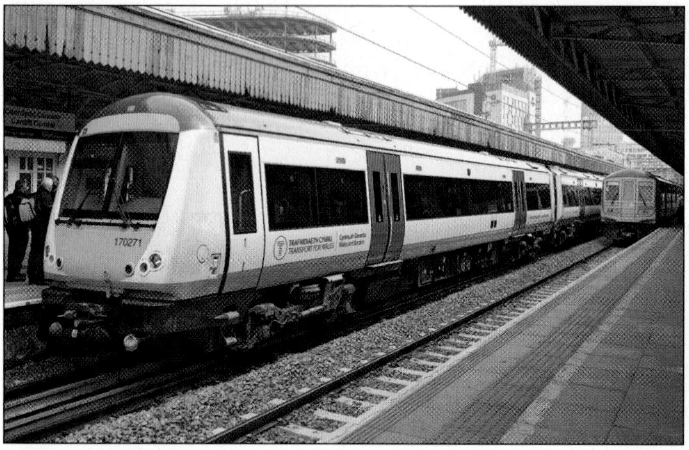

In spring 2022, 11 members of the Class 170/2 fleet were based at Cardiff and operated by Transport for Wales, but as new stock is delivered the sets will transfer to East Midlands Railway. Two-car set No. 170271 is seen at Cardiff in April 2021. **CJM**

170/3	Formation: DMSL+MS+DMSL or DMSL+MS+DMCL				
170393	50393+56393+79393	HA	SCR	PTR	ASR
170394	50394+56394+79394	HA	SCR	PTR	ASR
170395	50395+56395+79395	HA	SCR	PTR	ASR
170396	50396+56396+79396	HA	SCR	PTR	ASR
170397	50397+56397+79397	TS	AXC	PTR	AXC
170398	50398+56398+79398	TS	AXC	PTR	AXC

170/4	Formation: DMCL+MS+DMCL or DMSL+MS+DMSL					
170401	50401+56401+79401		HA	SCR	PTR	ASR
170402	50402+56402+79402		HA	SCR	PTR	ASR
170403	50403+56403+79403		HA	SCR	PTR	ASR
170404	50404+56404+79404		HA	SCR	PTR	ASR
170405	50405+56405+79405		HA	SCR	PTR	ASR
170406	50406+56406+79406		HA	SCR	PTR	ASR
170407	50407+56407+79407		HA	SCR	PTR	ASR
170408	50408+56408+79408		HA	SCR	PTR	ASR
170409	50409+56409+79409		HA	SCR	PTR	ASR
170410	50410+56410+79410		HA	SCR	PTR	ASR
170411	50411+56411+79411		HA	SCR	PTR	ASR
170412	50412+56412+79412		HA	SCR	PTR	ASR
170413	50413+56413+79413		HA	SCR	PTR	ASR
170414	50414+56414+79414		HA	SCR	PTR	ASR
170415	50415+56415+79415		HA	SCR	PTR	ASR
170416	50416+56416+79416		DY	EMP	EVL	EMR
170417	50417+56417+79417	*The Key Worker*	DY	EMP	EVL	EMR
170418	50418+56418+79418		DY	EMP	EVL	EMR
170419	50419+56419+79419		DY	EMP	EVL	EMR
170420	50420+56420+79420		DY	EMP	EVL	EMR
170425	50425+56425+79425		HA	SCR	PTR	ASR
170426	50426+56426+79426		HA	SCR	PTR	ASR
170427	50427+56427+79427		HA	SCR	PTR	ASR
170428	50428+56428+79428		HA	SCR	PTR	ASR
170429	50429+56429+79429		HA	SCR	PTR	ASR
170430	50430+56430+79430		HA	SCR	PTR	ASR
170431	50431+56431+79431		HA	SCR	PTR	ASR
170432	50432+56432+79432		HA	SCR	PTR	ASR
170433	50433+56433+79433		HA	SCR	PTR	ASR
170434	50434+56434+79434		HA	SCR	PTR	ASR
170450	50450+56450+79450		HA	SCR	PTR	ASR
170451	50451+56451+79451		HA	SCR	PTR	ASR
170452	50452+56452+79452		HA	SCR	PTR	ASR
170453	50453+56453+79453		NL	NNR	PTR	NOR
170454	50454+56454+79454		NL	NNR	PTR	NOR
170455	50455+56455+79455		NL	NNR	PTR	NOR
170456	50456+56456+79456		NL	NNR	PTR	NOR
170457	50457+56457+79457		NL	NNR	PTR	NOR
170458	50458+56458+79458		NL	NNR	PTR	NOR
170459	50459+56459+79459		NL	NNR	PTR	NOR
170460	50460+56460+79460		NL	NNR	PTR	NOR
170461	50461+56461+79461		NL	NNR	PTR	NOR
170470	50470+56470+79470		NL	NNR	PTR	NOR
170471	50471+56471+79471		NL	NNR	PTR	NOR
170472	50472+56472+79472		NL	NNR	PTR	NOR
170473	50473+56473+79473		NL	NNR	PTR	NOR
170474	50474+56474+79474		NL	NNR	PTR	NOR
170475	50475+56475+79475		NL	NNR	PTR	NOR
170476	50476+56476+79476		NL	NNR	PTR	NOR
170477	50477+56477+79477		NL	NNR	PTR	NOR
170478	50478+56478+79478		NL	NNR	PTR	NOR

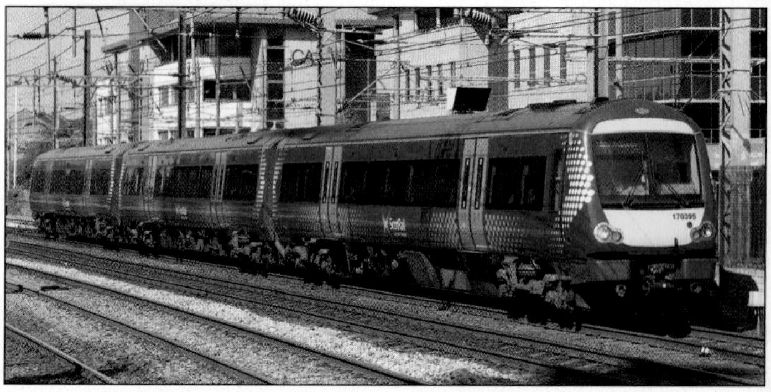

In spring 2022, 32 three-car Class 170s were operated by Scottish Railways, based at Haymarket depot in Edinburgh. In the main the fleet sports the blue/white Saltire colours as shown on set No. 170395 approaching Edinburgh Haymarket in June 2021. **CJM**

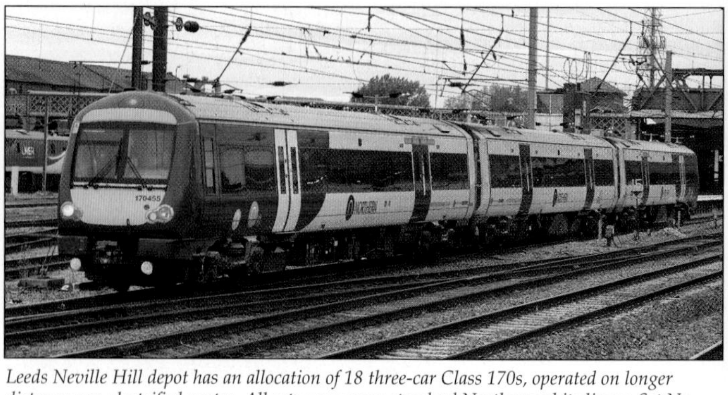

Leeds Neville Hill depot has an allocation of 18 three-car Class 170s, operated on longer distance non-electrified routes. All sets now carry standard Northern white livery. Set No. 170455 is seen departing from Doncaster with a Sheffield bound service. All sets meet PRM regulations and have a universal access toilet compartment. **CJM**

170/5	Formation: DMSL+DMS				
170501	50501+79501	TS	WMT	PTR	WMR
170502	50502+79502	DY	EMP	PTR	EMR
170503	50503+79503	DY	EMP	PTR	EMR
170504	50504+79504	DY	EMP	PTR	EMR
170505	50505+79505	DY	EMP	PTR	EMR
170506	50506+79506	DY	EMP	PTR	EMR
170507	50507+79507	DY	EMP	PTR	EMR
170508	50508+79508	DY	EMP	PTR	EMR
170509	50509+79509	DY	EMP	PTR	EMR
170510	50510+79510	DY	EMP	PTR	EMR
170511	50511+79511	DY	EMP	PTR	EMR
170512	50512+79512	DY	EMP	PTR	EMR

170513	50513+79513	DY	EMP	PTR	EMR
170514	50514+79514	DY	EMP	PTR	EMR
170515	50515+79515	DY	EMP	PTR	EMR
170516	50516+79516	TS	WMT	PTR	WMR
170517	50517+79517	DY	EMP	PTR	EMR
170530 (170630)	50630+79630	NM	EMP	PTR	EMR
170531 (170631)	50631+79631	NM	EMP	PTR	EMR
170532 (170632)	50632+79632	DY	EMP	PTR	EMR
170533 (170633)	50633+79633	DY	EMP	PTR	EMR
170534 (170634)	50634+79634	DY	EMP	PTR	EMR
170535 (170635)	50635+79635	DY	EMP	PTR	EMR

170/6 Formation: DMSL+MS+DMS

170618 (170518)	50518+56630+79518	TS	AXC	PTR	AXC
170619 (170519)	50519+56631+79519	TS	AXC	PTR	AXC
170620 (170520)	50520+56632+79520	TS	AXC	PTR	AXC
170621 (170521)	50521+56633+79521	TS	AXC	PTR	AXC
170622 (170522)	50522+56634+79522	TS	AXC	PTR	AXC
Pride of Leicester					
170623 (170523)	50523+56635+79523	TS	AXC	PTR	AXC
170636	50636+56636+79636	TS	AXC	PTR	AXC
170637	50637+56637+79637	TS	AXC	PTR	AXC
170638	50638+56638+79638	TS	AXC	PTR	AXC
170639	50639+56639+79639	TS	AXC	PTR	AXC

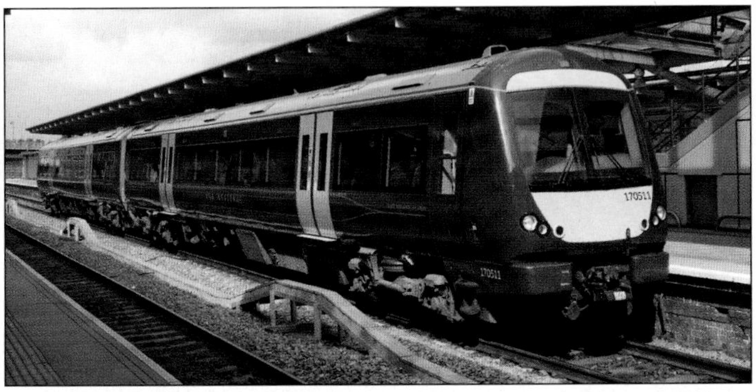

East Midlands Railway Regional services are concentating on Class 170s, many of which have recently been drafted in from West Midlands. Carrying the stylish EMT Regional maroon livery, two-car set No. 170511 is shown at Derby. **Adrian Paul**

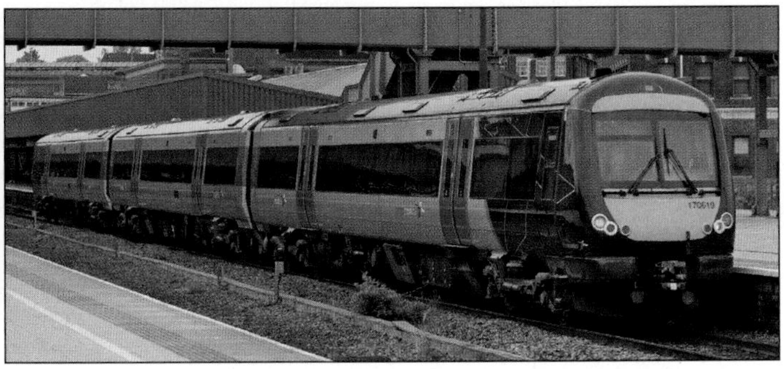

To provide CrossCountry with three-car Class 170s, some re-marshalling of sets took place in 2021, with the MS vehicles of West Midlands sets being formed in two-car XC Class 170/5 sets, with suitable renumbering. No. 170619 (170519) is shown at Leicester. **Antony Christie**

Class 171
Bombardier 2 and 4-car 'Turbostar'

Built: 2000-2004
Vehicle length: 76ft 6in (23.62m)
Height: 12ft 4½in (3.77m)
Width: 8ft 10in (2.69m)
Engine: 1 x MTU 6R 183TD 13H per car
Horsepower: 422hp (315kW)
Transmission: Hydraulic

171/2 Formation: DMCL+DMSL

171201§ (170421)	50421+79421	SU	SOU	EVL	GTR
171202§ (170423)	50423+79423	SU	SOU	EVL	GTR

171/4 Formation: DMCL+MS+MS+DMCL

171401§ (170422)	50422+56421+56422+79422	SU	SOU	EVL	GTR
171402§ (170424)	50424+56423+56424+79424	SU	SOU	EVL	GTR

171/7 Formation: DMCL+DMSL

171721	50721+79721	SU	SOU	PTR	GTR
171722	50722+79722	SU	SOU	PTR	GTR
171723	50723+79723	SU	SOU	PTR	GTR
171724	50724+79724	SU	SOU	PTR	GTR
171725	50725+79725	SU	SOU	PTR	GTR
171726	50726+79726	SU	SOU	PTR	GTR
171727	50727+79727	SU	SOU	PTR	GTR
171728	50728+79728	SU	SOU	PTR	GTR
171729	50729+79729	SU	SOU	PTR	GTR
171730 (170392)	50392+79392	SU	SOU	PTR	GTR

171/8 Formation: DMCL+MS+MS+DMCL

171801	50801+54801+56801+79801	SU	SOU	PTR	GTR
171802	50802+54802+56802+79802	SU	SOU	PTR	GTR
171803	50803+54803+56803+79803	SU	SOU	PTR	GTR
171804	50804+54804+56804+79804	SU	SOU	PTR	GTR
171805	50805+54805+56805+79805	SU	SOU	PTR	GTR
171806	50806+54806+56806+79806	SU	SOU	PTR	GTR

§ 171201/202, 171401/402 to be reformed as 3-car Class 170 sets for EMR in autumn 2022

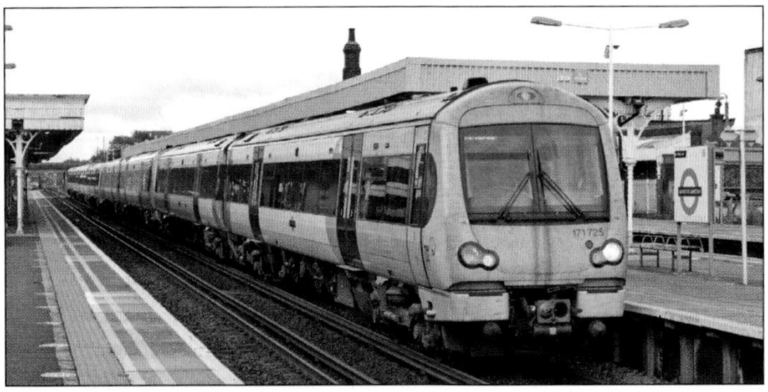

GTR Southern operates Class 171 Turbostar sets on non-electrified routes. These sets, based at Selhurst, have Dellner auto couplers. Two-car sets have one driving car and four car units have both driving cars with a first class seating area. Two-car set No. 171725, with its DMCL leading is seen at Norwood Junction. **Antony Christie**

Class 172
Bombardier 2 and 3-car 'Turbostar'

Built: 2010-2011
Vehicle length: Driving 76ft 3in (23.27m)
Intermediate 76ft 6in (23.36m)
Height: 12ft 4½in (3.77m)
Width: 8ft 8in (2.69m)
Engine: 1 x MTU 6H1800R83 per car
Horsepower: 484hp (360kW)
Transmission: Mechanical

172/0 Formation: DMSL+DMS

172001	59311+59411	TS	WMR	ANG	WMR
172002	59312+59412	TS	WMR	ANG	WMR
172003	59313+59413	TS	WMR	ANG	WMR
172004	59314+59414	TS	WMR	ANG	WMR
172005	59315+59415	TS	WMR	ANG	WMR
172006	59316+59416	TS	WMR	ANG	WMR
172007	59317+59417	TS	WMR	ANG	WMR
172008	59318+59418	TS	WMR	ANG	WMR

172/1 Formation: DMSL+DMS

172101	59111+59211	TS	WMR	ANG	WMR
172102	59112+59212	TS	WMR	ANG	WMR
172103	59113+59213	TS	WMR	ANG	WMR
172104	59114+59214	TS	WMR	ANG	WMR

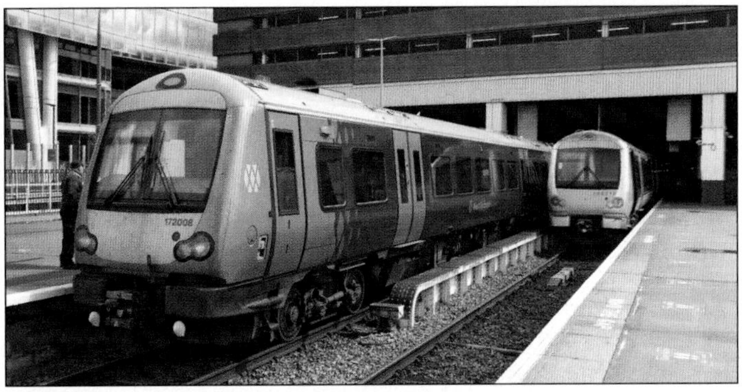

Class 172/0 and 172/2 two-car sets are non-end gangwayed, and have the same front style as a Class 170/171. Previously with TfL and Chiltern, all sets are now operated from Tyseley by West Midlands Railway. Unit 172008, one of the original TfL sets, is recorded at Birmingham Snow Hill next to a Chiltern Class 168. **CJM**

172/2 Formation: DMSL+DMS

172211	50211+79211	TS	WMR	PTR	WMR
172212	50212+79212	TS	WMR	PTR	WMR
172213	50213+79213	TS	WMR	PTR	WMR
172214	50214+79214	TS	WMR	PTR	WMR
172215	50215+79215	TS	WMR	PTR	WMR
172216	50216+79216	TS	WMR	PTR	WMR
172217	50217+79217	TS	WMR	PTR	WMR
172218	50218+79218	TS	WMR	PTR	WMR
172219	50219+79219	TS	WMR	PTR	WMR
172220	50220+79220	TS	WMR	PTR	WMR
172221	50221+79221	TS	WMR	PTR	WMR
172222	50222+79222	TS	WMR	PTR	WMR

172/3 Formation: DMSL+MS+DMS

172331	50331+56331+79331	TS	WMR	PTR	WMR
172332	50332+56332+79332	TS	WMR	PTR	WMR
172333	50333+56333+79333	TS	WMR	PTR	WMR
172334	50334+56334+79334	TS	WMR	PTR	WMR
172335	50335+56335+79335	TS	WMR	PTR	WMR
172336	50336+56336+79336	TS	WMR	PTR	WMR
172337	50337+56337+79337	TS	WMR	PTR	WMR
172338	50338+56338+79338	TS	WMR	PTR	WMR
172339	50339+56339+79339	TS	WMR	PTR	WMR
172340	50340+56340+79340	TS	WMR	PTR	WMR
172341	50341+56341+79341	TS	WMR	PTR	WMR

172342	50342+56342+79342	TS	WMR	PTR	WMR
172343	50343+56343+79343	TS	WMR	PTR	WMR
172344	50344+56344+79344	TS	WMR	PTR	WMR
172345	50345+56345+79345	TS	WMR	PTR	WMR

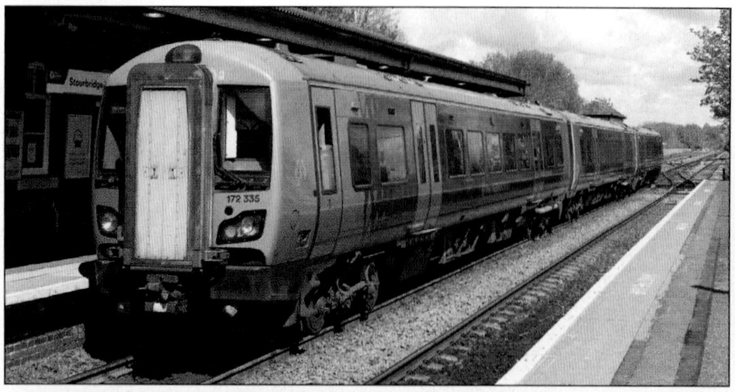

When the Class 170/2 (two-car) and 172/3 (three-car) sets for West Midlands were built, end gangways were incorporated. Three-car unit No. 172335 is shown departing from Stourbridge Junction on 6 May 2021. **CJM**

Class 175
Alstom 2 and 3-car 'Coradia'

Built: 1999-2001
Vehicle length: Driving 75ft 7in (23.03m)
Height: 12ft 4in (3.75m)
Width: 9ft 2in (2.79m)
Engine: 1 x Cummins N14 per car
Horsepower: 450hp (335kW)
Transmission: Hydraulic

175/0 Formation: DMSL+DMSL

175001	50701+79701	CH	TFW	ANG	TFW
175002	50702+79702	CH	TFW	ANG	TFW
175003	50703+79703	CH	TFW	ANG	TFW
175004	50704+79704	CH	TFW	ANG	TFW
175005	50705+79705	CH	TFW	ANG	TFW
175006	50706+79706	CH	TFW	ANG	TFW
175007	50707+79707	CH	TFW	ANG	TFW
175008	50708+79708	CH	TFW	ANG	TFW
175009	50709+79709	CH	TFW	ANG	TFW
175010	50710+79710	CH	TFW	ANG	TFW
175011	50711+79711	CH	TFW	ANG	TFW

175/1 Formation: DMSL+MSL+DMS

175101	50751+56751+79751	CH	TFW	ANG	TFW
175102	50752+56752+79752	CH	TFW	ANG	TFW
175103	50753+56753+79753	CH	TFW	ANG	TFW
175104	50754+56754+79754	CH	TFW	ANG	TFW
175105	50755+56755+79755	CH	TFW	ANG	TFW
175106	50756+56756+79756	CH	TFW	ANG	TFW
175107	50757+56757+79757	CH	TFW	ANG	TFW
175108	50758+56758+79758	CH	TFW	ANG	TFW
175109	50759+56759+79759	CH	TFW	ANG	TFW
175110	50760+56760+79760	CH	TFW	ANG	TFW
175111	50761+56761+79761	CH	TFW	ANG	TFW
175112	50762+56762+79762	CH	TFW	ANG	TFW
175113	50763+56763+79763	CH	TFW	ANG	TFW
175114	50764+56764+79764	CH	TFW	ANG	TFW
175115	50765+56765+79765	CH	TFW	ANG	TFW
175116	50766+56766+79766	CH	TFW	ANG	TFW

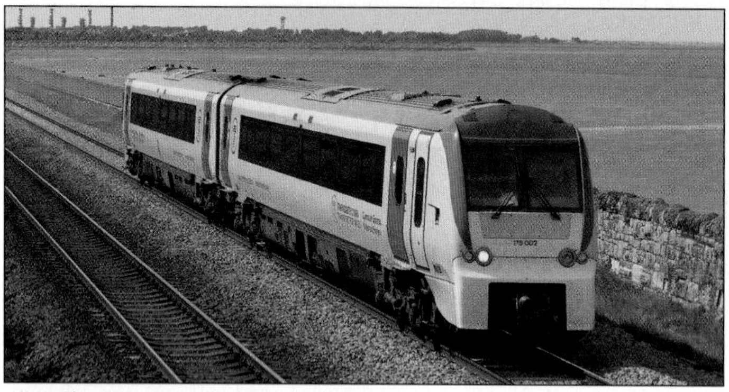

All 27 Class 175s operated by Transport for Wales have now been refreshed by Alstom and repainted in TfW grey, red and black livery. These sets will be displaced when new stock on order is delivered. Two-car set No. 175002 is seen near Mostyn. **CJM**

Class 180
Alstom 4/5-car 'Coradia'

Built: 2000-2001
Vehicle length: Driving 77ft 7in (23.71m)
Intermediate 75ft 5in (23.03m)
Height: 12ft 4in (3.75m)
Width: 9ft 2in (2.79m)
Engine: 1 x Cummins QSK19 per car
Horsepower: 750hp (560kW)
Transmission: Hydraulic

Formation: DMSL+MFL+MSL+MSLRB+DMSL

180101	50901+54901+55901+56901+59901	HT	GTO	ANG	GTL
180102	50902+54902+55902+56902+59902	HT	GTO	ANG	GTL
180103	50912+54903+55906+56903+59903	HT	GTO	ANG	GTL
180104	50904+54904+55904+56904+59904	HT	GTO	ANG	GTL
180105	50905+54905+55905+56905+59905 *The Yorkshire Artist Ashley Jackson*	HT	GTO	ANG	GTL
180106	50906+54906+55903+56906+59906	HT	GTO	ANG	GTL
180107	50907+54907+55907+56907+59907 *Hart of the North*	HT	GTO	ANG	GTL
180108§	50908+54908+55908+56908+59908 *William Shakespeare*	HT	GTO	ANG	GTL
180109	50909+54909+55913+56909+59909	DY	EMI	ANG	EMR
180110	50910+54910+55910+-+59910	DY	EMI	ANG	EMR
180111	50911+54911+55911+56911+59911	DY	EMI	ANG	EMR
180112	50903+54912+55912+56912+59912 *James Herriot Celebrating 100 Years 1916-2016*	HT	SPL	ANG	GTL
180113	50913+54913+55909+56913+59913	DY	EMI	ANG	EMR
180114	50914+54914+55914+56914+59914 *Kirkgate Calling*	HT	GTO	ANG	GTL

§ Fitted with ETCS for East Coast testing

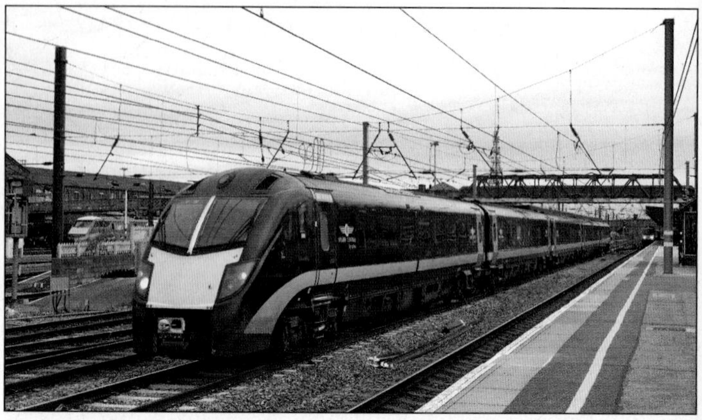

Ten five-car Alstom Class 180 sets are operated by Open Access operator Grand Central, they carry a black livery off-set by an orange train length band on the lower body. Based at Heaton, Newcastle the fleet operate Sunderland/Bradford to King's Cross services. **CJM**

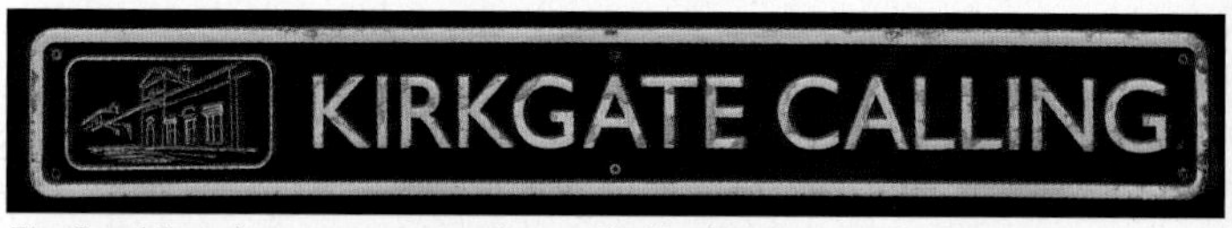

Five Grand Central sets carry cast nameplates on the side of driving cars. No. 180114 carries the name Kirkgate Calling, *marking the rejuvenation of Wakefield Kirkgate station in 2018.* **CJM**

Class 185
Siemens 3-car 'Desiro UK'

Built: 2005-2007
Vehicle length: Driving 77ft 11in (23.76m)
Intermediate 77ft 10in (23.75m)
Height: 12ft 4in (3.75m)
Width: 9ft 3in (2.84m)
Engine: 1 x Cummins QSK19 per car
Horsepower: 750hp (560kW)
Transmission: Hydraulic

Formation: DMCL+MSL+DMS

185101	51101+53101+54101	AK	FTN	EVL	FTP
185102	51102+53102+54102	AK	FTN	EVL	FTP
185103	51103+53103+54103	AK	FTN	EVL	FTP
185104	51104+53104+54104	AK	FTN	EVL	FTP
185105	51105+53105+54105	AK	FTN	EVL	FTP
185106	51106+53106+54106	AK	FTN	EVL	FTP
185107	51107+53107+54107	AK	FTN	EVL	FTP
185108	51108+53108+54108	AK	FTN	EVL	FTP
185109	51109+53109+54109	AK	FTN	EVL	FTP
185110	51110+53110+54110	AK	FTN	EVL	FTP
185111	51111+53111+54111	AK	FTN	EVL	FTP
185112	51112+53112+54112	AK	FTN	EVL	FTP
185113	51113+53113+54113	AK	FTN	EVL	FTP
185114	51114+53114+54114	AK	FTN	EVL	FTP
185115	51115+53115+54115	AK	FTN	EVL	FTP
185116	51116+53116+54116	AK	FTN	EVL	FTP
185117	51117+53117+54117	AK	FTN	EVL	FTP
185118	51118+53118+54118	AK	FTN	EVL	FTP
185119	51119+53119+54119	AK	FTN	EVL	FTP
185120	51120+53120+54120	AK	FTN	EVL	FTP
185121	51121+53121+54121	AK	FTN	EVL	FTP
185122	51122+53122+54122	AK	FTN	EVL	FTP
185123	51123+53123+54123	AK	FTN	EVL	FTP
185124	51124+53124+54124	AK	FTN	EVL	FTP
185125	51125+53125+54125	AK	FTN	EVL	FTP
185126	51126+53126+54126	AK	FTN	EVL	FTP
185127	51127+53127+54127	AK	FTN	EVL	FTP
185128	51128+53128+54128	AK	FTN	EVL	FTP
185129	51129+53129+54129	AK	FTN	EVL	FTP
185130	51130+53130+54130	AK	FTN	EVL	FTP
185131	51131+53131+54131	AK	FTN	EVL	FTP
185132	51132+53132+54132	AK	FTN	EVL	FTP
185133	51133+53133+54133	AK	FTN	EVL	FTP
185134	51134+53134+54134	AK	FTN	EVL	FTP
185135	51135+53135+54135	AK	FTN	EVL	FTP
185136	51136+53136+54136	AK	FTN	EVL	FTP
185137	51137+53137+54137	AK	FTN	EVL	FTP
185138	51138+53138+54138	AK	FTN	EVL	FTP

185139	51139+53139+54139	AK	FTN	EVL	FTP
185140	51140+53140+54140	AK	FTN	EVL	FTP
185141	51141+53141+54141	AK	FTN	EVL	FTP
185142	51142+53142+54142	AK	FTN	EVL	FTP
185143	51143+53143+54143	AK	FTN	EVL	FTP
185144	51144+53144+54144	AK	FTN	EVL	FTP
185145	51145+53145+54145	AK	FTN	EVL	FTP
185146	51146+53146+54146	AK	FTN	EVL	FTP
185147	51147+53147+54147	AK	FTN	EVL	FTP
185148	51148+53148+54148	AK	FTN	EVL	FTP
185149	51149+53149+54149	AK	FTN	EVL	FTP
185150	51150+53150+54150	AK	FTN	EVL	FTP
185151	51151+53151+54151	AK	FTN	EVL	FTP

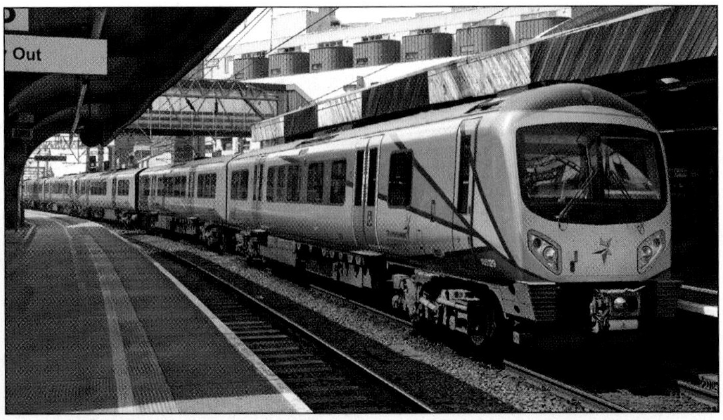

With introduction of Class 802 and Mk5 stock it was thought that some of the TransPennine Class 185s would go off-lease in 2021-2022, but it has now been announced all sets will remain with TPE. Set No. 185129 is shown at Manchester Oxford Road in summer 2021. **CJM**

Class 195
CAF 2 and 3-car 'Civity'

Built: 2018-2020
Vehicle length: Driving 78ft 6in (24.04m)
Intermediate 76ft 6in (23.35m)
Height: 12ft 7in (3.85m)
Width: 8ft 9in (2.71m)
Engine: 1 x Rolls Royce/MTU 6H1800R85L per car
Horsepower: 523hp (390kW)
Transmission: Hydraulic

195/0 Formation: DMSL+DMS

195001	101001+103001	NH	NNR	EVL	NOR
195002	101002+103002	NH	NNR	EVL	NOR
195003	101003+103003	NH	NNR	EVL	NOR
195004	101004+103004	NH	NNR	EVL	NOR
195005	101005+103005	NH	NNR	EVL	NOR
195006	101006+103006	NH	NNR	EVL	NOR
195007	101007+103007	NH	NNR	EVL	NOR
195008	101008+103008	NH	NNR	EVL	NOR
195009	101009+103009	NH	NNR	EVL	NOR
195010	101010+103010	NH	NNR	EVL	NOR
195011	101011+103011	NH	NNR	EVL	NOR
195012	101012+103012	NH	NNR	EVL	NOR
195013	101013+103013	NH	NNR	EVL	NOR
195014	101014+103014	NH	NNR	EVL	NOR
195015	101015+103015	NH	NNR	EVL	NOR
195016	101016+103016	NH	NNR	EVL	NOR
195017	101017+103017	NH	NNR	EVL	NOR
195018	101018+103018	NH	NNR	EVL	NOR
195019	101019+103019	NH	NNR	EVL	NOR
195020	101020+103020	NH	NNR	EVL	NOR
195021	101021+103021	NH	NNR	EVL	NOR
195022	101022+103022	NH	NNR	EVL	NOR
195023	101023+103023	NH	NNR	EVL	NOR
195024	101024+103024	NH	NNR	EVL	NOR
195025	101025+103025	NH	NNR	EVL	NOR

195/1 Formation: DMSL+MS+DMS

195101	101101+102101+103101		NH	NNR	EVL	NOR
195102	101102+102102+103102		NH	NNR	EVL	NOR
195103	101103+102103+103103		NH	NNR	EVL	NOR
195104	101104+102104+103104		NH	NNR	EVL	NOR
195105	101105+102105+103105	*Northern Powerhouse*	NH	NNR	EVL	NOR
195106	101106+102106+103106		NH	NNR	EVL	NOR
195107	101107+102107+103107		NH	NNR	EVL	NOR
195108	101108+102108+103108		NH	NNR	EVL	NOR
195109	101109+102109+103109	*Pride of Cumbria*	NH	NNR	EVL	NOR
195110	101110+102110+103110		NH	NNR	EVL	NOR
195111	101111+102111+103111	*Key Worker*	NH	NNR	EVL	NOR
195112	101112+102112+103112		NH	NNR	EVL	NOR
195113	101113+102113+103113		NH	NNR	EVL	NOR
195114	101114+102114+103114		NH	NNR	EVL	NOR
195115	101115+102115+103115		NH	NNR	EVL	NOR
195116	101116+102116+103116	*Proud to be Northern*	NH	NNR	EVL	NOR
195117	101117+102117+103117		NH	NNR	EVL	NOR
195118	101118+102118+103118		NH	NNR	EVL	NOR
195119	101119+102119+103119		NH	NNR	EVL	NOR
195120	101120+102120+103120		NH	NNR	EVL	NOR
195121	101121+102121+103121		NH	NNR	EVL	NOR
195122	101122+102122+103122		NH	NNR	EVL	NOR
195123	101123+102123+103123		NH	NNR	EVL	NOR
195124	101124+102124+103124		NH	NNR	EVL	NOR
195125	101125+102125+103125		NH	NNR	EVL	NOR
195126	101126+102126+103126		NH	NNR	EVL	NOR
195127	101127+102127+103127		NH	NNR	EVL	NOR
195128	101128+102128+103128	*Calder Champion*	NH	NNR	EVL	NOR
195129	101129+102129+103129		NH	NNR	EVL	NOR
195130	101130+102130+103130		NH	NNR	EVL	NOR
195131	101131+102131+103131		NH	NNR	EVL	NOR
195132	101132+102132+103132		NH	NNR	EVL	NOR
195133	101133+102133+103133		NH	NNR	EVL	NOR

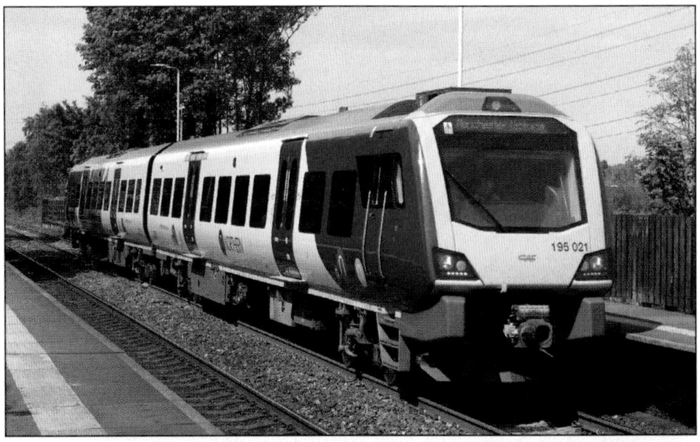

A total of 58 CAF-built Class 195s in both two and three-car form are in service with Northern. The sets are based at Manchester Newton Heath depot and operate over most of the western section of the Northern network. Two-car set No. 195021 is illustrated. **CJM**

Class 196
CAF 2 and 4-car 'Civity'

Built: 2018-2020
Vehicle length: Driving 78ft 6in (24.04m)
Intermediate 76ft 6in (23.35m)
Height: 12ft 7in (3.85m)
Width: 8ft 9in (2.71m)
Engine: 1 x Rolls Royce/MTU 6H1800R85L per car
Horsepower: 523hp (390kW)
Transmission: Hydraulic

196/0 Formation: DMSL+DMS

196001	121001+124001	TS	WMR	COR	WMR
196002	121002+124002	TS	WMR	COR	WMR
196003	121003+124003	TS	WMR	COR	WMR
196004	121004+124004	TS	WMR	COR	WMR
196005	121005+124005	TS	WMR	COR	WMR
196006	121006+124006	TS	WMR	COR	WMR
196007	121007+124007	TS	WMR	COR	WMR
196008	121008+124008	TS	WMR	COR	WMR
196009	121009+124009	TS	WMR	COR	WMR
196010	121010+124010	TS	WMR	COR	WMR
196011	121011+124011	TS	WMR	COR	WMR
196012	121012+124012	TS	WMR	COR	WMR

196/1 Formation: DMSL+MS+MS+DMS

196101	121101+122101+123101+124101	TS	WMR	COR	WMR
196102	121102+122102+123102+124102	TS	WMR	COR	WMR
196103	121103+122103+123103+124103	TS	WMR	COR	WMR
196104	121104+122104+123104+124104	TS	WMR	COR	WMR
196105	121105+122105+123105+124105	TS	WMR	COR	WMR
196106	121106+122106+123106+124106	TS	WMR	COR	WMR
196107	121107+122107+123107+124107	TS	WMR	COR	WMR
196108	121108+122108+123108+124108	TS	WMR	COR	WMR
196109	121109+122109+123109+124109	TS	WMR	COR	WMR
196110	121110+122110+123110+124110	TS	WMR	COR	WMR
196111	121111+122111+123111+124111	TS	WMR	COR	WMR
196112	121112+122112+123112+124112	TS	WMR	COR	WMR
196113	121113+122113+123113+124113	TS	WMR	COR	WMR
196114	121114+122114+123114+124114	TS	WMR	COR	WMR

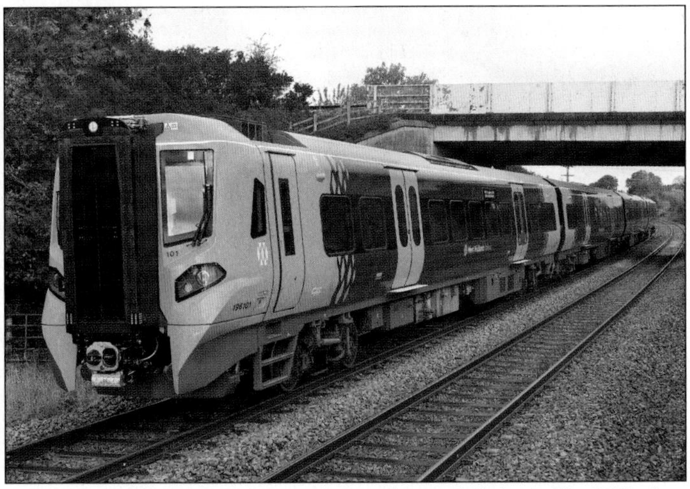

A fleet of two and four-car CAF 'Civity' units are under commissioning for West Midlands Railway, based at Tyseley. The sets are scheduled to go into service in spring 2022. Four-car set No. 196101 is illustrated on a commissioning run at Stratford Parkway. **CJM**

Class 197
CAF 2 and 3-car 'Civity'

Built: 2021-2023
Vehicle length: Driving 78ft 6in (24.04m)
Intermediate 76ft 6in (23.35m)
Height: 12ft 7in (3.85m)
Width: Width: 8ft 9in (2.71m)
Engine: 1 x Rolls Royce/MTU 6H1800R85L per car
Horsepower: 523hp (390kW)
Transmission: Hydraulic

197/0 Formation: DMSL+DMS

197001	131001+133001	TFW	TFW
197002	131002+133002	TFW	TFW
197003	131003+133003	TFW	TFW
197004	131004+133004	TFW	TFW
197005	131005+133005	TFW	TFW
197006	131006+133006	TFW	TFW
197007	131007+133007	TFW	TFW
197008	131008+133008	TFW	TFW
197009	131009+133009	TFW	TFW
197010	131010+133010	TFW	TFW
197011	131011+133011	TFW	TFW
197012	131012+133012	TFW	TFW
197013	131013+133013	TFW	TFW
197014	131014+133014	TFW	TFW
197015	131015+133015	TFW	TFW
197016	131016+133016	TFW	TFW
197017	131017+133017	TFW	TFW
197018	131018+133018	TFW	TFW
197019	131019+133019	TFW	TFW
197020	131020+133020	TFW	TFW
197021	131021+133021	TFW	TFW
197022	131022+133022	TFW	TFW
197023	131023+133023	TFW	TFW
197024	131024+133024	TFW	TFW
197025	131025+133025	TFW	TFW
197026	131026+133026	TFW	TFW
197027	131027+133027	TFW	TFW
197028	131028+133028	TFW	TFW
197029	131029+133029	TFW	TFW
197030	131030+133030	TFW	TFW
197031	131031+133031	TFW	TFW
197032	131032+133032	TFW	TFW
197033	131033+133033	TFW	TFW
197034	131034+133034	TFW	TFW
197035	131035+133035	TFW	TFW
197036	131036+133036	TFW	TFW
197037	131037+133037	TFW	TFW
197038	131038+133038	TFW	TFW
197039	131039+133039	TFW	TFW
197040	131040+133040	TFW	TFW
197041	131041+133041	TFW	TFW
197042	131042+133042	TFW	TFW
197043	131043+133043	TFW	TFW
197044	131044+133044	TFW	TFW
197045	131045+133045	TFW	TFW
197046	131046+133046	TFW	TFW
197047	131047+133047	TFW	TFW
197048	131048+133048	TFW	TFW
197049	131049+133049	TFW	TFW
197050	131050+133050	TFW	TFW
197051	131051+133051	TFW	TFW

197/1 Formation: DMSL+MS+DMS

197101	131101+132101+133101	TFW	TFW
197102	131102+132102+133102	TFW	TFW
197103	131103+132103+133103	TFW	TFW
197104	131104+132104+133104	TFW	TFW
197105	131105+132105+133105	TFW	TFW
197106	131106+132106+133106	TFW	TFW
197107	131107+132107+133107	TFW	TFW
197108	131108+132108+133108	TFW	TFW
197109	131109+132109+133109	TFW	TFW
197110	131110+132110+133110	TFW	TFW
197111	131111+132111+133111	TFW	TFW
197112	131112+132112+133112	TFW	TFW
197113	131113+132113+133113	TFW	TFW
197114	131114+132114+133114	TFW	TFW
197115	131115+132115+133115	TFW	TFW
197116	131116+132116+133116	TFW	TFW
197117	131117+132117+133117	TFW	TFW
197118	131118+132118+133118	TFW	TFW
197119	131119+132119+133119	TFW	TFW
197120	131120+132120+133120	TFW	TFW
197121	131121+132121+133121	TFW	TFW
197122	131122+132122+133122	TFW	TFW
197123	131123+132123+133123	TFW	TFW
197124	131124+132124+133124	TFW	TFW
197125	131125+132125+133125	TFW	TFW
197126	131126+132126+133126	TFW	TFW

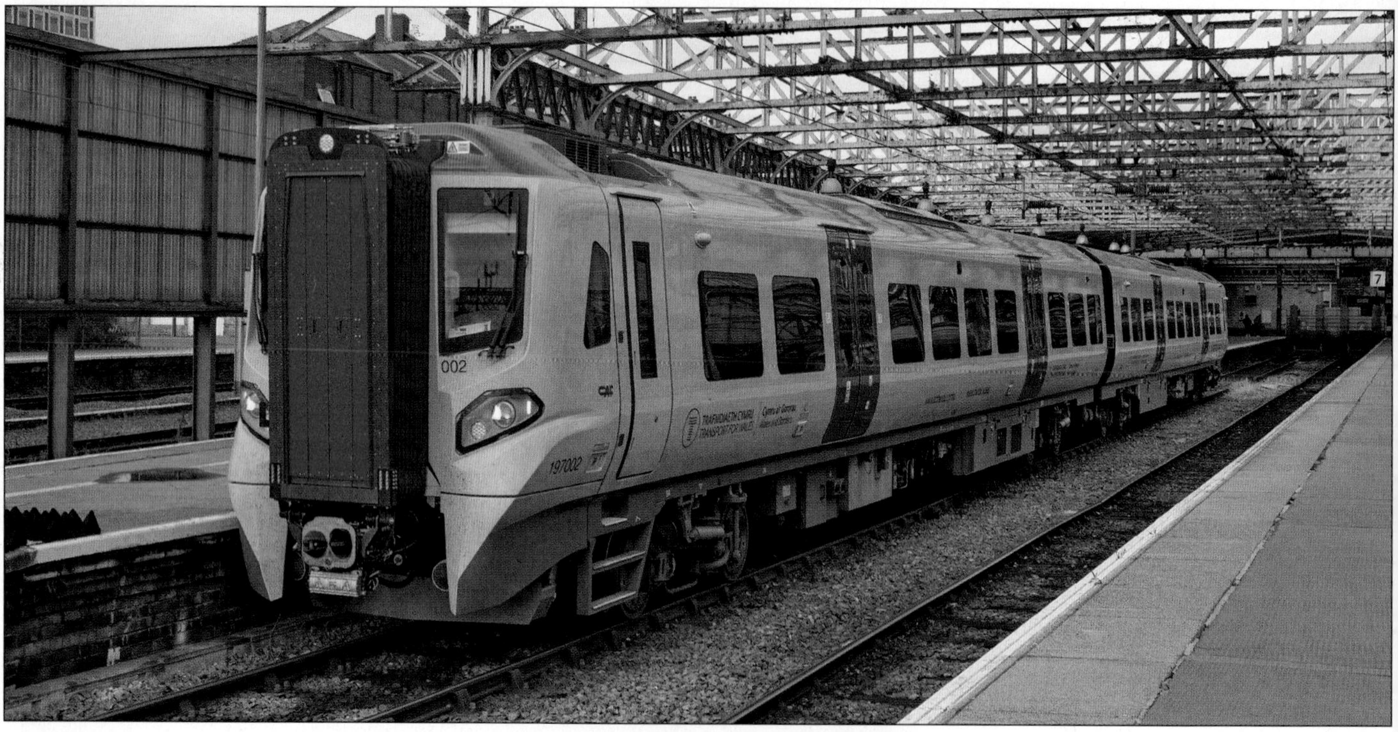

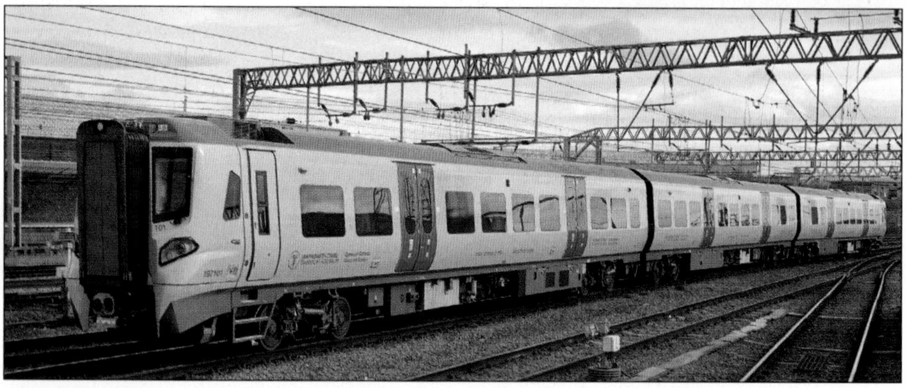

Very similar to the Class 196s for West Midlands Railway are a fleet of Class 197 CAF Civity sets for Transport for Wales, these come in two and three-car formations with the 77 sets scheduled to replace Class 150, 153, 158 and 175 sets from late 2022. In the above view 2-car set No. 197002 is seen at Crewe, during shake down and staff training. On the left, three-car set No.197101 departs from Crewe on a test run. Testing and training on the class was centered on Crewe in late 2021 early 2022. **Antony Christie / Spencer Conquest**

Diesel Electric Units

Class 201-210
DEMU stock

Class 201, 202, 203 (6S, 6L, 6B)

60000	1001	*Hastings*	DMBS	Hastings Diesels Ltd
60001	1001		DMBS	Hastings Diesels Ltd (S)
60016	1012	*Mountfield*	DMBS	Hastings Diesels Ltd (as 60116)
60018	1013	*Tunbridge Wells*	DMBS	Hastings Diesels Ltd (as 60118)
60019	1013		DMBS	Hastings Diesels Ltd
60500	1001		TS	Hastings Diesels Ltd (S)
60501	1001		TS	Hastings Diesels Ltd
60502	1001		TS	Hastings Diesels Ltd (S)
60527	1013		TS	Hastings Diesels Ltd (S)
60528	1013		TS	Hastings Diesels Ltd (S)
60529	1013		TS	Hastings Diesels Ltd§
60700	1001		TF	Hastings Diesels Ltd (S)
60708	1012		TF	Hastings Diesels Ltd (S)
60709	1013		TF	Hastings Diesels Ltd (S)
60750	1032		TBUF	Battleford Ltd (ex DB975386)

Class 205 (2H, 3H)

60108	1109	DMBSO	Eden Valley Railway
60110	1111	DMBSO	Epping & Ongar Railway
60117	1118	DMBSO	Lavender Line
60122	1123	DMBSO	Lavender Line
60124	1125	DMBSO	Mid Hants Railway
60145	1127	DMBSO	Hastings Diesels Ltd
60146	1128	DMBSO	Caledonian Railway, Brechin
60149	1131	DMBSO	Hastings Diesels Ltd (as 205031)
60150	1132	DMBSO	Caledonian Railway, Brechin
60151	1133	DMBSO	Lavender Line
60154	1101	DMBSO	East Kent Railway
60658	1109	TSO	Eden Valley Railway
60669	1120	TSO	Swindon & Cricklade Railway
60673	1128	TSO	Caledonian Railway, Brechin
60677	1132	TSO	Caledonian Railway, Brechin
60678	1133	TSO	Lavender Line
60800	1101	DTC	East Kent Railway
60808	1109	DTC	Eden Valley Railway
60810	1111	DTS	Epping & Ongar Railway
60820	1121	DTC	Hastings Diesels Ltd at Lavender Line
60822	1123	DTC	Swindon & Cricklade Railway
60824	1125	DTC	Mid Hants Railway
60827	1128	DTC	Caledonian Railway, Brechin
60828	1118	DTC	Lavender Line
60830	1131	DTC	Lavender Line
60831	1132	DTC	Caledonian Railway, Brechin
60832	1133	DTC	Lavender Line

Class 207 (3D)

60127	1302	DMBS	Swindon & Cricklade Railway
60130	1305	DMBS	COVES at MoD Bicester as 207202
60142	1317	DMBS	Spa Valley Railway
60616	1317	TC	Spa Valley Railway
60904	1305	DTS	COVES at MoD Bicester as 207202
60916	1317	DTS	Spa Valley Railway

Class 210

67300	210001	DMSO	East Kent Railway

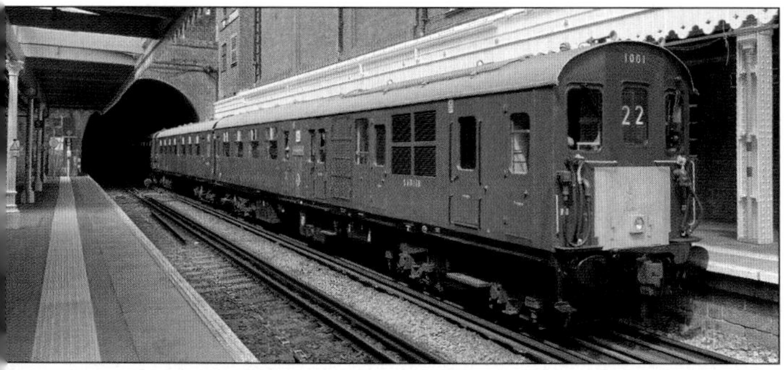

Hastings Diesels Ltd are the owner of a number of former 'Hastings' DEMU vehicles which are certified for main line operation. In immaculate condition 6L car 60118 running in set 1001 is shown at Tunbridge Wells. **Howard Lewsey**

Class 220
Bombardier 4-car 'Voyager'

Built: 2000-2001
Vehicle length: Driving 77ft 6in (23.62m)
Height: 12ft 4in (3.76m)
Width: 8ft 11in (2.72m)
Engine: 1 x Cummins QSK19 per car
Horsepower: 750hp (560kW)
Transmission: Electric

Formation: DMSL+MS+MSL+DMF

220001	60301+60701+60201+60401	CZ	AXC	BEA	AXC
220002	60302+60702+60202+60402	CZ	AXC	BEA	AXC
220003	60303+60703+60203+60403	CZ	AXC	BEA	AXC
220004	60304+60704+60204+60404	CZ	AXC	BEA	AXC
220005	60305+60705+60205+60405	CZ	AXC	BEA	AXC
220006	60306+60706+60206+60406	CZ	AXC	BEA	AXC
220007	60307+60707+60207+60407	CZ	AXC	BEA	AXC
220008	60308+60708+60208+60408	CZ	AXC	BEA	AXC
220009	60309+60709+60209+60409	CZ	AXC	BEA	AXC
	Hixon January 6th 1968				
220010	60310+60710+60210+60410	CZ	AXC	BEA	AXC
220011	60311+60711+60211+60411	CZ	AXC	BEA	AXC
220012	60312+60712+60212+60412	CZ	AXC	BEA	AXC
220013	60313+60713+60213+60413	CZ	AXC	BEA	AXC
220014	60314+60714+60214+60414	CZ	AXC	BEA	AXC
220015	60315+60715+60215+60415	CZ	AXC	BEA	AXC
220016	60316+60716+60216+60416	CZ	AXC	BEA	AXC
	Voyager 20				
220017	60317+60717+60217+60417	CZ	AXC	BEA	AXC
220018	60318+60718+60218+60418	CZ	AXC	BEA	AXC
220019	60319+60719+60219+60419	CZ	AXC	BEA	AXC
220020	60320+60720+60220+60420	CZ	AXC	BEA	AXC
220021	60321+60721+60221+60421	CZ	AXC	BEA	AXC
220022	60322+60722+60222+60422	CZ	AXC	BEA	AXC
220023	60323+60723+60223+60423	CZ	AXC	BEA	AXC
220024	60324+60724+60224+60424	CZ	AXC	BEA	AXC
220025	60325+60725+60225+60425	CZ	AXC	BEA	AXC
220026	60326+60726+60226+60426	CZ	AXC	BEA	AXC
220027	60327+60727+60227+60427	CZ	AXC	BEA	AXC
220028	60328+60728+60228+60428	CZ	AXC	BEA	AXC
220029	60329+60729+60229+60429	CZ	AXC	BEA	AXC
220030	60330+60730+60230+60430	CZ	AXC	BEA	AXC
220031	60331+60731+60231+60431	CZ	AXC	BEA	AXC
220032	60332+60732+60232+60432	CZ	AXC	BEA	AXC
220033	60333+60733+60233+60433	CZ	AXC	BEA	AXC
220034	60334+60734+60234+60434	CZ	AXC	BEA	AXC

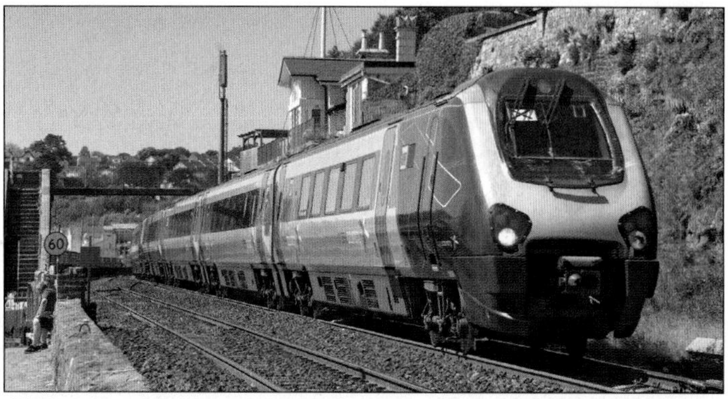

All 34 members of the 'Voyager' Class 220 fleet are operated by CrossCountry and based at Central Rivers, Burton-on-Trent. The sets operate along with the XC Class 221 fleet on all CrossCountry routes. With its first class driving car leading, set No. 220008 is seen passing Dawlish. **CJM**

Class 221
Bombardier 4 and 5-car 'Super Voyager'

Built: 2000-2001
Vehicle length: Driving 77ft 6in (23.62m)
Height: 12ft 4in (3.76m)
Width: 8ft 11in (2.72m)
Engine: 1 x Cummins QSK19 per car
Horsepower: 750hp (560kW)
Transmission: Electric

Formation: DMSL+MS+MS+MSL+DMF or DMSL+MS+MSL+DMF

221101	60351+60951+60851+60751+60451	CZ	AWG	BEA	AWC
221102	60352+60952+60852+60752+60452	CZ	AWG	BEA	AWC
221103	60353+60953+60853+60753+60453	CZ	AWG	BEA	AWC
221104	60354+60954+60854+60754+60454	CZ	AWG	BEA	AWC
221105	60355+60955+60855+60755+60455	CZ	AWG	BEA	AWC
221106	60356+60956+60856+60756+60456	CZ	AWG	BEA	AWC
221107	60357+60957+60857+60757+60457	CZ	AWG	BEA	AWC
221108	60358+60958+60858+60758+60458	CZ	AWG	BEA	AWC
221109	60359+60959+60859+60759+60459	CZ	AWG	BEA	AWC
221110	60360+60960+60860+60760+60460	CZ	AWG	BEA	AWC
221111	60361+60961+60861+60761+60461	CZ	AWG	BEA	AWC
221112	60362+60962+60862+60762+60462	CZ	AWG	BEA	AWC
221113	60363+60963+60863+60763+60463	CZ	AWG	BEA	AWC
221114	60364+60964+60864+60764+60464	CZ	AWG	BEA	AWC
221115	60365+60965+60865+60765+60465	CZ	AWG	BEA	AWC
221116	60366+60966+60866+60766+60466	CZ	AWG	BEA	AWC
221117	60367+60967+60867+60767+60467	CZ	AWG	BEA	AWC
221118	60368+60968+60868+60768+60468	CZ	AWG	BEA	AWC
221119	60369+60769+60969+60869+60469	CZ	AXG	BEA	AXC
221120	60370+60770+60970+60870+60470	CZ	AXC	BEA	AXC
221121	60371+60771+60971+60871+60471	CZ	AXC	BEA	AXC
221122	60372+60772+60972+60872+60472	CZ	AXC	BEA	AXC
221123	60373+60773+60973+60873+60473	CZ	AXC	BEA	AXC
221124	60374+60774+60974+60874+60474	CZ	AXC	BEA	AXC
221125	60375+60775+60975+60875+60475	CZ	AXC	BEA	AXC
221126	60376+60776+60976+60876+60476	CZ	AXC	BEA	AXC
221127	60377+60777+60977+60877+60477	CZ	AXC	BEA	AXC
221128	60378+60778+60978+60878+60478	CZ	AXC	BEA	AXC
221129	60379+60779+60979+60879+60479	CZ	AXC	BEA	AXC
221130	60380+60780+60980+60880+60480	CZ	AXC	BEA	AXC
221131	60381+60781+60981+60881+60481	CZ	AXC	BEA	AXC
221132	60382+60782+60982+60882+60482	CZ	AXC	BEA	AXC
221133	60383+60783+60983+60883+60483	CZ	AXC	BEA	AXC

221134	60384+60784+60984+60884+60484	CZ	AXC	BEA	AXC
221135	60385+60785+60985+60885+60485	CZ	AXC	BEA	AXC
221136	60386+60786+- +60886+60486	CZ	AXC	BEA	AXC
221137	60387+60787+60987+60887+60487	CZ	AXC	BEA	AXC
221138	60388+60788+60988+60888+60488	CZ	AXC	BEA	AXC
221139	60389+60789+60989+60889+60489	CZ	AXC	BEA	AXC
221140	60390+60790+- +60890+60490	CZ	AXC	BEA	AXC
221141	60391+60791+60991+- +60491	CZ	AXC	BEA	AXC
221142	60392+60992+60986+60792+60492	CZ	AWG	BEA	AWC
221143	60393+60993+60994+60793+60493	CZ	AWG	BEA	AWC
221144	60394+60794+60990+- +60494	CZ	AXC	BEA	AXC

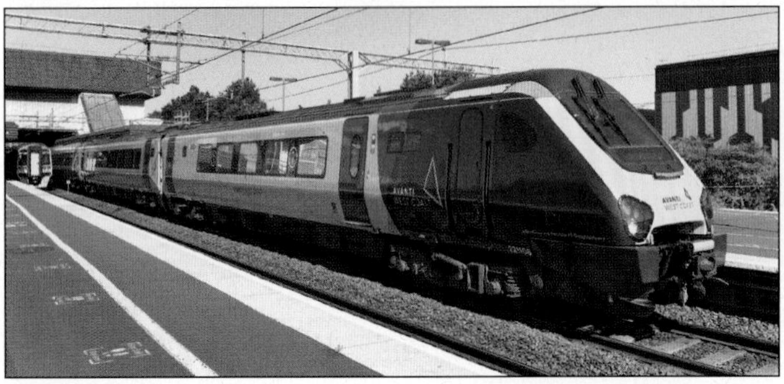

The Class 221 'Super Voyager' sets are operated by both Avanti West Coast and Cross Country, with sets based at Central Rivers depot. In the above image No. 221108 from the Avanti fleet is shown at Birmingham International, while below, CrossCountry set No. 221127 is seen at Leamington Spa. The yellow coupling cover box, indicates the first class end of the train. Both: **CJM**

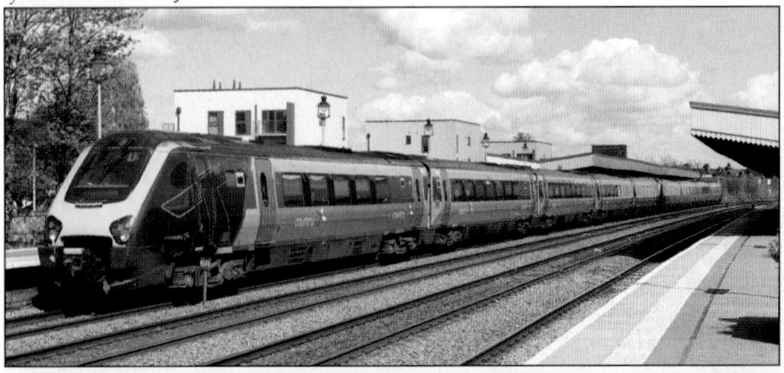

Class 222/0
Bombardier 7 and 5-car 'Meridian'

Built: 2004-2005
Vehicle length: Driving - 78ft 2in (23.85m)
Intermediate - 77ft 2in (23.00m)
Height: 12ft 4in (3.76m)
Width: 8ft 11in (2.72m)
Engine: 1 x Cummins QSK19 per car
Horsepower: 750hp (560kW) per car
Transmission: Electric

Formation: DMS+MS+MS+MSRMB+MF+MF+DMRFO

222001	60161+60551+60561+60621+60341+60445+60241	DY	EMI	EVL	EMR
	The Entrepreneur Express				
222002	60162+60544+60562+60622+60342+60346+60242	DY	EMI	EVL	EMR
	The Cutlers' Company				
222003	60163+60553+60563+60623+60343+60446+60243	DY	EMI	EVL	EMR
222004	60164+60554+60564+60624+60344+60345+60244	DY	EMI	EVL	EMR
	Childrens Hospital Sheffield				

Formation: DMS+MS+MSRMB+MC+DMRFO

222005	60165+60565+60625+60347+60245	DY	EMI	EVL	EMR
222006	60166+60566+60626+60447+60246	DY	EMI	EVL	EMR
	The Carbon Cutter				
222007	60167+60567+60627+60442+60247	DY	EMI	EVL	EMR
222008	60168+60545+60628+60918+60248	DY	EMI	EVL	EMR
	Derby Etches Park				
222009	60169+60557+60629+60919+60249	DY	EMI	EVL	EMR
222010	60170+60546+60630+60920+60250	DY	EMI	EVL	EMR

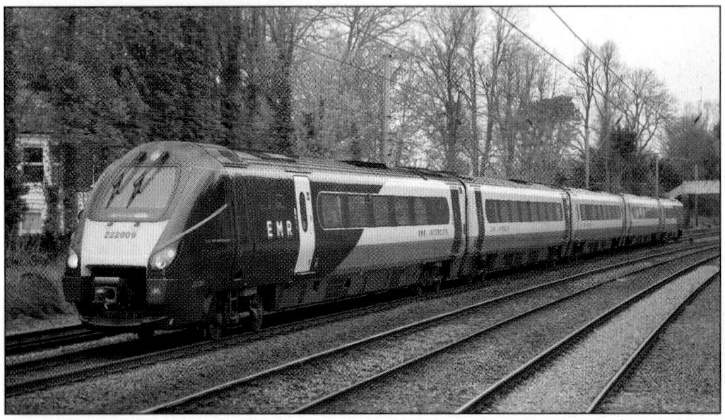

Soon to be replaced on East Midlands Railway by IET style trains, the Class 222/0 sets operate in both five and seven-car formation, but some reformations are on the cards. Sets now all display the latest EMR aubergine, grey and white livery. Five-car set No. 222009 is shown. **Antony Christie**

222011	60171+60531+60631+60921+60251	DY	EMI	EVL	EMR
222012	60172+60532+60632+60922+60252	DY	EMI	EVL	EMR
222013	60173+60536+60633+60923+60253	DY	EMI	EVL	EMR
222014	60174+60534+60634+60924+60254	DY	EMI	EVL	EMR
222015	60175+60535+60635+60925+60255	DY	EMI	EVL	EMR
	175 Years of Derby's Railways 1839-2014				
222016	60176+60533+60636+60926+60256	DY	EMI	EVL	EMR
222017	60177+60537+60637+60927+60257	DY	EMI	EVL	EMR
222018	60178+60444+60638+60928+60258	DY	EMI	EVL	EMR
222019	60179+60547+60639+60929+60259	DY	EMI	EVL	EMR
222020	60180+60543+60640+60930+60260	DY	EMI	EVL	EMR
222021	60181+60552+60641+60931+60261	DY	EMI	EVL	EMR
222022	60182+60542+60642+60932+60262	DY	EMI	EVL	EMR
	Invest in Nottingham				
222023	60183+60541+60643+60933+60263	DY	EMI	EVL	EMR

Class 222/1
Bombardier 5-car 'Meridian' (originally 'Pioneer')

Built: 2004-2005
Vehicle length: Driving - 78ft 2in (23.85m)
Intermediate - 77ft 2in (23.00m)
Height: 12ft 4in (3.76m)
Width: 8ft 11in (2.72m)
Engine: 1 x Cummins QSK19 per car
Horsepower: 750hp (560kW) per car
Transmission: Electric

Formation: DMF+MF+MC+MSRMB+DMS or DMF+MC+MSRMB+MS+DMS

222101	60271+60571+60681+60555+60191	DY	EMI	EVL	EMR
222102	60272+60572+60682+60556+60192	DY	EMI	EVL	EMR
222103	60273+60573+60683+60443+60193	DY	EMI	EVL	EMR
222104	60274+60574+60684+60441+60194	DY	EMP	EVL	EMR

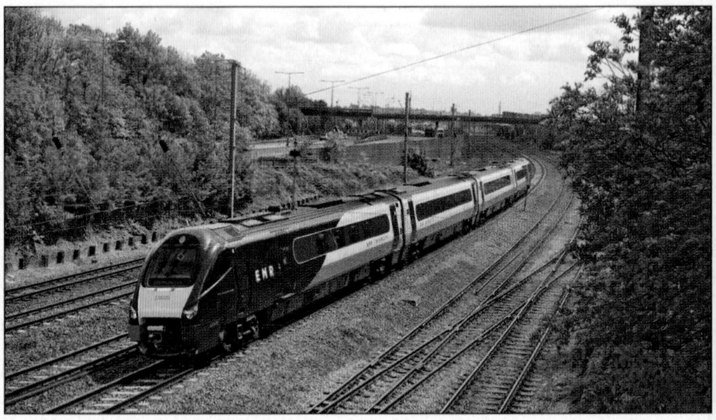

The Class 222/1 sub-class of four-car sets were originally operated with First Hull Trains, but when replaced by Class 802s were transferred to join the Class 222/0s on the Midland Main Line. Set No. 222101 is seen with its first class end nearest the camera in summer 2021. Set now reformed as five-car set. **Antony Christie**

Class 231
Stadler 4-car 'Flirt'

Built: 2021-2022
Vehicle length: Driving 74ft 3in (20.81m)
Intermediate 50ft 0in (15.22m)
Power Pack 21ft 9in (6.69m)
Height: 13ft 0in (3.95m)
Width: 9ft 1in (2.78m)
Power: 4 x Duetz V8/16
Horsepower: 2,575hp (1,920kW)
Transmission: Electric

Formation: DMS+TS+PP+TS+DMS

231001	381001+381201+381401+381301+381101	CV	TFW	SMB	TFW
231002	381002+381202+381402+381302+381102	CV	TFW	SMB	TFW
231003	381003+381203+381403+381303+381103	CV	TFW	SMB	TFW
231004	381004+381204+381404+381304+381105	CV	TFW	SMB	TFW
231005	381005+381205+381405+381305+381105	CV	TFW	SMB	TFW
231006	381006+381206+381406+381306+381106	CV	TFW	SMB	TFW
231007	381007+381207+381407+381307+381107	CV	TFW	SMB	TFW
231008	381008+381208+381408+381308+381108	CV	TFW	SMB	TFW
231009	381009+381209+381409+381309+381109	CV	TFW	SMB	TFW
231010	381010+381210+381410+381310+381110	CV	TFW	SMB	TFW
231011	381011+381211+381411+381311+381111	CV	TFW	SMB	TFW

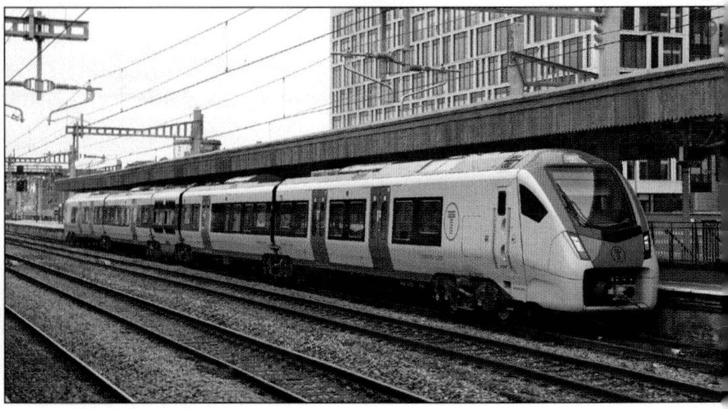

The first two of the 11 strong fleet of Class 231 five section 'Flirt' sets for Transport for Wales were delivered at the end of 2021 and commenced test and staff training runs soon after. On 1 March 2022, set No. 231004 is seen at Cardiff Central. **CJM**

Bi-Mode 'D' Stock Rebuids

Class 230
Vivarail 'D-Stock'

Built: 2016-2021
Vehicle length: Driving - 60ft 3in (18.37m)
Intermediate - 59ft 5in (18.12m)
Height: 11ft 11in (3.62m)
Width: 9ft 4in (2.85m)

Power: Ford Diesel, Battery or Gensets
230001 - 6 Hoppecke batteries below driving cars
Horsepower: 800-1,200hp (596-895-kW)
Transmission: Electric

	Formation: DMS+DMS or DMS+TS+DMS				
230001	300001 (7058)+300201 (17128)+300101 (7511) *Viva Venturer*	LM	SPL	VIV	VIV
230002	300002 (7122)+300202 (17091)+300102 (7067)	In USA as 2-car (Note 1)			
230003	300003 (7069)+300103 (7127)	BY	WMG	WMR	WMT
230004	300004 (7100)+300104 (7500)	BY	WMG	WMR	WMT
230005	300005 (7066)+300105 (7128)	BY	WMG	WMR	WMT
230006	300006 (7098)+300206 (17066)+300106 (7510)	BD	TFW	TFW	TFW
230007	300007 (7103)+300207 (17063)+300107 (7529)	BD	TFW	TFW	TFW
230008	300008 (7120)+300208 (17050)+300108 (7065)	BD	TFW	TFW	TFW
230009	300009 (7055)+300209 (17084)+300109 (7523)	BD	TFW	TFW	TFW
230010	300010 (7090)+300210 (17071)+300110 (7017)	BD	TFW	TFW	TFW
Car 7501	Vivarail battery development at Ecclesbourne Valley Railway				

Set 230001 battery only, was COP26 demonstration set, now for Great Western on West Ealing to Greenford route
Note 1 - 230002 at Rockhill, Pennsylvania as demonstrator with Railroad Development Corporation, two further trailer cars have been exported to form two 2-car sets

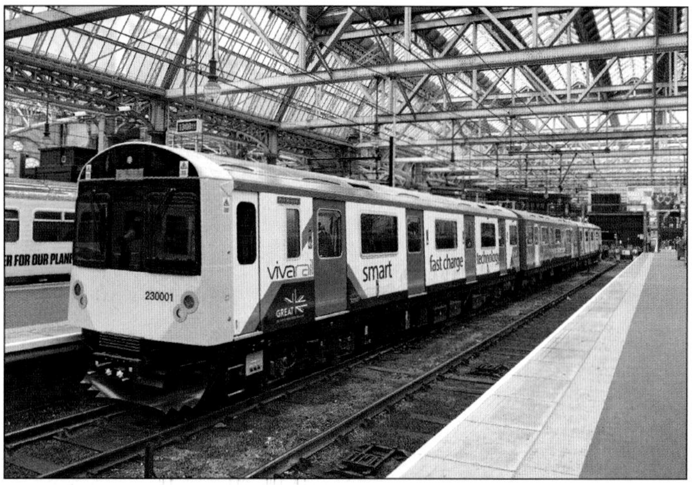

One of the most remarkable rolling stock events of recent time has been the rebuilding of former London Underground 'D' Stock into main line trains, a project masterminded by Vivarail. Various designs of two and three-car train using different propulsion systems have been used. In this view the all-battery set No. 230001 is seen taking part in the COP26 climate event held in Glasgow in November 2021. This three-car demonstrator set was previously a diesel powered unit. It is fitted with various concept interiors. The set is seen stabled under the roof at Glasgow Central. From mid-2022 the set will be used by Great Western on the West Ealing to Greenford route using 'fast-charge' facilities installed at West Ealing. **CJM**

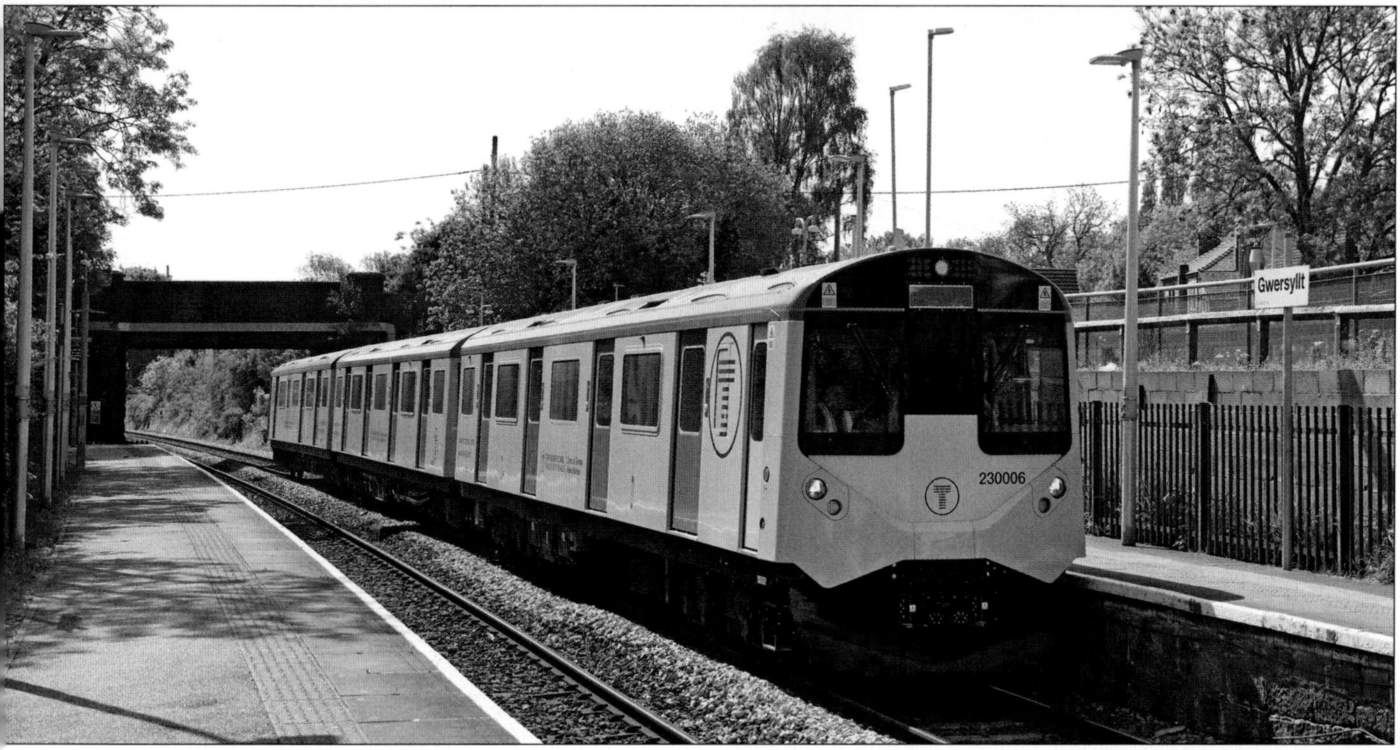

A fleet of five three-car Class 230s are awaiting entry into service between Wrexham and Bidston, based at Birkenhead. These sets with a slightly different front end design have been delayed entering service due to a small fire and delayed driver training due to Covid-19. Set No. 230006 is seen at Gwersyllt in June 2021. **CJM**

The following ex-London Underground 'D' Stock coaches are owned by Vivarail and stored at various sites in the Midlands and could be used in the rebuild project.

Driving Motor		7073	7109	7517	17025	17082	17510
7000	7035	7075	7110	7518	17026	17083	17520
7001	7038	7076	7112	7519	17029	17085	17522
7003	7039	7077	7113	7520	17035	17086	17528
7004	7041	7078	7114	7521	17036	17087	
7005	7043	7079	7115	7522	17043	17088	
7006	7044	7080	7116	7524	17045	17089	
7008	7045	7081	7117	7525	17047	17090	
7009	7046	7082	7118	7528	17049	17091	
7013	7047	7084	7119	7530	17052	17092	
7014	7048	7085	7121	7532	17053	17096	
7015	7049	7087	7125	7533	17054	17098	
7016	7050	7088	7126	7534	17055	17100	
7019	7052	7089	7129	7535	17056	17101	
7020	7053	7091	7501	7536	17058	17103	
7021	7054	7092	7502	7537	17059	17104	
7022	7056	7094	7503	7538	17062	17106	
7023	7057	7095	7504	7539	17064	17110	
7024	7059	7096	7505		17065	17112	
7025	7060	7097	7506	**Trailer**	17067	17113	
7026	7061	7099	7507	17003	17068	17114	
7028	7062	7101	7509	17011	17069	17116	
7029	7063	7102	7512	17013	17073	17117	
7030	7064	7104	7513	17015	17076	17120	
7031	7070	7105	7514	17020	17077	17124	
7033	7071	7106	7515	17021	17078	17127	
7034	7072	7108	7516	17023	17080	17129	

The first Class 230s to enter service were three two-car sets for West Midlands Railway working on the Bedford-Bletchley line, based at Bletchley. During the Covid-19 pandemic with a reduced service and numbers of train crew these sets were largely sidelined, but are now returning to traffic. Set No. 230005 is seen at Bletchley. **Adrian Paul**

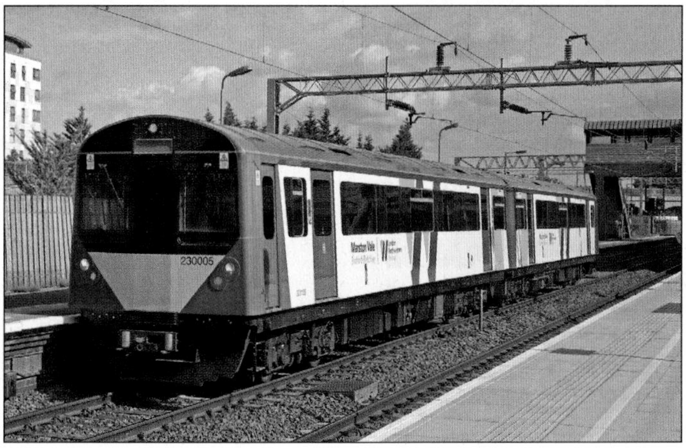

Electric Multiple Units

Electric Multiple Units - AC

Class 300 Series
Preserved Stock

AM2 (Class 302)

75033	302201	BR/ER	DTSO	Mangapps Farm
75250	302277	BR/ER	DTSO	Mangapps Farm

AM3 (Class 303)

61503	303023	BR/ScR	MBS	Bo'ness & Kinneil Railway
75597	303032	BR/ScR	DTSO	Bo'ness & Kinneil Railway
75632	303032	BR/ScR	BDTSO	Bo'ness & Kinneil Railway

AM6 (Class 306)

65217	306017	BR/ER	DMSO	National Railway Museum, Shildon
65417	306017	BR/ER	TBC	National Railway Museum, Shildon
65617	306017	BR/ER	DTSO	National Railway Museum, Shildon

AM7 (Class 307)

75023	307123	BR/ER	DTBSO	MoD Bicester (stored)

AM8 (Class 308)

75881	308136	BR/ER	DTCO	MoD Bicester (stored)

AM9 (Class 309)

61928	309624	BR/ER	MBSO	Lavender Line, Isfield
61937	309616	BR/ER	MBSO	Tanat Valley Railway
75642	309616	BR/ER	BDTC	Tanat Valley Railway
75965	309624	BR/ER	BDTC	Lavender Line, Isfield
75972	309624	BR/ER	DTSO	Lavender Line, Isfield
75981	309616	BR/ER	DTSO	Tanat Valley Railway

AM11 (Class 311)

62174	311103	BR/ScR	MBSO	Summerlee
76433	311103	BR/ScR	DTSO	Summerlee

AM12 (Class 312)

71205	312792	BR/ER	TS	Colne Valley Railway
78037	312792	BR/ER	DTS	Colne Valley Railway

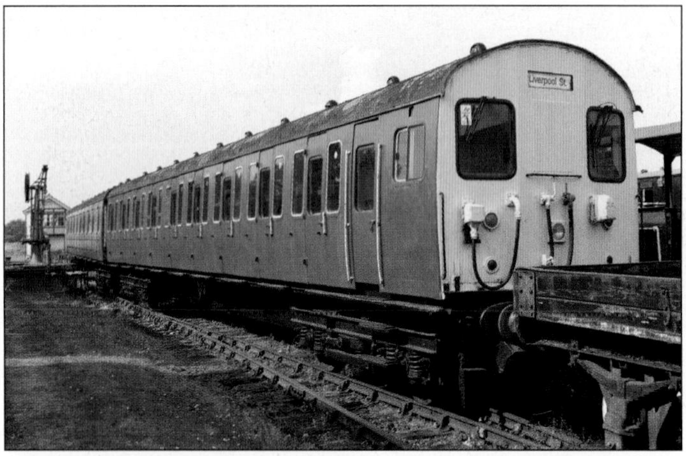

Two former Eastern Region Class AM2 (Class 302) vehicles are preserved at Mangapps farm Museum. DTC No. 75250 from set No. 302277 is shown. Both this and sister vehicle No. 75033 sport standard 1970s rail blue. **CJM**

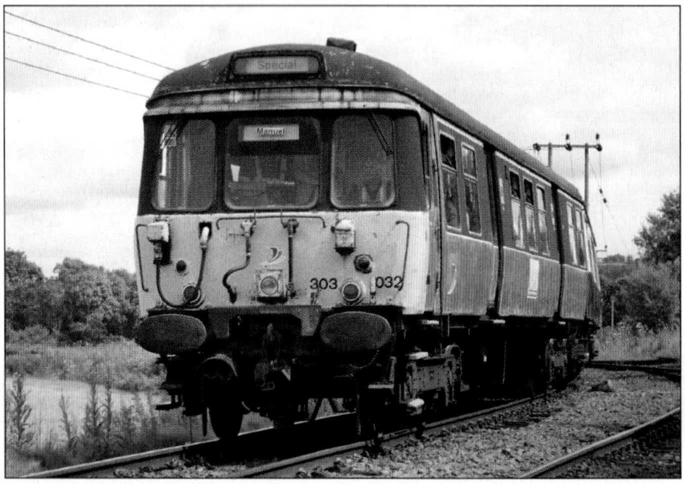

In Scotland, three former Class 303 'Glasgow Blue Train' vehicles are preserved at the Bo'ness & Kinneil Railway. The set has to be loco hauled but is used for passenger carrying. In 2021 the set was part painted in Glasgow orange and Carmine and cream livery. **Ian Lothian**

Class 313
BREL 3-Car Suburban

Built: 1976-1977
Vehicle length: Driving - 64ft 11½in (19.80m)
Intermediate - 65ft 4¼in (19.92m)
Height: 11ft 9in (3.58m)
Width: 9ft 3in (2.82m)
Power: 750V dc third rail (313/1 also 25kV ac)
Horsepower: 880hp (657kW)
Transmission: Electric

	Formaion: DMSO+TSO+BDMSO				
313121 (313021)	62549+71233+62613	ZG	NRL	BEA	NRL
313201 (313001/101)	62529+71213+62593	BI	BLG	BEA	GTR
313202 (313002/102)	62530+71214+62594	BI	SOU	BEA	GTR
313203 (313003/103)	62531+71215+62595	BI	SOU	BEA	GTR
313204 (313004/104)	62532+71216+62596	BI	SOU	BEA	GTR
313205 (313005/105)	62533+71217+62597	BI	SOU	BEA	GTR
313206 (313006/106)	62534+71218+62598	BI	SOU	BEA	GTR
313207 (313007/107)	62535+71219+62599	BI	SOU	BEA	GTR
313208 (313008/108)	62536+71220+62600	BI	SOU	BEA	GTR
313209 (313009/109)	62537+71221+62601	BI	SOU	BEA	GTR
313210 (313010/110)	62538+71222+62602	BI	SOU	BEA	GTR
313211 (313011/111)	62539+71223+62603	BI	SOU	BEA	GTR
313212 (313012/112)	62540+71224+62604	BI	SOU	BEA	GTR
313213 (313013/113)	62541+71225+62605	BI	SOU	BEA	GTR
313214 (313014/114)	62542+71226+62606	BI	SOU	BEA	GTR
313215 (313015/115)	62543+71227+62607	BI	SOU	BEA	GTR
313216 (313016/116)	62544+71228+62608	BI	SOU	BEA	GTR
313217 (313017/117)	62545+71229+61609	BI	SOU	BEA	GTR
313219 (313019/119)	62547+71231+61611	BI	SOU	BEA	GTR
313220 (313020/120)	62548+71232+61612	BI	SOU	BEA	GTR

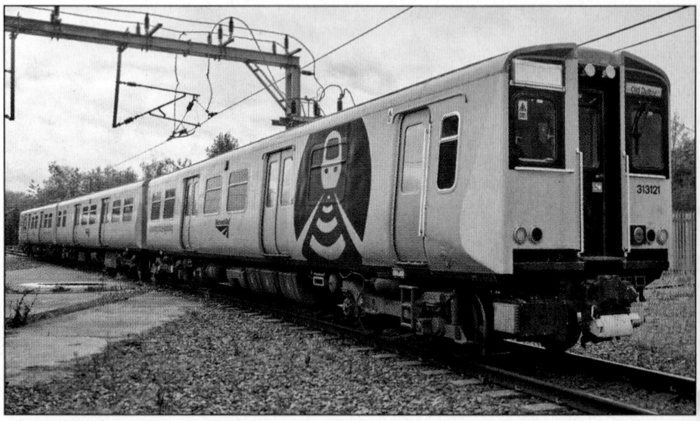

Network Rail operate the sole surviving member of Class 313/1, No. 313121 which is used for ETCS development and testing. The set is usually based at Eastleigh or at the Old Dalby test facility. It carries branded Network Rail yellow. **Network Rail**

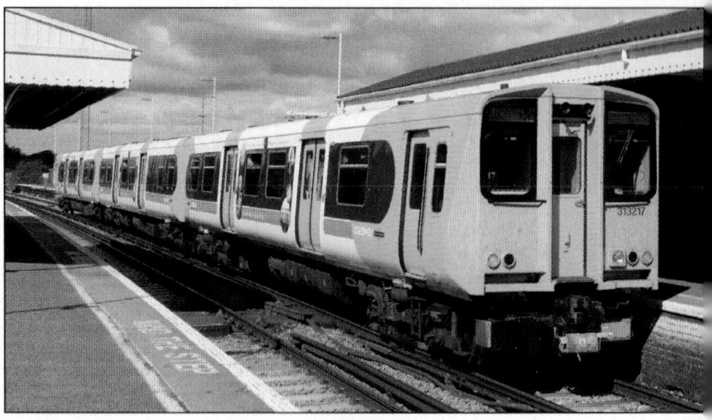

A fleet of 19 three-car Class 313/2s are based at Brighton and used on the Coastway services. The sets sport route branded GTR Southern green and white livery. These are the oldest EMUs currently in service having been introduced in 1976. Set No. 313217, the original No. 313017/117) is shown calling at Ford. **Nathan Williamson**

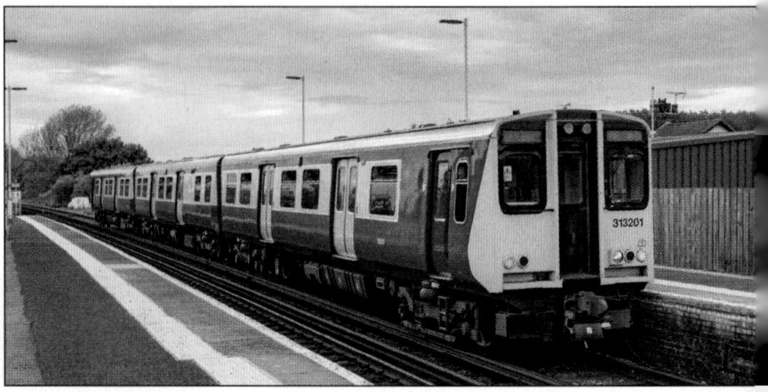

The first built Class 313 set for the Great Northern electrification of the 1970s, No. 313001 is now operated by GTR Southern as No. 313201. In is painted in 1970s rail blue and grey colours, illustrating the heritage of the pioneering 1972-design EMU stock. The set is seen at Ford on 17 May 2022 with a Coastway service. **CJM**

Class 315
BREL 4-Car Suburban

Built: 1980-1981
Vehicle length: Driving - 64ft 11½in (19.80m)
Intermediate - 65ft 4¼in (19.92m)
Height: 11ft 9in (3.58m)
Width: 9ft 3in (2.82m)
Power: 25kV ac overhead
Horsepower: 880hp (657kW)
Transmission: Electric

Formation: DMSO+TSO+PTSO+BDMSO

315837	64533+71317+71425+64534	IL	CRO	EVL	CRO
315838	64535+71318+71426+64536	IL	CRO	EVL	CRO
315847	64553+71327+71435+64554	IL	CRO	EVL	CRO
315853	64565+71333+71441+64566	IL	CRO	EVL	CRO
315856	64571+71336+71444+64572	IL	CRO	EVL	CRO
315857	64573+71337+71445+64574	IL	CRO	EVL	CRO

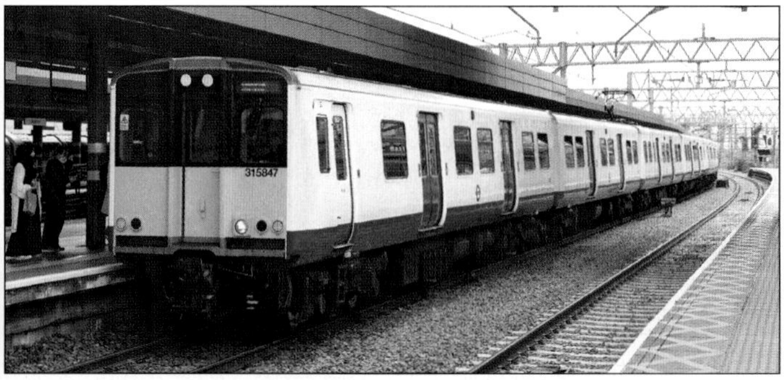

To be withdrawn by mid-2022, the remaining Class 315s, allocated to Ilford depot, operate on the Liverpool Street-Shenfield TfL (Elizabeth Line) route. Set No. 315847 is seen calling at Stratford bound for Shenfield. **CJM**

Class 317
BREL 4-Car Outer Suburban

Built: 1976-1977
Vehicle length: Driving - 65ft 0¾in (19.83m)
Intermediate - 65ft 4¼in (19.92m)
Height: 12ft 1½in (3.70m)
Width: 9ft 3in (2.82m)
Power: 25kV ac overhead
Horsepower: 1,328hp (990kW)
Transmission: Electric

317/3 Formation: DTSO+MSO+TSO+DTSO

317337	77036+62671+71613+77084	IL	TLK	ANG	GAR
317338	77037+62698+71614+77085	IL	TLK	ANG	GAR
317339	77038+62699+71615+77086	IL	TLK	ANG	GAR
317340	77039+62700+71616+77087	IL	TLK	ANG	GAR
317341	77040+62701+71617+77088	EL	AWT	ANG	(S)
317343	77042+62703+71619+77090	IL	TLK	ANG	GAR
317344	77029+62690+71620+77091	EL	AWT	ANG	OLS
317345	77092	East Anglian Railway Museum, Chappel & Wakes Colne			
	71621	The Depot, Caxton			
317347	77046+62707+71623+77094	IL	AWT	ANG	GAR

317/5 Formation: DTSO+MSO+TSO+DTSO

317501	(317301)	77024+62661+71577+77048	IL	AWT	ANG	GAR
317502	(317302)	77001+62662+71578+77049	IL	AWT	ANG	GAR
317504	(317304)	77003+62664+71580+77051	IL	AWT	ANG	GAR
317506	(317306)	77005+62666+71582+77053	IL	AWT	ANG	GAR
317507	(317307)	77006+62667+71583+77054	IL	AWT	ANG	GAR
		University of Cambridge 800 years 1209-2009				
317508	(317311)	77010+62697+71587+77058	IL	AWT	ANG	GAR
317510	(317313)	77012+62673+71589+77060	IL	AWT	ANG	GAR
317511	(317315)	77014+62675+71591+77062	IL	AWT	ANG	GAR
317512	(317316)	77015+62676+71592+77050	EL	AWT	ANG	(S)

317/8 Formation: DTSO+MSO+TSO+DTSO

317881	(317321)	77020+62681+71597+77068	IL	AWT	ANG	GAR
317882	(317324)	77023+62684+71600+77071	EL	NXU	ANG	(S)
317883	(317325)	77000+62685+71601+77072	EL	AWT	ANG	(S)
317884	(317326)	77025+62686+71602+77073	IL	AWT	ANG	GAR
317885	(317327)	77026+62687+71603+77074	EL	AWT	ANG	(S)
317886	(317328)	77027+62688+71604+77075	IL	AWT	ANG	GAR

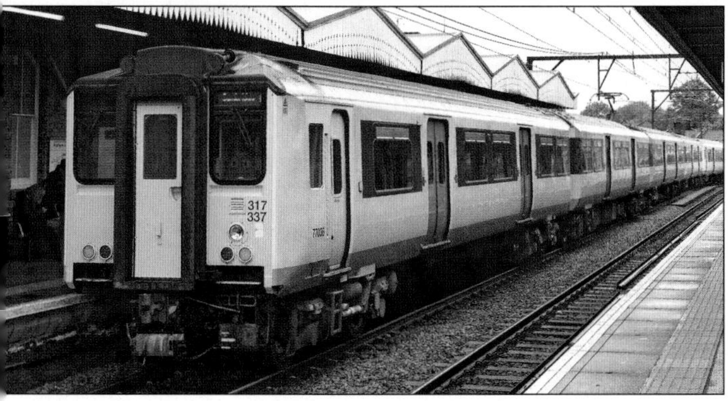

Another class soon to be withdrawn, following the full introduction of Class 720 stock on Greater Anglia, are the Class 317 sets. Currently working on the Greater Anglia 'West Anglia' routes, set No. 317337 is shown in unbranded GA white and blue livery. **CJM**

Class 318
BREL 3-Car Outer Suburban

Built: 1985-1986
Vehicle length: Driving - 65ft 0¾in (19.83m)
Intermediate - 65ft 4¼in (19.92m)
Height: 12ft 1½in (3.70m)
Width: 9ft 3in (2.82m)
Power: 25kV ac overhead
Horsepower: 1,438hp (1,072kW)
Transmission: Electric

Formation: DTSO+MSO+DTSO

318250	77240+62866+77260	GW	SCR	EVL	ASR
318251	77241+62867+77261	GW	SCR	EVL	ASR
318252	77242+62868+77262	GW	SCR	EVL	ASR
318253	77243+62869+77263	GW	SCR	EVL	ASR
318254	77244+62870+77264	GW	SCR	EVL	ASR
318255	77245+62871+77265	GW	SCR	EVL	ASR
318256	77246+62872+77266	GW	SCR	EVL	ASR
318257	77247+62873+77267	GW	SCR	EVL	ASR
318258	77248+62874+77268	GW	SCR	EVL	ASR
318259	77249+62875+77269	GW	SCR	EVL	ASR
318260	77250+62876+77270	GW	SCR	EVL	ASR
318261	77251+62877+77271	GW	SCR	EVL	ASR
318262	77252+62878+77272	GW	SCR	EVL	ASR
318263	77253+62879+77273	GW	SCR	EVL	ASR
318264	77254+62880+77274	GW	SCR	EVL	ASR
318265	77255+62881+77275	GW	SCR	EVL	ASR
318266	77256+62882+77276	GW	SCR	EVL	ASR
318267	77257+62883+77277	GW	SCR	EVL	ASR
318268	77258+62884+77278	GW	SCR	EVL	ASR
318269	77259+62885+77279	GW	SCR	EVL	ASR
318270	77288+62890+77289	GW	SCR	EVL	ASR

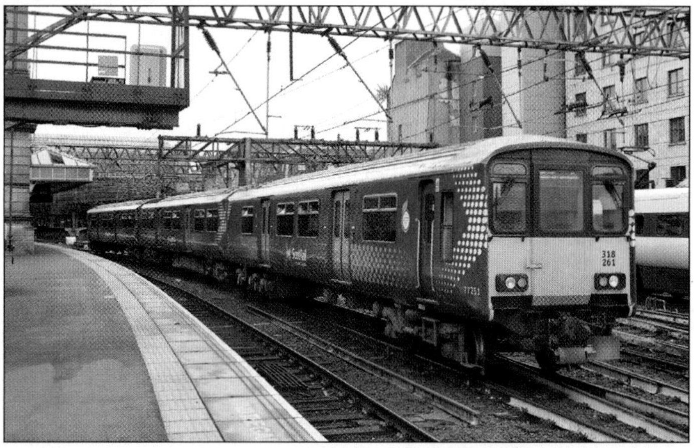

The 21 three-car Class 318 sets, which originally sported front end gangways are allocated to Glasgow Shields Road depot and operate suburban services in the Glasgow area. Set No. 318261 is seen arriving at Glasgow Central in November 2021. All sets sport Scottish Railways blue and white livery **CJM**

Class 319
BREL 4-Car Outer Suburban

Built: 1987-1989
Vehicle length: Driving - 65ft 0¾in (19.83m)
Intermediate - 65ft 4¼in (19.92m)
Height: 11ft 9in (3.58m)
Width: 9ft 3in (2.82m)
Power: 25kV ac overhead
Horsepower: 1,438hp (1,072kW)
Transmission: Electric

319/0 Formation: DTSO+MSO+TSO+DTSO

319005	77299+62895+71776+77298	NN	LMT	PTR	LMT
319011	77311+62901+71782+77310	ZG	ORI	PTR	ROG
319012	77313+62902+71783+77312	NN	LMT	PTR	LMT
319013	77315+62903+71784+77314	BU	LMI	PTR	(S)

319/2 Formation: DTSO+MSO+TSO+DTCO

319214	77317+62904+71785+77316	NN	LMT	PTR	LMT
319215	77319+62905+71786+77318	NN	LMT	PTR	LMT
319216	77321+62906+71787+77320	BU	LMT	PTR	(S)
319217	77323+62907+71788+77322	NN	WMT	PTR	LMT
319219	77327+62909+71790+77326	NN	WMT	PTR	LMT
319220	77329+62910+71791+77328	NN	LMT	PTR	LMT

319/3 Formation: DTSO+MSO+TSO+DTSO (§ DTLO+MLO+TLO+DTLO)

319361	77459+63043+71929+77458	AN	NNR	PTR	NOR
319365	77467+63047+71933+77466	LM	ORI	PTR	OLS
319366	77469+63048+71934+77468	AN	NNR	PTR	NOR
319367	77471+63049+71935+77470	AN	NNR	PTR	NOR
319368	77473+63050+71936+77472	AN	NNR	PTR	NOR
319369	77475+63051+71937+77474	AN	NNR	PTR	NOR
319370	77477+63052+71938+77476	AN	NNR	PTR	NOR
319371	77479+63053+71939+77478	LM	TLK	PTR	OLS
319372	77481+63054+71940+77480	AN	NNR	PTR	NOR
319375	77487+63057+71943+77486	AN	NNR	PTR	NOR
319378	77493+63060+71946+77492	AN	NNR	PTR	NOR
319379	77495+63061+71947+77494	AN	NNR	PTR	NOR
319381	77973+63093+71979+77974	AN	NNR	PTR	NOR
319383	77977+63096+71981+77978	AN	NNR	PTR	NOR
319384	77979+63096+71982+77980	LM	TLK	PTR	OLS
319385	77981+63097+71983+77982	AN	NNR	PTR	NOR
319386	77983+63098+71984+77984	AN	NNR	PTR	NOR

319/4 Formation: DTCO+MSO+TSO+DTSO

319429	77347+62919+71800+77346	NN	LMI	PTR	LMT
319433	77355+62923+71804+77354	NN	LMI	PTR	LMT
319454	77445+62968+71873+77444	LM	SPL	PTR	OLS
319457	77451+62971+71876+77450	NN	LMT	PTR	LMT
319460	77457+62974+71879+77456	BU	LMT	PTR	(S)

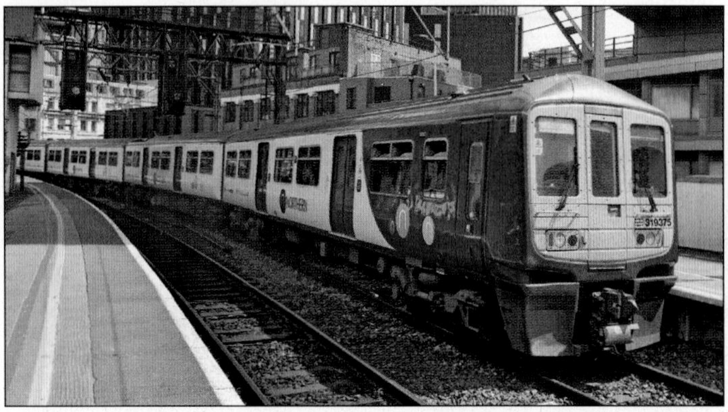

In 2022 the Class 319s are operated by Northern in passenger service. Many fleet members are stored for rebuilding to Class 326, 768 and 769 stock. Class 319 No. 319375 is seen at Manchester Oxford Road in June 2021 with a train from Manchester Airport to Blackpool North. **CJM**

Class 320
BREL 3-Car Outer Suburban

Built: 1990
Vehicle length: Driving - 65ft 0¾in (19.83m)
Intermediate - 65ft 4¼in (19.92m)
Height: 12ft ¾in (3.78m)
Width: 9ft 3in (2.82m)
Power: 25kV ac overhead
Horsepower: 1,438hp (1,072kW)
Transmission: Electric

320/3 Formation: DTSO+MSO+DTSO

320301	77899+63021+77921	GW	SCR	EVL	ASR
320302	77900+63022+77922	GW	SCR	EVL	ASR
320303	77901+63023+77923	GW	SCR	EVL	ASR
320304	77902+63024+77924	GW	SCR	EVL	ASR
320305	77903+63025+77925	GW	SCR	EVL	ASR
320306	77904+63026+77926	GW	SCR	EVL	ASR
320307	77905+63027+77927	GW	SCR	EVL	ASR
320308	77906+63028+77928	GW	SCR	EVL	ASR
320309	77907+63029+77929	GW	SCR	EVL	ASR
320310	77908+63030+77930	GW	SCR	EVL	ASR
320311	77909+63031+77931	GW	SCR	EVL	ASR
320312	77910+63032+77932	GW	SCR	EVL	ASR
320313	77911+63033+77933	GW	SCR	EVL	ASR
320314	77912+63034+77934	GW	SCR	EVL	ASR
320315	77913+63035+77935	GW	SCR	EVL	ASR
320316	77914+63036+77936	GW	SCR	EVL	ASR
320317	77915+63037+77937	GW	SCR	EVL	ASR
320318	77916+63038+77938	GW	SCR	EVL	ASR
320319	77917+63039+77939	GW	SCR	EVL	ASR
320320	77918+63040+77940	GW	SCR	EVL	ASR
320321	77919+63041+77941	GW	SCR	EVL	ASR
320322	77920+63042+77942	GW	SCR	EVL	ASR

320/4 Formation: DTSO+MSO+DTSO

320401 (321401)	78095+63063+77943	GW	SCR	EVL	ASR
320402 (321402)	78096+63064+77944	GW	SCR	EVL	ASR
320404 (321404)	78098+63066+77946	GW	SCR	EVL	ASR
320411 (321411)	78105+63073+77953	GW	SCR	EVL	ASR
320412 (321412)	78106+63074+77954	GW	SCR	EVL	ASR
320413 (321413)	78107+63075+77955	GW	SCR	EVL	ASR
320414 (321414)	78108+63076+77956	GW	SCR	EVL	ASR
320415 (321415)	78109+63077+77957	GW	SCR	EVL	ASR
320416 (321416)	78110+63078+77958	GW	SCR	EVL	ASR
320417 (321417)	78111+63079+77959	GW	SCR	EVL	ASR
320418 (321418)	78112+63080+77962	GW	SCR	EVL	ASR
320420 (321420)	78114+68032+77964	GW	SCR	EVL	ASR

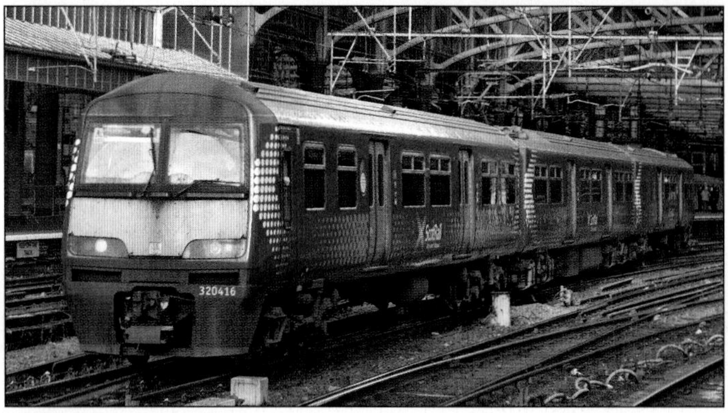

Modified from a four-car Class 321 to Class 320 three-car style for use in Scotland, set No. 320416 (321416), departs from Glasgow Central. These sets sport standard Scottish Railways blue and white livery and operate in a common pool with Class 320/3s. **CJM**

Class 321
BREL 4-Car Outer Suburban

Built: 1988-1991
Vehicle length: Driving - 65ft 0¾in (19.83m)
Intermediate - 65ft 4¼in (19.92m)
Height: 12ft 4¾in (3.78m)
Width: 9ft 3in (2.82m)
Power: 25kV ac overhead
Horsepower: 1,438hp (1,072kW)
Transmission: Electric

321/3 Formation: DTSO+MSO+TSO+DTSO

321301	78049+62975+71880+77853		IL	GAZ	EVL	GAR
321302	78050+62976+71881+77854		IL	GAZ	EVL	GAR
321303	78051+62977+71882+77855		IL	GAZ	EVL	GAR
321304	78052+62978+71883+77856		IL	GAZ	EVL	GAR
321305	78053+62979+71884+77857		IL	GAZ	EVL	GAR
321306	78054+62980+71885+77858		IL	GAZ	EVL	GAR
321307	78055+62981+71886+77859		IL	GAZ	EVL	GAR
321308	78056+62982+71887+77860		IL	GAZ	EVL	GAR
321309	78057+62983+71888+77861		IL	GAZ	EVL	GAR
321310	78058+62984+71889+77862		IL	GAZ	EVL	GAR
321311	78059+62985+71890+77863		IL	GAZ	EVL	GAR
321312	78060+62986+71891+77864		IL	GAZ	EVL	GAR
321313	78061+62987+71892+77865		IL	GAZ	EVL	GAR
321314	78062+62988+71893+77866		IL	GAZ	EVL	GAR
321315	78063+62989+71894+77867		IL	GAZ	EVL	GAR
321316	78064+62990+71895+77868		IL	GAZ	EVL	GAR
321317	78065+62991+71896+77869		IL	GAZ	EVL	GAR
321318	78066+62992+71897+77870		IL	GAZ	EVL	GAR
321319	78067+62993+71898+77871		IL	GAZ	EVL	GAR
321320	78068+62994+71899+77872		IL	GAZ	EVL	GAR
321321	78069+62995+71900+77873		IL	GAZ	EVL	GAR
321322	78070+62996+71901+77874		IL	GAZ	EVL	GAR
321323	78071+62997+71902+77875		IL	GAZ	EVL	GAR
321324	78072+62998+71903+77876		IL	GAZ	EVL	GAR
321325	78073+62999+71904+77877		IL	GAZ	EVL	GAR
321326	78074+63000+71905+77878		IL	GAZ	EVL	GAR
321327	78075+63001+71906+77879		IL	GAZ	EVL	GAR
321328	78076+63002+71907+77880		IL	GAZ	EVL	GAR
321329	78077+63003+71908+77881		IL	GAZ	EVL	GAR
321330	78078+63004+71909+77882		IL	GAR	EVL	GAR
321331	78079+63005+71910+77883		ZN	NXU	EVL	(S)
321332	78080+63006+71911+77884		ZN	NXU	EVL	OLS
321333	78081+63007+71912+77885		ZN	NXU	EVL	(S)
321334*	78082+63008+71913+77886	Swift Express set	-	SPL	-	EVL
321335	78083+63009+71914+77887		ZN	NXU	EVL	OLS
321336	78084+63010+71915+77888		ZN	NXU	EVL	OLS
321337	78085+63011+71916+77889		WS	NXU	EVL	OLS
321338	78086+63012+71917+77890		ZN	NXU	EVL	(S)
321339	78087+63013+71918+77891		ZN	NXU	EVL	(S)
321340	78088+63014+71919+77892		ZN	NXU	EVL	(S)
321341	78089+63015+71920+77893		ZN	NXU	EVL	(S)
321342	78090+63016+71921+77894	*R. Barnes*	ZN	NXU	EVL	(S)
321343	78091+63017+71922+77895		ZN	NXU	EVL	(S)

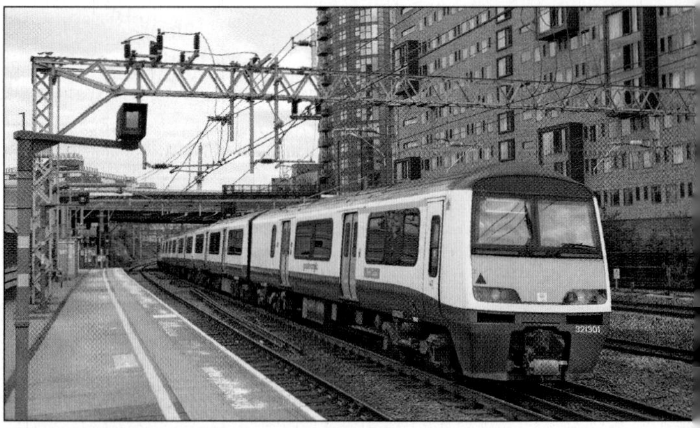

Another class which is rapidly disappearing is the Greater Anglia Class 321/322s, being replaced by new Class 720 stock. Refurbished 'Renatus' set No. 321301 departs from Stratford with its DTC coach nearest the camera. **CJM**

321/4 Formation: DTSO+MSO+TSO+DTSO

321403	78097+63065+71950+77945		IL	BLU	EVL	GAR
321405	78099+63067+71953+77947		GA	BLU	EVL	OLS
321406	78100+63068+71954+77948		WS	BLU	EVL	(S)
321407*	78101+63069+71955+77949	Swift Express set	ZN	SPL	-	EVL
321408	78102+63070+71956+77959		GA	BLU	EVL	OLS
321409	78103+63071+71957+77960	*Dame Alice Owen's School 400 Years of Learning*	WS	BLU	EVL	(S)
321410	78104+63072+71958+77961		GA	BLU	EVL	OLS
321419*	78113+63081+71969+77963	Swift Express set	ZN	SPL	-	EVL
321421	78115+63083+71969+77963		WS	NXU	EVL	OLS
321423	78117+63085+71971+77965		WS	NXU	EVL	(S)
321424	78118+63086+71972+77966		WS	NXU	EVL	(S)
321426	78120+63088+71974+77968		WS	NXU	EVL	OLS
321427	78121+63089+71975+77969		WS	NXU	EVL	OLS
321428*	78122+63090+71976+77970	Swift Express set	ZN	SPL	-	EVL
321429*	78123+62091+71977+77971	Swift Express set	ZN	SPL	-	EVL
321430	78124+63092+71978+77972		WS	NXU	EVL	OLS
321431	78151+63125+72011+78300		GA	NXU	EVL	OLS
321432	78152+63126+72012+78301		WS	NXU	EVL	OLS
321433	78153+63127+72013+78302		WS	NXU	EVL	OLS

321434	78154+63128+72014+78303	WS	NXU	EVL	(S)
321436	78156+63130+72016+78305	WS	NXU	EVL	(S)
321439	78159+63133+72019+78308	GA	AWT	EVL	OLS
321440	78160+63134+72020+78309	WS	AWT	EVL	OLS
321441	78161+63135+72021+78310	WS	AWT	EVL	OLS
321443	78125+63099+71985+78274	GA	AWT	EVL	OLS
321444	78126+63100+71986+78275	GA	AWT	EVL	OLS
321445	78127+63101+71987+78276	GA	AWT	EVL	OLS
321447	78129+63103+71989+78278	GA	AWT	EVL	OLS

* *Eversholt / Ricardo Rail 'Swift Express Freight' unit*

321/9 Formation: DTSO+MSO+TSO+DTSO

321901	77990+63153+72128+77993	IL	BLU	EVL	GAR
321902	77991+63154+72129+77994	IL	BLU	EVL	GAR
321903	77992+63155+72130+77995	IL	BLE	EVL	GAR

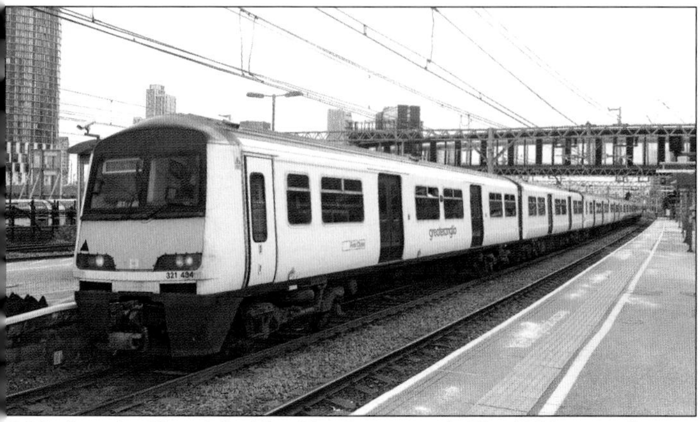

Originally used on Network SouthEast West Coast routes, the Class 321/4s now work on Greater Anglia. With the now declassified first class area leading set No. 321434 calls at Stratford with a Southend service in summer 2021. **CJM**

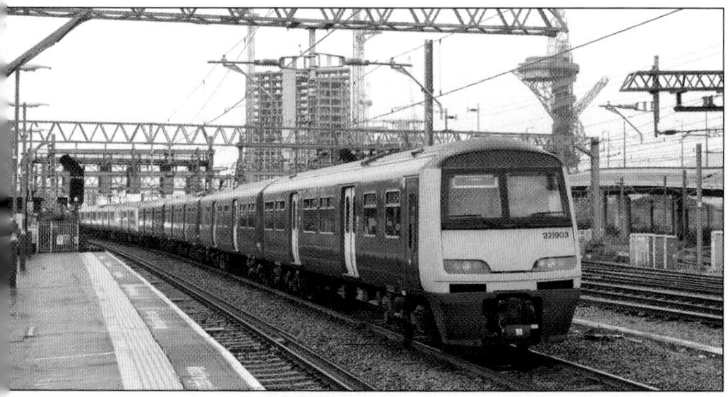

The three Class 321/9 units displaced from Leeds area use by the introduction of Class 331 stock, were transferred to Ilford to work alongside the Class 321s as they were closer to the required PRM standards. Set No. 321903 is seen at Stratford. **CJM**

Class 322
BREL 4-Car Outer Suburban

Built: 1990
Vehicle length: Driving - 65ft 0¾in (19.83m)
Intermediate - 65ft 4¼in (19.92m)
Height: 12ft 4¾in (3.78m)
Width: 9ft 3in (2.82m)
Power: 25kV ac overhead
Horsepower: 1,438hp (1,072kW)
Transmission: Electric

Formation: DTSOL+MSO+TSO+DTSO

322481	78163+63137+72023+77985	IL	BLU	EVL	GAR
322482	78164+63138+72024+77986	IL	BLU	EVL	GAR
322483	78165+63139+72025+77987	IL	BLU	EVL	GAR
322484	78166+63140+72026+77988	IL	BLU	EVL	GAR
322485	78167+63141+72027+77989	IL	BLU	EVL	GAR

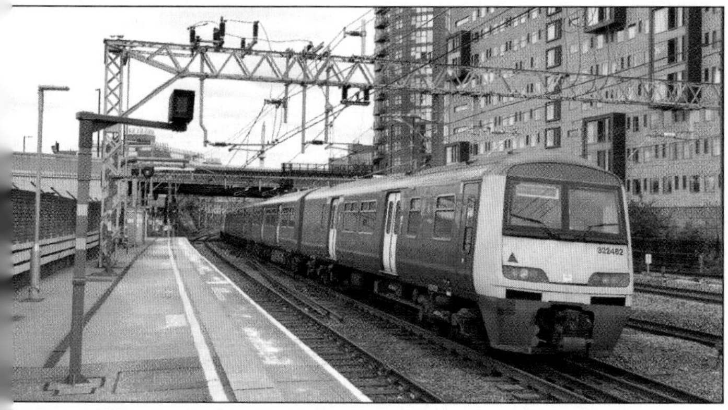

The Class 322 four-car fleet have operated in many different locations including the north west, Scotland and Yorkshire, they are finishing their days working on Greater Anglia alongside the Class 321s. Painted in all-over Northern blue No. 322482 with its DTSOL coach nearest the camera departs from Stratford. **CJM**

Class 323
Hunslet TPL 3-Car Suburban

Built: 1992-1993
Vehicle length: Driving - 76ft 8¾in (23.37m)
Intermediate - 76ft 10¾in (23.44m)
Height: 12ft 4¾in (3.78m)
Width: 9ft 2¼in (2.80m)
Power: 25kV ac overhead
Horsepower: 1,566hp (1,168kW)
Transmission: Electric

Formation: DMSO+PTSOL+DMSO

323201	64001+72201+65001	*Duddeston*	SI	WMT	PTR	WMR
323202	64002+72202+65002	*Butlers Lane*	SI	WMT	PTR	WMR
323203	64003+72203+65003	*Aston*	SI	WMT	PTR	WMR
323204	64004+72204+65004	*Selly Oak*	SI	WMT	PTR	WMR
323205	64005+72205+65005	*Blake Street*	SI	WMT	PTR	WMR
323206	64006+72206+65006	*Barnt Green*	SI	WMT	PTR	WMR
323207	64007+72207+65007	*Bournville*	SI	WMT	PTR	WMR
323208	64008+72208+65008	*Five Ways*	SI	WMT	PTR	WMR
323209	64009+72209+65009	*Birmingham New Street*	SI	WMT	PTR	WMR
323210	64010+72210+65010	*Shenstone*	SI	WMT	PTR	WMR
323211	64011+72211+65011	*Four Oaks*	SI	WMT	PTR	WMR
323212	64012+72212+65012	*Bromsgrove*	SI	WMT	PTR	WMR
323213	64013+72213+65013	*Sutton Coldfield*	SI	WMT	PTR	WMR
323214	64014+72214+65014	*Wylde Green*	SI	WMT	PTR	WMR
323215	64015+72215+65015	*Gravelly Hill*	SI	WMT	PTR	WMR
323216	64016+72216+65016	*University*	SI	WMT	PTR	WMR
323217	64017+72217+65017	*Chester Road*	SI	WMT	PTR	WMR
323218	64018+72218+65018	*Lichfield City*	SI	WMT	PTR	WMR
323219	64019+72219+65019	*Kings Norton*	SI	WMT	PTR	WMR
323220	64020+72220+65020	*Lichfield Trent Valley*	SI	WMT	PTR	WMR
323221	64021+72221+65021	*Northfield*	SI	WMT	PTR	WMR
323222	64022+72222+65022	*Redditch*	SI	WMT	PTR	WMR
323223	64023+72223+65023		AN	NNR	PTR	NOR
323224	64024+72224+65024		AN	NNR	PTR	NOR
323225	64025+72225+65025		AN	NNR	PTR	NOR
323226	64026+72226+65026		AN	NNR	PTR	NOR
323227	64027+72227+65027		AN	NNR	PTR	NOR
323228	64028+72228+65028		AN	NNR	PTR	NOR
323229	64029+72229+65029		AN	NNR	PTR	NOR
323230	64030+72230+65030		AN	NNR	PTR	NOR
323231	64031+72231+65031		AN	NNR	PTR	NOR
323232	64032+72232+65032		AN	NNR	PTR	NOR
323233	64033+72233+65033		AN	NNR	PTR	NOR
323234	64034+72234+65034		AN	NNR	PTR	NOR
323235	64035+72235+65035		AN	NNR	PTR	NOR
323236	64036+72236+65036		AN	NNR	PTR	NOR
323237	64037+72237+65037		AN	NNR	PTR	NOR
323238	64038+72238+65038		AN	NNR	PTR	NOR
323239	64039+72239+65039		AN	NNR	PTR	NOR
323240	64040+72340+65040	*Erdington*	SI	WMT	PTR	WMR
323241	64041+72341+65041	*Dave Pomroy 323 Fleet Engineer 40 Years Service*	SI	WMT	PTR	WMR
323242	64042+72342+65042	*Alvechurch*	SI	WMT	PTR	WMR
323243	64043+72343+65043	*Longbridge*	SI	WMT	PTR	WMR

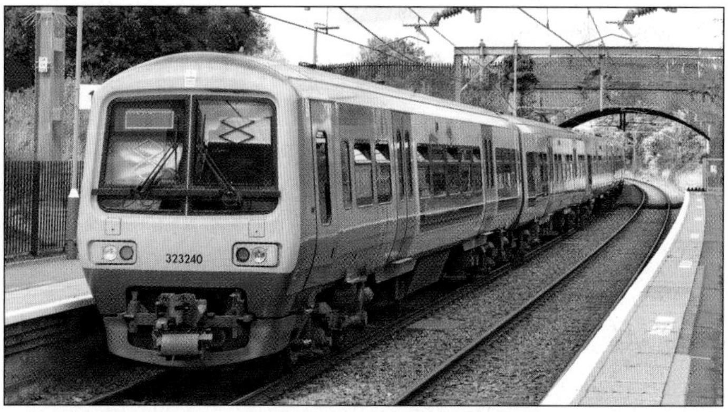

Soon to be replaced by Class 730 units, the West Midlands Class 323s remain the backbone of Cross-City electric services. Painted in WM gold, grey and grey livery, set No. 323240 departs from Alvechurch bound for Birmingham New Street. **CJM**

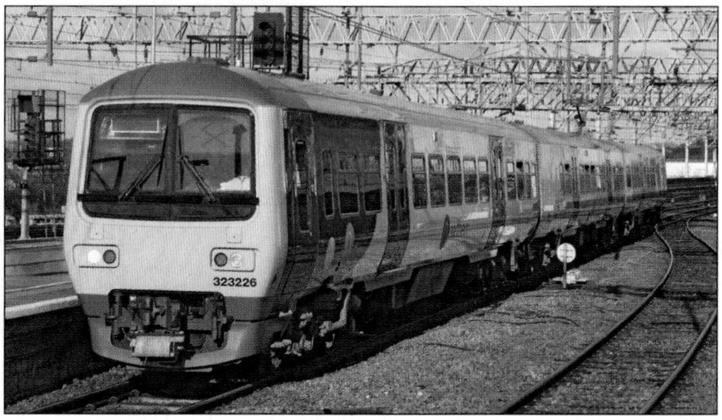

Northern operated Class 323s are based at Liverpool Allerton depot and sport Northern white and blue livery. Set No. 323226 is seen arriving at Stockport. A number of the West Midlands sets are due to transfer to Northern in 2022-2023. **CJM**

Class 325
AdTranz / Royal Mail 4-Car Parcels/Mail

Built: 1995-1996
Vehicle length: Driving - 65ft 0¾in (19.83m)
Intermediate - 65ft 4¼in (19.92m)
Height: 12ft 4¼in (3.77m)
Width: 9ft 3in (2.82m)
Power: 25kV ac overhead
Horsepower: 1,438hp (1,072kW)
Transmission: Electric

Formation: DTPMV+MPMV+TPMV+DTPMV

325001	68300+68340+68360+68301		CE	RMR	RML	DBC
325002	68302+68341+68361+68303		CE	RMR	RML	DBC
325003	68304+68342+68362+68305		CE	RMR	RML	DBC
325004	68306+68343+68363+68307		CE	RMR	RML	DBC
325005	68308+68344+68364+68309		CE	RMR	RML	DBC
325006	68310+68345+68365+68311		CE	RMR	RML	DBC
325007	68312+68346+68366+68313	*Peter Howarth C.B.E*	CE	RMR	RML	DBC
325008	68314+68347+68367+68315		CE	RMR	RML	DBC
325009	68316+68348+68368+68317		CE	RMR	RML	DBC
325011	68320+68350+68370+68321		CE	RMR	RML	DBC
325012	68322+68351+68371+68323		CE	RMR	RML	DBC
325013	68324+68352+68372+68325		CE	RMR	RML	DBC
325014	68326+68353+68373+68327		CE	RMR	RML	DBC
325015	68328+68354+68374+68329		CE	RMR	RML	DBC
325016	68330+68355+68375+68331		CE	RMR	RML	DBC

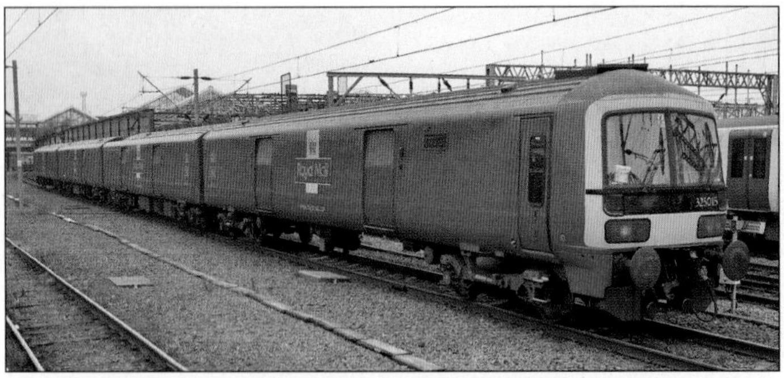

Operated by DB Cargo for Royal Mail, the Class 325 sets operate limited long distance mail services between Shieldmuir in Scotland and Wembley in London calling at some north eastern mail hubs. Set No. 325015 is seen at Crewe, carrying the latest Royal Mail colours in August 2021. **Spencer Conquest**

Class 326
BREL 4-Car Parcels & Mail

Built: 1987-1989
Vehicle length: Driving - 65ft 0¾in (19.83m)
Intermediate - 65ft 4¼in (19.92m)
Height: 11ft 9in (3.58m)
Width: 9ft 3in (2.82m)
Power: 25kV ac overhead
Horsepower: 1,438hp (1,072kW)
Transmission: Electric

Formation: DTPMV+MPMV+TPMV+DTPMV

326001	(319373)	77483+63055+71941+77482	ZG	ORI	PTR	ROG
326xxx	(319377)§	77491+63059+71945+77490	ZG	ORI	PTR	ROG
326xxx	(319380)§	77497+63062+71948+77496	ZG	ORI	PTR	ROG
326xxx	(319441)§	77371+62931+71812+77370	ZG	ORI	PTR	ROG

Nine sets for conversion § Awaiting conversion
In spring 2022 sets were awaiting renumbering to the 326xxx series

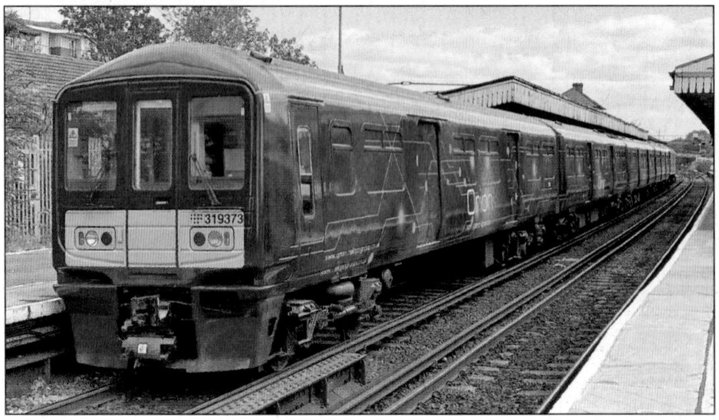

Rebuilt by Arlington at Eastleigh for light freight transport with Rail Operations Group under their Orion business, set No. 319373, soon to be renumbered as 326001 is seen hauled through Basingstoke. These sets have lost their 750V dc power collection. **Spencer Conquest**

Class 331
CAF 3 and 4-car 'Civity'

Built: 2017-2020
Vehicle length: Driving - 78ft 8in (24.02m)
Intermediate - 76ft 6in (23.35m)
Height: 12ft 7in (3.85m)
Width: 8ft 9in (2.71m)
Power: 25kV ac overhead
Horsepower: 1,475hp (1,100kW)
Transmission: Electric

331/0 Formation: DMSL+PTSO+DMS

331001	463001+464001+466001	AN	NNR	EVL	NOR
331002	463002+464002+466002	AN	NNR	EVL	NOR
331003	463003+464003+466003	AN	NNR	EVL	NOR
331004	463004+464004+466004	AN	NNR	EVL	NOR
331005	463005+464005+466005	AN	NNR	EVL	NOR
331006	463006+464006+466006	AN	NNR	EVL	NOR
331007	463007+464007+466007	AN	NNR	EVL	NOR
331008	463008+464008+466008	AN	NNR	EVL	NOR
331009	463009+464009+466009	AN	NNR	EVL	NOR
331010	463010+464010+466010	AN	NNR	EVL	NOR
331011	463011+464011+466011	AN	NNR	EVL	NOR
331012	463012+464012+466012	AN	NNR	EVL	NOR
331013	463013+464013+466013	AN	NNR	EVL	NOR
331014	463014+464014+466014	AN	NNR	EVL	NOR
331015	463015+464015+466015	AN	NNR	EVL	NOR
331016	463016+464016+466016	AN	NNR	EVL	NOR
331017	463017+464017+466017	AN	NNR	EVL	NOR
331018	463018+464018+466018	AN	NNR	EVL	NOR
331019	463019+464019+466019	AN	NNR	EVL	NOR
331020	463020+464020+466020	AN	NNR	EVL	NOR
331021	463021+464021+466021	AN	NNR	EVL	NOR
331022	463022+464022+466022	AN	NNR	EVL	NOR
331023	463023+464023+466023	AN	NNR	EVL	NOR
331024	463024+464024+466024	AN	NNR	EVL	NOR
331025	463025+464025+466025	AN	NNR	EVL	NOR
331026	463026+464026+466026	AN	NNR	EVL	NOR
331027	463027+464027+466027	AN	NNR	EVL	NOR
331028	463028+464028+466028	AN	NNR	EVL	NOR
331029	463029+464029+466029	AN	NNR	EVL	NOR
331030	463030+464030+466030	AN	NNR	EVL	NOR
331031	463031+464031+466031	AN	NNR	EVL	NOR

331/1 Formation: DMSL+PTSO+TSO+DMS

331101	463101+464101+465101+466101		NL	NNR	EVL	NOR
331102	463102+464102+465102+466102		NL	NNR	EVL	NOR
331103	463103+464103+465103+466103		NL	NNR	EVL	NOR
331104	463104+464104+465104+466104		AN	NNR	EVL	NOR
331105	463105+464105+465105+466105		NL	NNR	EVL	NOR
331106	463106+464106+465106+466106	*Proud to be Northern*	AN	NNR	EVL	NOR
331107	463107+464107+465107+466107		NL	NNR	EVL	NOR
331108	463108+464108+465108+466108		NL	NNR	EVL	NOR
331109	463109+464109+465109+466109		NL	NNR	EVL	NOR
331110	463110+464110+465110+466110	*Proud to be Northern*	NL	NNR	EVL	NOR
331111	463111+464111+465111+466111		NL	NNR	EVL	NOR
331112	463112+464112+465112+466112		NL	NNR	EVL	NOR

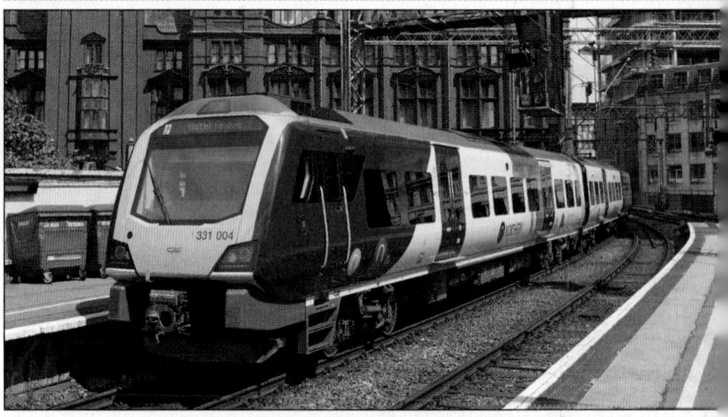

The electric version of the Class 195, is the Class 331, built by CAF in three and four-car formations for Northern. Three-car Class 331/0 No. 331004 departs from Manchester Oxford Road bound for Manchester Piccadilly. **CJM**

Class 332
CAF 'Heathrow Express'

Formation: DMS+TSO+PTSO

332001	78400+72412+63400	Siemens Training School, Goole

Class 333
CAF 4-Car Surburban

Built: 2000-2003
Vehicle length: Driving - 77ft 10¾in (23.74m)
Intermediate - 75ft 11in (23.14m)
Height: 12ft 1½in (3.70m)
Width: 9ft 1in (2.75m)
Power: 25kV ac overhead
Horsepower: 1,877hp (1,400kW)
Transmission: Electric

Formation: DMSO+PTSO+TSO+DMSO

333001	78451+74461+74477+78452	NL	NNR	ANG	NOR
333002	78453+74462+74478+78454	NL	NNR	ANG	NOR
333003	78455+74463+74479+78456	NL	NNR	ANG	NOR
333004	78457+74464+74480+78458	NL	NNR	ANG	NOR
333005	78459+74465+74481+78460	NL	NNR	ANG	NOR
333006	78461+74466+74482+78462	NL	NNR	ANG	NOR
333007	78463+74467+74483+78464	NL	NNR	ANG	NOR
333008	78465+74468+74484+78466	NL	NNR	ANG	NOR
333009	78467+74469+74485+78468	NL	NNR	ANG	NOR
333010	78469+74470+74486+78470	NL	NNR	ANG	NOR
333011	78471+74471+74487+78472	NL	NNR	ANG	NOR
333012	78473+74472+74488+78474	NL	NNR	ANG	NOR
333013	78475+74473+74489+78476	NL	NNR	ANG	NOR
333014	78477+74474+74490+78478	NL	NNR	ANG	NOR
333015	78479+74475+74491+78480	NL	NNR	ANG	NOR
333016	78481+74476+74492+78482	NL	NNR	ANG	NOR

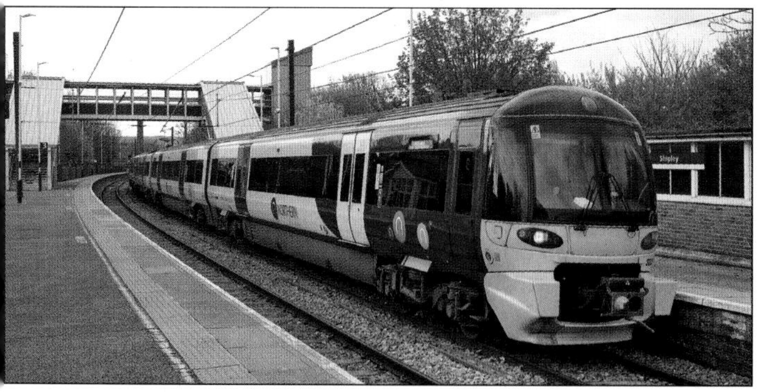

Aire Valley electric services in the Leeds, Bradford, Skipton area are operated by a fleet of CAF/ Siemens Class 333 four-car sets. All are refurbished and carry white/blue Northern livery and are based at Neville Hill depot. No. 333001 is seen at Shipley in May 2021. **Antony Christie**

Class 334
Alstom 4-car Outer-Suburban 'Juniper'

Built: 1999-2002
Vehicle length: Driving - 69ft 0¼in (21.05m)
Intermediate - 65ft 4¼in (19.92m)
Height: 12ft 3in (3.73m)
Width: 9ft 2¾in (2.81m)
Power: 25kV ac overhead
Horsepower: 1,448hp (1,080kW)
Transmission: Electric

	Formation: DMSO+PTSO+DMSO				
334001	64101+74301+65101	GW	SCR	EVL	ASR
334002	64102+74302+65102	GW	SCR	EVL	ASR
334003	64103+74303+65103	GW	SCR	EVL	ASR
334004	64104+74304+65104	GW	SCR	EVL	ASR
334005	64105+74305+65105	GW	SCR	EVL	ASR
334006	64106+74306+65106	GW	SCR	EVL	ASR
334007	64107+74307+65107	GW	SCR	EVL	ASR
334008	64108+74308+65108	GW	SCR	EVL	ASR
334009	64109+74309+65109	GW	SCR	EVL	ASR
334010	64110+74310+65110	GW	SCR	EVL	ASR
334011	64111+74311+65111	GW	SCR	EVL	ASR
334012	64112+74312+65112	GW	SCR	EVL	ASR
334013	64113+74313+65113	GW	SCR	EVL	ASR
334014	64114+74314+65114	GW	SCR	EVL	ASR
334015	64115+74315+65115	GW	SCR	EVL	ASR
334016	64116+74316+65116	GW	SCR	EVL	ASR
334017	64117+74317+65117	GW	SCR	EVL	ASR
334018	64118+74318+65118	GW	SCR	EVL	ASR
334019	64119+74319+65119	GW	SCR	EVL	ASR
334020	64120+74320+65120	GW	SCR	EVL	ASR
334021	64121+74321+65121	GW	SCR	EVL	ASR
334022	64122+74322+65122	GW	SCR	EVL	ASR
334023	64123+74323+65123	GW	SCR	EVL	ASR
334024	64124+74324+65124	GW	SCR	EVL	ASR
334025	64125+74325+65125	GW	SCR	EVL	ASR
334026	64126+74326+65126	GW	SCR	EVL	ASR
334027	64127+74327+65127	GW	SCR	EVL	ASR
334028	64128+74328+65128	GW	SCR	EVL	ASR
334029	64129+74329+65129	GW	SCR	EVL	ASR
334030	64130+74330+65130	GW	SCR	EVL	ASR
334031	64131+74331+65131	GW	SCR	EVL	ASR
334032	64132+74332+65132	GW	SCR	EVL	ASR
334033	64133+74333+65133	GW	SCR	EVL	ASR
334034	64134+74334+65134	GW	SCR	EVL	ASR
334035	64135+74335+65135	GW	SCR	EVL	ASR
334036	64136+74336+65136	GW	SCR	EVL	ASR
334037	64137+74337+65137	GW	SCR	EVL	ASR
334038	64138+74338+65138	GW	SCR	EVL	ASR
334039	64139+74339+65139	GW	SCR	EVL	ASR
334040	64140+74340+65140	GW	SCR	EVL	ASR

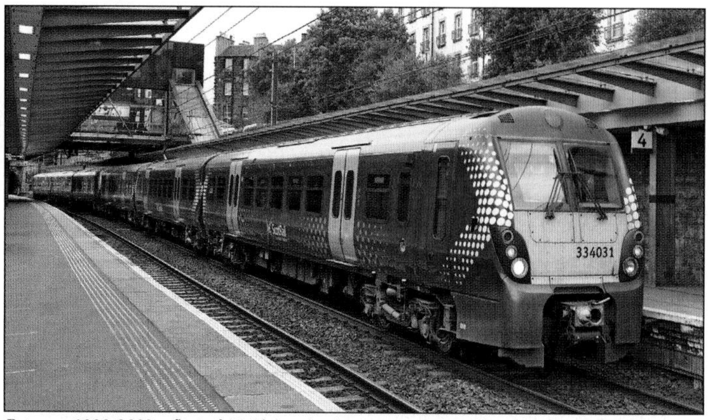

Between 1999-2002 a fleet of 40 Alstom Juniper sets were introduced by ScotRail. Allocated to Glasgow Shields Road depot, the three car sets operate in the Edinburgh-Glasgow area. No. 334031 arrives at Edinburgh Haymarket in November 2021. **CJM**

Class 345
Bombardier 9-car 'Elizabeth Line' 'Aventra'

Built: 2017-2020
Vehicle length: 73ft 9in (22.50m)
Height: 12ft 3in (3.73m)
Width: 9ft 2in (2.78m)
Power: 25kV ac overhead
Horsepower: 6,798hp (5,000kW)
Transmission: Electric

	Formation: DMS+PMS+MS+MS+TS+MS+MS+PMS+DMS				
345001	340101+340201+340301+340401+340501+340601+340701+340801+340901	OC	ELZ	3RL	ELZ
345002	340102+340202+340302+340402+340502+340602+340702+340802+340902	OC	ELZ	3RL	ELZ
345003	340103+340203+340303+340403+340503+340603+340703+340803+340903	OC	ELZ	3RL	ELZ
345004	340104+340204+340304+340404+340504+340604+340704+340804+340904	OC	ELZ	3RL	ELZ
345005	340105+340205+340305+340405+340505+340605+340705+340805+340905	OC	ELZ	3RL	ELZ
345006	340106+340206+340306+340406+340506+340606+340706+340806+340906	OC	ELZ	3RL	ELZ
345007	340107+340207+340307+340407+340507+340607+340707+340807+340907	OC	ELZ	3RL	ELZ
345008	340108+340208+340308+340408+340508+340608+340708+340808+340908	OC	ELZ	3RL	ELZ
345009	340109+340209+340309+340409+340509+340609+340709+340809+340909	OC	ELZ	3RL	ELZ
345010	340110+340210+340310+340410+340510+340610+340710+340810+340910	OC	ELZ	3RL	ELZ
345011	340111+340211+340311+340411+340511+340611+340711+340811+340911	OC	ELZ	3RL	ELZ
345012	340112+340212+340312+340412+340512+340612+340712+340812+340912	OC	ELZ	3RL	ELZ
345013	340113+340213+340313+340413+340513+340613+340713+340813+340913	OC	ELZ	3RL	ELZ
345014	340114+340214+340314+340414+340514+340614+340714+340814+340914	OC	ELZ	3RL	ELZ
345015	340115+340215+340315+340415+340515+340615+340715+340815+340915	OC	ELZ	3RL	ELZ
345016	340116+340216+340316+340416+340516+340616+340716+340816+340916	OC	ELZ	3RL	ELZ
345017	340117+340217+340317+340417+340517+340617+340717+340817+340917	OC	ELZ	3RL	ELZ
345018	340118+340218+340318+340418+340518+340618+340718+340818+340918	OC	ELZ	3RL	ELZ
345019	340119+340219+340319+340419+340519+340619+340719+340819+340919	OC	ELZ	3RL	ELZ
345020	340120+340220+340320+340420+340520+340620+340720+340820+340920	OC	ELZ	3RL	ELZ
345021	340121+340221+340321+340421+340521+340621+340721+340821+340921	OC	ELZ	3RL	ELZ
345022	340122+340222+340322+340422+340522+340622+340722+340822+340922	OC	ELZ	3RL	ELZ
345023	340123+340223+340323+340423+340523+340623+340723+340823+340923	OC	ELZ	3RL	ELZ
345024	340124+340224+340324+340424+340524+340624+340724+340824+340924	OC	ELZ	3RL	ELZ
345025	340125+340225+340325+340425+340525+340625+340725+340825+340925	OC	ELZ	3RL	ELZ
345026	340126+340226+340326+340426+340526+340626+340726+340826+340926	OC	ELZ	3RL	ELZ
345027	340127+340227+340327+340427+340527+340627+340727+340827+340927	OC	ELZ	3RL	ELZ
345028	340128+340228+340328+340428+340528+340628+340728+340828+340928	OC	ELZ	3RL	ELZ
345029	340129+340229+340329+340429+340529+340629+340729+340829+340929	OC	ELZ	3RL	ELZ
345030	340130+340230+340330+340430+340530+340630+340730+340830+340930	OC	ELZ	3RL	ELZ
345031	340131+340231+340331+340431+340531+340631+340731+340831+340931	OC	ELZ	3RL	ELZ
345032	340132+340232+340332+340432+340532+340632+340732+340832+340932	OC	ELZ	3RL	ELZ
345033	340133+340233+340333+340433+340533+340633+340733+340833+340933	OC	ELZ	3RL	ELZ
345034	340134+340234+340334+340434+340534+340634+340734+340834+340934	OC	ELZ	3RL	ELZ
345035	340135+340235+340335+340435+340535+340635+340735+340835+340935	OC	ELZ	3RL	ELZ
345036	340136+340236+340336+340436+340536+340636+340736+340836+340936	OC	ELZ	3RL	ELZ
345037	340137+340237+340337+340437+340537+340637+340737+340837+340937	OC	ELZ	3RL	ELZ
345038	340138+340238+340338+340438+340538+340638+340738+340838+340938	OC	ELZ	3RL	ELZ
345039	340139+340239+340339+340439+340539+340639+340739+340839+340939	OC	ELZ	3RL	ELZ
345040	340140+340240+340340+340440+340540+340640+340740+340840+340940	OC	ELZ	3RL	ELZ
345041	340141+340241+340341+340441+340541+340641+340741+340841+340941	OC	ELZ	3RL	ELZ
345042	340142+340242+340342+340442+340542+340642+340742+340842+340942	OC	ELZ	3RL	ELZ
345043	340143+340243+340343+340443+340543+340643+340743+340843+340943	OC	ELZ	3RL	ELZ
345044	340144+340244+340344+340444+340544+340644+340744+340844+340944	OC	ELZ	3RL	ELZ
345045	340145+340245+340345+340445+340545+340645+340745+340845+340945	OC	ELZ	3RL	ELZ

345046	340146+340246+340346+340446+340546+340646+340746+340846+340946	OC	ELZ	3RL	ELZ
345047	340147+340247+340347+340447+340547+340647+340747+340847+340947	OC	ELZ	3RL	ELZ
345048	340148+340248+340348+340448+340548+340648+340748+340848+340948	OC	ELZ	3RL	ELZ
345049	340149+340249+340349+340449+340549+340649+340749+340849+340949	OC	ELZ	3RL	ELZ
345050	340150+340250+340350+340450+340550+340650+340750+340850+340950	OC	ELZ	3RL	ELZ
345051	340151+340251+340351+340451+340551+340651+340751+340851+340951	OC	ELZ	3RL	ELZ
345052	340152+340252+340352+340452+340552+340652+340752+340852+340952	OC	ELZ	3RL	ELZ
345053	340153+340253+340353+340453+340553+340653+340753+340853+340953	OC	ELZ	3RL	ELZ
345054	340154+340254+340354+340454+340554+340654+340754+340854+340954	OC	ELZ	3RL	ELZ
345055	340155+340255+340355+340455+340555+340655+340755+340855+340955	OC	ELZ	3RL	ELZ
345056	340156+340256+340356+340456+340556+340656+340756+340856+340956	OC	ELZ	3RL	ELZ
345057	340157+340257+340357+340457+340557+340657+340757+340857+340957	OC	ELZ	3RL	ELZ
345058	340158+340258+340358+340458+340558+340658+340758+340858+340958	OC	ELZ	3RL	ELZ
345059	340159+340259+340359+340459+340559+340659+340759+340859+340959	OC	ELZ	3RL	ELZ
345060	340160+340260+340360+340460+340560+340660+340760+340860+340960	OC	ELZ	3RL	ELZ
345061	340161+340261+340361+340461+340561+340661+340761+340861+340961	OC	ELZ	3RL	ELZ
345062	340162+340262+340362+340462+340562+340662+340762+340862+340962	OC	ELZ	3RL	ELZ
345063	340163+340263+340363+340463+340563+340663+340763+340863+340963	OC	ELZ	3RL	ELZ
345064	340164+340264+340364+340464+340564+340664+340764+340864+340964	OC	ELZ	3RL	ELZ
345065	340165+340265+340365+340465+340565+340665+340765+340865+340965	OC	ELZ	3RL	ELZ
345066	340166+340266+340366+340466+340566+340666+340766+340866+340966	OC	ELZ	3RL	ELZ
345067	340167+340267+340367+340467+340567+340667+340767+340867+340967	OC	ELZ	3RL	ELZ
345068	340168+340268+340368+340468+340568+340668+340768+340868+340968	OC	ELZ	3RL	ELZ
345069	340169+340269+340369+340469+340569+340669+340769+340869+340969	OC	ELZ	3RL	ELZ
345070	340170+340270+340370+340470+340570+340670+340770+340870+340970	OC	ELZ	3RL	ELZ

Some sets are temporally reduced to seven-car formation, by the removal of two MS vehicles

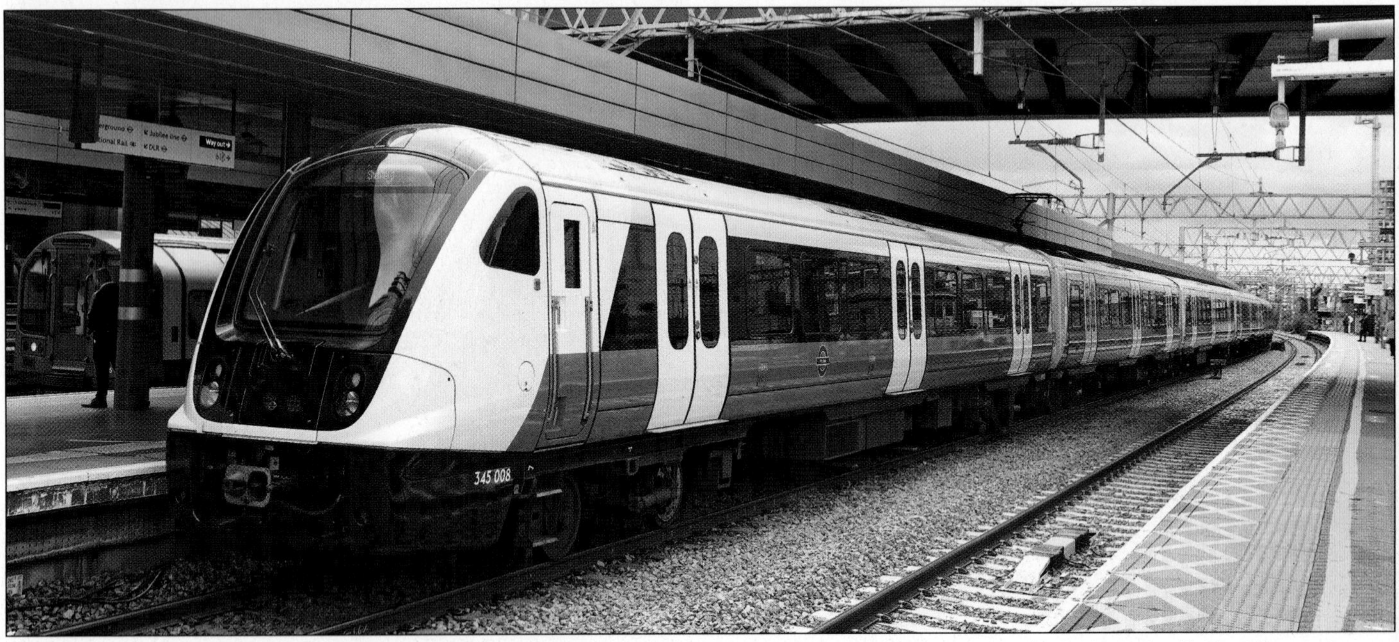

The Elizabeth Line linking east and west London commenced operation in the core section from Paddington to Abby Wood under central London in May 2022, with Class 345s operating Elizabeth Line services on the western end between Reading/Heathrow and Paddington, between Paddington and Abbey Wood and on the eastern end between Liverpool Street and Shenfield. Through running should start towards the end of 2022. Set 345008 arrives at Stratford in June 2021 with a service for Shenfield. **CJM**

Class 350
Siemens 4-car Main Line 'Desiro'

Built: 2004-2014
Vehicle length: 66ft 9in (20.34m)
Height: 12ft 1½in (3.70m)
Width: 9ft 2in (2.79m)
Power: 25kV ac overhead
Horsepower: 1,341hp (1,000kW)
Transmission: Electric

350/1 Formation: DMS+TC+PTSO+DMS

350101	63761+66811+66861+63711	NN	LNW	ANG	WMR
350102	63762+66812+66862+63712	NN	LNW	ANG	WMR
350103	63765+66813+66863+63713	NN	LNW	ANG	WMR
350104	63764+66814+66864+63714	NN	LNW	ANG	WMR
350105	63763+66815+66868+63715	NN	LNW	ANG	WMR
350106	63766+66816+66866+63716	NN	LNW	ANG	WMR
350107	63767+66817+66867+63717	NN	LNW	ANG	WMR
350108	63768+66818+66865+63718	NN	SPL	ANG	WMR
350109	63769+66819+66869+63719	NN	LNW	ANG	WMR
350110	63770+66820+66870+63720	NN	LNW	ANG	WMR
350111	63771+66821+66871+63721	NN	LNW	ANG	WMR
350112	63772+66822+66872+63722	NN	LNW	ANG	WMR
350113	63773+66823+66873+63723	NN	LNW	ANG	WMR
350114	63774+66824+66874+63724	NN	LNW	ANG	WMR
350115	63775+66825+66875+63725	NN	LNW	ANG	WMR
350116	63776+66826+66876+63726	NN	LNW	ANG	WMR
350117	63777+66827+66877+63727	NN	LNW	ANG	WMR
350118	63778+66828+66878+63728	NN	LNW	ANG	WMR
350119	63779+66829+66879+63729	NN	LNW	ANG	WMR
350120	63780+66830+66880+63730	NN	LNW	ANG	WMR
350121	63781+66831+66881+63731	NN	LNW	ANG	WMR
350122	63782+66832+66882+63732	NN	LNW	ANG	WMR
350123	63783+66833+66883+63733	NN	LNW	ANG	WMR
350124	63784+66834+66884+63734	NN	LNW	ANG	WMR
350125	63785+66835+66885+63735	NN	LNW	ANG	WMR
350126	63786+66836+66886+63736	NN	LNW	ANG	WMR
350127	63787+66837+66887+63737	NN	LNW	ANG	WMR
350128	63788+66838+66888+63738	NN	LNW	ANG	WMR
350129	63789+66839+66889+63739	NN	LNW	ANG	WMR
350130	63790+66840+66890+63740	NN	LNW	ANG	WMR

350/2 Formation: DMS+TC+PTSO+DMS

350231	61431+65231+67531+61531	NN	LNW	PTR	WMR
350232	61432+65232+67532+61532	NN	LNW	PTR	WMR
350233	61433+65233+67533+61546	NN	LMI	PTR	WMR
350234	61434+65234+67534+61534	NN	LNW	PTR	WMR
350235	61435+65235+67535+61535	NN	LMI	PTR	WMR
350236	61436+65236+67536+61536	NN	LMI	PTR	WMR
350237	61437+65237+67537+61537	NN	LMI	PTR	WMR
350238	61438+65238+67538+61538	NN	LMI	PTR	WMR
350239	61439+65239+67539+61539	NN	LNW	PTR	WMR
350240	61440+65240+67540+61540	NN	LNW	PTR	WMR
350241	61441+65241+67541+61541	NN	LMI	PTR	WMR
350242	61442+65242+67542+61542	NN	LMI	PTR	WMR

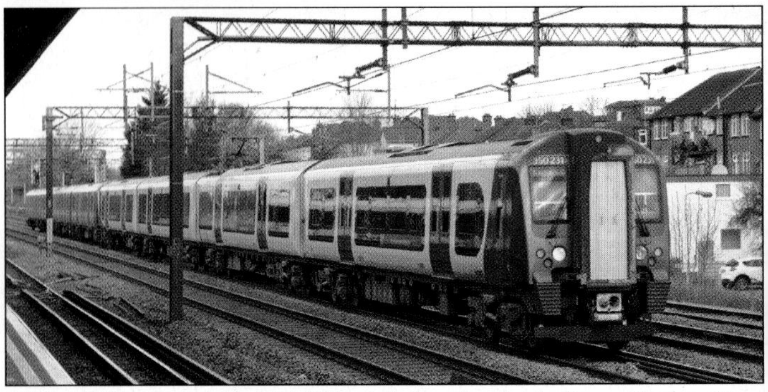

All Class 350s are operated by West Midlands Railway, based at the Siemens Northampton depot. The Class 350/2 sets owned by Porterbrook are due to be taken off lease when Class 730s enter service. Set No. 350231 passes South Kenton. **CJM**

350243	61443+65243+67543+61543	NN	LMI	PTR	WMR
350244	61444+65244+67544+61544	NN	LNW	PTR	WMR
350245	61445+65245+67545+61545	NN	LNW	PTR	WMR
350246	61446+65246+67546+61533	NN	LMI	PTR	WMR
350247	61447+65247+67547+61547	NN	LMI	PTR	WMR
350248	61448+65248+67548+61548	NN	LMI	PTR	WMR
350249	61449+65249+67549+61549	NN	LMI	PTR	WMR
350250	61450+65250+67550+61550	NN	LMI	PTR	WMR
350251	61451+65251+67551+61551	NN	LMI	PTR	WMR
350252	61452+65252+67552+61552	NN	LNW	PTR	WMR
350253	61453+65253+67553+61553	NN	LNW	PTR	WMR
350254	61454+65254+67554+61554	NN	LNW	PTR	WMR
350255	61455+65255+67555+61555	NN	LMI	PTR	WMR
350256	61456+65256+67556+61556	NN	LMI	PTR	WMR
350257	61457+65257+67557+61557	NN	LNW	PTR	WMR
350258	61458+65258+67558+61558	NN	LNW	PTR	WMR
350259	61459+65259+67559+61559	NN	LNW	PTR	WMR
350260	61460+65260+67560+61560	NN	LMI	PTR	WMR
350261	61461+65261+67561+61561	NN	LMI	PTR	WMR
350262	61462+65262+67562+61562	NN	LNW	PTR	WMR
350263	61463+65263+67563+61563	NN	LNW	PTR	WMR
350264	61464+65264+67564+61564	NN	LMI	PTR	WMR
350265	61465+65265+67565+61565	NN	LMI	PTR	WMR
350266	61466+65266+67566+61566	NN	LMI	PTR	WMR
350267	61467+65267+67567+61567	NN	LNW	PTR	WMR

350/3 Formation: DMS+TC+PTSO+DMS

350368	60141+60511+60651+60151		NN	LNW	ANG	WMR
350369	60142+60512+60652+60152		NN	LNW	ANG	WMR
350370	60143+60513+60653+60153		NN	LNW	ANG	WMR
350371	60144+60514+60654+60154		NN	LNW	ANG	WMR
350372	60145+60515+60655+60155		NN	LNW	ANG	WMR
350373	60146+60516+60656+60156		NN	LNW	ANG	WMR
350374	60147+60517+60657+60157		NN	LNW	ANG	WMR
350375	60148+60518+60658+60158	*Vic Hall*	NN	LNW	ANG	WMR
350376	60149+60519+60659+60159		NN	LNW	ANG	WMR
350377	60150+60520+60660+60160	*Graham Taylor OBE*	NN	LNW	ANG	WMR

350/4 Formation: DMS+TC+PTSO+DMS

350401	60691+60901+60941+60671	NN	LNW	ANG	WMR
350402	60692+60902+60942+60672	NN	LNW	ANG	WMR
350403	60693+60903+60943+60673	NN	LNW	ANG	WMR
350404	60694+60904+60944+60674	NN	LNW	ANG	WMR
350405	60695+60905+60945+60675	NN	LNW	ANG	WMR
350406	60696+60906+60946+60676	NN	LNW	ANG	WMR
350407	60697+60907+60947+60677	NN	LNW	ANG	WMR
350408	60698+60908+60948+60678	NN	LNW	ANG	WMR
350409	60699+60909+60949+60679	NN	LNW	ANG	WMR
350410	60700+60910+60950+60680	NN	LNW	ANG	WMR

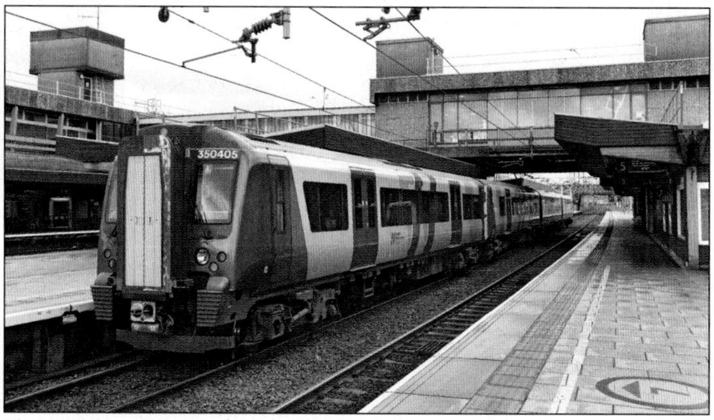

The 10 members of Class 350/4 were originally operated by TransPennine Express before transfer to WMR. They now sport standard WMR livery and operate in a common fleet pool. No. 350405 awaits departure from Stafford towards Birmingham. **CJM**

Class 357
Bombardier 4-car Outer Suburban 'Electrostar'

Built: 1999-2002
Vehicle length: Driving - 68ft 1in (20.75m)
Intermediate - 65ft 11½in (20.10m)
Height: 12ft 4½in (3.77m)
Width: 9ft 2¼in (2.80m)
Power: 25kV ac overhead
Horsepower: 2,010hp (1,500kW)
Transmission: Electric

357/0 Formation: DMS+MS+PTSOL+DMS

357001	67651+74151+74051+67751	*Barry Flaxman*	EM	C2C	PTR	c2c
357002	67652+74152+74052+67752	*Arthur Lewis Stride 1841-1922*	EM	C2C	PTR	c2c
357003	67653+74153+74053+67753	*Southend city.on.sea*	EM	C2C	PTR	c2c
357004	67654+74154+74054+67754	*Tony Amos*	EM	C2C	PTR	c2c
357005	67655+74155+74055+67755	*Southend : 2017 Alternative City of Culture*	EM	C2C	PTR	c2c
357006	67656+74156+74056+67756	*Diamond Jubilee 1952 - 2012*	EM	C2C	PTR	c2c
357007	67657+74157+74057+67757	*Sir Andrew Foster*	EM	C2C	PTR	c2c
357008	67658+74158+74058+67758		EM	C2C	PTR	c2c
357009	67659+74159+74059+67759		EM	C2C	PTR	c2c
357010	67660+74160+74060+67760		EM	C2C	PTR	c2c
357011	67661+74161+74061+67761	*John Lowing*	EM	C2C	PTR	c2c
357012	67662+74162+74062+67762		EM	C2C	PTR	c2c
357013	67663+74163+74063+67763		EM	C2C	PTR	c2c
357014	67664+74164+74064+67764		EM	C2C	PTR	c2c
357015	67665+74165+74065+67765		EM	C2C	PTR	c2c
357016	67666+74166+74066+67766		EM	C2C	PTR	c2c
357017	67667+74167+74067+67767		EM	C2C	PTR	c2c
357018	67668+74168+74068+67768	*Remembering our Fallen 88 1914-1918*	EM	C2C	PTR	c2c
357019	67669+74169+74069+67769		EM	C2C	PTR	c2c
357020	67670+74170+74070+67770		EM	C2C	PTR	c2c
357021	67671+74171+74071+67771		EM	C2C	PTR	c2c
357022	67672+74172+74072+67772		EM	C2C	PTR	c2c
357023	67673+74173+74073+67773		EM	C2C	PTR	c2c
357024	67674+74174+74074+67774		EM	C2C	PTR	c2c
357025	67675+74175+74075+67775		EM	C2C	PTR	c2c
357026	67676+74176+74076+67776		EM	C2C	PTR	c2c
357027	67677+74177+74077+67777		EM	C2C	PTR	c2c
357028	67678+74178+74078+67778	*London, Tilbury & Southend Railway 1854-2004*	EM	C2C	PTR	c2c
357029	67679+74179+74079+67779	*Thomas Whitelegg 1840-1922*	EM	C2C	PTR	c2c
357030	67680+74180+74080+67780	*Robert Harben Whitelegg 1871-1957*	EM	C2C	PTR	c2c
357031	67681+74181+74081+67781		EM	C2C	PTR	c2c
357032	67682+74182+74082+67782		EM	C2C	PTR	c2c
357033	67683+74183+74083+67783		EM	C2C	PTR	c2c
357034	67684+74184+74084+67784		EM	C2C	PTR	c2c
357035	67685+74185+74085+67785		EM	C2C	PTR	c2c
357036	67686+74186+74086+67786		EM	C2C	PTR	c2c
357037	67687+74187+74087+67787		EM	C2C	PTR	c2c
357038	67688+74188+74088+67788		EM	C2C	PTR	c2c
357039	67689+74189+74089+67789		EM	C2C	PTR	c2c
357040	67690+74190+74090+67790		EM	C2C	PTR	c2c
357041	67691+74191+74091+67791		EM	C2C	PTR	c2c
357042	67692+74192+74092+67792		EM	C2C	PTR	c2c
357043	67693+74193+74093+67793		EM	C2C	PTR	c2c
357044	67694+74194+74094+67794		EM	C2C	PTR	c2c
357045	67695+74195+74095+67795		EM	C2C	PTR	c2c
357046	67696+74196+74096+67796		EM	C2C	PTR	c2c

357/2 Formation: DMS+MS+PTSOL+DMS

357201	68601+74701+74601+68701	*Ken Bird*	EM	C2C	ANG	c2c
357202	68602+74702+74602+68702	*Kenny Mitchell*	EM	C2C	ANG	c2c
357203	68603+74703+74603+68703	*Henry Pumfrett*	EM	C2C	ANG	c2c
357204	68604+74704+74604+68704	*Derek Flowers*	EM	C2C	ANG	c2c
357205	68605+74705+74605+68705	*John D'Silva*	EM	C2C	ANG	c2c
357206	68606+74706+74606+68706	*Martin Aungier*	EM	C2C	ANG	c2c
357207	68607+74707+74607+68707	*John Page*	EM	C2C	ANG	c2c
357208	68608+74708+74608+68708	*Dave Davis*	EM	C2C	ANG	c2c
357209	68609+74709+74609+68709	*James Snelling*	EM	C2C	ANG	c2c
357210	68610+74710+74610+68710		EM	C2C	ANG	c2c
357211	68611+74711+74611+68711		EM	C2C	ANG	c2c

357/3 Formation: DMS+MS+PTSOL+DMS

357312 (357212)	68612+74712+74612+68712		EM	C2C	ANG	c2c
357313 (357213)	68613+74713+74613+68713	*Upminster IECC*	EM	C2C	ANG	c2c
357314 (357214)	68614+74714+74614+68714		EM	C2C	ANG	c2c
357315 (357215)	68615+74715+74615+68715		EM	C2C	ANG	c2c
357316 (357216)	68616+74716+74616+68716		EM	C2C	ANG	c2c
357317 (357217)	68617+74717+74617+68717	*Allan Burnell*	EM	C2C	ANG	c2c
357318 (357218)	68618+74718+74618+68718		EM	C2C	ANG	c2c
357319 (357219)	68619+74719+74619+68719		EM	C2C	ANG	c2c
357320 (357220)	68620+74720+74620+68720		EM	C2C	ANG	c2c
357321 (357221)	68621+74721+74621+68721		EM	C2C	ANG	c2c
357322 (357222)	68622+74722+74622+68722		EM	C2C	ANG	c2c
357323 (357223)	68623+74723+74623+68723		EM	C2C	ANG	c2c
357324 (357224)	68624+74724+74624+68724		EM	C2C	ANG	c2c
357325 (357225)	68625+74725+74625+68725		EM	C2C	ANG	c2c
357326 (357226)	68626+74726+74626+68726		EM	C2C	ANG	c2c
357327 (357227)	68627+74727+74627+68727	*Southend United*	EM	C2C	ANG	c2c
357328 (357228)	68628+74728+74628+68728		EM	C2C	ANG	c2c

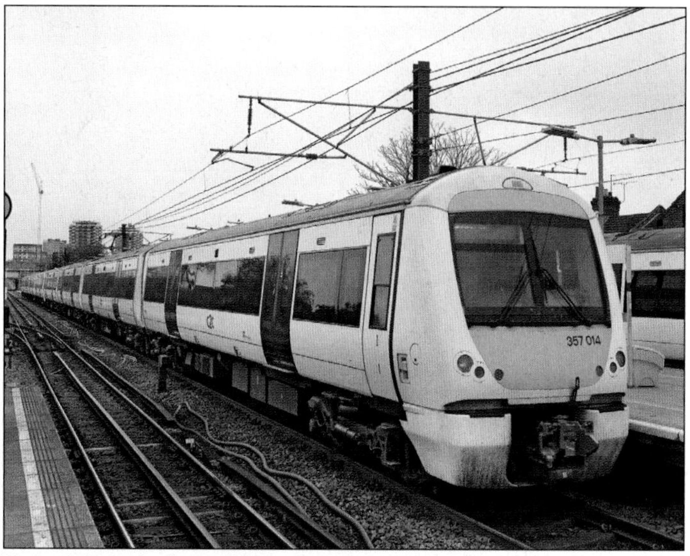

The late 1990s modernisation of the London Tilbury & Southend route operated by c2c saw two batches of Bombardier 'Electrostar' units introduced. Class 357/0 and 357/2s have a common interior design, while the 357/3s have a reduced seating 'Metro' interior. Set No. 357014 is seen at West Ham. **CJM**

Class 360
Siemens 4 and 5-car Main Line 'Desiro'

Built: 2002-2006
Vehicle length: 66ft 9in (20.34m)
Height: 12ft 1½in (3.95m)
Width: 9ft 2in (2.79m)
Power: 25kV ac overhead
Horsepower: 1,341hp (1,000kW)
Transmission: Electric

360/0 Formation: DMS+PTSO+TSO+DMS

360101	65551+72551+74551+68551	BF	EMP	ANG	GAR
360102	65552+72552+74552+68552	BF	EMP	ANG	GAR
360103	65553+72553+74553+68553	BF	EMP	ANG	EMR
360104	65554+72554+74554+68554	BF	EMP	ANG	EMR
360105	65555+72555+74555+68555	BF	FNA	ANG	GAR
360106	65556+72556+74556+68556	BF	FNO	ANG	GAR
360107	65557+72557+74557+68557	BF	EMP	ANG	GAR
360108	65558+72558+74558+68558	BF	FNA	ANG	GAR
360109	65559+72559+74559+68559	BF	EMP	ANG	GAR
360110	65560+72560+74560+68560	BF	FNA	ANG	GAR
360111	65561+72561+74561+68561	BF	FNA	ANG	GAR
360112	65562+72562+74562+68562	BF	EMP	ANG	GAR
360113	65563+72563+74563+68563	BF	EMP	ANG	EMR
360114	65564+72564+74564+68564	BF	EMP	ANG	GAR
360115	65565+72565+74565+68565	BF	FNA	ANG	GAR
360116	65566+72566+74566+68566	BF	EMP	ANG	EMR
360117	65567+72567+74567+68567	BF	FNA	ANG	GAR
360118	65568+72568+74568+68568	BF	EMP	ANG	GAR
360119	65569+72569+74569+68569	BF	FNA	ANG	GAR
360120	65570+72570+74570+68570	BF	EMP	ANG	EMR
360121	65571+72571+74571+68571	BF	EMP	ANG	EMR

360/2 Formation: DMS+PTSO+TSO+TSO+DMS (Former Heathrow Connect)

360201	78431+63421+72431+72421+78441	MB	HEC	ROG	(S)
360202	78432+63422+72432+72422+78442	MB	HEC	ROG	(S)
360203	78433+63423+72433+72423+78443	MB	HEC	ROG	(S)
360204	78434+63424+72434+72424+78444	MB	HEC	ROG	(S)
360205	78435+63425+72435+72425+78445	MB	HEL	ROG	(S)

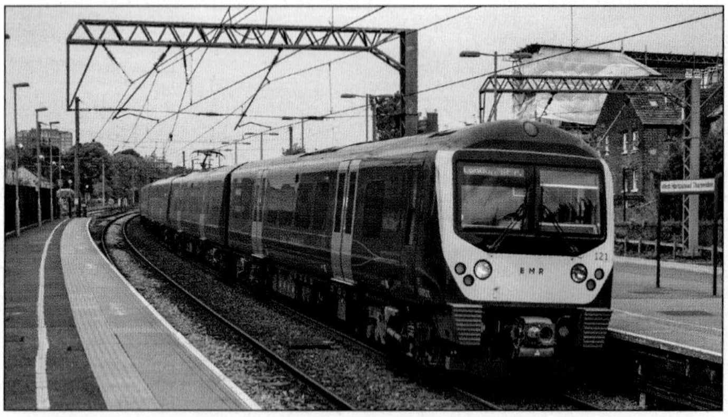

Originally operated on the Anglia main line, the 21 4-car 'Desiro' 360/1s are now operated by East Midlands Railway on 'Connect' services, including the St Pancras to Corby route. In aubergine livery. No. 360121 is seen at West Hampstead Thameslink. **Antony Christie**

Class 365
ABB 4-car Main Line 'Networker Express'

Built: 1994-1995
Vehicle length: 68ft 6½in (20.89m)
Height: 12ft 4½in (3.77m)
Width: 9ft 2½in (2.81m)
Power: 25kV ac overhead
Horsepower: 1,680hp (1,256kW)
Transmission: Electric

Formation: DMCO+TSO+PTSO+DMCO

365524	65917+72287		Preserved East Kent Railway
365526	65919		Stored Wolverton Works
365540		65974	Preserved East Kent Railway

Class 370 (APT)
BR / BREL Advanced Passenger Train

Built: 1978-1979
Vehicle length: DTS - 70ft 4in (21.44m),
M - 66ft 9in (20.4m)
Trailers - 70ft 4in (21.44m)
Height: 11ft 6in (3.51m)
Width: 8ft 11in (2.72m)
Power: 25kV ac overhead
Horsepower: 4,000hp (2,983kW) half-train
Transmission: Electric

Half train formation: DTA+TS+TRSB+TU+TF+TBF+M +

48103	DTSOL	Crewe Heritage Centre
48106	DTSOL	Crewe Heritage Centre
48602	TBFOL	Crewe Heritage Centre
48603	TBFOL	Crewe Heritage Centre
48404	TSRBL	Crewe Heritage Centre
49002	M	Crewe Heritage Centre
49006	M	Crewe Heritage Centre

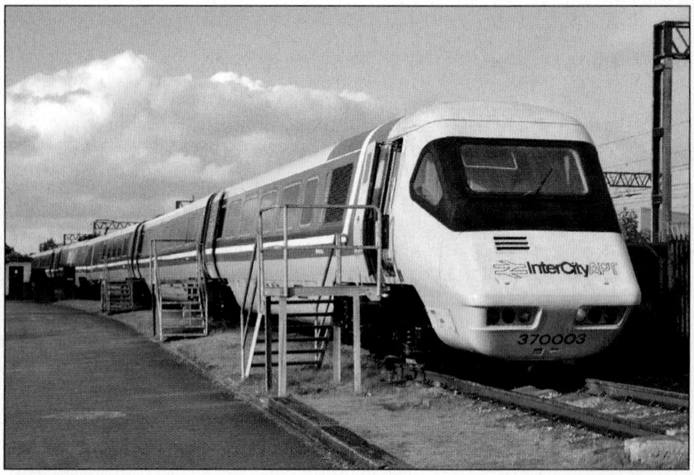

While it is highly unlikely that any of the Class 370 electric APT stock will ever be restored to main line conditions, seven vehicles are preserved static at Crewe Heritage Centre, where the set can be seen from passing main line services. Two driving cars, two power cars and three intermediate vehicles are available for inspection. **Cliff Beeton**

Class 373 (Eurostar)
GEC-Alstom International Train (e300)

Built: 1992-1996
Vehicle length: DM - 72ft 8in (22.15m),
MS - 71ft 8in (21.84m)
Trailers - 61ft 4in (18.69m)
Height: 12ft 4½in (3.77m)
Width: 9ft 3in (2.82m)
Power: 25kV ac overhead
Horsepower: 16,400hp (12,249kW) half-train
Transmission: Electric

Formation: DM+MS+TS+TS+TS+TS+TBK+TF+TF+TBF (half train)

UK sets 373/0 (half sets)

373007	3730070+3730071+3730072+3730073+3730074+3730075+3730076+3730077+3730078+3730079	TI	EUB	EUS	EUS
373008	3730080+3730081+3730082+3730083+3730084+3730085+3730086+3730087+3730088+3730089	TI	EUB	EUS	EUS
373015	3730150+3730151+3730152+3730153+3730154+3730155+3730156+3730157+3730158+3730159	TI	EUB	EUS	EUS
373016	3730160+3730161+3730162+3730163+3730164+3730165+3730166+3730167+3730168+3730169	TI	EUB	EUS	EUS

Belgian sets Class 373/1 (half sets)

3101	DM only	Training vehicle at Doncaster Training Academy
3102	DM only	Training vehicle stored at HNRC, Worksop
3106	DM, plus car 9	Train World, Brussels

French sets Class 373/2 (half sets)

373205	3732050+3732051+3732052+3732053+3732054+3732055+3732056+3732057+3732058+3732059	LY	EUB	SNF	EUS
373206	3732060+3732061+3732062+3732063+3732064+3732065+3732066+3732067+3732068+3732069	LY	EUB	SNF	EUS
373209	3732090+3732091+3732092+3732093+3732094+3732095+3732096+3732097+3732098+3732099	LY	EUB	SNF	EUS
373210	3732100+3732101+3732102+3732103+3732104+3732105+3732106+3732107+3732108+3732109	LY	EUB	SNF	EUS
373211	3732030+3732031+3732032+3732033+3732034+3732035+3732036+3732037+3732038+3732039	LY	EUB	SNF	EUS
373212	3732040+3732041+3732042+3732043+3732044+3732045+3732046+3732047+3732048+3732049	LY	EUB	SNF	EUS
373219	3732190+3732191+3732192+3732193+3732194+3732195+3732196+3732197+3732198+3732199	LY	EUB	SNF	EUS
373220	3732200+3732201+3732202+3732203+3732204+3732205+3732206+3732207+3732208+3732209	LY	EUB	SNF	EUS
373221	3732210+3732211+3732212+3732213+3732214+3732215+3732216+3732217+3732218+3732219	LY	EUB	SNF	EUS
373222	3732220+3732221+3732222+3732223+3732224+3732225+3732226+3732227+3732228+3732229	LY	EUB	SNF	EUS
373229	3732290+3732291+3732292+3732293+3732294+3732295+3732296+3732297+3732298+3732299	LY	EUS	SNF	EUS
373230	3732300+3732301+3732302+3732303+3732304+3732305+3732306+3732307+3732308+3732309	LY	EUS	SNF	EUS

3999	Spare driving vehicle used as required	LY	EUB	EUS	Under test for Belgian TBL1+

North of London sets Class 373/3

3304	DM+R1	One:One Railway Museum, Margate
3308	DM only	National Railway Museum, York
3314	DM only	Temple Mills depot - to be plinthed

Only eight full length Class 373 sets remain, with several sets stored due to a downturn in business due to Covid-19. One spare power car No. 3999 is maintained and can operate in any set as required for maintenance requirements. French sets No. 373211 and 373212 pass Stratford International station on 21 January 2022 with a test run from St Pancras to Ashford. **Jacob Tyne**

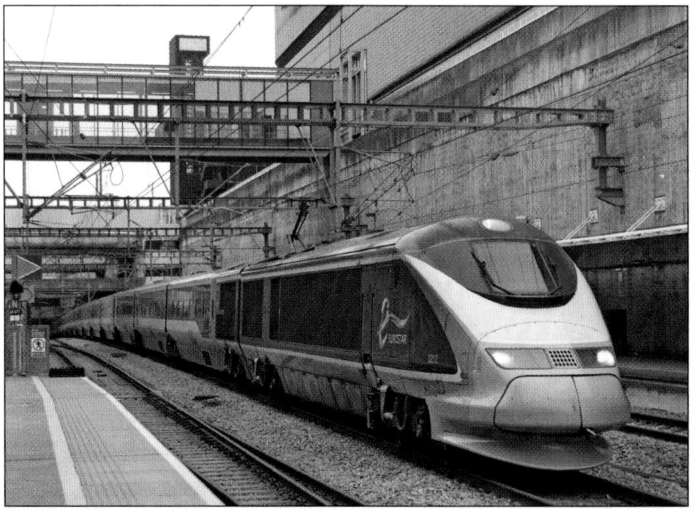

Class 374 (Eurostar)
Siemens International Train 'Velaro' (e320)

Built: 1992-1996
Vehicle length: DM - 72ft 8in (22.15m), MS - 71ft 8in (21.84m), Trailers - 61ft 4in (18.69m)
Height: 12ft 4½in (3.77m)
Width: 9ft 3in (2.82m)
Power: 25kV ac overhead
Horsepower: 16,400hp (12,249kW) half-train
Transmission: Electric

	Formation: DMF+TBF+MF+TS+TS+MS+TS+MSRB (half train)				
374001	93 70 3740 011+93 70 3740 012+93 70 3740 013+93 70 3740 014+93 70 3740 015+93 70 3740 016+93 70 3740 017+93 70 3740 018	TI	EUB	EUS	EUS
374002	93 70 3740 021+93 70 3740 022+93 70 3740 023+93 70 3740 024+93 70 3740 025+93 70 3740 026+93 70 3740 027+93 70 3740 028	TI	EUB	EUS	EUS
374003	93 70 3740 031+93 70 3740 032+93 70 3740 033+93 70 3740 034+93 70 3740 035+93 70 3740 036+93 70 3740 037+93 70 3740 038	TI	EUB	EUS	EUS
374004	93 70 3740 041+93 70 3740 042+93 70 3740 043+93 70 3740 044+93 70 3740 045+93 70 3740 046+93 70 3740 047+93 70 3740 048	TI	EUB	EUS	EUS
374005	93 70 3740 051+93 70 3740 052+93 70 3740 053+93 70 3740 054+93 70 3740 055+93 70 3740 056+93 70 3740 057+93 70 3740 058	TI	EUB	EUS	EUS
374006	93 70 3740 061+93 70 3740 062+93 70 3740 063+93 70 3740 064+93 70 3740 065+93 70 3740 066+93 70 3740 067+93 70 3740 068	TI	EUB	EUS	EUS
374007	93 70 3740 071+93 70 3740 072+93 70 3740 073+93 70 3740 074+93 70 3740 075+93 70 3740 076+93 70 3740 077+93 70 3740 078	TI	EUB	EUS	EUS
374008	93 70 3740 081+93 70 3740 082+93 70 3740 083+93 70 3740 084+93 70 3740 085+93 70 3740 086+93 70 3740 087+93 70 3740 088	TI	EUB	EUS	EUS
374009	93 70 3740 091+93 70 3740 092+93 70 3740 093+93 70 3740 094+93 70 3740 095+93 70 3740 096+93 70 3740 097+93 70 3740 098	TI	EUB	EUS	EUS
374010	93 70 3740 101+93 70 3740 102+93 70 3740 103+93 70 3740 104+93 70 3740 105+93 70 3740 106+93 70 3740 107+93 70 3740 101	TI	EUB	EUS	EUS
374011	93 70 3740 111+93 70 3740 112+93 70 3740 113+93 70 3740 114+93 70 3740 115+93 70 3740 116+93 70 3740 117+93 70 3740 118	TI	EUB	EUS	EUS
374012	93 70 3740 121+93 70 3740 122+93 70 3740 123+93 70 3740 124+93 70 3740 125+93 70 3740 126+93 70 3740 127+93 70 3740 128	TI	EUB	EUS	EUS
374013	93 70 3740 131+93 70 3740 132+93 70 3740 133+93 70 3740 134+93 70 3740 135+93 70 3740 136+93 70 3740 137+93 70 3740 138	TI	EUB	EUS	EUS
374014	93 70 3740 141+93 70 3740 142+93 70 3740 143+93 70 3740 144+93 70 3740 145+93 70 3740 146+93 70 3740 147+93 70 3740 148	TI	EUB	EUS	EUS
374015	93 70 3740 151+93 70 3740 152+93 70 3740 153+93 70 3740 154+93 70 3740 155+93 70 3740 156+93 70 3740 157+93 70 3740 158	TI	EUB	EUS	EUS
374016	93 70 3740 161+93 70 3740 162+93 70 3740 163+93 70 3740 164+93 70 3740 165+93 70 3740 166+93 70 3740 167+93 70 3740 168	TI	EUB	EUS	EUS
374017	93 70 3740 171+93 70 3740 172+93 70 3740 173+93 70 3740 174+93 70 3740 175+93 70 3740 176+93 70 3740 177+93 70 3740 178	TI	EUB	EUS	EUS
374018	93 70 3740 181+93 70 3740 182+93 70 3740 183+93 70 3740 184+93 70 3740 185+93 70 3740 186+93 70 3740 187+93 70 3740 188	TI	EUB	EUS	EUS
374019	93 70 3740 191+93 70 3740 192+93 70 3740 193+93 70 3740 194+93 70 3740 195+93 70 3740 196+93 70 3740 197+93 70 3740 198	TI	EUB	EUS	EUS
374020	93 70 3740 201+93 70 3740 202+93 70 3740 203+93 70 3740 204+93 70 3740 205+93 70 3740 206+93 70 3740 207+93 70 3740 208	TI	EUB	EUS	EUS
374021	93 70 3740 211+93 70 3740 212+93 70 3740 213+93 70 3740 214+93 70 3740 215+93 70 3740 216+93 70 3740 217+93 70 3740 218	TI	EUB	EUS	EUS
374022	93 70 3740 221+93 70 3740 222+93 70 3740 223+93 70 3740 224+93 70 3740 225+93 70 3740 226+93 70 3740 227+93 70 3740 228	TI	EUB	EUS	EUS
374023	93 70 3740 231+93 70 3740 232+93 70 3740 233+93 70 3740 234+93 70 3740 235+93 70 3740 236+93 70 3740 237+93 70 3740 238	TI	EUB	EUS	EUS
374024	93 70 3740 241+93 70 3740 242+93 70 3740 243+93 70 3740 244+93 70 3740 245+93 70 3740 246+93 70 3740 247+93 70 3740 248	TI	EUB	EUS	EUS
374025	93 70 3740 251+93 70 3740 252+93 70 3740 253+93 70 3740 254+93 70 3740 255+93 70 3740 256+93 70 3740 257+93 70 3740 258	TI	EUB	EUS	EUS
374026	93 70 3740 261+93 70 3740 262+93 70 3740 263+93 70 3740 264+93 70 3740 265+93 70 3740 266+93 70 3740 267+93 70 3740 268	TI	EUB	EUS	EUS
374027	93 70 3740 271+93 70 3740 272+93 70 3740 273+93 70 3740 274+93 70 3740 275+93 70 3740 276+93 70 3740 277+93 70 3740 278	TI	EUB	EUS	EUS
374028	93 70 3740 281+93 70 3740 282+93 70 3740 283+93 70 3740 284+93 70 3740 285+93 70 3740 286+93 70 3740 287+93 70 3740 288	TI	EUB	EUS	EUS
374029	93 70 3740 291+93 70 3740 292+93 70 3740 293+93 70 3740 294+93 70 3740 295+93 70 3740 296+93 70 3740 297+93 70 3740 298	TI	EUB	EUS	EUS
374030	93 70 3740 301+93 70 3740 302+93 70 3740 303+93 70 3740 304+93 70 3740 305+93 70 3740 306+93 70 3740 307+93 70 3740 308	TI	EUB	EUS	EUS
374031	93 70 3740 311+93 70 3740 312+93 70 3740 313+93 70 3740 314+93 70 3740 315+93 70 3740 316+93 70 3740 317+93 70 3740 318	TI	EUB	EUS	EUS
374032	93 70 3740 321+93 70 3740 322+93 70 3740 323+93 70 3740 324+93 70 3740 325+93 70 3740 326+93 70 3740 327+93 70 3740 328	TI	EUB	EUS	EUS
374033	93 70 3740 331+93 70 3740 332+93 70 3740 333+93 70 3740 334+93 70 3740 335+93 70 3740 336+93 70 3740 337+93 70 3740 338	TI	EUB	EUS	EUS
374034	93 70 3740 341+93 70 3740 342+93 70 3740 343+93 70 3740 344+93 70 3740 345+93 70 3740 346+93 70 3740 347+93 70 3740 348	TI	EUB	EUS	EUS

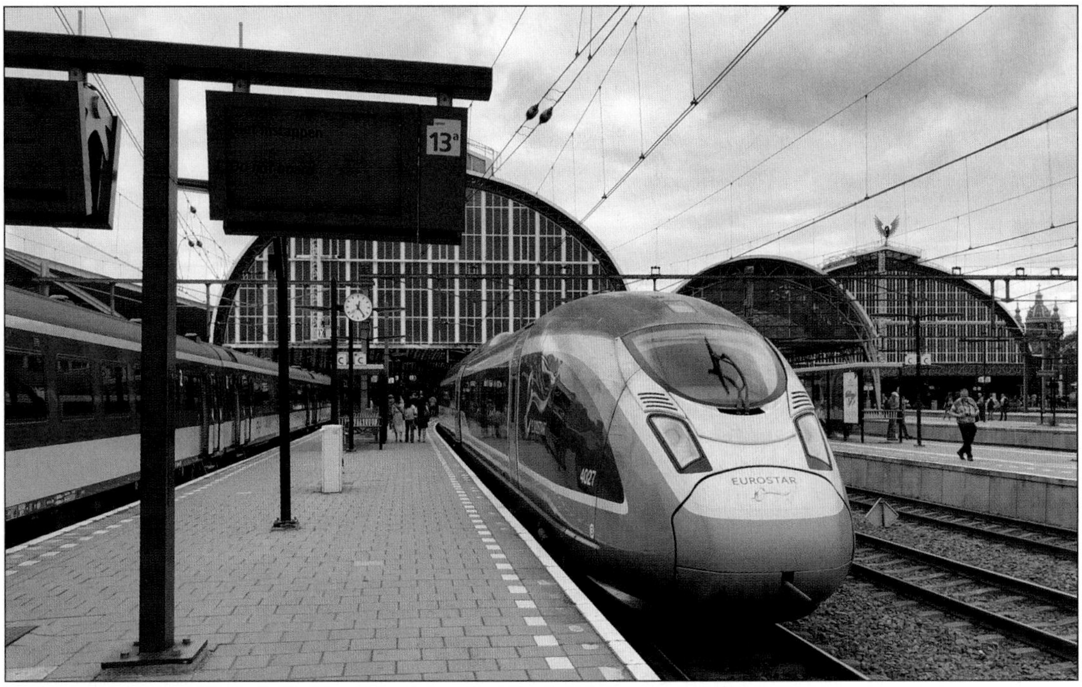

The 17 2-section Class 374 Eurostar sets operate the majority of St Pancras International to Paris/Brussels services, as well as the through trains to Amsterdam. Set (37)4027 is seen at Amsterdam Central after arrival from London. These train sets are part of the Siemens 'Valero' platform and are deemed as e320 sets with a top speed of 320kmh. **Howard Lewsey**

Class 375
Bombardier 3 and 4-car Main Line 'Electrostar'

Built: 1999-2004
Vehicle length: Driving 66ft 11in (20.40m)
Intermediate 65ft 6in (19.99m)
Height: 12ft 4in (3.78m)
Width: 9ft 2in (2.80m)
*Power: 750V dc third rail**
Horsepower: 3-car 1,341hp (1,000kW), 4-car 2,012hp (1,500kW)
Transmission: Electric
** Class 375/6 fitted for 25kV ac overhead operation*

375/3 Formation: DMS+TS+DMC

375301	67921+74351+67931	RM	SEB	EVL	SET
375302	67922+74352+67932	RM	SEB	EVL	SET
375303	67923+74353+67933	RM	SEB	EVL	SET
375304	67924+74354+67934	RM	SEB	EVL	SET
375305	67925+74355+67935	RM	SEB	EVL	SET
375306	67926+74356+67936	RM	SEB	EVL	SET
375307	67927+74357+67937	RM	SEB	EVL	SET
375308	67928+74358+67938	RM	SEB	EVL	SET
375309	67929+74359+67939	RM	SEB	EVL	SET
375310	67930+74360+67940	RM	SEB	EVL	SET

375/6 Formation: DMS+MC+PTS+DMS

375601	67801+74251+74201+67851		RM	SEB	EVL	SET
375602	67802+74252+74202+67852		RM	SEB	EVL	SET
375603	67803+74253+74203+67853		RM	SEB	EVL	SET
375604	67804+74254+74204+67854		RM	SEB	EVL	SET
375605	67805+74255+74205+67855		RM	SEB	EVL	SET
375606	67806+74256+74206+67856		RM	SEB	EVL	SET
375607	67807+74257+74207+67857		RM	SEB	EVL	SET
375608	67808+74258+74208+67858		RM	SEB	EVL	SET
375609	67809+74259+74209+67859		RM	SEB	EVL	SET
375610	67810+74260+74210+67860		RM	SEB	EVL	SET
375611	67811+74261+74211+67861		RM	SEB	EVL	SET
375612	67812+74262+74212+67862		RM	SEB	EVL	SET
375613	67813+74263+74213+67863		RM	SEB	EVL	SET
375614	67814+74264+74214+67864		RM	SEB	EVL	SET
375615	67815+74265+74215+67865		RM	SEB	EVL	SET
375616	67816+74266+74216+67866		RM	SEB	EVL	SET
375617	67817+74267+74217+67867		RM	SEB	EVL	SET
375618	67818+74268+74218+67868		RM	SEB	EVL	SET
375619	67819+74269+74219+67869	*Driver John Neve*	RM	SEB	EVL	SET
375620	67820+74270+74220+67870		RM	SEB	EVL	SET
375621	67821+74271+74221+67871		RM	SEB	EVL	SET
375622	67822+74272+74222+67872		RM	SEB	EVL	SET
375623	67823+74273+74223+67873	*Hospital in the Weald*	RM	SEB	EVL	SET
375624	67824+74274+74224+67874		RM	SEB	EVL	SET
375625	67825+74275+74225+67875		RM	SEB	EVL	SET
375626	67826+74276+74226+67876		RM	SEB	EVL	SET
375627	67827+74277+74227+67877		RM	SEB	EVL	SET
375628	67828+74278+74228+67878		RM	SEB	EVL	SET
375629	67829+74279+74229+67879		RM	SEB	EVL	SET
375630	67830+74280+74230+67880		RM	SEB	EVL	SET

375/7 Formation: DMS+MC+TS+DMS

375701	67831+74281+74231+67881	*Kent Air Ambulance Explorer*	RM	SEB	EVL	SET
375702	67832+74282+74232+67882		RM	SEB	EVL	SET
375703	67833+74283+74233+67883		RM	SEB	EVL	SET
375704	67834+74284+74234+67884		RM	SEB	EVL	SET
375705	67835+74285+74235+67885		RM	SEB	EVL	SET
375706	67836+74286+74236+67886		RM	SEB	EVL	SET
375707	67837+74287+74237+67887		RM	SEB	EVL	SET
375708	67838+74288+74238+67888		RM	SEB	EVL	SET
375709	67839+74289+74239+67889		RM	SEB	EVL	SET
375710	67840+74290+74240+67890	*Rochester Castle*	RM	SEB	EVL	SET
375711	67841+74291+74241+67891		RM	SEB	EVL	SET
375712	67842+74292+74242+67892		RM	SEB	EVL	SET
375713	67843+74293+74243+67893		RM	SEB	EVL	SET
375714	67844+74294+74244+67894	*Rochester Cathedral*	RM	SEB	EVL	SET
375715	67845+74295+74245+67895		RM	SEB	EVL	SET

375/8 Formation: DMS+MC+TS+DMS

375801	73301+79001+78201+73701		RM	SEB	EVL	SET
375802	73302+79002+78202+73702		RM	SEB	EVL	SET
375803	73303+79003+78203+73703		RM	SEB	EVL	SET
375804	73304+79004+78204+73704		RM	SEB	EVL	SET
375805	73305+79005+78205+73705		RM	SEB	EVL	SET
375806	73306+79006+78206+73706		RM	SEB	EVL	SET
375807	73307+79007+78207+73707		RM	SEB	EVL	SET
375808	73308+79008+78208+73708		RM	SEB	EVL	SET
375809	73309+79009+78209+73709		RM	SEB	EVL	SET
375810	73310+79010+78210+73710		RM	SEB	EVL	SET
375811	73311+79011+78211+73711		RM	SEB	EVL	SET
375812	73312+79012+78212+73712		RM	SEB	EVL	SET
375813	73313+79013+78213+73713		RM	SEB	EVL	SET
375814	73314+79014+78214+73714		RM	SEB	EVL	SET
375815	73315+79015+78215+73715		RM	SEB	EVL	SET
375816	73316+79016+78216+73716		RM	SEB	EVL	SET
375817	73317+79017+78217+73717		RM	SEB	EVL	SET
375818	73318+79018+78218+73718		RM	SEB	EVL	SET
375819	73319+79019+78219+73719		RM	SEB	EVL	SET
375820	73320+79020+78220+73720		RM	SEB	EVL	SET
375821	73321+79021+78221+73721		RM	SEB	EVL	SET
375822	73322+79022+78222+73722		RM	SEB	EVL	SET
375823	73323+79023+78223+73723	*Ashford Proudly Served by Rail for 175 Years*	RM	SEB	EVL	SET
375824	73324+79024+78224+73724		RM	SEB	EVL	SET
375825	73325+79025+78225+73725		RM	SEB	EVL	SET
375826	73326+79026+78226+73726		RM	SEB	EVL	SET
375827	73327+79027+78227+73727		RM	SEB	EVL	SET
375828	73328+79028+78228+73728		RM	SEB	EVL	SET
375829	73329+79029+78229+73729		RM	SEB	EVL	SET
375830	73330+79030+78230+73730		RM	SEB	EVL	SET

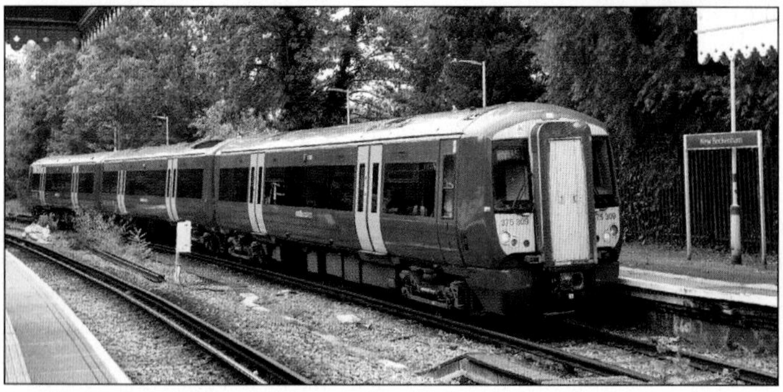

SouthEastern operate a fleet of 10 three-car Class 375/3 sets, allocated to Ramsgate depot. These are used to strengthen four or eight car trains or operate on their own on lightly used services. Set No. 375309 is seen passing New Beckenham. **CJM**

375/9 Formation: DMC+MS+TS+DMC

375901	73331+79031+79061+73731	RM	SEB	EVL	SET
375902	73332+79032+79062+73732	RM	SEB	EVL	SET
375903	73333+79033+79063+73733	RM	SEB	EVL	SET
375904	73334+79034+79064+73734	RM	SEB	EVL	SET
375905	73335+79035+79065+73735	RM	SEB	EVL	SET
375906	73336+79036+79066+73736	RM	SEB	EVL	SET
375907	73337+79037+79067+73737	RM	SEB	EVL	SET
375908	73338+79038+79068+73738	RM	SEB	EVL	SET
375909	73339+79039+79069+73739	RM	SEB	EVL	SET
375910	73340+79040+79070+73740	RM	SEB	EVL	SET
375911	73341+79041+79071+73741	RM	SEB	EVL	SET
375912	73342+79042+79072+73742	RM	SEB	EVL	SET
375913	73343+79043+79073+73743	RM	SEB	EVL	SET
375914	73344+79044+79074+73744	RM	SEB	EVL	SET
375915	73345+79045+79075+73745	RM	SEB	EVL	SET
375916	73346+79046+79076+73746	RM	SEB	EVL	SET
375917	73347+79047+79077+73747	RM	SEB	EVL	SET
375918	73348+79048+79078+73748	RM	SEB	EVL	SET
375919	73349+79049+79079+73749	RM	SEB	EVL	SET
375920	73350+79050+79080+73750	RM	SEB	EVL	SET
375921	73351+79051+79081+73751	RM	SEB	EVL	SET
375922	73352+79052+79082+73752	RM	SEB	EVL	SET
375923	73353+79053+79083+73753	RM	SEB	EVL	SET
375924	73354+79054+79084+73754	RM	SEB	EVL	SET
375925	73355+79055+79085+73755	RM	SEB	EVL	SET
375926	73356+79056+79086+73756	RM	SEB	EVL	SET
375927	73357+79057+79087+73757	RM	SEB	EVL	SET

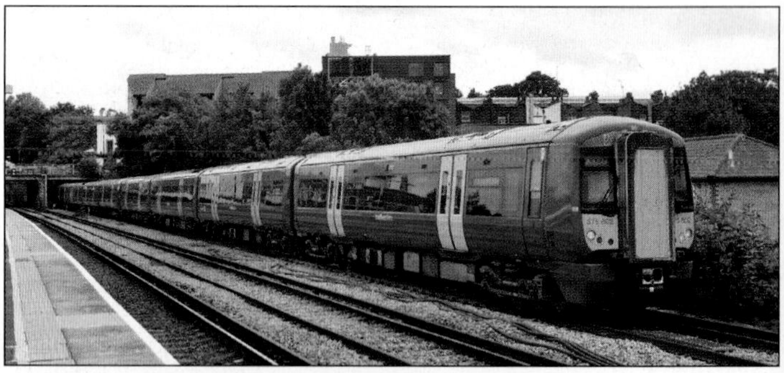

Members of Class 375/6, 375/7 and 375/8 are formed with first class accommodation in the intermediate Motor Composite, identifiable by the yellow band above window height. Set No. 375602 leads another set through New Cross in September 2021. **CJM**

Class 376
Bombardier 5-car Suburban 'Electrostar'

Built: 2004-2005
Vehicle length: Driving 66ft 11in (20.40m)
Intermediate 65ft 6in (19.99m)
Height: 12ft 4in (3.78m)
Width: 9ft 2in (2.80m)
Power: 750V dc third rail
Horsepower: 2,145hp (1,600kW)
Transmission: Electric

Formation: DMS+MS+TS+MS+DMS

376001	61101+63301+64301+63501+61601	*Alan Doggett*	SG	SET	EVL	SET
376002	61102+63302+64302+63502+61602		SG	SET	EVL	SET
376003	61103+63303+64303+63503+61603		SG	SET	EVL	SET
376004	61104+63304+64304+63504+61604		SG	SET	EVL	SET
376005	61105+63305+64305+63505+61605		SG	SET	EVL	SET
376006	61106+63306+64306+63506+61606		SG	SET	EVL	SET
376007	61107+63307+64307+63507+61607		SG	SET	EVL	SET
376008	61108+63308+64308+63508+61608		SG	SET	EVL	SET
376009	61109+63309+64309+63509+61609		SG	SET	EVL	SET
376010	61110+63310+64310+63510+61610		SG	SET	EVL	SET
376011	61111+63311+64311+63511+61611		SG	SET	EVL	SET
376012	61112+63312+64312+63512+61612		SG	SET	EVL	SET
376013	61113+63313+64313+63513+61613		SG	SET	EVL	SET
376014	61114+63314+64314+63514+61614		SG	SET	EVL	SET

376015	61115+63315+64315+63515+61615	SG	SET	EVL	SET
376016	61116+63316+64316+63516+61616	SG	SET	EVL	SET
376017	61117+63317+64317+63517+61617	SG	SET	EVL	SET
376018	61118+63318+64318+63518+61618	SG	SET	EVL	SET
376019	61119+63319+64319+63519+61619	SG	SET	EVL	SET
376020	61120+63320+64320+63520+61620	SG	SET	EVL	SET
376021	61121+63321+64321+63521+61621	SG	SET	EVL	SET
376022	61122+63322+64322+63522+61622	SG	SET	EVL	SET
376023	61123+63323+64323+63523+61623	SG	SET	EVL	SET
376024	61124+63324+64324+63524+61624	SG	SET	EVL	SET
376025	61125+63325+64325+63525+61625	SG	SET	EVL	SET
376026	61126+63326+64326+63526+61626	SG	SET	EVL	SET
376027	61127+63327+64327+63527+61627	SG	SET	EVL	SET
376028	61128+63328+64328+63528+61628	SG	SET	EVL	SET
376029	61129+63329+64329+63529+61629	SG	SET	EVL	SET
376030	61130+63330+64330+63530+61630	SG	SET	EVL	SET
376031	61131+63331+64331+63531+61631	SG	SET	EVL	SET
376032	61132+63332+64332+63532+61632	SG	SET	EVL	SET
376033	61133+63333+64333+63533+61633	SG	SET	EVL	SET
376034	61134+63334+64334+63534+61634	SG	SET	EVL	SET
376035	61135+63335+64335+63535+61635	SG	SET	EVL	SET
376036	61136+63336+64336+63536+61636	SG	SET	EVL	SET

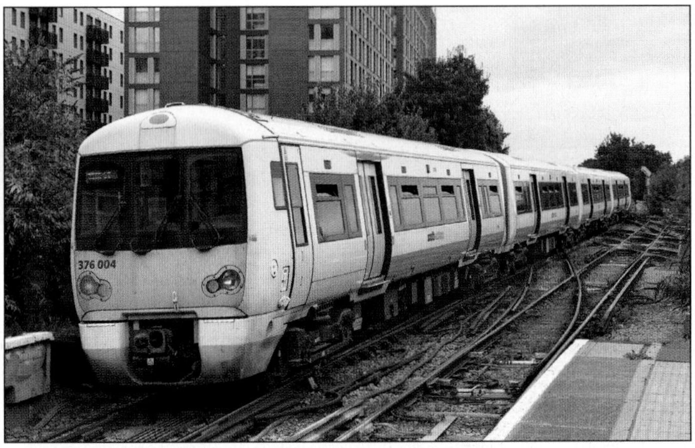

SouthEastern 'Metro' services are operated by a fleet of 36 Bombardier-built five-car non gangwayed 'Electrostar' set based at Slade Green. These are very basic sets without toilet compartments and have standard sliding doors. No. 376004 is seen departing from Lewisham. **CJM**

Class 377
Bombardier 3, 4 and 5-car 'Electrostar'

Built: 2001-2013
Vehicle length: Driving 66ft 11in (20.40m)
Intermediate 65ft 6in (19.99m)
Height: 12ft 4in (3.78m)
Width: 9ft 2in (2.80m)
*Power: 750V dc third rail**
Horsepower: 3-car 1,341hp (1,000kW)
4/5-car 2,012hp (1,500kW)
Transmission: Electric
** Class 375/2, 375/5, 375/7 also fitted for 25kV ac overhead operation*

377/1 Formation: DMCO(A)+MSO+TSO+DMCO(B)

377101	78501+77101+78901+78701	SU	SOU	PTR	GTR
377102	78502+77102+78902+78702	SU	SOU	PTR	GTR
377103	78503+77103+78903+78703	SU	SOU	PTR	GTR
377104	78504+77104+78904+78704	SU	SOU	PTR	GTR
377105	78505+77105+78905+78705	SU	SOU	PTR	GTR
377106	78506+77106+78906+78706	SU	SOU	PTR	GTR
377107	78507+77107+78907+78707	SU	SOU	PTR	GTR
377108	78508+77108+78908+78708	SU	SOU	PTR	GTR
377109	78509+77109+78909+78709	SU	SOU	PTR	GTR
377110	78510+77110+78910+78710	SU	SOU	PTR	GTR
377111	78511+77111+78911+78711	SU	SOU§	PTR	GTR
377112	78512+77112+78912+78712	SU	SOU	PTR	GTR
377113	78513+77113+78913+78713	SU	SOU	PTR	GTR
377114	78514+77114+78914+78714	SU	SOU	PTR	GTR
377115	78515+77115+78915+78715	SU	SOU	PTR	GTR
377116	78516+77116+78916+78716	SU	SOU	PTR	GTR
377117	78517+77117+78917+78717	SU	SOU	PTR	GTR
377118	78518+77118+78918+78718	SU	SOU	PTR	GTR
377119	78519+77119+78919+78719	SU	SOU	PTR	GTR
377120	78520+77120+78920+78720	SU	SOU	PTR	GTR
377121	78521+77121+78921+78721	SU	SOU	PTR	GTR
377122	78522+77122+78922+78722	SU	SOU	PTR	GTR
377123	78523+77123+78923+78723	SU	SOU	PTR	GTR
377124	78524+77124+78924+78724	SU	SOU	PTR	GTR
377125	78525+77125+78925+78725	SU	SOU	PTR	GTR
377126	78526+77126+78926+78726	SU	SOU	PTR	GTR
377127	78527+77127+78927+78727	SU	SOU	PTR	GTR
377128	78528+77128+78928+78728	SU	SOU	PTR	GTR
377129	78529+77129+78929+78729	SU	SOU	PTR	GTR
377130	78530+77130+78930+78730	SU	SOU	PTR	GTR
377131	78531+77131+78931+78731	SU	SOU	PTR	GTR
377132	78532+77132+78932+78732	SU	SOU	PTR	GTR
377133	78533+77133+78933+78733	SU	SOU	PTR	GTR
377134	78534+77134+78934+78734	SU	SOU	PTR	GTR
377135	78535+77135+78935+78735	SU	SOU	PTR	GTR
377136	78536+77136+78936+78736	SU	SOU	PTR	GTR
377137	78537+77137+78937+78737	SU	SOU	PTR	GTR
377138	78538+77138+78938+78738	SU	SOU	PTR	GTR

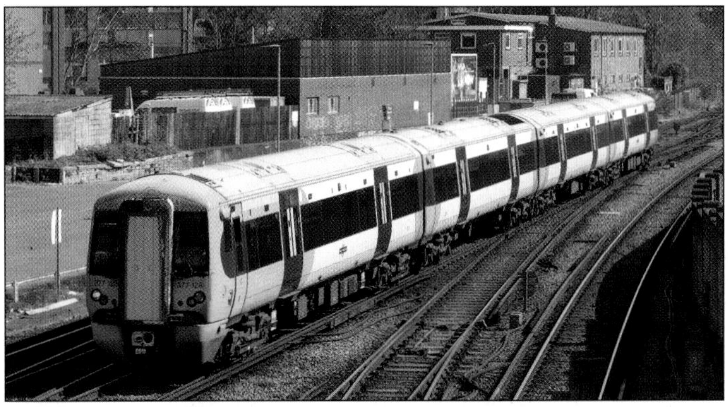

The mainstay of GTR Southern operations is operated by various fleets of Class 377 'Electrostar' units formed as 3, 4 and 5-car formations. Class 377/1 set No. 377128 is recorded arriving at Southampton with a service from Victoria. All sets have a pantograph well is the roof of the TSO, but only Class 377/2, 377/5 and 377/7 are ac fitted. **CJM**

377139	78539+77139+78939+78739	SU	SOU	PTR	GTR
377140	78540+77140+78940+78740	SU	SOU	PTR	GTR
377141	78541+77141+78941+78741	SU	SOU	PTR	GTR
377142	78542+77142+78942+78742	SU	SOU	PTR	GTR
377143	78543+77143+78943+78743	SU	SOU	PTR	GTR
377144	78544+77144+78944+78744	SU	SOU	PTR	GTR
377145	78545+77145+78945+78745	SU	SOU	PTR	GTR
377146	78546+77146+78946+78746	SU	SOU	PTR	GTR
377147	78547+77147+78947+78747	SU	SOU	PTR	GTR
377148	78548+77148+78948+78748	SU	SOU	PTR	GTR
377149	78549+77149+78949+78749	SU	SOU	PTR	GTR
377150	78550+77150+78950+78750	SU	SOU	PTR	GTR
377151	78551+77151+78951+78751	SU	SOU	PTR	GTR
377152	78552+77152+78952+78752	SU	SOU	PTR	GTR
377153	78553+77153+78953+78753	SU	SOU	PTR	GTR
377154	78554+77154+78954+78754	SU	SOU	PTR	GTR
377155	78555+77155+78955+78755	SU	SOU	PTR	GTR
377156	78556+77156+78956+78756	SU	SOU	PTR	GTR
377157	78557+77157+78957+78757	SU	SOU	PTR	GTR
377158	78558+77158+78958+78758	SU	SOU	PTR	GTR
377159	78559+77159+78959+78759	SU	SOU	PTR	GTR
377160	78560+77160+78960+78760	SU	SOU	PTR	GTR
377161	78561+77161+78961+78761	SU	SOU	PTR	GTR
377162	78562+77162+78962+78762	SU	SOU	PTR	GTR
377163	78563+77163+78963+78763	SU	SOU	PTR	GTR
377164	78564+77164+78964+78764	SU	SOU	PTR	GTR

§ Carries NHS/Key Workers branding

377/2 Formation: DMCO(A)+MSO+TSO+DMCO(B)

377201	78571+77171+78971+78771	SU	SOU	PTR	GTR
377202	78572+77172+78972+78772	SU	SOU	PTR	GTR
377203	78573+77173+78973+78773	SU	SOU	PTR	GTR
377204	78574+77174+78974+78774	SU	SOU	PTR	GTR
377205	78575+77175+78975+78775	SU	SOU	PTR	GTR
377206	78576+77176+78976+78776	SU	SOU	PTR	GTR
377207	78577+77177+78977+78777	SU	SOU	PTR	GTR
377208	78578+77178+78978+78778	SU	SOU	PTR	GTR
377209	78579+77179+78979+78779	SU	SOU	PTR	GTR
377210	78580+77180+78980+78780	SU	SOU	PTR	GTR
377211	78581+77181+78981+78781	SU	SOU	PTR	GTR
377212	78582+77182+78982+78782	SU	SOU	PTR	GTR
377213	78583+77183+78983+78783	SU	SOU	PTR	GTR
377214	78584+77184+78984+78784	SU	SOU	PTR	GTR
377215	78585+77185+78985+78785	SU	SOU	PTR	GTR

377/3 Formation: DMCO(A)+TSO+DMCO(B)

377301	(375311)	68201+74801+68401	SU	SOU	PTR	GTR
377302	(375312)	68202+74802+68402	SU	SOU	PTR	GTR
377303	(375313)	68203+74803+68403	SU	SOU	PTR	GTR
377304	(375314)	68204+74804+68404	SU	SOU	PTR	GTR
377305	(375315)	68205+74805+68405	SU	SOU	PTR	GTR
377306	(375316)	68206+74806+68406	SU	SOU	PTR	GTR
377307	(375317)	68207+74807+68407	SU	SOU	PTR	GTR

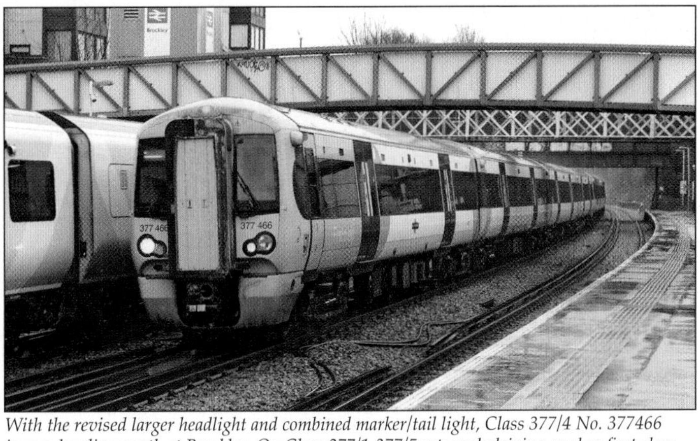

With the revised larger headlight and combined marker/tail light, Class 377/4 No. 377466 is seen heading south at Brockley. On Class 377/1-377/5 sets each driving car has first class accommodation directly inward of the cab. **CJM**

377308	(375318)	68208+74808+68408	SU	SOU	PTR	GTR
377309	(375319)	68209+74809+68409	SU	SOU	PTR	GTR
377310	(375320)	68210+74810+68410	SU	SOU	PTR	GTR
377311	(375321)	68211+74811+68411	SU	SOU	PTR	GTR
377312	(375322)	68212+74812+68412	SU	SOU	PTR	GTR
377313	(375323)	68213+74813+68413	SU	SOU	PTR	GTR
377314	(375324)	68214+74814+68414	SU	SOU	PTR	GTR
377315	(375325)	68215+74815+68415	SU	SOU	PTR	GTR
377316	(375326)	68216+74816+68416	SU	SOU	PTR	GTR
377317	(375327)	68217+74817+68417	SU	SOU	PTR	GTR
377318	(375328)	68218+74818+68418	SU	SOU	PTR	GTR
377319	(375329)	68219+74819+68419	SU	SOU	PTR	GTR
377320	(375330)	68220+74820+68420	SU	SOU	PTR	GTR
377321	(375331)	68221+74821+68421	SU	SOU	PTR	GTR
377322	(375332)	68222+74822+68422	SU	SOU	PTR	GTR
377323	(375333)	68223+74823+68423	SU	SOU	PTR	GTR
377324	(375334)	68224+74824+68424	SU	SOU	PTR	GTR
377325	(375335)	68225+74825+68425	SU	SOU	PTR	GTR
377326	(375336)	68226+74826+68426	SU	SOU	PTR	GTR
377327	(375337)	68227+74827+68427	SU	SOU	PTR	GTR
377328	(375338)	68228+74828+68428	SU	SOU	PTR	GTR

377/4 Formation: DMCO(A)+MSO+TSO+DMCO(B)

377401	73401+78801+78601+73801	SU	SOU	PTR	GTR
377402	73402+78802+78602+73802	SU	SOU	PTR	GTR
377403	73403+78803+78603+73803	SU	SOU	PTR	GTR
377404	73404+78804+78604+73804	SU	SOU	PTR	GTR
377405	73405+78805+78605+73805	SU	SOU	PTR	GTR
377406	73406+78806+78606+73806	SU	SOU	PTR	GTR
377407	73407+78807+78607+73807	SU	SOU	PTR	GTR
377408	73408+78808+78608+73808	SU	SOU	PTR	GTR
377409	73409+78809+78609+73809	SU	SOU	PTR	GTR
377410	73410+78810+78610+73810	SU	SOU	PTR	GTR
377411	73411+78811+78611+73811	SU	SOU	PTR	GTR
377412	73412+78812+78612+73812	SU	SOU	PTR	GTR
377413	73413+78813+78613+73813	SU	SOU	PTR	GTR
377414	73414+78814+78614+73814	SU	SOU	PTR	GTR
377415	73415+78815+78615+73815	SU	SOU	PTR	GTR
377416	73416+78816+78616+73816	SU	SOU	PTR	GTR
377417	73417+78817+78617+73817	SU	SOU	PTR	GTR
377418	73418+78818+78618+73818	SU	SOU	PTR	GTR
377419	73419+78819+78619+73819	SU	SOU	PTR	GTR
377420	73420+78820+78620+73820	SU	SOU	PTR	GTR
377421	73421+78821+78621+73821	SU	SOU	PTR	GTR
377422	73422+78822+78622+73822	SU	SOU	PTR	GTR
377423	73423+78823+78623+73823	SU	SOU	PTR	GTR
377424	73424+78824+78624+73824	SU	SOU	PTR	GTR
377425	73425+78825+78625+73825	SU	SOU	PTR	GTR
377426	73426+78826+78626+73826	SU	SOU	PTR	GTR
377427	73427+78827+78627+73827	SU	SOU	PTR	GTR
377428	73428+78828+78628+73828	SU	SOU	PTR	GTR
377429	73429+78829+78629+73829	SU	SOU	PTR	GTR
377430	73430+78830+78630+73830	SU	SOU	PTR	GTR
377431	73431+78831+78631+73831	SU	SOU	PTR	GTR
377432	73432+78832+78632+73832	SU	SOU	PTR	GTR
377433	73433+78833+78633+73833	SU	SOU	PTR	GTR
377434	73434+78834+78634+73834	SU	SOU	PTR	GTR
377435	73435+78835+78635+73835	SU	SOU	PTR	GTR
377436	73436+78836+78636+73836	SU	SOU	PTR	GTR
377437	73437+78837+78637+73837	SU	SOU	PTR	GTR
377438	73438+78838+78638+73838	SU	SOU	PTR	GTR
377439	73439+78839+78639+73839	SU	SOU	PTR	GTR
377440	73440+78840+78640+73840	SU	SOU	PTR	GTR
377441	73441+78841+78641+73841	SU	SOU	PTR	GTR
377442	73442+78842+78642+73842	SU	SOU	PTR	GTR
377443	73443+78843+78643+73843	SU	SOU	PTR	GTR
377444	73444+78844+78644+73844	SU	SOU	PTR	GTR
377445	73445+78845+78645+73845	SU	SOU	PTR	GTR
377446	73446+78846+78646+73846	SU	SOU	PTR	GTR
377447	73447+78847+78647+73847	SU	SOU	PTR	GTR
377448	73448+78848+78648+73848	SU	SOU	PTR	GTR
377449	73449+78849+78649+73849	SU	SOU	PTR	GTR
377450	73450+78850+78650+73850	SU	SOU	PTR	GTR
377451	73451+78851+78651+73851	SU	SOU	PTR	GTR
377452	73452+78852+78652+73852	SU	SOU	PTR	GTR
377453	73453+78853+78653+73853	SU	SOU	PTR	GTR
377454	73454+78854+78654+73854	SU	SOU	PTR	GTR
377455	73455+78855+78655+73855	SU	SOU	PTR	GTR
377456	73456+78856+78656+73856	SU	SOU	PTR	GTR
377457	73457+78857+78657+73857	SU	SOU	PTR	GTR
377458	73458+78858+78658+73858	SU	SOU	PTR	GTR
377459	73459+78859+78659+73859	SU	SOU	PTR	GTR
377460	73460+78860+78660+73860	SU	SOU	PTR	GTR
377461	73461+78861+78661+73861	SU	SOU	PTR	GTR
377462	73462+78862+78662+73862	SU	SOU	PTR	GTR
377463	73463+78863+78663+73863	SU	SOU	PTR	GTR
377464	73464+78864+78664+73864	SU	SOU	PTR	GTR
377465	73465+78865+78665+73865	SU	SOU	PTR	GTR
377466	73466+78866+78666+73866	SU	SOU	PTR	GTR
377467	73467+78867+78667+73867	SU	SOU	PTR	GTR
377468	73468+78868+78668+73868	SU	SOU	PTR	GTR
377469	73469+78869+78669+73869	SU	SOU	PTR	GTR
377470	73470+78870+78670+73870	SU	SOU	PTR	GTR
377471	73471+78871+78671+73871	SU	SOU	PTR	GTR
377472	73472+78872+78672+73872	SU	SOU	PTR	GTR
377473	73473+78873+78673+73873	SU	SOU	PTR	GTR
377474	73474+78874+78674+73874	SU	SOU	PTR	GTR
377475	73475+78875+78675+73875	SU	SOU	PTR	GTR

377/5 Formation: DMCO(A)+MSO+TSO+DMCO(B)

377501	73501+75901+74901+73601	RM	SEB	PTR	SET
377502	73502+75902+74902+73602	RM	SEB	PTR	SET
377503	73503+75903+74903+73603	RM	SEB	PTR	SET
377504	73504+75904+74904+73604	RM	SEB	PTR	SET
377505	73505+75905+74905+73605	RM	SEB	PTR	SET
377506	73506+75906+74906+73606	RM	SEB	PTR	SET
377507	73507+75907+74907+73607	RM	SEB	PTR	SET
377508	73508+75908+74908+73608	RM	SEB	PTR	SET
377509	73509+75909+74909+73609	RM	SEB	PTR	SET
377510	73510+75910+74910+73610	RM	SEB	PTR	SET
377511	73511+75911+74911+73611	RM	SEB	PTR	SET
377512	73512+75912+74912+73612	RM	SEB	PTR	SET
377513	73513+75913+74913+73613	RM	SEB	PTR	SET
377514	73514+75914+74914+73614	RM	SEB	PTR	SET
377515	73515+75915+74915+73615	RM	SEB	PTR	SET
377516	73516+75916+74916+73616	RM	SEB	PTR	SET
377517	73517+75917+74917+73617	RM	SEB	PTR	SET
377518	73518+75918+74918+73618	RM	SEB	PTR	SET
377519	73519+75919+74919+73619	RM	SEB	PTR	SET
377520	73520+75920+74920+73620	RM	SEB	PTR	SET
377521	73521+75921+74921+73621	RM	SEB	PTR	SET
377522	73522+75922+74922+73622	RM	SEB	PTR	SET
377523	73523+75923+74923+73623	RM	SEB	PTR	SET

377/6 Formation: DMCO+MSO+PTSO+MSO+DMSO

377601	70101+70201+70301+70401+70501	SU	SOU	PTR	GTR
377602	70102+70202+70302+70402+70502	SU	SOU	PTR	GTR
377603	70103+70203+70303+70403+70503	SU	SOU	PTR	GTR
377604	70104+70204+70304+70404+70504	SU	SOU	PTR	GTR
377605	70105+70205+70305+70405+70505	SU	SOU	PTR	GTR
377606	70106+70206+70306+70406+70506	SU	SOU	PTR	GTR
377607	70107+70207+70307+70407+70507	SU	SOU	PTR	GTR
377608	70108+70208+70308+70408+70508	SU	SOU	PTR	GTR
377609	70109+70209+70309+70409+70509	SU	SOU	PTR	GTR
377610	70110+70210+70310+70410+70510	SU	SOU	PTR	GTR
377611	70111+70211+70311+70411+70511	SU	SOU	PTR	GTR
377612	70112+70212+70312+70412+70512	SU	SOU	PTR	GTR
377613	70113+70213+70313+70413+70513	SU	SOU	PTR	GTR
377614	70114+70214+70314+70414+70514	SU	SOU	PTR	GTR
377615	70115+70215+70315+70415+70515	SU	SOU	PTR	GTR
377616	70116+70216+70316+70416+70516	SU	SOU	PTR	GTR
377617	70117+70217+70317+70417+70517	SU	SOU	PTR	GTR
377618	70118+70218+70318+70418+70518	SU	SOU	PTR	GTR
377619	70119+70219+70319+70419+70519	SU	SOU	PTR	GTR
377620	70120+70220+70320+70420+70520	SU	SOU	PTR	GTR
377621	70121+70221+70321+70421+70521	SU	SOU	PTR	GTR
377622	70122+70222+70322+70422+70522	SU	SOU	PTR	GTR
377623	70123+70223+70323+70423+70523	SU	SOU	PTR	GTR
377624	70124+70224+70324+70424+70524	SU	SOU	PTR	GTR
377625	70125+70225+70325+70425+70525	SU	SOU	PTR	GTR
377626	70126+70226+70326+70426+70526	SU	SOU	PTR	GTR

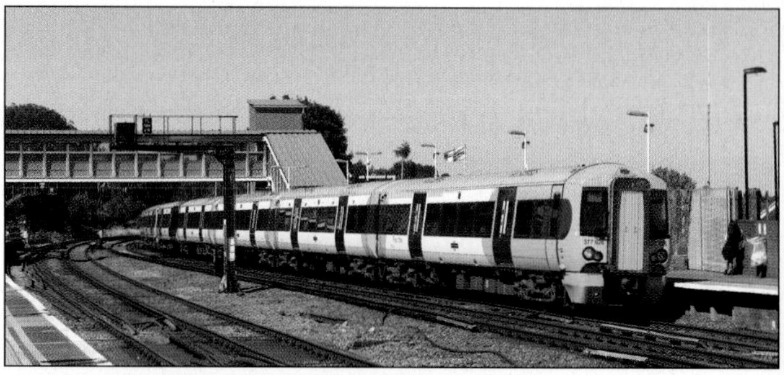

The five-car Class 377/6 and 377/7 sets have first class at the inner end of one driving car, as seen in this view of set No. 377626 passing Forest Hill. These sets are allocated to Selhurst and usually operate suburban routes. **CJM**

377/7 Formation: DMCO+MSO+TSO+MSO+DMSO

377701	65201+70601+65601+70701+65401	SU	SOU	PTR	GTR
377702	65202+70602+65602+70702+65402	SU	SOU	PTR	GTR
377703	65203+70603+65603+70703+65403	SU	SOU	PTR	GTR
377704	65204+70604+65604+70704+65404	SU	SOU	PTR	GTR
377705	65205+70605+65605+70705+65405	SU	SOU	PTR	GTR
377706	65206+70606+65606+70706+65406	SU	SOU	PTR	GTR
377707	65207+70607+65607+70707+65407	SU	SOU	PTR	GTR
377708	65208+70608+65608+70708+65408	SU	SOU	PTR	GTR

Class 378
Bombardier 5-car Suburban 'Capitalstar'

Built: 2009-2011
Vehicle length: Driving 66ft 2in (20.46m)
Intermediate 66ft 1in (20.14m)
Height: 12ft 4½in (3.77m)
Width: 9ft 2in (2.80m)
Power: 378/1 - 750V dc third rail
378/2 - 750V dc third rail and 25kV ac overhead
Horsepower: 2,145hp (1,600kW),
Transmission: Electric

378/1 Formation: DMS+MS+TS+MS+DMS

378135	38035+38235+38335+38435+38135	*Daks Hamilton*	NG	LON	QWR	LOG
378136	38036+38236+38336+38436+38136	*Transport for London*	NG	LON	QWR	LOG
378137	38037+38237+38337+38437+38137		NG	LOG	QWR	LOG
378138	38038+38238+38338+38438+38138		NG	LOG	QWR	LOG
378139	38039+38239+38339+38439+38139		NG	LOG	QWR	LOG
378140	38040+38240+38340+38440+38140		NG	LOG	QWR	LOG
378141	38041+38241+38341+38441+38141		NG	LOG	QWR	LOG

378142	38042+38242+38342+38442+38142	NG	LOG	QWR	LOG
378143	38043+38243+38343+38443+38143	NG	LOG	QWR	LOG
378144	38044+38244+38344+38444+38144	NG	LOG	QWR	LOG
378145	38045+38245+38345+38445+38145	NG	LOG	QWR	LOG
378146	38046+38246+38346+38446+38146	NG	LOG	QWR	LOG
378147	38047+38247+38347+38447+38147	NG	LON	QWR	LOG
378148	38048+38248+38348+38448+38148	NG	LOG	QWR	LOG
378149	38049+38249+38349+38449+38149	NG	LOG	QWR	LOG
378150	38050+38250+38350+38450+38150	NG	LON	QWR	LOG
378151	38051+38251+38351+38451+38151	NG	LOG	QWR	LOG
378152	38052+38252+38352+38452+38152	NG	LOG	QWR	LOG
378153	38053+38253+38353+38453+38153	NG	LOG	QWR	LOG
378154	38054+38254+38354+38454+38154	NG	LOG	QWR	LOG

378/2	Formation: DMS+MS+TS+MS+DMS				
378201 (378001)	38001+38201+38301+38401+38101	NG	LOG	QWR	LOG
378202 (378002)	38002+38202+38302+38402+38102	NG	LOG	QWR	LOG
378203 (378003)	38003+38203+38303+38403+38103	NG	LOG	QWR	LOG
378204 (378004)	38004+38204+38304+38404+38104	NG	LON	QWR	LOG
	Professor Sir Peter Hall				
378205 (378005)	38005+38205+38305+38405+38105	NG	LOG	QWR	LOG
378206 (378006)	38006+38206+38306+38406+38106	NG	LON	QWR	LOG
378207 (378007)	38007+38207+38307+38407+38107	NG	LOG	QWR	LOG
378208 (378008)	38008+38208+38308+38408+38108	NG	LOG	QWR	LOG
378209 (378009)	38009+38209+38309+38409+38109	NG	LOG	QWR	LOG
378210 (378010)	38010+38210+38310+38410+38110	NG	LOG	QWR	LOG
378211 (378011)	38011+38211+38311+38411+38111	NG	LON	QWR	LOG
	Gary Hunter				
378212 (378012)	38012+38212+38312+38412+38112	NG	LOG	QWR	LOG
378213 (378013)	38013+38213+38313+38413+38113	NG	LOG	QWR	LOG
378214 (378014)	38014+38214+38314+38414+38114	NG	LOG	QWR	LOG
378215 (378015)	38015+38215+38315+38415+38115	NG	LOG	QWR	LOG
378216 (378016)	38016+38216+38316+38416+38116	NG	LOG	QWR	LOG
378217 (378017)	38017+38217+38317+38417+38117	NG	LOG	QWR	LOG
378218 (378018)	38018+38218+38318+38418+38118	NG	LOG	QWR	LOG
378219 (378019)	38019+38219+38319+38419+38119	NG	LOG	QWR	LOG
378220 (378020)	38020+38220+38320+38420+38120	NG	LOG	QWR	LOG
378221 (378021)	38021+38221+38321+38421+38121	NG	LOG	QWR	LOG
378222 (378022)	38022+38222+38322+38422+38122	NG	LOG	QWR	LOG
378223 (378023)	38023+38223+38323+38423+38123	NG	LOG	QWR	LOG
378224 (378024)	38024+38224+38324+38424+38124	NG	LOG	QWR	LOG
378225	38025+38225+38325+38425+38125	NG	LOG	QWR	LOG
378226	38026+38226+38326+38426+38126	NG	LOG	QWR	LOG
378227	38027+38227+38327+38427+38127	NG	LOG	QWR	LOG
378228	38028+38228+38328+38428+38128	NG	LOG	QWR	LOG
378229	38029+38229+38329+38429+38129	NG	LOG	QWR	LOG
378230	38030+38230+38330+38430+38130	NG	LOG	QWR	LOG
378231	38031+38231+38331+38431+38131	NG	LOG	QWR	LOG
378232	38032+38232+38332+38432+38132 *Jeff Langston*	NG	LON	QWR	LOG
378233	38033+38233+38333+38433+38133 *Ian Brown CBE*	NG	LOG	QWR	LOG
378234	38034+38234+38334+38434+38134	NG	LOG	QWR	LOG
378255	38055+38255+38355+38455+38155	NG	LOG	QWR	LOG
378256	38056+38256+38356+38456+38156	NG	LOG	QWR	LOG
378257	38057+38257+38357+38457+38157	NG	LOG	QWR	LOG

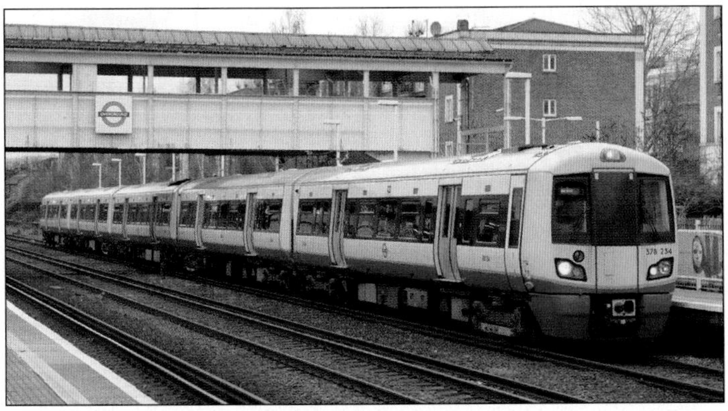

The Class 378 'Capitalstar' Class 378/1 (dc only) and 378/2 (ac/dc) sets operate on London Overground services. Sets are in the process of being repainted in the new LOG colours. In the above view set No. 378234 at Kensington Olympia shows the as delivered livery style of white, blue and orange. The picture below shows set No. 378204 at Clapham Junction carrying the latest colours of black, white and blue. **CJM / Antony Christie**

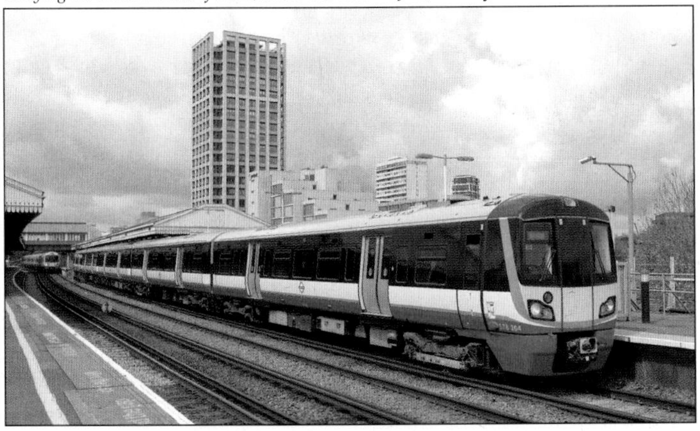

Class 379
Bombardier 4-car Main Line 'Electrostar'

Built: 2010-2011
Vehicle length: Driving 66ft 9in (20.40m)
Intermediate 65ft 6in (19.99m)
Height: 12ft 4in (3.78m)
Width: 9ft 2in (2.80m)
Power: 25kV ac overhead
Horsepower: 1,609hp (1,200kW),
Transmission: Electric

	Formation: DMS+MS+PTS+DMC				
379001	61201+61701+61901+62101	IL	NXU	AKI	OLS
379002	61202+61702+61902+62102	IL	NXU	AKI	OLS
379003	61203+61703+61903+62103	IL	NXU	AKI	OLS
379004	61204+61704+61904+62104	IL	NXU	AKI	OLS
379005	61205+61705+61905+62105	IL	NXU	AKI	OLS
379006	61206+61706+61906+62106	IL	NXU	AKI	OLS
379007	61207+61707+61907+62107	IL	NXU	AKI	OLS
379008	61208+61708+61908+62108	IL	NXU	AKI	OLS
379009	61209+61709+61909+62109	IL	NXU	AKI	OLS
379010	61210+61710+61910+62110	IL	NXU	AKI	OLS
379011	61211+61711+61911+62111	IL	NXU	AKI	OLS
379012	61212+61712+61912+62112	IL	NXU	AKI	OLS
379013	61213+61713+61913+62113	IL	NXU	AKI	OLS
379014	61214+61714+61914+62114	IL	NXU	AKI	OLS
379015	61215+61715+61915+62115	IL	NXU	AKI	OLS
379016	61216+61716+61916+62116	IL	NXU	AKI	OLS
379017	61217+61717+61917+62117	IL	NXU	AKI	OLS
379018	61218+61718+61918+62118	IL	NXU	AKI	OLS
379019	61219+61719+61919+62119	IL	NXU	AKI	OLS
379020	61220+61720+61920+62120	IL	NXU	AKI	OLS
379021	61221+61721+61921+62121	IL	NXU	AKI	OLS
379022	61222+61722+61922+62122	IL	NXU	AKI	OLS
379023	61223+61723+61923+62123	IL	NXU	AKI	OLS
379024	61224+61724+61924+62124	IL	NXU	AKI	OLS
379025	61225+61725+61925+62125	IL	NXU	AKI	OLS
379026	61226+61726+61926+62126	IL	NXU	AKI	OLS
379027	61227+61727+61927+62127	IL	NXU	AKI	OLS
379028	61228+61728+61928+62128	IL	NXU	AKI	OLS
379029	61229+61729+61929+62129	IL	NXU	AKI	OLS
379030	61230+61730+61930+62130	IL	NXU	AKI	OLS

All sets stored

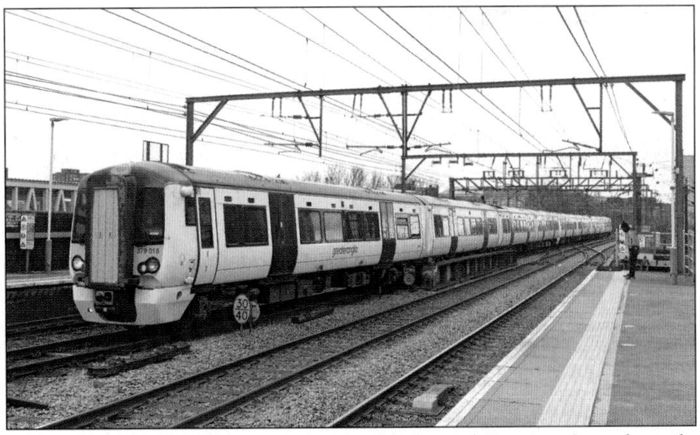

The four-car Class 379 'Electrostar' sets introduced for Stansted Airport services and recently used on West Anglia routes are stored, following the introduction of Class 720s. Set No. 379018 is captured approaching Hackney Downs. **CJM**

Class 380
Siemens 3 and 4-car Main Line 'Desiro'

Built: 2010-2011
Vehicle length: Driving 75ft 5in (23.00m)
Height: 12ft 4in (3.78m)
Width: 9ft 2in (2.80m)
Power: 25kV ac overhead
Horsepower: 1,341hp (1,000kW),
Transmission: Electric

380/0	Formation: DMS+PTS+DMS				
380001	38501+38601+38701	GW	SCR	EVL	ASR
380002	38502+38602+38702	GW	SCR	EVL	ASR
380003	38503+38603+38703	GW	SCR	EVL	ASR
380004	38504+38604+38704	GW	SCR	EVL	ASR
380005	38505+38605+38705	GW	SCR	EVL	ASR
380006	38506+38606+38706	GW	SCR	EVL	ASR
380007	38507+38607+38707	GW	SCR	EVL	ASR
380008	38508+38608+38708	GW	SCR	EVL	ASR
380009	38509+38609+38709	GW	SCR	EVL	ASR
380010	38510+38610+38710	GW	SCR	EVL	ASR
380011	38511+38611+38711	GW	SCR	EVL	ASR
380012	38512+38612+38712	GW	SCR	EVL	ASR
380013	38513+38613+38713	GW	SCR	EVL	ASR
380014	38514+38614+38714	GW	SCR	EVL	ASR
380015	38515+38615+38715	GW	SCR	EVL	ASR
380016	38516+38616+38716	GW	SCR	EVL	ASR
380017	38517+38617+38717	GW	SCR	EVL	ASR
380018	38518+38618+38718	GW	SCR	EVL	ASR
380019	38519+38619+38719	GW	SCR	EVL	ASR
380020	38520+38620+38720	GW	SCR	EVL	ASR
380021	38521+38621+38721	GW	SCR	EVL	ASR
380022	38522+38622+38722	GW	SCR	EVL	ASR

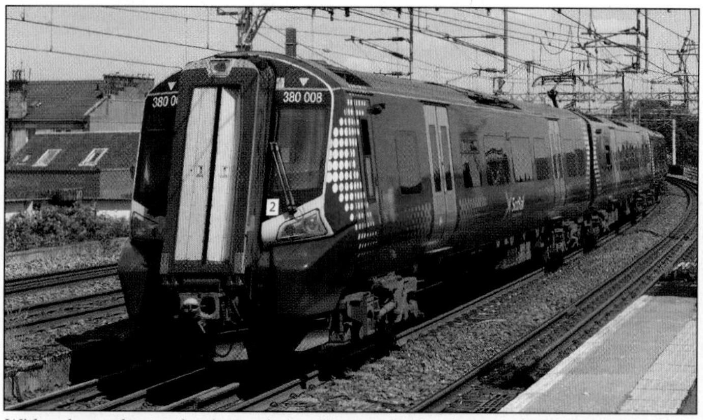

With a clumsy front end gangway design, Siemens 'Desiro' three-car set No. 380008 departs from Paisley Gilmour Street with an Ayr to Glasgow working in June 2021. These sets are based at Glasgow Shields Road and are not compatible with any other fleet. **CJM**

380/1 Formation: DMS+PTS+TSO+DMS

380101	38551+38651+38851+38751	GW	SCR	EVL	ASR
380102	38552+38652+38852+38752	GW	SCR	EVL	ASR
380103	38553+38653+38853+38753	GW	SCR	EVL	ASR
380104	38554+38654+38854+38754	GW	SCR	EVL	ASR
380105	38555+38655+38855+38755	GW	SCR	EVL	ASR
380106	38556+38656+38856+38756	GW	SCR	EVL	ASR
380107	38557+38657+38857+38757	GW	SCR	EVL	ASR
380108	38558+38658+38858+38758	GW	SCR	EVL	ASR
380109	38559+38659+38859+38759	GW	SCR	EVL	ASR
380110	38560+38660+38860+38760	GW	SCR	EVL	ASR
380111	38561+38661+38861+38761	GW	SCR	EVL	ASR
380112	38562+38662+38862+38762	GW	SCR	EVL	ASR
380113	38563+38663+38863+38763	GW	SCR	EVL	ASR
380114	38564+38664+38864+38764	GW	SCR	EVL	ASR
380115	38565+38665+38865+38765	GW	SCR	EVL	ASR
380116	38566+38666+38866+38766	GW	SCR	EVL	ASR

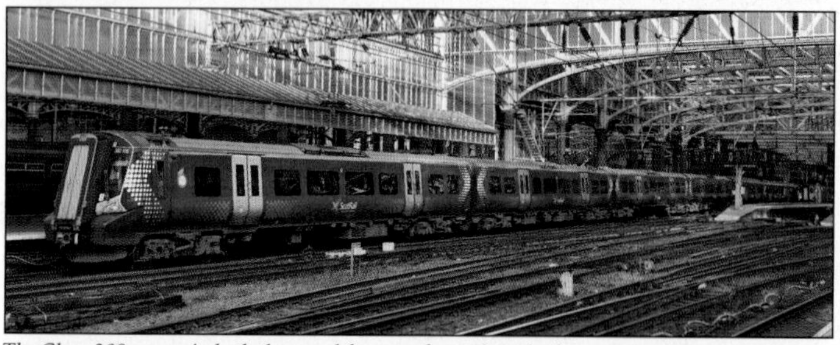

The Class 380s come in both three and four-car formation, the four car sets have an additional Trailer Standard with 74 seats. One universal access toilet is located in the pantograph coach, marshalled second in this view of set No. 380108 at Glasgow Central. **CJM**

Class 385
Hitachi 3 and 4-car Main Line 'AT200'

Built: 2017-2019
Vehicle length: Driving 76ft 4in (23.18m)
Intermediate 72ft 4in (22.08m)
Height: 12ft 2in (3.79m)
Width: 8ft 10in (2.74m)
Power: 25kV ac overhead
Horsepower: 3-car - 2,010hp (1499kW),
4-car - 2,680hp (2,000kW)
Transmission: Electric

385/0 Formation: DMS+PTS+DMS

385001	441001+442001+444001	EC	SCR	CAL	ASR
385002	441002+442002+444002	EC	SCR	CAL	ASR
385003	441003+442003+444003	EC	SCR	CAL	ASR
385004	441004+442004+444004	EC	SCR	CAL	ASR
385005	441005+442005+444005	EC	SCR	CAL	ASR
385006	441006+442006+444006	EC	SCR	CAL	ASR
385007	441007+442007+444007	EC	SCR	CAL	ASR
385008	441008+442008+444008	EC	SCR	CAL	ASR
385009	441009+442009+444009	EC	SCR	CAL	ASR
385010	441010+442010+444010	EC	SCR	CAL	ASR
385011	441011+442011+444011	EC	SCR	CAL	ASR
385012	441012+442012+444012	EC	SCR	CAL	ASR
385013	441013+442013+444013	EC	SCR	CAL	ASR
385014	441014+442014+444014	EC	SCR	CAL	ASR
385015	441015+442015+444015	EC	SCR	CAL	ASR
385016	441016+442016+444016	EC	SCR	CAL	ASR
385017	441017+442017+444017	EC	SCR	CAL	ASR
385018	441018+442018+444018	EC	SCR	CAL	ASR
385019	441019+442019+444019	EC	SCR	CAL	ASR
385020	441020+442020+444020	EC	SCR	CAL	ASR
385021	441021+442021+444021	EC	SCR	CAL	ASR
385022	441022+442022+444022	EC	SCR	CAL	ASR
385023	441023+442023+444023	EC	SCR	CAL	ASR
385024	441024+442024+444024	EC	SCR	CAL	ASR
385025	441025+442025+444025	EC	SCR	CAL	ASR
385026	441026+442026+444026	EC	SCR	CAL	ASR
385027	441027+442027+444027	EC	SCR	CAL	ASR
385028	441028+442028+444028	EC	SCR	CAL	ASR
385029	441029+442029+444029	EC	SCR	CAL	ASR
385030	441030+442030+444030	EC	SCR	CAL	ASR
385031	441031+442031+444031	EC	SCR	CAL	ASR
385032	441032+442032+444032	EC	SCR	CAL	ASR
385033	441033+442033+444033	EC	SCR	CAL	ASR
385034	441034+442034+444034	EC	SCR	CAL	ASR
385035	441035+442035+444035	EC	SCR	CAL	ASR
385036	441036+442036+444036	EC	SCR	CAL	ASR
385037	441037+442037+444037	EC	SCR	CAL	ASR
385038	441038+442038+444038	EC	SCR	CAL	ASR
385039	441039+442039+444039	EC	SCR	CAL	ASR
385040	441040+442040+444040	EC	SCR	CAL	ASR
385041	441041+442041+444041	EC	SCR	CAL	ASR
385042	441042+442042+444042	EC	SCR	CAL	ASR
385043	441043+442043+444043	EC	SCR	CAL	ASR
385044	441044+442044+444044	EC	SCR	CAL	ASR
385045	441045+442045+444045	EC	SCR	CAL	ASR
385046	441046+442046+444046	EC	SCR	CAL	ASR

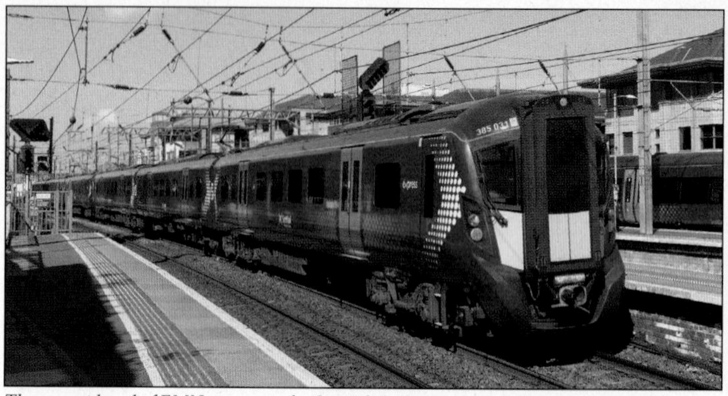

The newest breed of EMU to operate for Scottish Railways are the Class 385s, part of the AT200 platform built by Hitachi. A fleet of 46 three-car sets classified as 385/0 are in use, No. 385033 is shown arriving at Edinburgh Haymarket in June 2021. **CJM**

385/1 Formation: DMC+PTS+TSO+DMS

385101	441101+442101+443101+444101		EC	SCR	CAL	ASR
385102	441102+442102+443102+444102		EC	SCR	CAL	ASR
385103	441103+442103+443103+444103	*ScotRail**	EC	SCR	CAL	ASR
385104	441104+442104+443104+444104		EC	SCR	CAL	ASR
385105	441105+442105+443105+444105		EC	SCR	CAL	ASR
385106	441106+442106+443106+444106		EC	SCR	CAL	ASR
385107	441107+442107+443107+444107		EC	SCR	CAL	ASR
385108	441108+442108+443108+444108		EC	SCR	CAL	ASR
385109	441109+442109+443109+444109		EC	SCR	CAL	ASR
385110	441110+442110+443110+444110		EC	SCR	CAL	ASR
385111	441111+442111+443111+444111		EC	SCR	CAL	ASR
385112	441112+442112+443112+444112		EC	SCR	CAL	ASR
385113	441113+442113+443113+444113		EC	SCR	CAL	ASR
385114	441114+442114+443114+444114		EC	SCR	CAL	ASR
385115	441115+442115+443115+444115		EC	SCR	CAL	ASR
385116	441116+442116+443116+444116		EC	SCR	CAL	ASR
385117	441117+442117+443117+444117		EC	SCR	CAL	ASR
385118	441118+442118+443118+444118		EC	SCR	CAL	ASR
385119	441119+442119+443119+444119		EC	SCR	CAL	ASR
385120	441120+442120+443120+444120		EC	SCR	CAL	ASR
385121	441121+442121+443121+444121		EC	SCR	CAL	ASR
385122	441122+442122+443121+444122		EC	SCR	CAL	ASR
385123	441123+442123+443123+444123		EC	SCR	CAL	ASR
385124	441124+442124+443124+444124		EC	SCR	CAL	ASR

* ScotRail Government owned branding

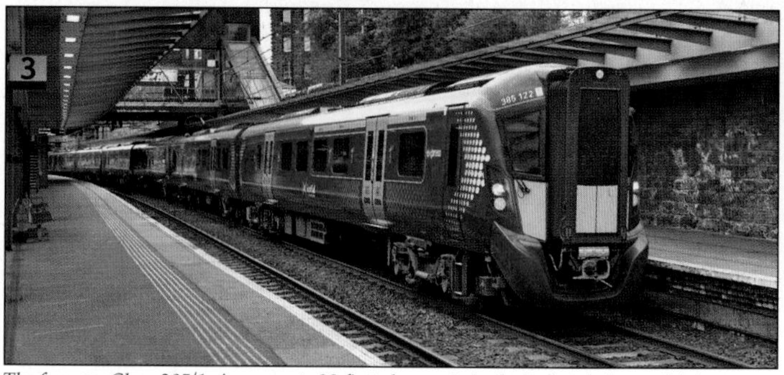

The four-car Class 385/1s incorporate 20 first class seats in the 2+1 style in one driving car. These sets, in addition to other routes, are used on the Edinburgh-Glasgow high speed service. Set No. 385122 with its DMC vehicle leading arrives at Edinburgh Haymarket with a Glasgow Queen Street service. **CJM**

Class 387
Bombardier 4-car Main Line 'Electrostar'

Built: 2014-2017
Vehicle length: Driving 66ft 11in (20.40m)
Intermediate 65ft 6in (19.99m)
Height: 12ft 4in (3.78m)
Width: 9ft 2in (2.80m)
Power: 25kV ac overhead
Horsepower: 2,012hp (1,500kW),
Transmission: Electric

387/0 Formation: DMC+MS+PTS+DMS or DMS+MS+PTS+DMS

387101	421101+422101+423101+424101	HE	GOV	PTR	GTR
387102	421102+422102+423102+424102	HE	GOV	PTR	GTR
387103	421103+422103+423103+424103	HE	GOV	PTR	GTR
387104	421104+422104+423104+424104	HE	GOV	PTR	GTR

387105	421105+422105+423105+424105		HE	GOV	PTR	GTR
387106	421106+422106+423106+424106		HE	GOV	PTR	GTR
387107	421107+422107+423107+424107		HE	GOV	PTR	GTR
387108	421108+422108+423108+424108		HE	GOV	PTR	GTR
387109	421109+422109+423109+424109		HE	GOV	PTR	GTR
387110	421110+422110+423110+424110		HE	GOV	PTR	GTR
387111	421111+422111+423111+424111		HE	GOV	PTR	GTR
387112	421112+422112+423112+424112		HE	GOV	PTR	GTR
387113	421113+422113+423113+424113		HE	GOV	PTR	GTR
387114	421114+422114+423114+424114		HE	GOV	PTR	GTR
387115	421115+422115+423115+424115		HE	GOV	PTR	GTR
387116	421116+422116+423116+424116		HE	GOV	PTR	GTR
387117	421117+422117+423117+424117		HE	GOV	PTR	GTR
387118	421118+422118+423118+424118		HE	GOV	PTR	GTR
387119	421119+422119+423119+424119		HE	GOV	PTR	GTR
387120	421120+422120+423120+424120		HE	GOV	PTR	GTR
387121	421121+422121+423121+424121		HE	GOV	PTR	GTR
387122	421122+422122+423122+424122		HE	GOV	PTR	GTR
387123	421123+422123+423123+424123		HE	GOV	PTR	GTR
387124	421124+422124+423124+424124		HE	GOV	PTR	GTR
387125	421125+422125+423125+424125		HE	GOV	PTR	GTR
387126	421126+422126+423126+424126		HE	GOV	PTR	GTR
387127	421127+422127+423127+424127		HE	GOV	PTR	GTR
387128	421128+422128+423128+424128		HE	GOV	PTR	GTR
387129	421129+422129+423129+424129		HE	GOV	PTR	GTR
387130	421130+422130+423130+424130	*San Francisco*	RG	HEX	PTR	GWR
387131	421131+422131+423131+424131	*Sydney*	RG	HEX	PTR	GWR
387132	421132+422132+423132+424132	*New York*	RG	HEX	PTR	GWR
387133	421133+422133+423133+424133	*Tokyo*	RG	HEX	PTR	GWR
387134	421134+422134+423134+424134	*Barcelona*	RG	HEX	PTR	GWR
387135	421135+422135+423135+424135	*Rome*	RG	HEX	PTR	GWR
387136	421136+422136+423136+424136	*Paris*	RG	HEX	PTR	GWR
387137	421137+422137+423137+424137	*Amsterdam*	RG	HEX	PTR	GWR
387138	421138+422138+423138+424138	*Las Vegas*	RG	HEX	PTR	GWR
387139	421139+422139+423139+424139	*Dublin*	RG	HEX	PTR	GWR
387140	421140+422140+423140+424140	*London*	RG	HEX	PTR	GWR
387141	421141+422141+423141+424141	*Prague*	RG	HEX	PTR	GWR
387142	421142+422142+423142+424142		RG	GWG	PTR	GWR
387143	421143+422143+423143+424143		RG	GWG	PTR	GWR
387144	421144+422144+423144+424144		RG	GWG	PTR	GWR
387145	421145+422145+423145+424145		RG	GWG	PTR	GWR
387146	421146+422146+423146+424146		RG	GWG	PTR	GWR
387147	421147+422147+423147+424147		RG	GWG	PTR	GWR
387148	421148+422148+423148+424148		RG	GWG	PTR	GWR
387149	421149+422149+423149+424149		RG	GWG	PTR	GWR
387150	421150+422150+423150+424150		RG	GWG	PTR	GWR
387151	421151+422151+423151+424151		RG	GWG	PTR	GWR
387152	421152+422152+423152+424152		RG	GWG	PTR	GWR
387153	421153+422153+423153+424153		RG	GWG	PTR	GWR
387154	421154+422154+423154+424154		RG	GWG	PTR	GWR
387155	421155+422155+423155+424155		RG	GWG	PTR	GWR
387156	421156+422156+423156+424156		RG	GWG	PTR	GWR
387157	421157+422157+423157+424157		RG	GWG	PTR	GWR
387158	421158+422158+423158+424158		RG	GWG	PTR	GWR
387159	421159+422159+423159+424159		RG	GWG	PTR	GWR
387160	421160+422160+423160+424160		RG	GWG	PTR	GWR
387161	421161+422161+423161+424161		RG	GWG	PTR	GWR
387162	421162+422162+423162+424162		RG	GWG	PTR	GWR
387163	421163+422163+423163+424163		RG	GWG	PTR	GWR
387164	421164+422164+423164+424164		RG	GWG	PTR	GWR
387165	421165+422166+423165+424165		RG	GWG	PTR	GWR
387166	421166+422166+423166+424166		RG	GWG	PTR	GWR
387167	421167+422167+423167+424167		RG	GWG	PTR	GWR
387168	421168+422168+423168+424168		RG	GWG	PTR	GWR
387169	421169+422169+423169+424169		RG	GWG	PTR	GWR
387170	421170+422170+423170+424170		RG	GWG	PTR	GWR
387171	421171+422171+423171+424171		RG	GWG	PTR	GWR
387172	421172+422172+423172+424172		RG	GWG	PTR	GWR
387173	421173+422173+423173+424173		RG	GWG	PTR	GWR
387174	421174+422174+423174+424174		RG	GWG	PTR	GWR

387/2 Formation: DMC+MS+PTS+DMS

387201	421201+422201+423201+424201	HE	RED	PTR	GTR
387202	421202+422202+423202+424202	HE	RED	PTR	GTR
387203	421203+422203+423203+424203	HE	RED	PTR	GTR
387204	421204+422204+423204+424204	HE	RED	PTR	GTR
387205	421205+422205+423205+424205	HE	RED	PTR	GTR
387206	421206+422206+423206+424206	HE	RED	PTR	GTR
387207	421207+422207+423207+424207	HE	RED	PTR	GTR
387208	421208+422208+423208+424208	HE	RED	PTR	GTR
387209	421209+422209+423209+424209	HE	RED	PTR	GTR
387210	421210+422210+423210+424210	SL	GAT	PTR	GTR
387211	421211+422211+423211+424211	SL	GAT	PTR	GTR
387212	421212+422212+423212+424212	SL	GAT	PTR	GTR
387213	421213+422213+423213+424213	SL	GAT	PTR	GTR
387214	421214+422214+423214+424214	SL	GAT	PTR	GTR
387215	421215+422215+423215+424215	SL	GAT	PTR	GTR
387216	421216+422216+423216+424216	SL	GAT	PTR	GTR
387217	421217+422217+423217+424217	SL	GAT	PTR	GTR
387218	421218+422218+423218+424218	SL	GAT	PTR	GTR
387219	421219+422219+423219+424219	SL	GAT	PTR	GTR
387220	421220+422220+423220+424220	SL	GAT	PTR	GTR
387221	421221+422221+423221+424221	SL	GAT	PTR	GTR
387222	421222+422222+423222+424222	SL	GAT	PTR	GTR
387223	421223+422223+423223+424223	SL	GAT	PTR	GTR
387224	421224+422224+423224+424224	SL	GAT	PTR	GTR
387225	421225+422225+423225+424225	SL	GAT	PTR	GTR
387226	421226+422226+423226+424226	SL	GAT	PTR	GTR
387227	421227+422227+423227+424227	SL	GAT	PTR	GTR

387/3 Formation: DMS+MS+PTS+DMS

387301	421301+422301+423301+424301	RG	C2C	PTR	GWR
387302	421302+422302+423302+424302	RG	C2C	PTR	GWR
387303	421303+422303+423303+424303	EM	C2C	PTR	C2C
387304	421304+422304+423304+424304	EM	C2C	PTR	C2C
387305	421305+422305+423305+424305	RG	C2C	PTR	C2C
387306	421306+422306+423306+424306	EM	C2C	PTR	GWR

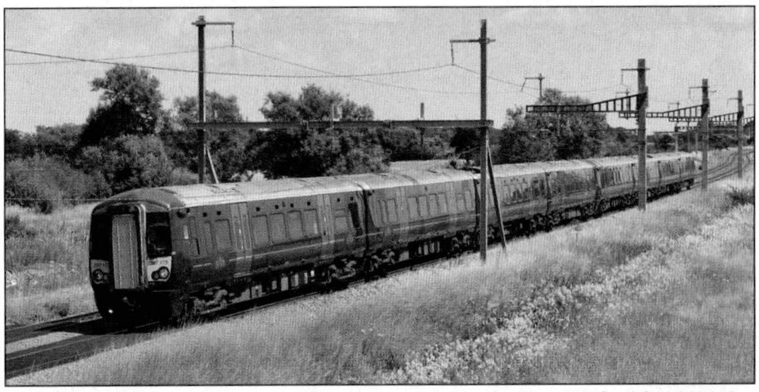

A number of different sub-classes and liveries are carried by the Class 387 fleet. Sets 387142-387174 are painted in Great Western green and operate GW Thames Valley electric services, as well as some Paddington-Cardiff 'stand-in' services while IETs are under repair. Set No. 387173 is seen on the outskirts of Swindon at Shrivenham **CJM**

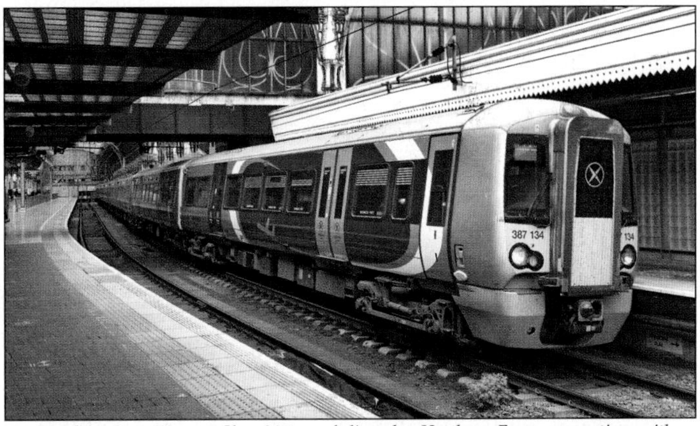

Twelve of the Great Western Class 387s are dedicated to Heathrow Express operations with a revised interior and airport livery, sets are also named after destinations served by London Heathrow Airport. Set No. 387134 now named Barcelona *is seen at Paddington displaying the colour Airport livery. These sets are based at Reading depot with the rest of the Great Western '387' fleet.* **CJM**

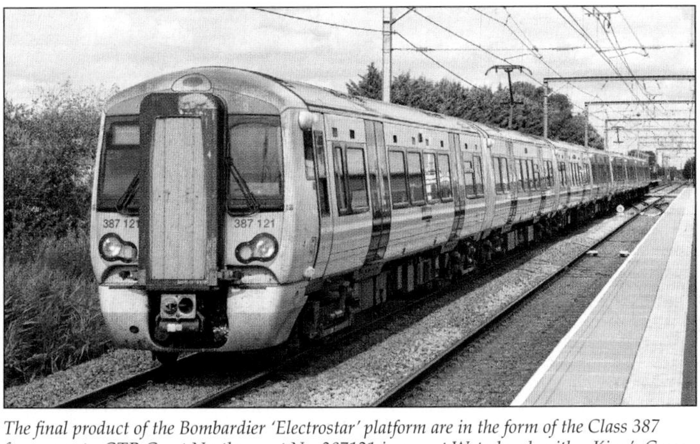

The final product of the Bombardier 'Electrostar' platform are in the form of the Class 387 four-car sets. GTR Great Northern set No. 387121 is seen at Waterbeach with a King's Cross to Kings Lynn service. **CJM**

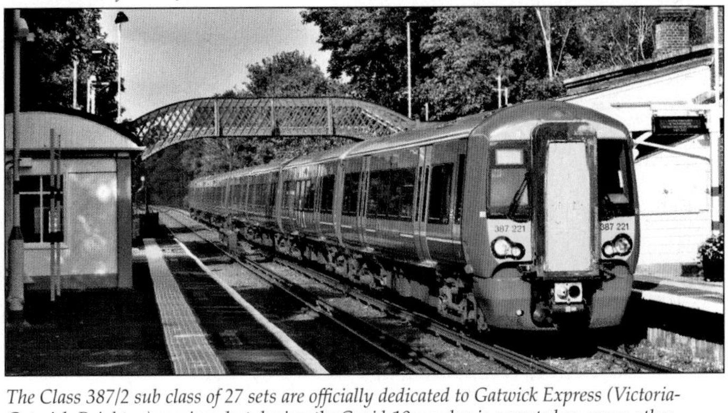

The Class 387/2 sub class of 27 sets are officially dedicated to Gatwick Express (Victoria-Gatwick-Brighton) services, but during the Covid-19 pandemic operated on many other routes. Set No. 387221 is shown. **John Vaughan**

Class 390
Alstom 9 or 11-car Main Line 'Pendolino'

Built: 2001-2011
Vehicle length: Driving 81ft 3in (24.80m)
Intermediate 78ft 4in (23.90m)
Height: 11ft 6in (3.56m)
Width: 8ft 9in (2.73m)

Power: 25kV ac overhead
Horsepower: 9-car 6,839hp (5,100kW),
11-car 9,120hp (6,803kW
Transmission: Electric

Formation: 9-car DMRFO+MF+PTF+MS+TS+MS+PTRMB+MS+DMSO
11-car DMRFO+MF+PTF+MF(MS*)+TS+MS+TS+MS+PTRMB+MS+DMSO

390001	69101+69401+69501+69601*+68801+69701+69801+69901+69201	*Bee Together*	MA	AWC	ANG	AWC
390002	69102+69402+69502+69602*+68802+69702+69802+69902+69202	*Stephen Sutton*	MA	AWC	ANG	AWC
390103	69103+69403+69503+69603+65303+68903+68803+69703+69803+69903+69203		MA	AWC	ANG	AWC
390104	69104+69404+69504+69604+65304+68904+68804+69704+69804+69904+69204	*Alstom Pendolino*	MA	AWC	ANG	AWC
390005	69105+69405+69505+69605*+68805+69705+69805+69905+69205	*City of Wolverhampton*	MA	AWC	ANG	AWC
390006	69106+69406+69506+69606*+68806+69706+69806+69906+69206	*Rethink Mental Illness*	MA	AWC	ANG	AWC
390107	69107+69407+69507+69607+65307+68907+68807+69707+69807+69907+69207		MA	AWC	ANG	AWC
390008	69108+69408+69508+69608*+68808+69708+69808+69908+69208	*Charles Rennie Mackintosh*	MA	AWC	ANG	AWC
390009	69109+69409+69509+69609*+68809+69709+69809+69909+69209	*Treaty of Union*	MA	AWC	ANG	AWC
390010	69110+69410+69510+69610*+68810+69710+69810+69910+69210	*Cumbrian Spirit*	MA	AWC	ANG	AWC
390011	69111+69411+69511+69611*+68811+69711+69811+69911+69211	*City of Lichfield*	MA	AWC	ANG	AWC
390112	69112+69412+69512+69612+65312+68912+68812+69712+69812+69912+69212		MA	AWC	ANG	AWC
390013	69113+69413+69513+69613*+68813+69713+69813+69913+69213	*Blackpool Belle*	MA	AWC	ANG	AWC
390114	69114+69414+69514+69614+65314+68914+68814+69714+69814+69914+69214	*City of Manchester*	MA	AWC	ANG	AWC
390115	69115+69415+69515+69615+65315+68915+68815+69715+69815+69915+69215	*Crewe - All Change (Alison)*	MA	AWC	ANG	AWC
390016	69116+69416+69516+69616*+68816+69716+69816+69916+69216		MA	AWC	ANG	AWC
390117	69117+69417+69517+69617+65317+68917+68817+69717+69817+69917+69217	*Blue Peter*	MA	AWC	ANG	AWC
390118	69118+69418+69518+69618+65318+68918+68818+69718+69818+69918+69218		MA	AWC	ANG	AWC
390119	69119+69419+69519+69619+65319+68919+68819+69719+69819+69919+69219	*Progress*	MA	SPL	ANG	AWC
390020	69120+69420+69520+69620*+68820+69720+69820+69920+69220		MA	AWC	ANG	AWC
390121	69121+69421+69521+69621+65321+68921+68821+69721+69821+69921+69221	*Opportunity*	MA	SPL	ANG	AWC
390122	69122+69422+69522+69622+65322+68922+68822+69722+69822+69922+69222	*Penny the Pendolino*	MA	AWC	ANG	AWC
390123§	69123+69423+69523+69623+69323+68923+68823+69723+69823+69923+69223		MA	AWC	ANG	AWC
390124	69124+69424+69524+69624+65324+68924+68824+69724+69824+69924+69224		MA	AWC	ANG	AWC
390125§	69125+69425+69525+69625+65325+68925+68825+69725+69825+69925+69225	*Virgin Stagecoach*	MA	AWC	ANG	AWC
390126	69126+69426+69526+69626+65326+68926+68826+69726+69826+69926+69226		MA	AWC	ANG	AWC
390127	69127+69427+69527+69627+65327+68927+68827+69727+69827+69927+69227		MA	AWC	ANG	AWC
390128	69128+69428+69528+69628+65328+68928+68828+69728+69828+69928+69228	*City of Preston*	MA	AWC	ANG	AWC
390129	69129+69429+69529+69629+65329+68929+68829+69729+69829+69929+69229	*City of Stoke-on-Trent (Brett)*	MA	AWC	ANG	AWC
390130	69130+69430+69530+69630+65330+68930+68830+69730+69830+69930+69230	*City of Edinburgh*	MA	AWC	ANG	AWC
390131	69131+69431+69531+69631+65331+68931+68831+69731+69831+69931+69231	*City of Liverpool*	MA	AWC	ANG	AWC
390132	69132+69432+69532+69632+65332+68932+68832+69732+69832+69932+69232	*City of Birmingham*	MA	AWC	ANG	AWC
390033	Cars 61933 and 69833 at Avanti Training School, Crewe					
390134	69134+69434+69534+69634+65334+68934+68834+69734+69834+69934+69234	*City of Carlisle*	MA	AWC	ANG	AWC
390135	69135+69435+69535+69635+65335+68935+68835+69735+69835+69935+69235	*City of Lancaster*	MA	AWC	ANG	AWC
390136	69136+69436+69536+69636+65336+68936+68836+69736+69836+69936+69236	*City of Coventry*	MA	AWC	ANG	AWC
390137	69137+69437+69537+69637+65337+68937+68837+69737+69837+69937+69237		MA	AWC	ANG	AWC
390138	69138+69438+69538+69638+65338+68938+68838+69738+69838+69938+69238	*City of London*	MA	AWC	ANG	AWC
390039	69139+69439+69539+69639*+68839+69739+69839+69939+69239	*Lady Godiva*	MA	AWC	ANG	AWC
390040	69140+69440+69540+69640*+68840+69740+69840+69940+69240		MA	AWC	ANG	AWC
390141	69141+69441+69541+69641+65341+68941+68841+69741+69841+69941+69241		MA	AWC	ANG	AWC
390042	69142+69442+69542+69642*+68842+69742+69842+69942+69242		MA	AWC	ANG	AWC
390043	69143+69443+69543+69643*+68843+69743+69843+69943+69243		MA	AWC	ANG	AWC
390044	69144+69444+69544+69644*+68844+69744+69844+69944+69244	*Royal Scot*	MA	AWC	ANG	AWC
390045	69145+69445+69545+69645*+68845+69745+69845+69945+69245		MA	AWC	ANG	AWC
390046	69146+69446+69546+69646*+68846+69746+69846+69946+69246		MA	AWC	ANG	AWC
390047	69147+69447+69547+69647*+68847+69747+69847+69947+69247	*Clic Sargent*	MA	AWC	ANG	AWC
390148	69148+69448+69548+69648+65348+68948+68848+69748+69848+69948+69248	*Flying Scouseman*	MA	AWC	ANG	AWC
390049	69149+69449+69549+69649*+68849+69749+69849+69949+69249		MA	AWC	ANG	AWC
390050	69150+69450+69550+69650*+68850+69750+69850+69950+69250		MA	AWC	ANG	AWC
390151	69151+69451+69551+69651+65351+68951+68851+69751+69851+69951+69251	*Unknown Soldier*	MA	AWC	ANG	AWC
390152	69152+69452+69552+69652+65352+68952+68852+69752+69852+69952+69252		MA	AWC	ANG	AWC
390153	69153+69453+69553+69653+65353+68953+68853+69753+69853+69953+69253		MA	AWC	ANG	AWC
390154	69154+69454+69554+69654+65354+68954+68854+69754+69854+69954+69254	*Matthew Flinders*	MA	AWC	ANG	AWC
390155§	69155+69455+69555+69655+68355+68955+68855+69755+69855+69955+69255	*Railway Benefit Fund*	MA	AWC	ANG	AWC
390156§	69156+69456+69556+69656+68356+68956+68856+69756+69856+69956+69256		MA	AWC	ANG	AWC
390157	69157+69457+69557+69657+68357+68957+68857+69757+69857+69957+69257	*Chad Varah*	MA	AWC	ANG	AWC

§ Refurbished train

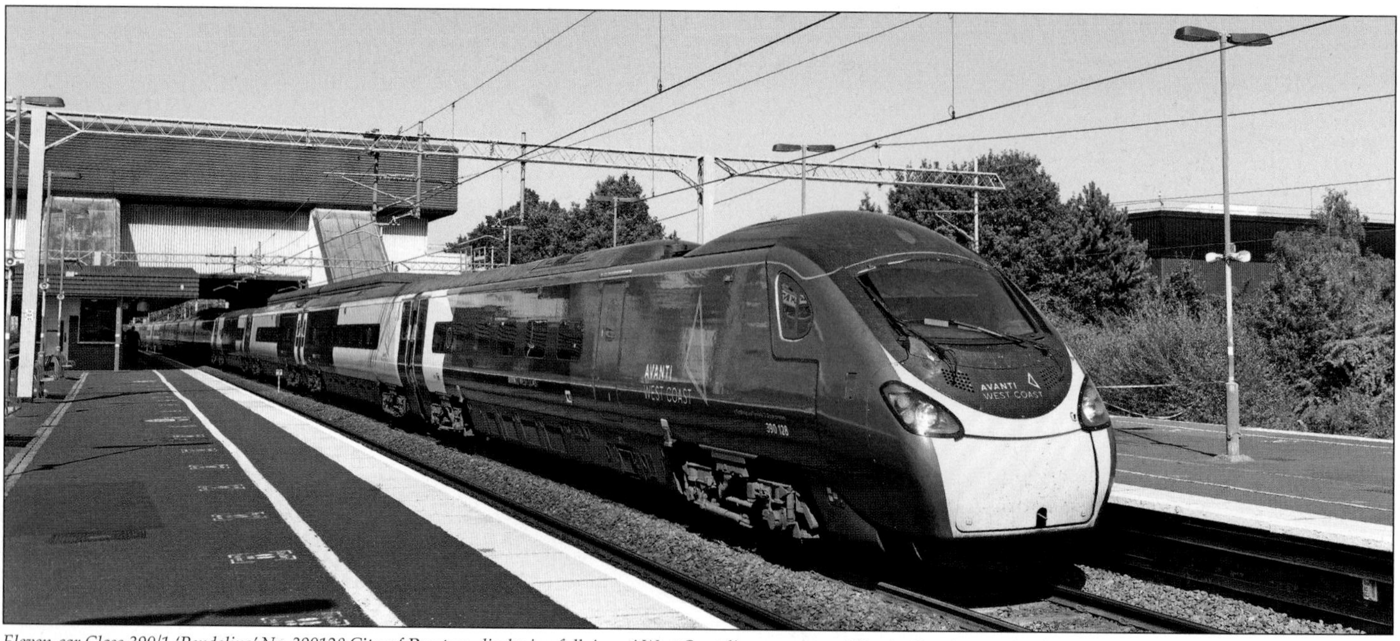

Eleven-car Class 390/1 'Pendolino' No. 390128 City of Preston, *displaying full Avanti West Coast livery, arrives at Birmingham International on 7 September 2021 with the 09.47 Blackpool North to Euston. A major refurbishment of the 'Pendolino' fleet commenced at Alstom, Widnes in autumn 2021.* **CJM**

Class 395
Hitachi 6-car Main Line 'Javelin'

Built: 2007-2009
Vehicle length: Driving 68ft 5in (20.88m)
Intermediate 65ft 6in (20m)
Height: 12ft 6in (3.81m)
Width: 9ft 2in (2.80m)
Power: 750Vdc third rail and 25kV ac overhead
Horsepower: 2,253hp (1,680kW),
Transmission: Electric

Formation: DMS+MS+MS+MS+MS+DMS

395001	39011+39012+39013+39014+39015+39016	*Dame Kelly Holmes*	AD	HS1	EVL	SET
395002	39021+39022+39023+39024+39025+39026	*Sebastian Coe*	AD	HS1§	EVL	SET
395003	39031+39032+39033+39034+39035+39036	*Sir Steve Redgrave*	AD	HS1	EVL	SET
395004	39041+39042+39043+39044+39045+39046	*Sir Chris Hoy*	AD	HS1	EVL	SET
395005	39051+39052+39053+39054+39055+39056	*Dame Tanni Grey-Thompson*	AD	HS1	EVL	SET
395006	39061+39062+39063+39064+39065+39066	*Daley Thompson*	AD	HS1	EVL	SET
395007	39071+39072+39073+39074+39075+39076	*Steve Backley*	AD	HS1	EVL	SET
395008	39081+39082+39083+39084+39085+39086	*Ben Ainslie*	AD	HS1	EVL	SET
395009	39091+39092+39093+39094+39095+39096	*Rebecca Adlington*	AD	HS1	EVL	SET
395010	39101+39102+39103+39104+39105+39106	*Duncan Goodhew*	AD	HS1	EVL	SET
395011	39111+39112+39113+39114+39115+39116	*Katherine Grainger*	AD	HS1	EVL	SET
395012	39121+39122+39123+39124+39125+39126		AD	HS1	EVL	SET
395013	39131+39132+39133+39134+39135+39136	*Hornby Visitor Centre Margate Kent*	AD	HS1§	EVL	SET
395014	39141+39142+39143+39144+39145+39146		AD	HS1	EVL	SET
395015	39151+39152+39153+39154+39155+39156		AD	HS1	EVL	SET
395016	39161+39162+39163+39164+39165+39166		AD	HS1	EVL	SET
395017	39171+39172+39173+39174+39175+39176		AD	HS1	EVL	SET
395018	39181+39182+39183+39184+39185+39186	*The Victory Javelin*	AD	HS1	EVL	SET
395019	39191+39192+39193+39194+39195+39196	*Jessica Ennis*	AD	HS1	EVL	SET
395020	39201+39202+39203+39204+39205+39206	*Jason Kenny*	AD	HS1	EVL	SET
395021	39211+39212+39213+39214+39215+39216	*Ed Clancy MBE*	AD	HS1	EVL	SET
395022	39221+39222+39223+39224+39225+39226	*Alistair Brownlee*	AD	HS1	EVL	SET
395023	39231+39232+39233+39234+39235+39236	*Ellie Simmonds*	AD	HS1	EVL	SET
395024	39241+39242+39243+39244+39245+39246	*Jonnie Peacock*	AD	HS1	EVL	SET
395025	39251+39252+39253+39254+39255+39256	*Victoria Pendleton*	AD	HS1	EVL	SET
395026	39261+39262+39263+39264+39265+39266	*Marc Woods*	AD	HS1	EVL	SET
395027	39271+39272+39273+39274+39275+39276	*Hannah Cockcroft*	AD	HS1	EVL	SET
395028	39281+39282+39283+39284+39285+39286	*Laura Trott*	AD	HS1	EVL	SET
395029	39291+39292+39293+39294+39295+39296	*David Weir*	AD	HS1	EVL	SET

§ carries facemask

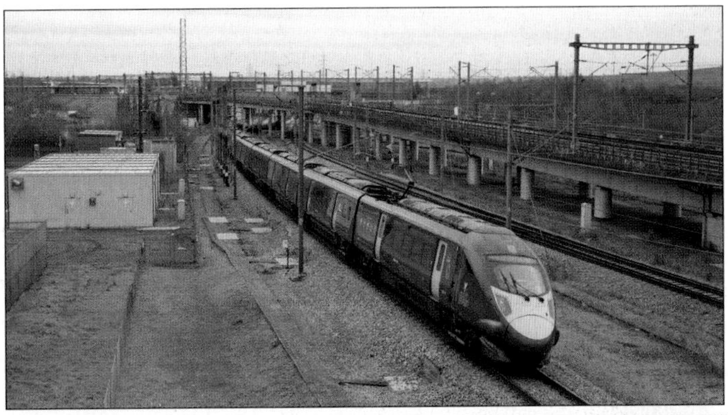

The SouthEastern operated 'Javelin' high speed service linking London St Pancras with Kent via HS1, uses a fleet of 29 six car Class 395 sets, built by Hitachi and maintained at a purpose-built Hitachi depot in Ashford, Kent. On 27 January 2022, set No. 395018 in Poppy livery, passes Ebbsfleet International. **Antony Christie**

Class 397
CAF 5-car Main Line 'Civity' 'Nova 2'

Built: 2017-2019
Vehicle length: Driving 78ft 10in (24.02m)
Intermediate 76ft 4in (20.35m)
Height: 12ft 6in (3.80m)
Width: 8ft 10in (2.71m)
Power: 25kV ac overhead
Horsepower: 3,540hp (2,640kW),
Transmission: Electric

Formation: DMF+PTS+MS+PTS+DMS

397001	471001+472001+473001+474001+475001	MA	FTN	EVL	FTP
397002	471001+472002+473002+474002+475002	MA	FTN	EVL	FTP
397003	471003+472003+473003+474003+475003	MA	FTN	EVL	FTP
397004	471004+472004+473004+474004+475004	MA	FTN	EVL	FTP
397005	471005+472005+473005+474005+475005	MA	FTN	EVL	FTP
397006	471006+472006+473006+474006+475006	MA	FTN	EVL	FTP
397007	471007+472007+473007+474007+475007	MA	FTN	EVL	FTP
397008	471008+472008+473008+474008+475008	MA	FTN	EVL	FTP
397009	471009+472009+473009+474009+475009	MA	FTN	EVL	FTP
397010	471010+472010+473010+474010+475010	MA	FTN	EVL	FTP
397011	471011+472011+473011+474011+475011	MA	FTN	EVL	FTP
397012	471012+472012+473012+474012+475012	MA	FTN	EVL	FTP

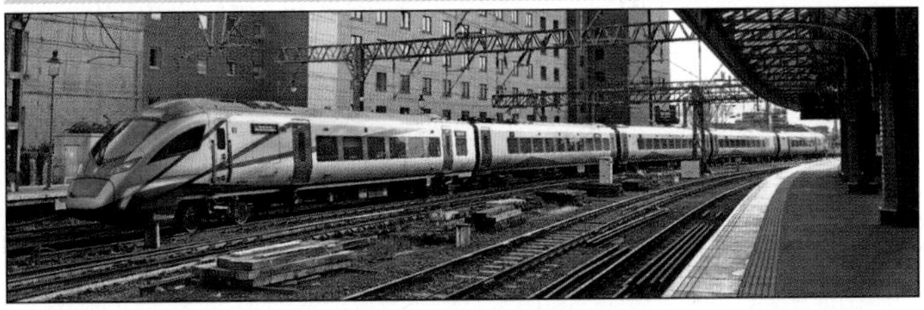

CAF-built five-car main line 'Civity' sets are operated by TransPennine Express on main line services on the West Coast Main Line. The streamlined units are based at Manchester International depot. Set No. 397012 is seen arriving at Glasgow Central. **CJM**

Class 398
Stadler 3-car BMU 'Citylink' Tram-Train

Built: 2021-2023
Vehicle length: Driving awaited
Intermediate awaited
Height: awaited
Width: awaited
Power: 25kV ac overhead and battery
Horsepower: awaited
Transmission: Electric

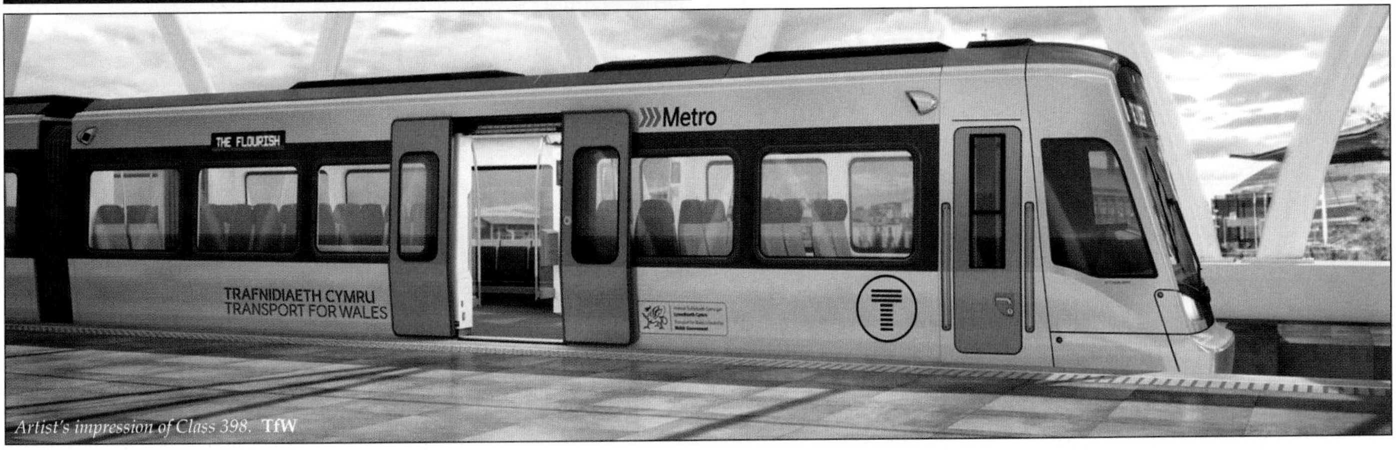

Artist's impression of Class 398. **TfW**

	Formation: DMS+TS+DMS				
398001	999051+999151+999251	CV	TFW	TFW	TFW
398002	999052+999152+999252	CV	TFW	TFW	TFW
398003	999053+999153+999253	CV	TFW	TFW	TFW
398004	999054+999154+999254	CV	TFW	TFW	TFW
398005	999055+999155+999255	CV	TFW	TFW	TFW
398006	999056+999156+999256	CV	TFW	TFW	TFW
398007	999057+999157+999257	CV	TFW	TFW	TFW
398008	999058+999158+999258	CV	TFW	TFW	TFW
398009	999059+999159+999259	CV	TFW	TFW	TFW
398010	999060+999160+999260	CV	TFW	TFW	TFW
398011	999061+999161+999261	CV	TFW	TFW	TFW
398012	999062+999162+999262	CV	TFW	TFW	TFW
398013	999063+999163+999263	CV	TFW	TFW	TFW
398014	999064+999164+999264	CV	TFW	TFW	TFW
398015	999065+999165+999265	CV	TFW	TFW	TFW
398016	999066+999166+999266	CV	TFW	TFW	TFW
398017	999067+999167+999267	CV	TFW	TFW	TFW
398018	999068+999168+999268	CV	TFW	TFW	TFW
398019	999069+999169+999269	CV	TFW	TFW	TFW
398020	999070+999170+999270	CV	TFW	TFW	TFW
398021	999071+999171+999271	CV	TFW	TFW	TFW
398022	999072+999172+999272	CV	TFW	TFW	TFW
398023	999073+999173+999273	CV	TFW	TFW	TFW
398024	999074+999174+999274	CV	TFW	TFW	TFW
398025	999075+999175+999275	CV	TFW	TFW	TFW
398026	999076+999176+999276	CV	TFW	TFW	TFW
398027	999077+999177+999277	CV	TFW	TFW	TFW
398028	999078+999178+999278	CV	TFW	TFW	TFW
398029	999079+999179+999279	CV	TFW	TFW	TFW
398030	999080+999180+999280	CV	TFW	TFW	TFW
398031	999081+999181+999281	CV	TFW	TFW	TFW
398032	999082+999182+999282	CV	TFW	TFW	TFW
398033	999083+999183+999283	CV	TFW	TFW	TFW
398034	999084+999184+999284	CV	TFW	TFW	TFW
398035	999085+999185+999285	CV	TFW	TFW	TFW
398036	999086+999186+999286	CV	TFW	TFW	TFW

Class 399
Vossloh 3-car EMU 'Citylink' Tram-Train

Built: 2015-2016
Length: 122ft 1in (37.2m)
Height: 12ft 2in (3.71m)
Width: 8ft 7in (2.65m)
Power: 750V dc overhead
Horsepower: 1,166hp (870kW)
Transmission: Electric

	Formation: DMS+MS+DMS				
399201 (201)*	999001+999101+999201	§	SST	SST	SST
399202 (202)*	999002+999102+999204 *Theo The Childrens Hospital Charity*	§	SST	SST	SST
399203 (203)*	999003+999103+999203	§	SST	SST	SST
399204 (204)*	999004+999104+999202	§	SST	SST	SST
399205 (205)	999005+999105+999205	§	SST	SST	SST
399206 (206)	999006+999106+999206	§	SST	SST	SST
399207 (207)	999007+999107+999207	§	SST	SST	SST

* Authorised for Tram-Train/Network Rail operation

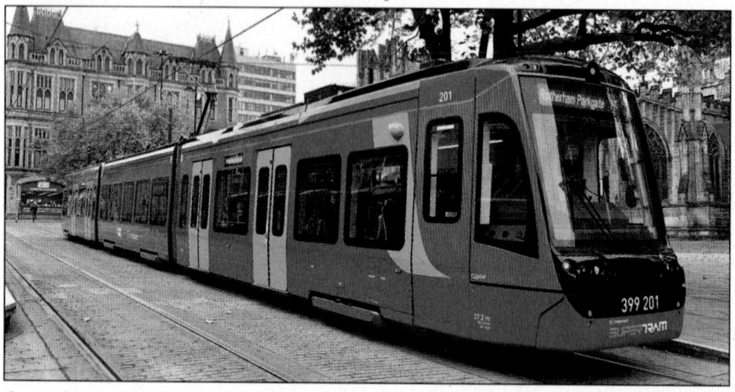

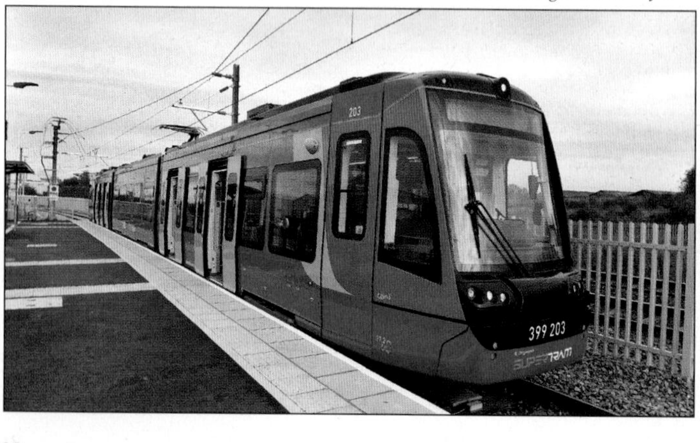

Seven three-section Vossloh 'Tram-Trains' operate in Sheffield, working over the Sheffield Super Tram network as well as Network Rail metals between Meadowhall and Rotherham Parkgate. Above set No. 399201 stands in Sheffield city centre at Sheffield Cathedral with a service heading to Parkgate. Below, No. 399203 is seen at Rotherham Parkgate. Both: **CJM**

Electric Multiple Units - DC

Class 400 Series
Preserved Stock

5BEL

Number	Set	Origin	Type	Location
279	3051	SR	TFK	5-BEL Trust stored at Peak Rail
281	3053	SR	TFK	VSOE Stewarts Lane
280	3052	SR	TFK	VSOE Stewarts Lane
282	3051	SR	TFK	5-BEL Trust
283	3053	SR	TFK	VSOE Stewarts Lane
284	3052	SR	TFK	VSOE Stewarts Lane
285	3053	SR	TPT	5-BEL Trust
286	3051	SR	TPT	VSOE Stewarts Lane
287	3052	SR	TPT	5-BEL Trust stored at Peak Rail
288	3051	SR	DMBPT	5-BEL Trust
289	3051	SR	DMBPT	Little Mill Inn, Rowarth, Derbyshire
291	3052	SR	DMBPT	5-BEL Trust
292	3053	SR	DMBPT	VSOE Stewarts Lane
293	3053	SR	DMBPT	VSOE Stewarts Lane
6PUL				
264	3012	SR	TKC	VSOE Stewarts Lane
278	3017	SR	TKC	VSOE Stewarts Lane
2BIL (Class 401)				
10656	2090	SR	DMBS	National Railway Museum Shildon
12123	2090	SR	DTC	National Railway Museum Shildon
4COR (Class 404)				
10096	3142	SR	TSK	East Kent Railway
11161	3142	SR	DMBS	Sellinge
11179	3131	SR	DMBS	National Railway Museum York
11187	3135	SR	DMBS	East Kent Railway
11201	3142	SR	DMBS	Sellinge
11825	3142	SR	TC	Sellinge
4DD				
13003	4002	SR	DMBT	4DD Group, Sellinge
13004	4002	SR	DMBT	4DD Group, Sellinge
4 SUB (Class 405)				
8143	4308	SR	DMBS	National Railway Museum, York
10239	4732	BR/SR	TS	One:One Railway Museum, Margate
12354	4732	BR/SR	TSO	One:One Railway Museum, Margate
12795	4732	BR/SR	DMBS	One:One Railway Museum, Margate
12796	4732	BR/SR	DMBS	One:One Railway Museum, Margate
4CEP/BEP (Class 411/412)				
61229	7105	BR/SR	DMBSO	Southall (NR No. 99229)
61230	7105	BR/SR	DMBSO	Southall (NR No. 99230)
61736	2304	BR/SR	DMBSO	Chinnor & Princess Risborough Rly
61737	2304	BR/SR	DMBSO	Chinnor & Princess Risborough Rly
61798	2315	BR/SR	DMBSO	Eden Valley Railway
61799	2315	BR/SR	DMBSO	Eden Valley Railway
61804	2311	BR/SR	DMBSO	Eden Valley Railway
61805	2311	BR/SR	DMBSO	Eden Valley Railway
69013	7012	BR/SR	TBS	Epping and Ongar Railway
70229	2315	BR/SR	TSO	Eden Valley Railway
70235	7107	BR/SR	TBCK	Epping and Ongar Railway
70262	1524	BR/SR	TSO	Hastings Diesels Ltd
70273	1392	BR/SR	TSO	East Kent Railway
70284	1520	BR/SR	TSO	Northampton Ironstone Railway
70292	1554	BR/SR	TSO	Speyside Railway, Grantown
70296	1559	BR/SR	TSO	Northampton Ironstone Railway
70300	1698	BR/SR	TSO	Fighting Cocks Pub, Middleton St George
70345	1500	BR/SR	TBCK	Hydraulic Hse, Sutton Bridge, Cambs
70354	2315	BR/SR	TBCK	Eden Valley Railway
70510	1597	BR/SR	TSO	Northampton Ironstone Railway
70527	1589	BR/SR	TSO	Great Central Railway
70531	1610	BR/SR	TSO	Speyside Railway, Grantown
70539	2311	BR/SR	TBCK	Eden Valley Railway
70547	1569	BR/SR	TSO	Private in Hungerford

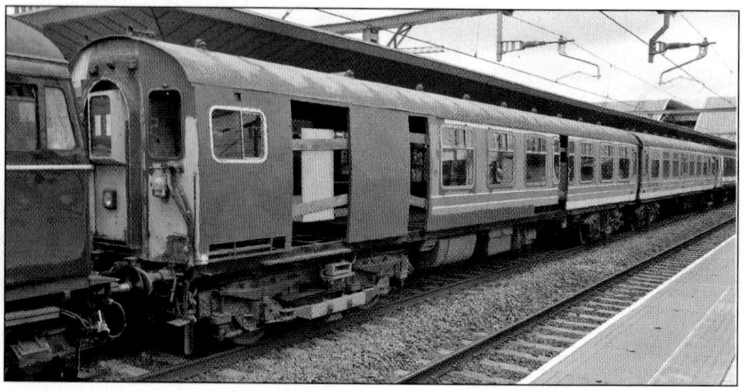

Considering no preserved electric multiple units can operate under their own power, a large number are preserved. The two driving cars from CEP No. 7105 are seen in transit from Eastleigh to Southall for restoration back to their original 1950s style. **Spencer Conquest**

70549	1567	BR/SR	TSO	East Lancs Railway, Bury
70573	2304	BR/SR	TBCK	Chinnor & Princess Risborough Rly
70576	1589	BR/SR	TBCK	Great Central Railway
70607	2311	BR/SR	TSO	Eden Valley Railway

2HAP (Class 414)

61275	4308	BR/SR	DMBS	National Railway Museum, Shildon
61287	4311	BR/SR	DMBS	Private in Clipstone, Nottinghamshire
75395	4308	BR/SR	DTC	National Railway Museum, Shildon
75407	4311	BR/SR	DTS	Private in Clipstone, Nottinghamshire

4EPB (Class 415)

14351	5176	BR/SR	DMBSO	Northampton Ironstone Railway
14352	5176	BR/SR	DMBSO	Northampton Ironstone Railway
15254	5176	BR/SR	TSO	1:1 Museum, Margate
15396	5176	BR/SR	TSO	Northampton Ironstone Railway

2EPB (Class 416)

14573	6307	BR/SR	DMBS	Hope Farm, Sellindge
16117	6307	BR/SR	DTS	Hope Farm, Sellindge
65321	5791	BR/SR	DMBS	Peak Rail, Darley Dale
65373	5759	BR/SR	DMBS	Southall
77112	5793	BR/SR	DTS	Peak Rail, Darley Dale
77558	5759	BR/SR	DTS	Southall

MLV (Class 419)

68001	9001	BR/SR	DMBL	Southall
68002	9002	BR/SR	DMBL	Southall
68003	9003	BR/SR	DMBL	Eden Valley Railway
68004	9004	BR/SR	DMBL	Mid-Norfolk Railway
68005	9005	BR/SR	DMBL	Eden Valley Railway
68008	9008	BR/SR	DMBL	Southall
68009	9009	BR/SR	DMBL	Southall
68010	9010	BR/SR	DMBL	Eden Valley Railway

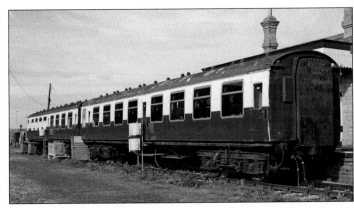

Originally preserved as a cafe near Bridport, CEP vehicles 70531 (unit 1610) and 70292 (unit 1554) are now under preservation at the Speyside Railway. The two coaches are seen in their early days in Dorset, painted in a non railway style livery. **Antony Christie**

4CIG (Class 421)

62043	1753	BR/SR	MBSO	Nemesis Rail, Burton-on-Trent
62364	1373	BR/SR	MBSO	400 Series Group, at Barrow Hill
62385	1399	BR/SR	MBSO	East Kent Railway
62402	1497	BR/SR	MBSO	Spa Valley Railway
70721	1753	BR/SR	TSO	Nemesis Rail, Burton-on-Trent
71041	1306	BR/SR	TSO	Private in Hever
71080	1881	BR/SR	TSO	Dean Forest Railway
71085	1884	BR/SR	TSO	Private Morden Wharf, Grenwich
76048	1753	BR/SR	DTC	Nemesis Rail, Burton-on-Trent
76102	1753	BR/SR	DTC	Nemesis Rail, Burton-on-Trent
76740	1392	BR/SR	DTC	Southall
76747	1399	BR/SR	DTC	400 Series Group at EKR
76762	1881	BR/SR	DTC	Barrow Hill
76764	1497	BR/SR	DTC	Spa Valley Railway
76835	1497	BR/SR	DTC	Spa Valley Railway

4BIG (Class 422)

69302	2251	BR/SR	TRSB	Abbey View Centre, Neath
69304	2260	BR/SR	TRSB	Northampton Ironstone Railway
69306	2254	BR/SR	TRSB	Spa Valley Railway
69316	2258	BR/SR	TRSB	Waverley Heritage Centre
69318	2259	BR/SR	TRSB	Last Moorings, Stickney, Lincolnshire
69332	2257	BR/SR	TRSB	Eden Valley, Warcop
69333	2262	BR/SR	TRSB	Lavender Line (for sale)
69335	2209	BR/SR	TRSB	Wensleydale Railway
69337	2210	BR/SR	TRSB	Hastings Diesels Ltd
69338	2211	BR/SR	TRSB	Station Rest, Gulf Corporation, Bahrain
69339	2205	BR/SR	TRSB	Nemesis Rail, Burton-on-Trent

4VEP/VOP (Class 423)

62236	3417	BR/SR	MBSO	Strawberry Hill
62321	3918	BR/SR	MBSO	Baroow Hill
70797	3417	BR/SR	TSO	Strawberry Hill
70904	3905	BR/SR	TSO	East Kent Railway
76262	3417	BR/SR	DTCO	Strawberry Hill
76263	3417	BR/SR	DTCO	Strawberry Hill
76397	3905	BR/SR	DTC	East Kent Railway
76398	3905	BR/SR	DTC	East Kent Railway
76875	3545	BR/SR	DTC	East Kent Railway
76887	3568	BR/SR	DTC	Woking Miniature Railway

TC (Class 438)

70823	428	BR/SR	TBSK	London Transport set
70824	413	BR/SR	TBSK	Swanage Railway
70826	415	BR/SR	TBSK	Sandford & Barnwell Station
70855	412	BR/SR	TFK	Swanage Railway
70859	416	BR/SR	TFK	Stravithie Station
70860	417	BR/SR	TFK	Cambridge North Road
71163	428	BR/SR	TFK	London Transport set
76275	404	BR/SR	DTSO	Swanage Railway
76277	405	BR/SR	DTSO	(977335) Dartmoor Railway
76297	428	BR/SR	DTSO	London Transport set
76298	415	BR/SR	DTSO	Swanage Railway
76301	417	BR/SR	DTSO	Bellingham, Northumberland
76302	417	BR/SR	DTSO	Bellingham, Northumberland
76322	413	BR/SR	DTSO	Swanage Railway
76324	428	BR/SR	DTSO	London Transport set

Class 442

77382	442401	BR/SR	DTC	Private at Arlington, Eastleigh

Class 457

67300	7001	BR/WR	DMSO	East Kent Railway

Class 483

122+225	(483)002	RSS Wishaw, (stored)
124+224	(483)004	Holliers Park Farm, Hale Common, Isle of Wight
126+226	(483)006	LT Group at Llanelli and Mynydd Mawr Railway
127+227	(483)007	Isle of Wight Steam Railway, Haven Street
128+228	(483)008	LT Group at Llanelli and Mynydd Mawr Railway
129	(483)009	Restoration at East Somerset Railway
229	(483009)	Rail Freight Services, Stoke (stored)

Class 487 1940 Waterloo & City

61		SR	DMSO	LT Museum, Acton

GLV (Class 489)

68500	489101	BR/IC	DMBL	Ecclesbourne Valley Railway
68503	489104	BR/IC	DMBL	Spa Valley Railway
68506	489106	BR/IC	DMBL	Ecclesbourne Valley Railway
68507	489108	BR/IC	DMBL	Great Central Railway
68509	489110	BR/IC	DMBL	Vale of Glamorgan Railway

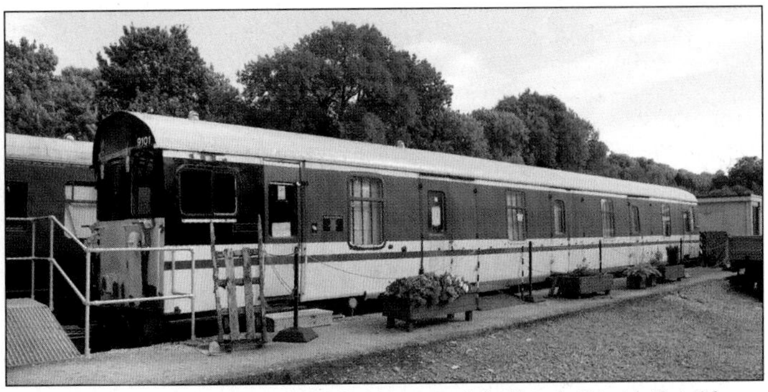

Five of the Gatwick Luggage Vans (GLVs) which operated the Victoria-Gatwick 'Gatwick Express' service are preserved. No. 68500, set No. 489101 is painted in Gatwick Express livery and is at the Ecclesbourne Valley Railway. **Nathan Williamson**

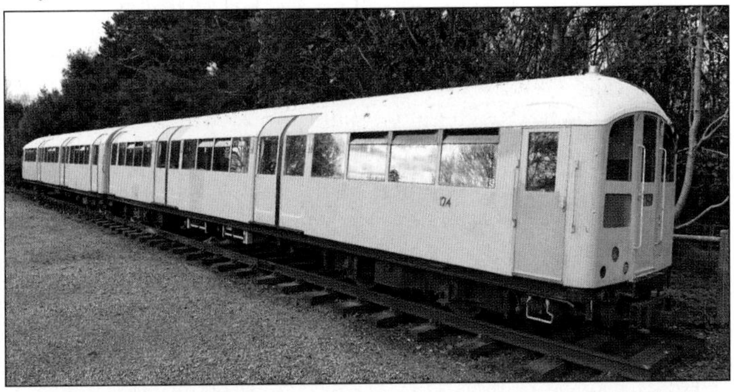

Former Isle of Wight set No. 004 is now located in the carpark of Holliers Park Farm, Hale Common, Branstone near Sandown, where it is planned to use at least one vehicle as an on site cafe, with external restoration into LU red. In November 2021 it is seen painted in a silver grey livery. **CJM**

Class 444
Siemens 5-car EMU Main Line 'Desiro'

Built: 2003-2004
Vehicle length: Driving 77ft 3in (23.57m)
Height: 12ft 1½in (3.74m)
Width: 8ft 9in (2.74m)
Power: 750V dc third rail
Horsepower: 2,682hp (2,000kW)
Transmission: Electric

Formation: DMSO+TSO+TSO+TSO+DMCO

444001	63801+67101+67151+67201+63851 *Naomi House*	NT	SWN	ANG	SWR
444002	63802+67102+67152+67202+63852	NT	SWR	ANG	SWR
444003	63803+67103+67153+67203+63853	NT	SWR	ANG	SWR
444004	63804+67104+67154+67204+63854	NT	SWN	ANG	SWR

444005	63805+67105+67155+67205+63855		NT	SWR	ANG	SWR
444006	63806+67106+67156+67206+63856		NT	SWR	ANG	SWR
444007	63807+67107+67157+67207+63857		NT	SWR	ANG	SWR
444008	63808+67108+67158+67208+63858		NT	SWN	ANG	SWR
444009	63809+67109+67159+67209+63859		NT	SWN	ANG	SWR
444010	63810+67110+67160+67210+63860		NT	SWN	ANG	SWR
444011	63811+67111+67161+67211+63861		NT	SWR	ANG	SWR
444012	63812+67112+67162+67212+63862	*Destination Weymouth*	NT	SWR	ANG	SWR
444013	63813+67113+67163+67213+63863		NT	SWN	ANG	SWR
444014	63814+67114+67164+67214+63864		NT	SWR	ANG	SWR
444015	63815+67115+67165+67215+63865		NT	SWR	ANG	SWR
444016	63816+67116+67166+67216+63866		NT	SWR	ANG	SWR
444017	63817+67117+67167+67217+63867		NT	SWR	ANG	SWR
444018	63818+67118+67168+67218+63868	*The Fab 444*	NT	SWR	ANG	SWR
444019	63819+67119+67169+67219+63869		NT	SWR	ANG	SWR
444020	63820+67120+67170+67220+63870		NT	SWR	ANG	SWR
444021	63821+67121+67171+67221+63871		NT	SWR	ANG	SWR
444022	63822+67122+67172+67222+63872		NT	SWN	ANG	SWR
444023	63823+67123+67173+67223+63873		NT	SWR	ANG	SWR
444024	63824+67124+67174+67224+63874		NT	SWR	ANG	SWR
444025	63825+67125+67175+67225+63875		NT	SWR	ANG	SWR
444026	63826+67126+67176+67226+63876		NT	SWN	ANG	SWR
444027	63827+67127+67177+67227+63877		NT	SWR	ANG	SWR
444028	63828+67128+67178+67228+63878		NT	SWN	ANG	SWR
444029	63829+67129+67179+67229+63879		NT	SWR	ANG	SWR
444030	63830+67130+67180+67230+63880		NT	SWR	ANG	SWR
444031	63831+67131+67181+67231+63881		NT	SWR	ANG	SWR
444032	63832+67132+67182+67232+63882		NT	SWR	ANG	SWR
444033	63833+67133+67183+67233+63883		NT	SWN	ANG	SWR
444034	63834+67134+67184+67234+63884		NT	SWN	ANG	SWR
444035	63835+67135+67185+67235+63885		NT	SWN	ANG	SWR
444036	63836+67136+67186+67236+63886		NT	SWN	ANG	SWR
444037	63837+67137+67187+67237+63887		NT	SWR	ANG	SWR
444038	63838+67138+67188+67238+63888		NT	SWR	ANG	SWR
444039	63839+67139+67189+67239+63889		NT	SWN	ANG	SWR
444040	63840+67140+67190+67240+63890	*The D-Day Story Portsmouth*	NT	SWR	ANG	SWR
444041	63841+67141+67191+67241+63891		NT	SWN	ANG	SWR
444042	63842+67142+67192+67242+63892		NT	SWR	ANG	SWR
444043	63843+67143+67193+67243+63893		NT	SWR	ANG	SWR
444044	63844+67144+67194+67244+63894		NT	SWN	ANG	SWR
444045	63845+67145+67195+67245+63895		NT	SWN	ANG	SWR

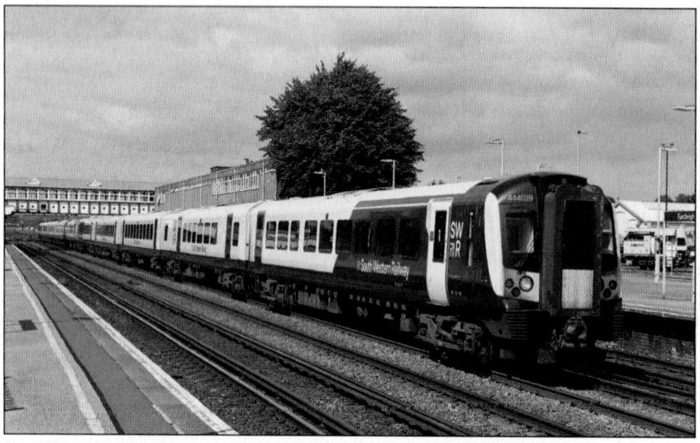

South Western Railway main line Class 444 units operate the main express services on the Waterloo to Portsmouth Harbour and Weymouth route. Most sets now carry the latest SWR grey and blue livery. No. 444029 is seen passing Eastleigh in July 2021. **CJM**

Class 450
Siemens 4-car EMU Outer Suburban 'Desiro'

Built: 2002-2007
Vehicle length: Driving 66ft 9in (20.40m)
Height: 12ft 1½in (3.74m)
Width: 8ft 9in (2.74m)
Power: 750V dc third rail
Horsepower: 2,682hp (2,000kW)
Transmission: Electric

Formation: DMCO+TSO+TSO+DMCO

450001		63201+64201+68101+63601		NT	SWO	ANG	SWR
450002		63202+64202+68102+63602		NT	SWO	ANG	SWR
450003		63203+64203+68103+63603		NT	SWR	ANG	SWR
450004		63204+64204+68104+63604		NT	SWO	ANG	SWR
450005		63205+64205+68105+63605		NT	SWR	ANG	SWR
450006		63206+64206+68106+63606		NT	SWR	ANG	SWR
450007		63207+64207+68107+63607		NT	SWR	ANG	SWR
450008		63208+64208+68108+63608		NT	SWO	ANG	SWR
450009		63209+64209+68109+63609		NT	SWR	ANG	SWR
450010		63210+64210+68110+63610		NT	SWR	ANG	SWR
450011		63211+64211+68111+63611		NT	SWR	ANG	SWR
450012		63212+64212+68112+63612		NT	SWR	ANG	SWR
450013		63213+64213+68113+63613		NT	SWR	ANG	SWR
450014		63214+64214+68114+63614		NT	SWR	ANG	SWR
450015		63215+64215+68115+63615	*Desiro*	NT	SWR	ANG	SWR
450016		63216+64216+68116+63616		NT	SWR	ANG	SWR
450017		63217+64217+68117+63617		NT	SWR	ANG	SWR
450018		63218+64218+68118+63618		NT	SWR	ANG	SWR
450019		63219+64219+68119+63619		NT	SWO	ANG	SWR
450020		63220+64220+68120+63620		NT	SWR	ANG	SWR
450021		63221+64221+68121+63621		NT	SWR	ANG	SWR
450022		63222+64222+68122+63622		NT	SWR	ANG	SWR
450023		63223+64223+68123+63623		NT	SWR	ANG	SWR
450024		63224+64224+68124+63624		NT	SWR	ANG	SWR
450025		63225+64225+68125+63625		NT	SWR	ANG	SWR
450026		63226+64226+68126+63626		NT	SWR	ANG	SWR
450027		63227+64227+68127+63627		NT	SWR	ANG	SWR
450028		63228+64228+68128+63628		NT	SWO	ANG	SWR
450029		63229+64229+68129+63629		NT	SWR	ANG	SWR
450030		63230+64230+68130+63630		NT	SWR	ANG	SWR
450031		63231+64231+68131+63631		NT	SWR	ANG	SWR
450032		63232+64232+68132+63632		NT	SWO	ANG	SWR
450033		63233+64233+68133+63633		NT	SWR	ANG	SWR
450034		63234+64234+68134+63634		NT	SWR	ANG	SWR
450035		63235+64235+68135+63635		NT	SWO	ANG	SWR
450036		63236+64236+68136+63636		NT	SWR	ANG	SWR
450037		63237+64237+68137+63637		NT	SWR	ANG	SWR
450038		63238+64238+68138+63638		NT	SWR	ANG	SWR
450039		63239+64239+68139+63639		NT	SWR	ANG	SWR
450040		63240+64240+68140+63640		NT	SWO	ANG	SWR
450041		63241+64241+68141+63641		NT	SWR	ANG	SWR
450042		63242+64242+68142+63642	*Treloar College*	NT	SWR	ANG	SWR
450043	(450543)	63243+64243+68143+63643		NT	SWR	ANG	SWR
450044	(450544)	63244+64244+68144+63644		NT	SWO	ANG	SWR
450045	(450545)	63245+64245+68145+63645		NT	SWO	ANG	SWR
450046	(450546)	63246+64246+68146+63646		NT	SWO	ANG	SWR
450047	(450547)	63247+64247+68147+63647		NT	SWR	ANG	SWR
450048	(450548)	63248+64248+68148+63648		NT	SWR	ANG	SWR
450049	(450549)	63249+64249+68149+63649		NT	SWR	ANG	SWR
450050	(450550)	63250+64250+68150+63650		NT	SWO	ANG	SWR
450051	(450551)	63251+64251+68151+63651		NT	SWR	ANG	SWR
450052	(450552)	63252+64252+68152+63652		NT	SWR	ANG	SWR
450053	(450553)	63253+64253+68153+63653		NT	SWR	ANG	SWR
450054	(450554)	63254+64254+68154+63654		NT	SWR	ANG	SWR
450055	(450555)	63255+64255+68155+63655		NT	SWR	ANG	SWR
450056	(450556)	63256+64256+68156+63656		NT	SWR	ANG	SWR
450057	(450557)	63257+64257+68157+63657		NT	SWR	ANG	SWR
450058	(450558)	63258+64258+68158+63658		NT	SWR	ANG	SWR
450059	(450559)	63259+64259+68159+63659		NT	SWO	ANG	SWR
450060	(450560)	63260+64260+68160+63660		NT	SWO	ANG	SWR
450061	(450561)	63261+64261+68161+63661		NT	SWR	ANG	SWR
450062	(450562)	63262+64262+68162+63662		NT	SWO	ANG	SWR
450063	(450563)	63263+64263+68163+63663		NT	SWR	ANG	SWR
450064	(450564)	63264+64264+68164+63664		NT	SWO	ANG	SWR
450065	(450565)	63265+64265+68165+63665		NT	SWO	ANG	SWR
450066	(450566)	63266+64266+68166+63666		NT	SWR	ANG	SWR
450067	(450567)	63267+64267+68167+63667		NT	SPL	ANG	SWR
450068	(450568)	63268+64268+68168+63668		NT	SWR	ANG	SWR
450069	(450569)	63269+64269+68169+63669		NT	SWO	ANG	SWR
450070	(450570)	63270+64270+68170+63670		NT	SWO	ANG	SWR
450071		63271+64271+68171+63671		NT	SWO	ANG	SWR
450072		63272+64272+68172+63672		NT	SWR	ANG	SWR
450073		63273+64273+68173+63673		NT	SWR	ANG	SWR
450074		63274+64274+68174+63674		NT	SWO	ANG	SWR
450075		63275+64275+68175+63675		NT	SWR	ANG	SWR
450076		63276+64276+68176+63676		NT	SWO	ANG	SWR
450077		63277+64277+68177+63677		NT	SWR	ANG	SWR
450078		63278+64278+68178+63678		NT	SWO	ANG	SWR
450079		63279+64279+68179+63679		NT	SWO	ANG	SWR
450080		63280+64280+68180+63680		NT	SWO	ANG	SWR
450081		63281+64281+68181+63681		NT	SWR	ANG	SWR
450082		63282+64282+68182+63682		NT	SWO	ANG	SWR
450083		63283+64283+68183+63683		NT	SWO	ANG	SWR
450084		63284+64284+68184+63684		NT	SWO	ANG	SWR
450085		63285+64285+68185+63685		NT	SWO	ANG	SWR
450086		63286+64286+68186+63686		NT	SWO	ANG	SWR
450087		63287+64287+68187+63687		NT	SWO	ANG	SWR
450088		63288+64288+68188+63688		NT	SWR	ANG	SWR
450089		63289+64289+68189+63689		NT	SWR	ANG	SWR
450090		63290+64290+68190+63690		NT	SWO	ANG	SWR
450091		63291+64291+68191+63691		NT	SWO	ANG	SWR
450092		63292+64292+68192+63692		NT	SWO	ANG	SWR
450093		63293+64293+68193+63693		NT	SWO	ANG	SWR

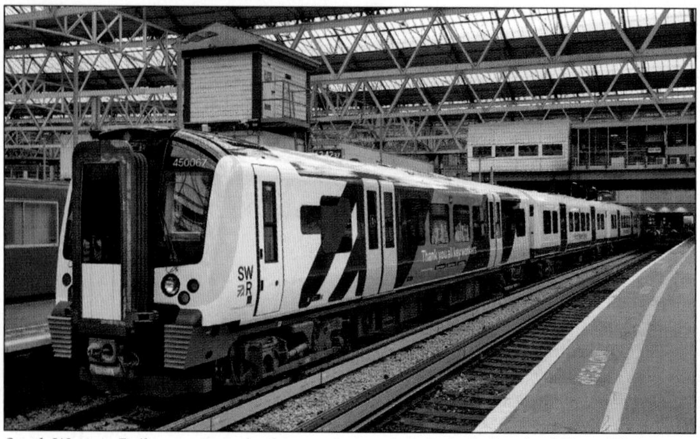

South Western Railway outer-suburban services are largely in the hands of Class 450 four-car 'Desiro' sets, the fleet carries a mix of older Stagecoach swirl and modern SWR grey and blue colours. Set No. 450067 sports a 'Thank You Key Workers' livery on its driving cars, as seen at Waterloo. **Antony Christie**

450094	63294+64294+68194+63694		NT	SWO	ANG	SWR
450095	63295+64295+68195+63695		NT	SWO	ANG	SWR
450096	63296+64296+68196+63696		NT	SWR	ANG	SWR
450097	63297+64297+68197+63697		NT	SWO	ANG	SWR
450098	63298+64298+68198+63698		NT	SWO	ANG	SWR
450099	63299+64299+68199+63699		NT	SWO	ANG	SWR
450100	63300+64300+68200+63700		NT	SWO	ANG	SWR
450101	63701+66851+66801+63751		NT	SWR	ANG	SWR
450102	63702+66852+66802+63752		NT	SWO	ANG	SWR
450103	63703+66853+66803+63753		NT	SWR	ANG	SWR
450104	63704+66854+66804+63754		NT	SWO	ANG	SWR
450105	63705+66855+66805+63755		NT	SWO	ANG	SWR
450106	63706+66856+66806+63756		NT	SWR	ANG	SWR
450107	63707+66857+66807+63757		NT	SWR	ANG	SWR
450108	63708+66858+66808+63758		NT	SWR	ANG	SWR
450109	63709+66859+66809+63759		NT	SWO	ANG	SWR
450110	63710+66860+66810+63750		NT	SWO	ANG	SWR
450111	63901+66921+66901+63921		NT	SWO	ANG	SWR
450112	63902+66922+66902+63922		NT	SWO	ANG	SWR
450113	63903+66923+66903+63923		NT	SWR	ANG	SWR
450114	63904+66924+66904+63924	*Fairbridge Investing in the Future*	NT	SWO	ANG	SWR
450115	63905+66925+66905+63925		NT	SWO	ANG	SWR
450116	63906+66926+66906+63926		NT	SWO	ANG	SWR
450117	63907+66927+66907+63927		NT	SWR	ANG	SWR
450118	63908+66928+66908+63928		NT	SWO	ANG	SWR
450119	63909+66929+66909+63929		NT	SWR	ANG	SWR
450120	63910+66930+66910+63930		NT	SWO	ANG	SWR
450121	63911+66931+66911+63931		NT	SWO	ANG	SWR
450122	63912+66932+66912+63932		NT	SWR	ANG	SWR
450123	63913+66933+66913+63933		NT	SWR	ANG	SWR
450124	63914+66934+66914+63934		NT	SWO	ANG	SWR
450125	63915+66935+66915+63935		NT	SWO	ANG	SWR
450126	63916+66936+66916+63936		NT	SWR	ANG	SWR
450127	63917+66937+66917+63937	*Dave Gunson*	NT	SWR	ANG	SWR

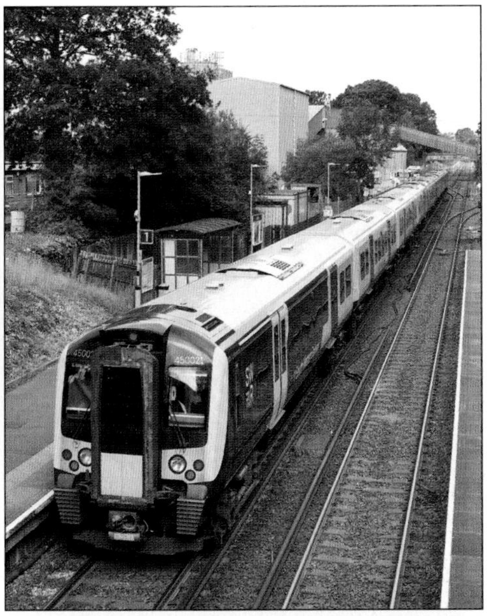

Set No. 450021 shows the standard South Western Railway grey and blue colours at Botley on the Portsmouth-Eastleigh route. After refurbishment these sets now sport a small first class seating area behind the driving cab in each driving car. **CJM**

Class 455
BREL 4-car EMU Suburban

Built: 1982-1985
Vehicle length: Driving 65ft 0½in (19.83m)
Intermediate: 65ft 4½in (19.92m)
Height: 12ft 1½in (3.74m)
Width: 9ft 3¼in (2.82m)
Power: 750V dc third rail
Horsepower: 1,000hp (746kW)
Transmission: Electric

455/7 Formation: DTS+MS+TS+DTS

(45)5701	77727+62783+71545+77728	WD	SWS	PTR	SWR
(45)5702	77729+62784+71547+77730	WD	SWS	PTR	SWR
(45)5703	77731+62785+71540+77732	WD	SWS	PTR	SWR
(45)5704	77733+62786+71548+77734	LM	SWS	PTR	(S)
(45)5705	77735+62787+71565+77736	WD	SWS	PTR	SWR
(45)5706	77737+62788+71534+77738	WD	SWS	PTR	SWR
(45)5707	77739+62789+71536+77740	WD	SWS	PTR	SWR
(45)5708	77741+62790+71560+77742	WD	SWS	PTR	(S)
(45)5709	77743+62791+71532+77744	WD	SWS	PTR	SWR
(45)5710	77745+62792+71566+77746	WD	SWS	PTR	SWR
(45)5711	77747+62793+71542+77748	WD	SWS	PTR	SWR
(45)5712	77749+62794+71546+77750	WD	SWS	PTR	SWR
(45)5713	77751+62795+71567+77752	WD	SWS	PTR	SWR
(45)5714	77753+62796+71539+77754	WD	SWS	PTR	SWR
(45)5715	77755+62797+71535+77756	WD	SWS	PTR	SWR
(45)5716	77757+62798+71564+77758	WD	SWS	PTR	SWR
(45)5717	77759+62799+71528+77760	WD	SWS	PTR	SWR
(45)5718	77761+62800+71557+77762	WD	SWS	PTR	SWR
(45)5719	77763+62801+71558+77764	WD	SWS	PTR	SWR
(45)5720	77765+62802+71568+77766	WD	SWS	PTR	SWR
(45)5721	77767+62803+71553+77768	WD	SWS	PTR	SWR
(45)5722	77769+62804+71533+77770	WD	SWS	PTR	SWR
(45)5723	77771+62805+71526+77772	WD	SWS	PTR	SWR

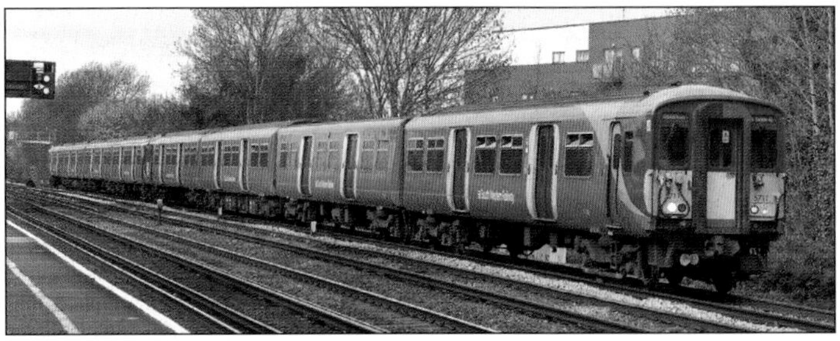

Soon to be displaced by Class 701 stock, the Class 455/7s are recognisable in having one vehicle (the TS) of a different body profile, that of a Class 508. Set No. (45)5711 is captured approaching Raynes Park, the ex-508 coach is the second vehicle. **CJM**

(45)5724	77773+62806+71561+77774	WD	SWS	PTR	SWR
(45)5725	77775+62807+71541+77776	WD	SWS	PTR	SWR
(45)5726	77777+62608+71556+77778	LM	SWS	PTR	(S)
(45)5727	77779+62809+71562+77780	WD	SWS	PTR	SWR
(45)5728	77781+62810+71527+77782	WD	SWS	PTR	SWR
(45)5729	77783+62811+71550+77784	WD	SWS	PTR	SWR
(45)5730	77785+62812+71551+77786	WD	SWS	PTR	SWR
(45)5731	77787+62813+71555+77788	WD	SWS	PTR	SWR
(45)5732	77789+62814+71552+77790	WD	SWS	PTR	SWR
(45)5733	77791+62815+71549+77792	WD	SWS	PTR	SWR
(45)5734	77793+62816+71531+77794	WD	SWS	PTR	SWR
(45)5735	77795+62817+71563+77796	WD	SWS	PTR	SWR
(45)5736	77797+62818+71554+77798	LM	SWS	PTR	(S)
(45)5737	77799+62819+71544+77800	WD	SWS	PTR	SWR
(45)5738	77801+62820+71529+77802	WD	SWS	PTR	SWR
(45)5739	77803+62821+71537+77804	WD	SWS	PTR	SWR
(45)5741	77807+62823+71559+77808	WD	SWS	PTR	SWR
(45)5742	77809+62824+71543+77810	WD	SWS	PTR	SWR
(45)5750§	77811+62825+71538+77812	WD	SWS	PTR	SWR

§ Originally numbered (45)5743

455/8 Formation: DTS+MS+TS+DTS

455801	77627+62709+71657+77580	SL	SOU	EVL	(S)
455802	77581+62710+71664+77582	SL	SOU	EVL	(S)
455803	77583+62711+71639+77584	SL	SOU	EVL	(S)
455804	77585+62712+71640+77586	SL	SOU	EVL	(S)
455805	77587+62713+71641+77588	SL	SOU	EVL	(S)
455806	77589+62714+71642+77590	SL	SOU	EVL	(S)
455807	77591+62715+71643+77592	SL	SOU	EVL	(S)
455808	77637+62716+71644+77594	SL	SOU	EVL	(S)
455812	77595+62720+71645+77626	SL	SOU	EVL	(S)
455813	77603+62721+71649+77604	SL	SOU	EVL	(S)
455814	77605+62722+71650+77606	SL	SOU	EVL	(S)
455815	77607+62723+71651+77608	SL	SOU	EVL	(S)
455817	77611+62725+71653+77612	SL	SOU	EVL	(S)
455819	77615+62727+71637+77616	SL	SOU	EVL	(S)
455820	77617+62728+71656+77618	SL	SOU	EVL	(S)
455822	77621+62730+71658+77622	SL	SOU	EVL	(S)
455823	77601+62731+71659+77596	SL	SOU	EVL	(S)
455826	77630+62734+71662+77629	SL	SOU	EVL	(S)
455829	77635+62737+71665+77636	SL	SOU	EVL	(S)
455830	77625+62743+71666+77638	SL	SOU	EVL	(S)
455833	77643+62741+71669+77644	SL	SOU	EVL	(S)
455834	77645+62742+71670+77646	SL	SOU	EVL	(S)
455836	77649+62744+71672+77650	SL	SOU	EVL	(S)
455837	77651+62745+71673+77652	SL	SOU	EVL	(S)
455840	77657+62748+71676+77658	SL	SOU	EVL	(S)
455842	77661+62750+71678+77662	SL	SOU	EVL	(S)
455843	77663+62751+71679+77664	SL	SOU	EVL	(S)
455844	77665+62752+71680+77666	SL	SOU	EVL	(S)
(45)5847	77671+62755+71683+77672	LM	SWS	PTR	(S)
(45)5848	77673+62756+71684+77674	WD	SWS	PTR	SWR
(45)5849	77675+62757+71685+77676	WD	SWS	PTR	SWR
(45)5850	77677+62758+71686+77678	WD	SWS	PTR	SWR
(45)5851	77679+62759+71687+77680	WD	SWS	PTR	SWR
(45)5852	77681+62760+71688+77682	WD	SWS	PTR	SWR
(45)5853	77683+62761+71689+77684	WD	SWS	PTR	SWR
(45)5854	77685+62762+71690+77686	WD	SWS	PTR	SWR
(45)5855	77687+62763+71691+77688	WD	SWS	PTR	(S)
(45)5856	77689+62764+71692+77690	WD	SWS	PTR	SWR
(45)5857	77691+62765+71693+77692	WD	SWS	PTR	SWR
(45)5858	77693+62766+71694+77694	WD	SWS	PTR	SWR
(45)5859	77695+62767+71695+77696	WD	SWS	PTR	SWR

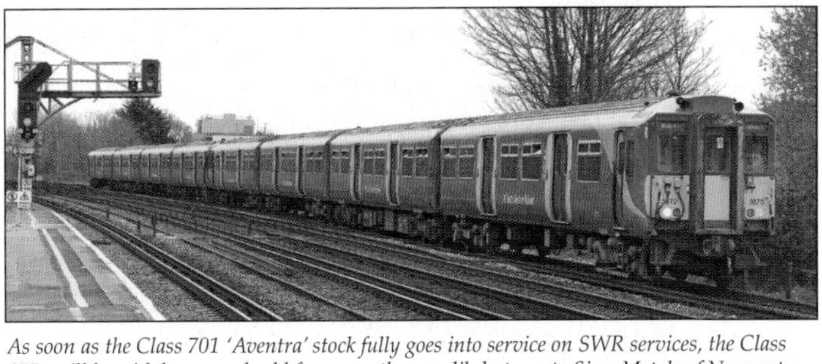

As soon as the Class 701 'Aventra' stock fully goes into service on SWR services, the Class 455s will be withdrawn and sold for scrap, they are likely to go to Sims Metals of Newport, Wales, where the first of the GTR sets were dealt with in May 2022. On 8 April 2021, set No. 455870 with No. 455853 approach Raynes Park, with the 10.57 Waterloo Main to Waterloo Windsor service. **CJM**

(45)5860	77697+62768+71696+77698	WD	SWS	PTR	SWR
(45)5861	77699+62769+71697+77700	WD	SWS	PTR	SWR
(45)5862	77701+62770+71698+77702	WD	SWS	PTR	SWR
(45)5863	77703+62771+71699+77704	WD	SWS	PTR	SWR
(45)5864	77705+62772+71700+77706	WD	SWS	PTR	SWR
(45)5865	77707+62773+71701+77708	WD	SWS	PTR	SWR
(45)5866	77709+62774+71702+77710	WD	SWS	PTR	SWR
(45)5867	77711+62775+71703+77712	WD	SWS	PTR	SWR
(45)5868	77713+62776+71704+77714	WD	SWS	PTR	SWR
(45)5869	77715+62777+71705+77716	WD	SWS	PTR	SWR
(45)5870	77717+62778+71706+77718	WD	SWS	PTR	SWR
(45)5871	77719+62779+71707+77720	WD	SWS	PTR	SWR
(45)5872	77721+62780+71708+77722	WD	SWS	PTR	SWR
(45)5873	77723+62781+71709+77724	WD	SWS	PTR	SWR
(45)5874	77725+62782+71710+77726	WD	SWS	PTR	SWR

455/9	Formation: DTS+MS+TS+DTS				
(45)5901	77813+62826+71714+77814	WD	SWS	PTR	SWR
(45)5902	77815+62827+71715+77816	WD	SWS	PTR	SWR
(45)5903	77817+62828+71716+77818	WD	SWS	PTR	SWR
(45)5904	77819+62829+71717+77820	WD	SWS	PTR	SWR
(45)5905	77821+62830+71725+77822	WD	SWS	PTR	(S)
(45)5906	77823+62831+71719+77824	WD	SWS	PTR	SWR
(45)5907	77825+62832+71720+77826	WD	SWS	PTR	(S)
(45)5908	77827+62833+71721+77828	WD	SWS	PTR	SWR
(45)5909	77829+62834+71722+77830	WD	SWS	PTR	SWR
(45)5910	77831+62835+71723+77832	WD	SWS	PTR	(S)
(45)5911	77833+62836+71724+77834	WD	SWS	PTR	SWR
(45)5912	77835+62837+67400+77836	WD	SWS	PTR	SWR
(45)5913	77837+67301+71726+77838	WD	SWS	PTR	SWR
(45)5914	77839+62839+71727+77840	WD	SWS	PTR	SWR
(45)5915	77841+62840+71728+77842	WD	SWS	PTR	SWR
(45)5916	77843+62841+71729+77844	WD	SWS	PTR	SWR
(45)5917	77845+62842+71730+77846	WD	SWS	PTR	SWR
(45)5918	77847+62843+71732+77848	WD	SWS	PTR	SWR
(45)5919	77849+62844+71718+77850	WD	SWS	PTR	SWR
(45)5920	77851+62845+71733+77852	WD	SWS	PTR	SWR

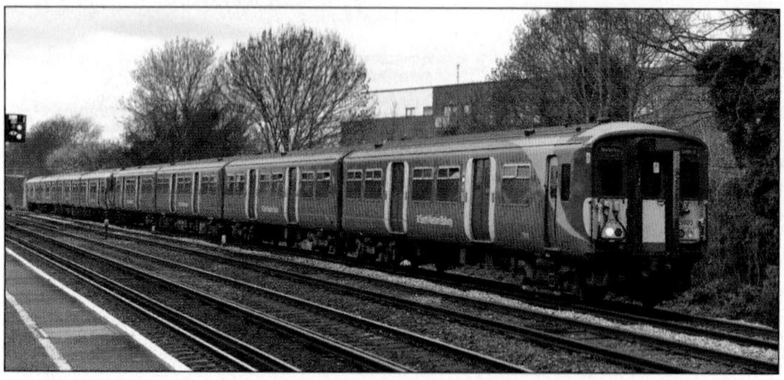

Like all Class 455 sub-classes, a number of 455/9s were stored in late 2021, early 2022 in readiness for withdrawal after Class 701s are introduced. Class 455/9 (45)5903 is captured at Raynes Park. These sets are identifiable by larger roof ventilators. **CJM**

Class 456
BREL 2-car EMU Suburban

Built: 1990-1991
Vehicle length: Driving 65ft 0½in (19.83m)
Height: 12ft 4½in (3.77m)
Width: 9ft 3¼in (2.82m)
Power: 750V dc third rail
Horsepower: 500hp (370kW)
Transmission: Electric

	Formation: DMS+DTS				
456002	64736+78251	LM	SWS	PTR	OLS
456003	64737+78252	LM	SWS	PTR	OLS
456004	64738+78253	LM	SWS	PTR	OLS
456006	64740+78255	LM	SWS	PTR	OLS
456007	64741+78256	LM	SWS	PTR	OLS
456008	64742+78257	LM	SWS	PTR	OLS
456009	64743+78258	LM	SWS	PTR	OLS
456010	64744+78259	LM	SWS	PTR	OLS
456011	64745+78260	LM	SWS	PTR	OLS
456012	64746+78261	LM	SWS	PTR	OLS
456013	64747+78262	LM	SWS	PTR	OLS
456014	64748+78263	LM	SWS	PTR	OLS
456015	64749+78264	LM	SWS	PTR	OLS
456016	64750+78265	LM	SWS	PTR	OLS
456018	64752+78267	LM	SWS	PTR	OLS
456019	64753+78268	LM	SWS	PTR	OLS
456020	64754+78269	LM	SWS	PTR	OLS
456021	64755+78270	LM	SWS	PTR	OLS
456022	64756+78271	LM	SWS	PTR	OLS
456023	64757+78272	LM	SWS	PTR	OLS
456024	64758+78273	LM	SWS	PTR	OLS

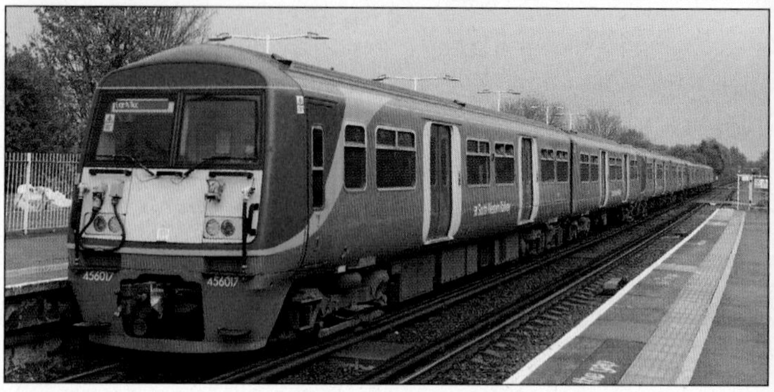

All 24 Class 456 units were stood down by operator South Western Railway in January 2022 as surplus to requirements in advance of Class 701s being introduced and due to a much reduced timetable operated. Sets have been moved to Porterbrook's Long Marston site for store. Set No. 456017 departs from Earlsfield in April 2021. **CJM**

Class 458
Alstom 5-car EMU Outer Suburban 'Juniper'

Built: 1990-1991
Vehicle length: Driving 69ft 6in (21.16m)
Intermediate 65ft 4in (19.94m)
Height: 12ft 3in (3.77m)
Width: 9ft 2in (2.80m)
Power: 750V dc third rail
Horsepower: 2,172hp (1,620kW)
Transmission: Electric

		Formation: DMS+TSO*+TSO+MSO+DMS (* ex Class 460)				
458501	(458001)	67601+74431+74001+74101+67701	WD	SWO	PTR	SWR
458502	(458002)	67602+74421+74002+74102+67702	WD	SWO	PTR	SWR
458503	(458003)	67603+74441+74003+74103+67703	WD	SWO	PTR	SWR
458504	(458004)	67604+74451+74004+74104+67704	WD	SWO	PTR	(S)
458505	(458005)	67605+74425+74005+74105+67705	WD	SWO	PTR	(S)
458506	(458006)	67606+74436+74006+74106+67706	WD	SWO	PTR	(S)
458507	(458007)	67607+74428+74007+74107+67707	LM	SWO	PTR	(S)
458508	(458008)	67608+74433+74008+74108+67708	WD	SWO	PTR	SWR
458509	(458009)	67609+74452+74009+74109+67709	WD	SWO	PTR	SWR
458510	(458010)	67610+74405+74010+74110+67710	WD	SWO	PTR	SWR
458511	(458011)	67611+74435+74011+74111+67711	WD	SWO	PTR	SWR
458512	(458012)	67612+74427+74012+74112+67712	WD	SWO	PTR	SWR
458513	(458013)	67613+74437+74013+74113+67713	WD	SWO	PTR	SWR
458514	(458014)	67614+74407+74014+74114+67714	WD	SWO	PTR	SWR
458515	(458015)	67615+74404+74015+74115+67715	WD	SWO	PTR	SWR
458516	(458016)	67616+74406+74016+74116+67716	WD	SWO	PTR	SWR
458517	(458017)	67617+74426+74017+74117+67717	LM	SWO	PTR	(S)
458518	(458018)	67618+74432+74018+74118+67718	WD	SWO	PTR	SWR
458519	(458019)	67619+74403+74019+74119+67719	WD	SWO	PTR	SWR
458520	(458020)	67620+74401+74020+74120+67720	WD	SWO	PTR	SWR
458521	(458021)	67621+74438+74021+74121+67721	WD	SWO	PTR	SWR

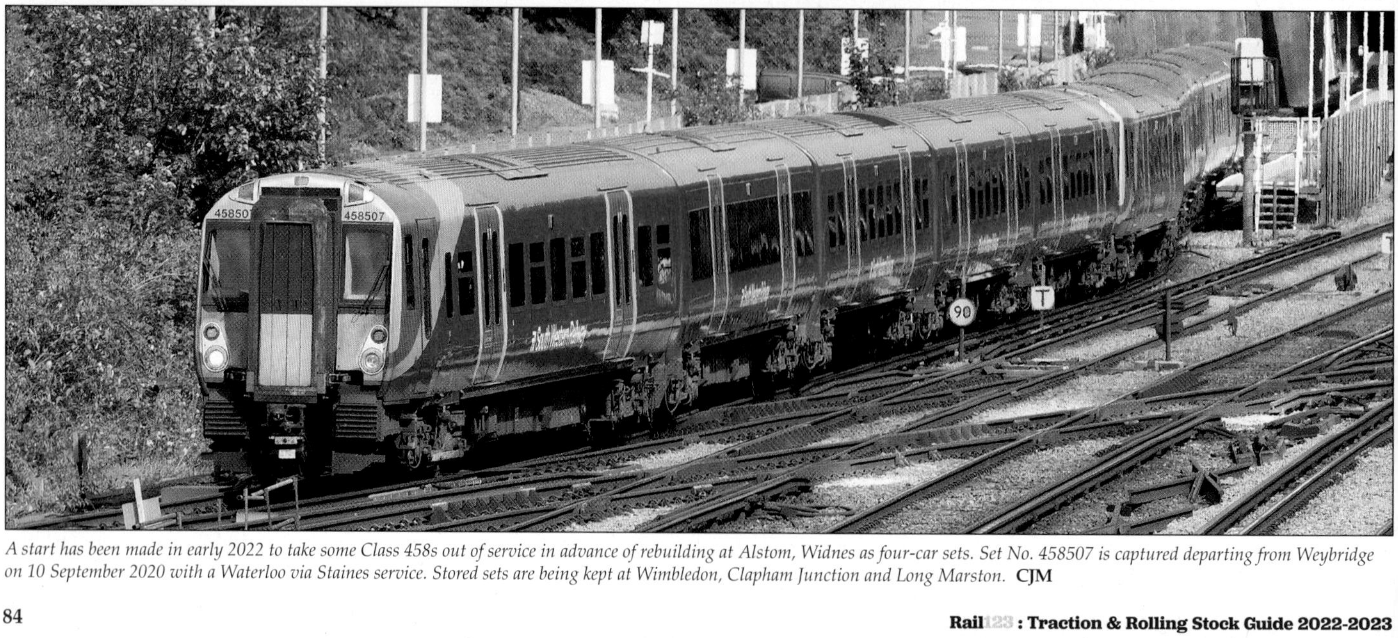

A start has been made in early 2022 to take some Class 458s out of service in advance of rebuilding at Alstom, Widnes as four-car sets. Set No. 458507 is captured departing from Weybridge on 10 September 2020 with a Waterloo via Staines service. Stored sets are being kept at Wimbledon, Clapham Junction and Long Marston. **CJM**

458522	(458022)	67622+74424+74022+74122+67722	WD	SWO	PTR	SWR
458523	(458023)	67623+74434+74023+74123+67723	WD	SWO	PTR	SWR
458524	(458024)	67624+74402+74024+74124+67724	WD	SWO	PTR	SWR
458525	(458025)	67625+74422+74025+74125+67725	WD	SWO	PTR	SWR
458526	(458026)	67626+74442+74026+74126+67726	WD	SWO	PTR	SWR
458527	(458027)	67627+74412+74027+74127+67727	WD	SWO	PTR	SWR
458528	(458028)	67628+74408+74028+74128+67728	WD	SWO	PTR	SWR
458529	(458029)	67629+74423+74029+74129+67729	WD	SWO	PTR	(S)
458530	(458030)	67630+74411+74030+74130+67730	WD	SWO	PTR	SWR
458531		67913+74418+74446+74458+67912	WD	SWO	PTR	SWR
458532		67904+74417+74447+74457+67905	WD	SWO	PTR	SWR
458533		67917+74413+74443+74453+67916	WD	SWO	PTR	SWR
458534		67914+74414+74444+74454+67918	WD	SWO	PTR	SWR
458535		67915+74415+74445+74455+67911	WD	SWO	PTR	(S)
458536		67906+74416+74448+74456+67902	WD	SWO	PTR	SWR

28 sets (458501-458528) to be reformed as four-car units, (less the ex-Class 460 TSO) overhauled for 100mph main line service and allocated to Bournemouth. Sets 458529-458536 will be withdrawn for disposal.

Class 465
ABB/Met Cam 4-car EMU Suburban 'Networker'

Built: 1991-1993
Vehicle length: Driving 68ft 6½in (20.89m)
Intermediate 65ft 9¾in (20.06m)
Height: 12ft 4½in (3.77m)
Width: 9ft 3in (2.82m)
Power: 750V dc third rail
Horsepower: 3,004hp (2,240kW)
Transmission: Electric

465/0 Formation: DMS+TSO+TSOL+DMS

465001	64759+72028+72029+64809	SG	SET	EVL	SET
465002	64760+72030+72031+64810	SG	SET	EVL	SET
465003	64761+72032+72033+64811	SG	SET	EVL	SET
465004	64762+72034+72035+64812	SG	SET	EVL	SET
465005	64763+72036+72037+64813	SG	SET	EVL	SET
465006	64764+72038+72039+64814	SG	SET	EVL	SET
465007	64765+72040+72041+64815	SG	SET	EVL	SET
465008	64766+72042+72043+64816	SG	SET	EVL	SET
465009	64767+72044+72045+64817	SG	SET	EVL	SET
465010	64768+72046+72047+64818	SG	SET	EVL	SET
465011	64769+72048+72049+64819	SG	SET	EVL	SET
465012	64770+72050+72051+64820	SG	SET	EVL	SET
465013	64771+72052+72053+64821	SG	SET	EVL	SET
465014	64772+72054+72055+64822	SG	SET	EVL	SET
465015	64773+72056+72057+64823	SG	SET	EVL	SET
465016	64774+72058+72059+64824	SG	SET	EVL	SET
465017	64775+72060+72061+64825	SG	SET	EVL	SET
465018	64776+72062+72063+64826	SG	SET	EVL	SET
465019	64777+72064+72065+64827	SG	SET	EVL	SET
465020	64778+72066+72067+64828	SG	SET	EVL	SET
465021	64779+72068+72069+64829	SG	SET	EVL	SET
465022	64780+72070+72071+64830	SG	SET	EVL	SET
465023	64781+72072+72073+64831	SG	SET	EVL	SET
465024	64782+72074+72075+64832	SG	SET	EVL	SET
465025	64783+72076+72077+64833	SG	SET	EVL	SET
465026	64784+72078+72079+64834	SG	SET	EVL	SET
465027	64785+72080+72081+64835	SG	SET	EVL	SET
465028	64786+72082+72083+64836	SG	SET	EVL	SET
465029	64787+72084+72085+64837	SG	SET	EVL	SET
465030	64788+72086+72087+64838	SG	SET	EVL	SET
465031	64789+72088+72089+64839	SG	SET	EVL	SET
465032	64790+72090+72091+64840	SG	SET	EVL	SET
465033	64791+72092+72093+64841	SG	SET	EVL	SET
465034	64792+72094+72095+64842	SG	SET	EVL	SET
465035	64793+72096+72097+64843	SG	SET	EVL	SET
465036	64794+72098+72099+64844	SG	SET	EVL	SET
465037	64795+72100+72101+64845	SG	SET	EVL	SET
465038	64796+72102+72103+64846	SG	SET	EVL	SET
465039	64797+72104+72105+64847	SG	SET	EVL	SET
465040	64798+72106+72107+64848	SG	SET	EVL	SET
465041	64799+72108+72109+64849	SG	SET	EVL	SET
465042	64800+72110+72111+64850	SG	SET	EVL	SET
465043	64801+72112+72113+64851	SG	SET	EVL	SET
465044	64802+72114+72115+64852	SG	SET	EVL	SET
465045	64803+72116+72117+64853	SG	SET	EVL	SET
465046	64804+72118+72119+64854	SG	SET	EVL	SET
465047	64805+72120+72121+64855	SG	SET	EVL	SET
465048	64806+72122+72123+64856	SG	SET	EVL	SET
465049	64807+72124+72125+64857	SG	SET	EVL	SET
465050	64808+72126+72127+64858	SG	SET	EVL	SET

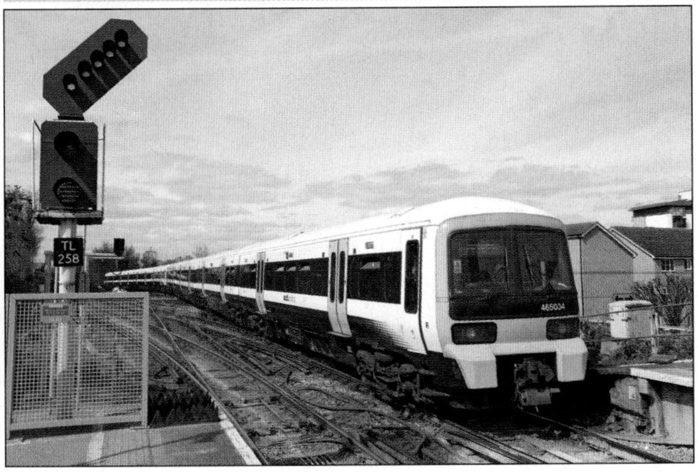

Now over 30 years old, the 'Networker' fleet introduced by Network SouthEast will soon be up for renewal. Class 465/0 No. 465034 built by ABB is seen approaching Lewisham. **CJM**

465/1 Formation: DMS+TSO+TSOL+DMS

465151	65800+72900+72901+65847	SG	SET	EVL	SET
465152	65801+72902+72903+65848	SG	SET	EVL	SET
465153	65802+72904+72905+65849	SG	SET	EVL	SET
465154	65803+72906+72907+65850	SG	SET	EVL	SET
465155	65804+72908+72909+65851	SG	SET	EVL	SET
465156	65805+72910+72911+65852	SG	SET	EVL	SET
465157	65806+72912+72913+65853	SG	SET	EVL	SET
465158	65807+72914+72915+65854	SG	SET	EVL	SET
465159	65808+72916+72917+65855	SG	SET	EVL	SET
465160	65809+72918+72919+65856	SG	SET	EVL	SET
465161	65810+72920+72921+65857	SG	SET	EVL	SET
465162	65811+72922+72923+65858	SG	SET	EVL	SET
465163	65812+72924+72925+65859	SG	SET	EVL	SET
465164	65813+72926+72927+65860	SG	SET	EVL	SET
465165	65814+72928+72929+65861	SG	SET	EVL	SET
465166	65815+72930+72931+65862	SG	SET	EVL	SET
465167	65816+72932+72933+65863	SG	SET	EVL	SET
465168	65817+72934+72935+65864	SG	SET	EVL	SET
465169	65818+72936+72937+65865	SG	SET	EVL	SET
465170	65819+72938+72939+65866	SG	SET	EVL	SET
465171	65820+72940+72941+65867	SG	SET	EVL	SET
465172	65821+72942+72943+65868	SG	SET	EVL	SET
465173	65822+72944+72945+65869	SG	SET	EVL	SET
465174	65823+72946+72947+65870	SG	SET	EVL	SET
465175	65824+72948+72949+65871	SG	SET	EVL	SET
465176	65825+72950+72951+65872	SG	SET	EVL	SET
465177	65826+72952+72953+65873	SG	SET	EVL	SET
465178	65827+72954+72955+65874	SG	SET	EVL	SET
465179	65828+72956+72957+65875	SG	SET	EVL	SET
465180	65829+72958+72959+65876	SG	SET	EVL	SET
465181	65830+72960+72961+65877	SG	SET	EVL	SET
465182	65831+72962+72963+65878	SG	SET	EVL	SET
465183	65832+72964+72965+65879	SG	SET	EVL	SET
465184	65833+72966+72967+65880	SG	SET	EVL	SET
465185	65834+72968+72969+65881	SG	SET	EVL	SET
465186	65835+72970+72971+65882	SG	SET	EVL	SET
465187	65836+72972+72973+65883	SG	SET	EVL	SET
465188	65837+72974+72975+65884	SG	SET	EVL	SET
465189	65838+72976+72977+65885	SG	SET	EVL	SET
465190	65839+72978+72979+65886	SG	SET	EVL	SET
465191	65840+72980+72981+65887	SG	SET	EVL	SET
465192	65841+72982+72983+65888	SG	SET	EVL	SET
465193	65842+72984+72985+65889	SG	SET	EVL	SET
465194	65843+72986+72987+65890	SG	SET	EVL	SET
465195	65844+72988+72989+65891	SG	SET	EVL	SET
465196	65845+72990+72991+65892	SG	SET	EVL	SET
465197	65846+72992+72993+65893	SG	SET	EVL	SET

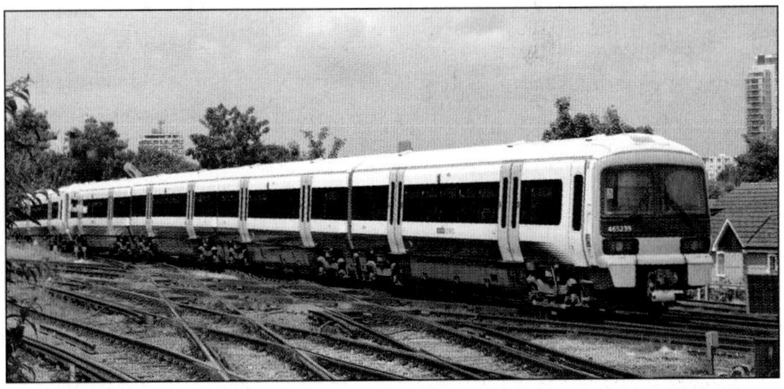

The Metro-Cammell built Class 465/2s were very similar to the ABB fleet, but with detail interior differences. Today they retain their full between bogie skirts on all vehicles. Set No. 465239 is recorded at Lewisham in June 2021. **CJM**

465/2 Formation: DMC+TSO+TSOL+DMC

465235	65734+72787+72788+65784	EL	SET	ANG	OLS
465236	65735+72789+72790+65785	EL	SET	ANG	OLS
465237	65736+72791+72792+65786	WS	SET	ANG	OLS
465238	65737+72793+72794+65787	EL	SET	ANG	OLS
465239	65738+72795+72796+65788	EL	SET	ANG	OLS
465240	65739+72797+72798+65789	EL	SET	ANG	OLS
465241	65740+72799+72800+65790	WS	SET	ANG	OLS
465242	65741+72801+72802+65791	WS	SET	ANG	OLS
465243	65742+72803+72804+65792	EL	SET	ANG	OLS
465244	65743+72805+72806+65793	EL	SET	ANG	OLS
465245	65744+72807+72808+65794	EL	SET	ANG	OLS
465246	65745+72809+72810+65795	EL	SET	ANG	OLS
465247	65746+72811+72812+65796	WS	SET	ANG	OLS
465248	65747+72813+72814+65797	EL	SET	ANG	OLS
465249	65748+72815+72816+65798	EL	SET	ANG	OLS
465250	65749+72817+72818+65799	EL	SET	ANG	OLS

465/9 Formation: DMC+TSO+TSOL+DMC

465901 (465201)	65700+72719+72720+65750	SG	SET	ANG	SET
465902 (465202)	65701+72721+72722+65751	SG	SET	ANG	SET
465903 (465203)	65702+72723+72724+65752	SG	SET	ANG	SET

465904 (465204)	65703+72725+72726+65753	SG	SET	ANG	SET
465905 (465205)	65704+72727+72728+65754	SG	SET	ANG	SET
465906 (465206)	65705+72729+72730+65755	SG	SET	ANG	SET
465907 (465207)	65706+72731+72732+65756	SG	SET	ANG	SET
465908 (465208)	65707+72733+72734+65757	SG	SET	ANG	SET
465909 (465209)	65708+72735+72736+65758	SG	SET	ANG	SET
465910 (465210)	65709+72737+72738+65759	SG	SET	ANG	SET
465911 (465211)	65710+72739+72740+65760	SG	SET	ANG	SET
465912 (465212)	65711+72741+72742+65761	SG	SET	ANG	SET
465913 (465213)	65712+72743+72744+65762	SG	SET	ANG	SET
465914 (465214)	65713+72745+72746+65763	SG	SET	ANG	SET
465915 (465215)	65714+72747+72748+65764	SG	SET	ANG	SET
465916 (465216)	65715+72749+72750+65765	SG	SET	ANG	SET
465917 (465217)	65716+72751+72752+65766	SG	SET	ANG	SET
465918 (465218)	65717+72753+72754+65767	SG	SET	ANG	SET
465919 (465219)	65718+72755+72756+65768	SG	SET	ANG	SET
465920 (465220)	65719+72757+72758+65769	SG	SET	ANG	SET
465921 (465221)	65720+72759+72760+65770	SG	SET	ANG	SET
465922 (465222)	65721+72761+72762+65771	SG	SET	ANG	SET
465923 (465223)	65722+72763+72764+65772	SG	SET	ANG	SET
465924 (465224)	65723+72765+72766+65773	SG	SET	ANG	SET
465925 (465225)	65724+72767+72768+65774	SG	SET	ANG	SET
465926 (465226)	65725+72769+72770+65775	SG	SET	ANG	SET
465927 (465227)	65726+72771+72772+65776	SG	SET	ANG	SET
465928 (465228)	65727+72773+72774+65777	SG	SET	ANG	SET
465929 (465229)	65728+72775+72776+65778	SG	SET	ANG	SET
465930 (465230)	65729+72777+72778+65779	SG	SET	ANG	SET
465931 (465231)	65730+72779+72780+65780	SG	SET	ANG	SET
465932 (465232)	65731+72781+72782+65781	SG	SET	ANG	SET
465933 (465233)	65732+72783+72784+65782	SG	SET	ANG	SET
465934 (465234)	65733+72785+72786+65783	SG	SET	ANG	SET

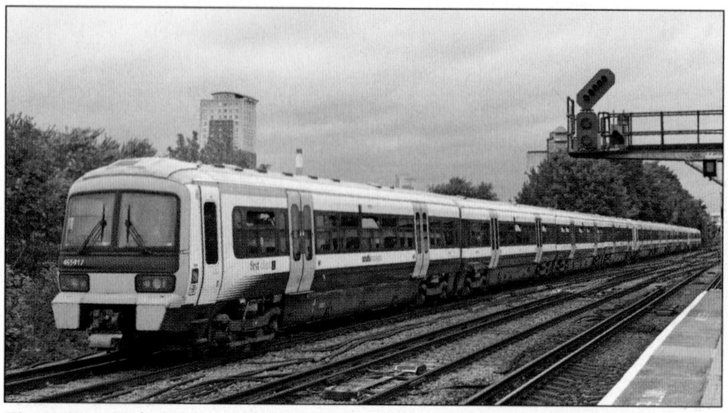

The 34 Class 465/9 sets were rebuilt from Class 465/2 by changing the interior design and installing first class seating in both driving cars just behind the cab end. Set No. 465917 is seen heading towards Charing Cross at New Cross in September 2021. **CJM**

Class 466
Met Cam 2-car EMU Suburban 'Networker'

Built: 1992-1994
Vehicle length: 68ft 6½in (20.89m)
Height: 12ft 4½in (3.77m)
Width: 9ft 3in (2.82m)
Power: 750V dc third rail
Horsepower: 1,502hp (1,120kW)
Transmission: Electric

Formation: DMS+DTS

466001	64860+78312	SG	SET	ANG	SET
466002	64861+78313	SG	SET	ANG	SET
466003	64862+78314	SG	SET	ANG	SET
466004	64863+78315	WS	SET	ANG	OLS
466005	64864+78316	SG	SET	ANG	SET
466006	64865+78317	SG	SET	ANG	SET
466007	64866+78318	SG	SET	ANG	SET
466008	64867+78319	SG	SET	ANG	SET
466009	64868+78320	SG	SET	ANG	SET
466010	64869+78321	WS	SET	ANG	OLS
466011	64870+78322	SG	SET	ANG	SET
466012	64871+78323	SG	SET	ANG	SET
466013	64872+78324	SG	SET	ANG	SET
466014	64873+78325	SG	SET	ANG	SET
466015	64874+78326	SG	SET	ANG	SET
466016	64875+78327	WS	SET	ANG	OLS
466017	64876+78328	SG	SET	ANG	SET
466018	64877+78329	SG	SET	ANG	SET
466019	64878+78330	SG	SET	ANG	SET
466020	64879+78331	SG	SET	ANG	SET
466021	64880+78332	SG	SET	ANG	SET
466022	64881+78333	SG	SET	ANG	SET
466023	64882+78334	SG	SET	ANG	SET
466024	64883+78335	WS	SET	ANG	OLS
466025	64884+78336	SG	SET	ANG	SET
466026	64885+78337	SG	SET	ANG	SET
466027	64886+78338	SG	SET	ANG	SET
466028	64887+78339	SG	SET	ANG	SET
466029	64888+78340	SG	SET	ANG	SET
466030	64889+78341	SG	SET	ANG	SET
466031	64890+78342	SG	SET	ANG	SET
466032	64891+78343	SG	SET	ANG	SET
466033	64892+78344	WS	SET	ANG	OLS
466034	64893+78345	SG	SET	ANG	SET
466035	64894+78346	SG	SET	ANG	SET
466036	64895+78347	SG	SET	ANG	SET
466037	64896+78348	SG	SET	ANG	SET
466038	64897+78349	SG	SET	ANG	SET
466039	64898+78350	SG	SET	ANG	SET
466040	64899+78351	SG	SET	ANG	SET
466041	64900+78352	SG	SET	ANG	SET
466042	64901+78353	SG	SET	ANG	SET
466043	64902+78354	WS	SET	ANG	OLS

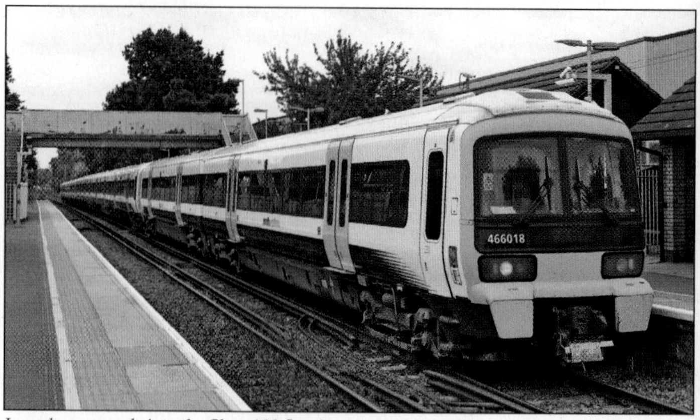

Inroads were made into the Class 466 fleet in autumn 2021 with several sets taken off lease and stored. These two-car sets are usually used to strengthen four or eight car trains to six or ten cars. No. 466018 is seen from its driving trailer vehicle at Lower Sydenham. **CJM**

Class 484
Vivarail 2-car EMU 'D-78'

Built: 2020-2021
Vehicle length: Driving - 60ft 3in (18.37m)
Intermediate - 59ft 5in (18.12m)
Height: 11ft 11in (3.62m)
Width: 9ft 4in (2.85m)
Power: 660V dc third rail
Horsepower: awaited
Transmission: Electric

Formation: DMS+DMS *(former LT identity in brackets)*

484001	131 (7086)+231 (7011)	RY	SWI	LOM	SWR
484002	132 (7068)+232 (7002)	RY	SWI	LOM	SWR
484003	133 (7051)+233 (7083)	RY	SWI	LOM	SWR
484004	134 (7074)+234 (7111)	RY	SWI	LOM	SWR
484005	135 (7124)+235 (7093)	RY	SWI	LOM	SWR

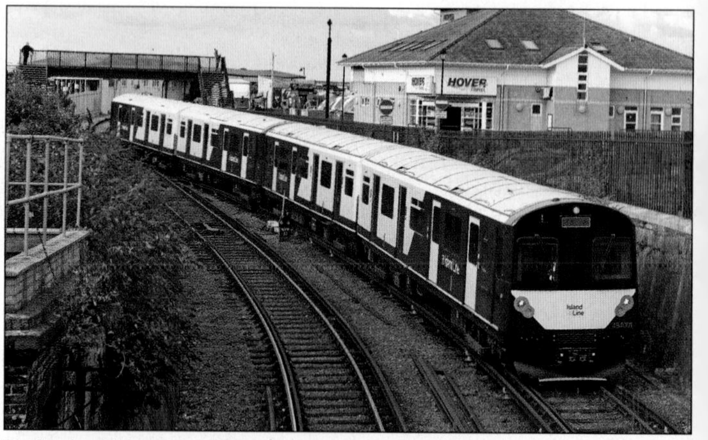

The first four of the Vivarail Class 484s for the Island Line were introduced in November 2021. Based at Ryde the sets operate between Ryde Pier Head and Shanklin. They are a huge change to the 1938 ex tube stock they replaced. Set No. 484001 departs from Ryde. **CJM**

Class 500 Series
Preserved Stock

Number	Set	Origin	Type	Location
Class 501				
61183	501183	BR/LM	DMBS	Stored at MoD Bicester
75186	501183	BR/LM	DTBS	Stored at MoD Bicester
Class 502				
28361	-	LMS	DMBS	Burscough
29896	-	LMS	DTC	Burscough
Class 503				
28690	-	LMS	DMBS	One:One Railway Museum, Margate
29282	-	LMS	DTS	One:One Railway Museum, Margate
29720	-	LMS	TCO	One:One Railway Museum, Margate
Class 504				
65451	-	BR/LM	DMBSO	East Lancashire Railway
77172	-	BR/LM	DTBSO	East Lancashire Railway
Class 505 (MSJ&AR)				
29666	-	LMS	TS	Midland Railway Centre
29670	-	LMS	TS	Midland Railway Centre

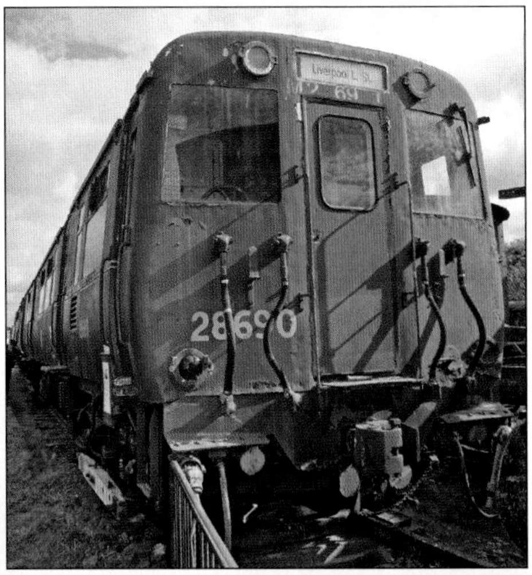

A three-car LMS-design Class 503 set is preserved, for many years it was kept in the open at the Coventry Electric Railway Museum, but is now preserved at the 1:1 Museum in Margate. Vehicle No. 28690, the DMBS vehicle is seen in its days stored at Coventry. **Adrian Paul**

Class 507
BREL 3-car EMU Suburban

Built: 1978-1980
Vehicle length: 64ft 11½in (19.80m)
Height: 11ft 6½in (3.58m)
Width: 9ft 3in (2.82m)
Power: 750V dc third rail
Horsepower: 880hp (657kW)
Transmission: Electric

Formation: DMS+TS+DMS

507001	64367+71342+64405		BD	MEY	ANG	MER
507002	64368+71343+64406		BD	ADV	ANG	MER
507003	64369+71344+64407		BD	MEY	ANG	MER
507004	64388+71345+64408	*Bob Paisley*	BD	MEY	ANG	MER
507005	64371+71346+64409		BD	MEY	ANG	MER
507007	64373+71348+64411		BD	MEY	ANG	MER
507008	64374+71349+64412	*Harold Wilson*	BD	MEY	ANG	MER
507009	64375+71350+64413	*Dixie Dean*	BD	MEY	ANG	MER
507010	64376+71351+64414		BD	MEY	ANG	MER
507011	64377+71352+64415		BD	MEY	ANG	MER
507012	64378+71353+64416		BD	MEY	ANG	MER
507013	64379+71354+64417		BD	MEY	ANG	MER
507014	64380+71355+64418		BD	MEY	ANG	MER
507015	64381+71356+64419		BD	MEY	ANG	MER
507016	64382+71357+64420	*Merseyrail - celebrating the first ten years 2003-2013*	BD	MEY	ANG	MER
507017	64383+71358+64421		BD	MEY	ANG	MER
507018	64384+71359+64422		BD	MEY	ANG	MER
507019	64385+71360+64423		BD	MEY	ANG	MER
507020	64386+71361+64424	*John Peel*	BD	MEY	ANG	MER
507021	64387+71362+64425	*Red Rum*	BD	MEY	ANG	MER
507023	64389+71364+64427	*Operating Inspector Stuart Mason*	BD	MEY	ANG	MER
507024	64390+71365+64428		BD	MEY	ANG	MER
507025	64391+71366+64429		BD	MEY	ANG	MER
507026	64392+71367+64430	*Councillor George Howard*	BD	MEY	ANG	MER
507027	64393+71368+64431		BD	MEY	ANG	MER
507028	64394+71369+64432		BD	MEY	ANG	MER
507029	64395+71370+64433		BD	MEY	ANG	MER
507030	64396+71371+64434		BD	MEY	ANG	MER
507031	64397+71372+64435		BD	MEY	ANG	MER
507032	64398+71373+64436		BD	MEY	ANG	MER
507033	64399+71374+64437	*Councillor Jack Spriggs*	BD	MEY	ANG	MER

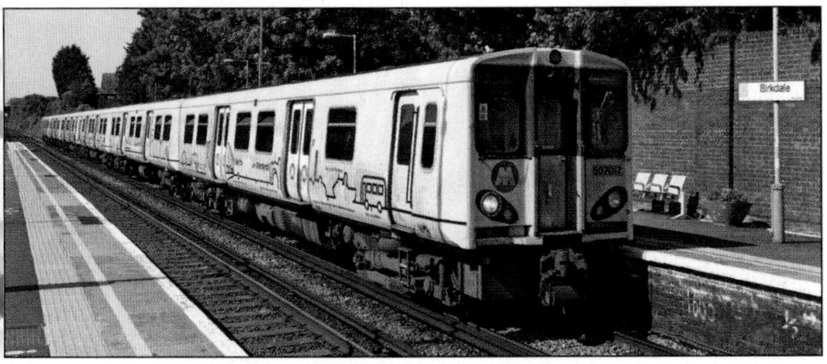

The days are numbered for the Class 507s, with the imminent introduction of Class 777 stock on the Merseyrail system. With its yellow side near, set No. 507017 is seen passing Birkdale en route to Southport on 2 June 2021. **CJM**

Class 508
BREL 3-car EMU Suburban

Built: 1978-1980
Vehicle length: 64ft 11½in (19.80m)
Height: 11ft 6½in (3.58m)
Width: 9ft 3in (2.82m)
Power: 750V dc third rail
Horsepower: 880hp (657kW)
Transmission: Electric

Formation: DMS+TS+DMS

508103	64651+71485+64694		BD	MEY	ANG	MER
508104	64652+71486+64964		BD	MEY	ANG	MER
508108	64656+71490+64699		BD	MEY	ANG	MER
508111	64659+71493+64702	*The Beatles*	BD	SPL	ANG	MER
508112	64660+71494+64703		BD	MEY	ANG	MER
508114	64662+71496+64705		BD	MEY	ANG	MER
508115	64663+71497+64708		BD	MEY	ANG	MER
508117	64665+71499+64908		BD	MEY	ANG	MER
508120	64668+71502+64711		BD	MEY§	ANG	MER
508122	64670+71504+64713	*William Roscoe*	BD	MEY	ANG	MER
508123	64671+71505+64714		BD	MEY§	ANG	MER
508124	64672+71506+64715		BD	MEY	ANG	MER
508125	64673+71507+64716		BD	MEY	ANG	MER
508126	64674+71508+64717		BD	MEY	ANG	MER
508127	64675+71509+64718		BD	MEY	ANG	MER
508128	64676+71510+64719		BD	MEY	ANG	MER
508130	64678+71512+64721		BD	MEY	ANG	MER
508131	64679+71513+64722		BD	MEY§	ANG	MER
508136	64684+71518+64727		BD	MEY	ANG	MER
508137	64685+71519+64728		BD	MEY	ANG	MER
508138	64686+71520+64729		BD	MEY	ANG	MER
508139	64687+71521+64730		BD	MEY	ANG	MER
508140	64688+71522+64731		BD	MEY§	ANG	MER
508141	64689+71523+64732		BD	MEY	ANG	MER
508143	64691+71525+64734		BD	MEY§	ANG	MER

§ Carries facemask

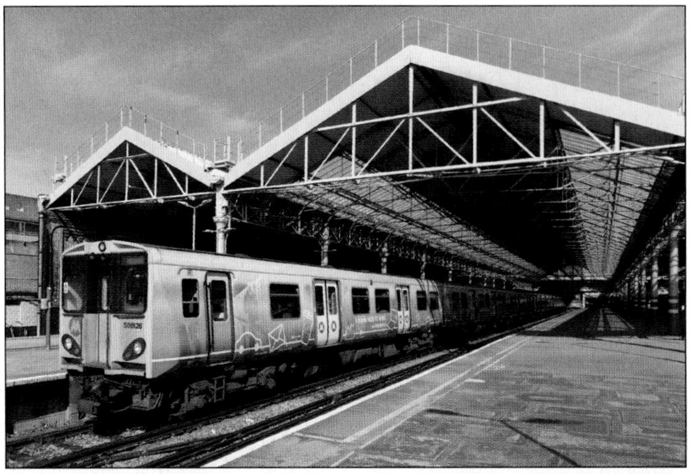

The Class 508 sets are likely to be withdrawn from Merseyrail service in advance of the '507s'. Viewed from its silver/grey side, No. 508126 is seen at Southport with a Liverpool City centre bound service. **CJM**

Class 600
Alstom 'Breeze' Hydrogen Multiple Unit (HMU)

The conversion of former Class 321 sets into three-car Hydrogen Multiple Units is now underway. The sets will be classified 600, but actual renumbering is yet to be announced, 10 sets have been set aside for this project. The first set sent for conversion is No. 321437, plus the previously used Alstom development set No. 321448 (See Class 321 section for details).

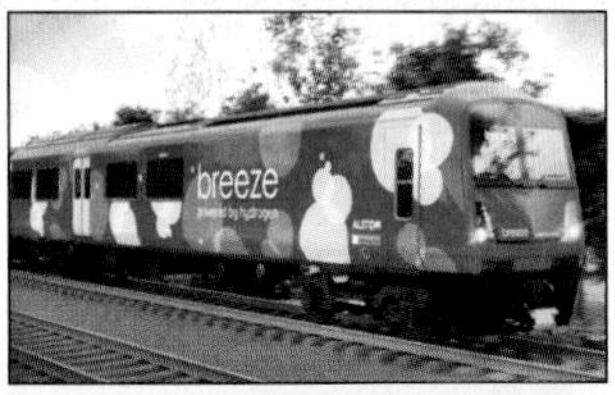

Class 614
BREL 3-Car Suburban 'Hydrogen' development

Built: 1979
Vehicle length: Driving - 64ft 11½in (19.80m)
Intermediate - 65ft 4¼in (19.92m)
Height: 11ft 9in (3.58m)
Width: 9ft 3in (2.82m)
Power: 25kV ac overhead
Horsepower: 880hp (657kW)
Transmission: Electric

Formation: DMSO+PTSO+BDMSO

614209 (314209) 64599+71458+64600 Hydrogen Development Unit at Bo'ness

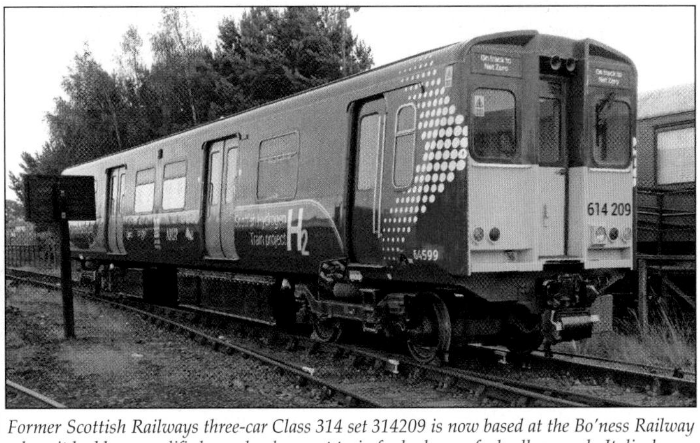

Former Scottish Railways three-car Class 314 set 314209 is now based at the Bo'ness Railway where it had been modified as a development train for hydrogen fuel cell research. It displays a joint livery of Scottish Railways and its development partners. **Ian Lothian**

Class 700
Siemens 8 and 12-car EMU Main Line 'Desiro City'

Built: 2015-2018
Vehicle length: 67ft 4in (20.52m)
Height: 12ft 1in (3.70m)
Width: 9ft 2in (2.80m)

Power: 25kV ac overhead and 750V dc third rail
Horsepower: 8-car 4,291hp (3,200kW)
12-car 6,439hp (4,800kW)
Transmission: Electric

700/0	Formation: 8-car DMC+PTS+MS+TS+TS+MS+PTS+DMC - Reduced Length Unit (RLU)				
700001	401001+402001+403001+406001+407001+410001+411001+412001	TB	TMK	CLT	GTR
700002	401002+402002+403002+406002+407002+410002+411002+412002	TB	TMK	CLT	GTR
700003	401003+402003+403003+406003+407003+410003+411003+412003	TB	TMK	CLT	GTR
700004	401004+402004+403004+406004+407004+410004+411004+412004	TB	TMK	CLT	GTR
700005	401005+402005+403005+406005+407005+410005+411005+412005	TB	TMK	CLT	GTR
700006	401006+402006+403006+406006+407006+410006+411006+412006	TB	TMK	CLT	GTR
700007	401007+402007+403007+406007+407007+410007+411007+412007	TB	TMK	CLT	GTR
700008	401008+402008+403008+406008+407008+410008+411008+412008	TB	TMK	CLT	GTR
700009	401009+402009+403009+406009+407009+410009+411009+412009	TB	TMK	CLT	GTR
700010	401010+402010+403010+406010+407010+410010+411010+412010	TB	TMK	CLT	GTR
700011	401011+402011+403011+406011+407011+410011+411011+412011	TB	TMK	CLT	GTR
700012	401012+402012+403012+406012+407012+410012+411012+412012	TB	TMK	CLT	GTR
700013	401013+402013+403013+406013+407013+410013+411013+412013	TB	TMK	CLT	GTR
700014	401014+402014+403014+406014+407014+410014+411014+412014	TB	TMK	CLT	GTR
700015	401015+402015+403015+406015+407015+410015+411015+412015	TB	TMK	CLT	GTR
700016	401016+402016+403016+406016+407016+410016+411016+412016	TB	TMK	CLT	GTR
700017	401017+402017+403017+406017+407017+410017+411017+412017	TB	TMK	CLT	GTR
700018	401018+402018+403018+406018+407018+410018+411018+412018	TB	TMK	CLT	GTR
700019	401019+402019+403019+406019+407019+410019+411019+412019	TB	TMK	CLT	GTR
700020	401020+402020+403020+406020+407020+410020+411020+412020	TB	TMK	CLT	GTR
700021	401021+402021+403021+406021+407021+410021+411021+412021	TB	TMK	CLT	GTR
700022	401022+402022+403022+406022+407022+410022+411022+412022	TB	TMK	CLT	GTR
700023	401023+402023+403023+406023+407023+410023+411023+412023	TB	TMK	CLT	GTR
700024	401024+402024+403024+406024+407024+410024+411024+412024	TB	TMK	CLT	GTR
700025	401025+402025+403025+406025+407025+410025+411025+412025	TB	TMK	CLT	GTR
700026	401026+402026+403026+406026+407026+410026+411026+412026	TB	TMK	CLT	GTR
700027	401027+402027+403027+406027+407027+410027+411027+412027	TB	TMK	CLT	GTR
700028	401028+402028+403028+406028+407028+410028+411028+412028	TB	TMK	CLT	GTR
700029	401029+402029+403029+406029+407029+410029+411029+412029	TB	TMK	CLT	GTR
700030	410030+402030+403030+406030+407030+410030+411030+412030	TB	TMK	CLT	GTR
700031	401031+402031+403031+406031+407031+410031+411031+412031	TB	TMK	CLT	GTR
700032	401032+402032+403032+406032+407032+410032+411032+412032	TB	TMK	CLT	GTR
700033	401033+402033+403033+406033+407033+410033+411033+412033	TB	TMK	CLT	GTR
700034	401034+402034+403034+406034+407034+410034+411034+412034	TB	TMK	CLT	GTR
700035	401035+402035+403035+406035+407035+410035+411035+412035	TB	TMK	CLT	GTR
700036	401036+402036+403036+406036+407036+410036+411036+412036	TB	TMK	CLT	GTR
700037	401037+402037+403037+406037+407037+410037+411037+412037	TB	TMK	CLT	GTR
700038	401038+402038+403038+406038+407038+410038+411038+412038	TB	TMK	CLT	GTR
700039	401039+402039+403039+406039+407039+410039+411039+412039	TB	TMK	CLT	GTR
700040	401040+402040+403040+406040+407040+410040+411040+412040	TB	TMK	CLT	GTR
700041	401041+402041+403041+406041+407041+410041+411041+412041	TB	TMK	CLT	GTR
700042	401042+402042+403042+406042+407042+410042+411042+412042	TB	TMK	CLT	GTR
700043	401043+402043+403043+406043+407043+410043+411043+412043	TB	TMK	CLT	GTR
700044	401044+402044+403044+406044+407044+410044+411044+412044	TB	TMK	CLT	GTR
700045	401045+402045+403045+406045+407045+410045+411045+412045	TB	TMK	CLT	GTR
700046	401046+402046+403046+406046+407046+410046+411046+412046	TB	TMK	CLT	GTR
700047	401047+402047+403047+406047+407047+410047+411047+412047	TB	TMK	CLT	GTR
700048	401048+402048+403048+406048+407048+410048+411048+412048	TB	TMK	CLT	GTR
700049	401049+402049+403049+406049+407049+410049+411049+412049	TB	TMK	CLT	GTR
700050	401050+402050+403050+406050+407050+410050+411050+412050	TB	TMK	CLT	GTR
700051	401051+402051+403051+406051+407051+410051+411051+412051	TB	TMK	CLT	GTR
700052	401052+402052+403052+406052+407052+410052+411052+412052	TB	TMK	CLT	GTR
700053	401053+402053+403053+406053+407053+410053+411053+412053	TB	TMK	CLT	GTR
700054	401054+402054+403054+406054+407054+410054+411054+412054	TB	TMK	CLT	GTR
700055	401055+402055+403055+406055+407055+410055+411055+412055	TB	TMK	CLT	GTR
700056	401056+402056+403056+406056+407056+410056+411056+412056	TB	TMK	CLT	GTR
700057	401057+402057+403057+406057+407057+410057+411057+412057	TB	TMK	CLT	GTR
700058	401058+402058+403058+406058+407058+410058+411058+412058	TB	TMK	CLT	GTR
700059	401059+402059+403059+406059+407059+410059+411059+412059	TB	TMK	CLT	GTR
700060	401060+402060+403060+406060+407060+410060+411060+412060	TB	TMK	CLT	GTR

700/1	12-car DMC+PTS+MS+MS+TS+TS+TS+TS+MS+MS+PTS+DMC - Full Length Unit (FLU)				
700101	401101+402101+403101+404101+405101+406101+407101+408101+409101+410101+411101+412101	TB	TMK	CLT	GTR
700102	401102+402102+403102+404102+405102+406102+407102+408102+409102+410102+411102+412102	TB	TMK	CLT	GTR
700103	401103+402103+403103+404103+405103+406103+407103+408103+409103+410103+411103+412103	TB	TMK	CLT	GTR
700104	401104+402104+403104+404104+405104+406104+407104+408104+409104+410104+411104+412104	TB	TMK	CLT	GTR
700105	401105+402105+403105+404105+405105+406105+407105+408105+409105+410105+411105+412105	TB	TMK	CLT	GTR
700106	401106+402106+403106+404106+405106+406106+407106+408106+409106+410106+411106+412106	TB	TMK	CLT	GTR
700107	401107+402107+403107+404107+405107+406107+407107+408107+409107+410107+411107+412107	TB	TMK	CLT	GTR
700108	401108+402108+403108+404108+405108+406108+407108+408108+409108+410108+411108+412108	TB	TMK	CLT	GTR
700109	401109+402109+403109+404109+405109+406109+407109+408109+409109+410109+411109+412109	TB	TMK	CLT	GTR
700110	401110+402110+403110+404110+405110+406110+407110+408110+409110+410110+411110+412110	TB	TMK	CLT	GTR
700111	401111+402111+403111+404111+405111+406111+407111+408111+409111+410111+411111+412111	TB	TMK§	CLT	GTR
700112	401112+402112+403112+404112+405112+406112+407112+408112+409112+410112+411112+412112	TB	TMK	CLT	GTR
700113	401113+402113+403113+404113+405113+406113+407113+408113+409113+410113+411113+412113	TB	TMK	CLT	GTR
700114	401114+402114+403114+404114+405114+406114+407114+408114+409114+410114+411114+412114	TB	TMK	CLT	GTR
700115	401115+402115+403115+404115+405115+406115+407115+408115+409115+410115+411105+412115	TB	TMK	CLT	GTR
700116	401116+402116+403116+404116+405116+406116+407116+408116+409116+410116+411116+412116	TB	TMK	CLT	GTR
700117	401117+402117+403117+404117+405117+406117+407117+408117+409117+410117+411107+412117	TB	TMK	CLT	GTR
700118	401118+402118+403118+404118+405118+406118+407118+408118+409118+410118+411108+412118	TB	TMK	CLT	GTR
700119	401119+402119+403119+404119+405119+406119+407119+408119+409119+410119+411109+412119	TB	TMK	CLT	GTR
700120	401120+402120+403120+404120+405120+406120+407120+408120+409120+410120+411120+412120	TB	TMK	CLT	GTR
700121	401121+402121+403121+404121+405121+406121+407121+408121+409121+410121+411121+412121	TB	TMK	CLT	GTR
700122	401122+402122+403122+404122+405122+406122+407122+408122+409122+410122+411122+412122	TB	TMK	CLT	GTR
700123	401123+402123+403123+404123+405123+406123+407123+408123+409123+410123+411123+412123	TB	TMK	CLT	GTR
700124	401124+402124+403124+404124+405124+406124+407124+408124+409124+410124+411124+412124	TB	TMK	CLT	GTR
700125	401125+402125+403125+404125+405125+406125+407125+408125+409125+410125+411125+412125	TB	TMK	CLT	GTR
700126	401126+402126+403126+404126+405126+406126+407126+408126+409126+410126+411126+412126	TB	TMK	CLT	GTR
700127	401127+402127+403127+404127+405127+406127+407127+408127+409127+410127+411127+412127	TB	TMK	CLT	GTR
700128	401128+402128+403128+404128+405128+406128+407128+408128+409128+410128+411128+412128	TB	TMK	CLT	GTR
700129	401129+402129+403129+404129+405129+406129+407129+408129+409129+410129+411129+412129	TB	TMK	CLT	GTR
700130	401130+402130+403130+404130+405130+406130+407130+408130+409130+410130+411130+412130	TB	TMK	CLT	GTR

700131	401131+402131+403131+404131+405131+406131+407131+408131+409131+410131+411131+412131	TB	TMK	CLT	GTR
700132	401132+402132+403132+404132+405132+406132+407132+408132+409132+410132+411132+412132	TB	TMK	CLT	GTR
700133	401133+402133+403133+404133+405133+406133+407133+408133+409133+410133+411133+412133	TB	TMK	CLT	GTR
700134	401134+402134+403134+404134+405134+406134+407134+408134+409134+410134+411134+412134	TB	TMK	CLT	GTR
700135	401135+402135+403135+404135+405135+406135+407135+408135+409135+410135+411135+412135	TB	TMK	CLT	GTR
700136	401136+402136+403136+404136+405136+406136+407136+408136+409136+410136+411136+412136	TB	TMK	CLT	GTR
700137	401137+402137+403137+404137+405137+406137+407137+408137+409137+410137+411137+412137	TB	TMK	CLT	GTR
700138	401138+402138+403138+404138+405138+406138+407138+408138+409138+410138+411138+412138	TB	TMK	CLT	GTR
700139	401139+402139+403139+404139+405139+406139+407139+408139+409139+410139+411139+412139	TB	TMK	CLT	GTR
700140	401140+402140+403140+404140+405140+406140+407140+408140+409140+410140+411140+412140	TB	TMK	CLT	GTR
700141	401141+402141+403141+404141+405141+406141+407141+408141+409141+410141+411141+412141	TB	TMK	CLT	GTR
700142	401142+402142+403142+404142+405142+406142+407142+408142+409142+410142+411142+412142	TB	TMK	CLT	GTR
700143	401143+402143+403143+404143+405143+406143+407143+408143+409143+410143+411143+412143	TB	TMK	CLT	GTR
700144	401144+402144+403144+404144+405144+406144+407144+408144+409144+410144+411144+412144	TB	TMK	CLT	GTR
700145	401145+402145+403145+404145+405145+406145+407145+408145+409145+410145+411145+412145	TB	TMK	CLT	GTR
700146	401146+402146+403146+404146+405146+406146+407146+408146+409146+410146+411146+412146	TB	TMK	CLT	GTR
700147	401147+402147+403147+404147+405147+406147+407147+408147+409147+410147+411147+412147	TB	TMK	CLT	GTR
700148	401148+402148+403148+404148+405148+406148+407148+408148+409148+410148+411148+412148	TB	TMK	CLT	GTR
700149	401149+402149+403149+404149+405149+406149+407149+408149+409149+410149+411149+412149	TB	TMK	CLT	GTR
700150	401150+402150+403150+404150+405150+406150+407150+408150+409150+410150+411150+412150	TB	TMK	CLT	GTR
700151	401151+402151+403151+404151+405151+406151+407151+408151+409151+410151+411151+412151	TB	TMK	CLT	GTR
700152	401152+402152+403152+404152+405152+406152+407152+408152+409152+410152+411152+412152	TB	TMK	CLT	GTR
700153	401153+402153+403153+404153+405153+406153+407153+408153+409153+410153+411153+412153	TB	TMK	CLT	GTR
700154	401154+402154+403154+404154+405154+406154+407154+408154+409154+410154+411154+412154	TB	TMK	CLT	GTR
700155	401155+402155+403155+404155+405155+406155+407155+408155+409155+410155+411155+412155	TB	SPL	CLT	GTR

§ Carries NHS/Key Workers branding

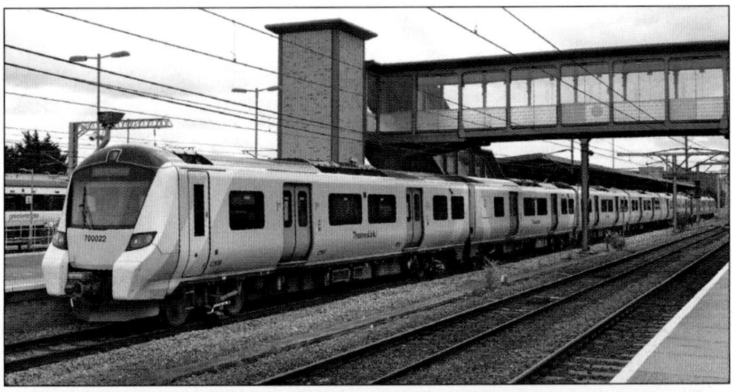

The Class 700 eight and twelve-car 'Desiro City' sets were designed for use on the north-south 'Thameslink' system, operated by GTR. Based at Three Bridges depot, the sets have a wide operating area. Each driving car has first class seating, and usually only operate as single sets. On the left, reduced length set (RLU) No. 700022 is viewed at Cambridge, while below PTS No. 411053 from set No. 700053 is shown, the pantograph fitted cars are coupled to the driving vehicles. **CJM / Antony Christie**

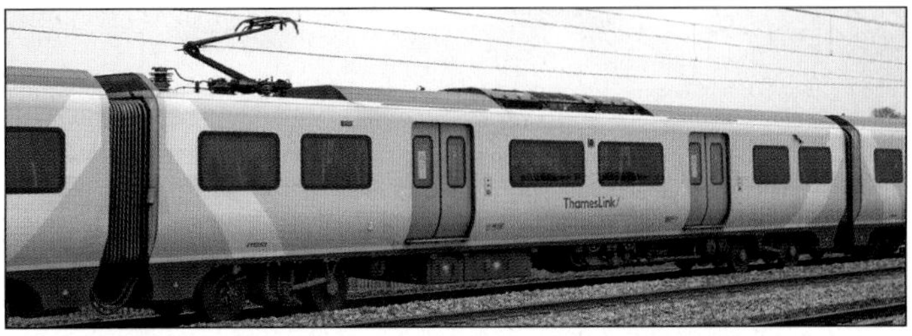

Class 701
Alstom 5 and 10-car EMU Suburban 'Aventra'

Built: 2019-2021
Vehicle length: Driving 20.88m
Intermediate 19.90m
Height: awaited
Width: 9ft 1in (2.78m)
Power: 25kV ac overhead and750V dc third rail
Horsepower: 5-car awaited
10-car awaited
Transmission: Electric

701/0 Formation: 10-car DMS+MS+TS+MS+MS+MS+MS+TS+MS+DMS

701001	480001+481001+482001+483001+484001+485001+486001+487001+488001+489001	WD	SWR	ROK	SWR
701002	480002+481002+482002+483002+484002+485002+486002+487002+488002+489002	WD	SWR	ROK	SWR
701003	480003+481003+482003+483003+484003+485003+486003+487003+488003+489003	WD	SWR	ROK	SWR
701004	480004+481004+482004+483004+484004+485004+486004+487004+488004+489004	WD	SWR	ROK	SWR
701005	480005+481005+482005+483005+484005+485005+486005+487005+488005+489005	WD	SWR	ROK	SWR
701006	480006+481006+482006+483006+484006+485006+486006+487006+488006+489006	WD	SWR	ROK	SWR
701007	480007+481007+482007+483007+484007+485007+486007+487007+488007+489007	WD	SWR	ROK	SWR
701008	480008+481008+482008+483008+484008+485008+486008+487008+488008+489008	WD	SWR	ROK	SWR
701009	480009+481009+482009+483009+484009+485009+486009+487009+488009+489009	WD	SWR	ROK	SWR
701010	480010+481010+482010+483010+484010+485010+486010+487010+488010+489010	WD	SWR	ROK	SWR
701011	480011+481011+482011+483011+484011+485011+486011+487011+488011+489011	WD	SWR	ROK	SWR
701012	480012+481012+482012+483012+484012+485012+486012+487012+488012+489012	WD	SWR	ROK	SWR
701013	480013+481013+482013+483013+484013+485013+486013+487013+488013+489013	WD	SWR	ROK	SWR

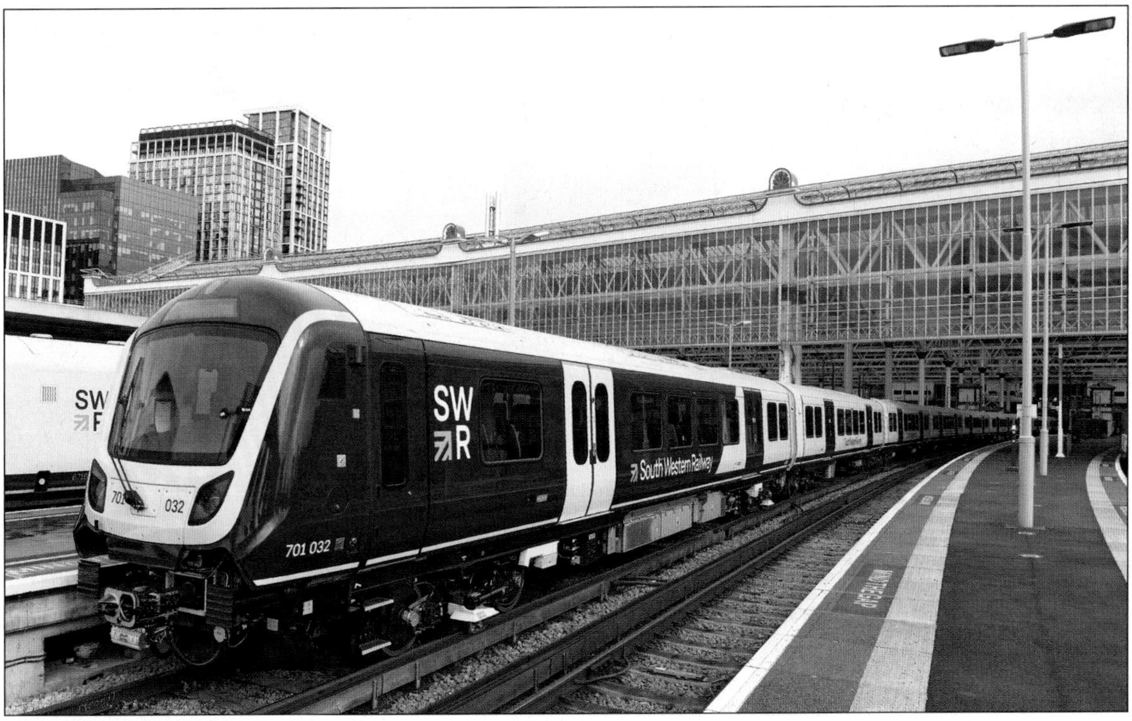

The original Bombardier, now Alstom (following the merger of the two builders) Class 701 are some of the most problematic sets ever seen on the railway, with by February 2022 not a single unit accepted by SWR as fit for purpose. Although the builders keep producing the sets, they are being stored at many sites and only a handful are on SWR under test based at Eastleigh. Devoid of its front skirt, set No. 701032 is seen at Waterloo on 30 September 2021 during a test run. It is hoped that some sets will be placed in passenger service by summer 2022, but the full fleet will not be in traffic until 2023. **CJM**

701014	480014+481014+482014+483014+484014+485014+486014+487014+488014+489014	WD	SWR	ROK	SWR
701015	480015+481015+482015+483015+484015+485015+486015+487015+488015+489015	WD	SWR	ROK	SWR
701016	480016+481016+482016+483016+484016+485016+486016+487016+488016+489016	WD	SWR	ROK	SWR
701017	480017+481017+482017+483017+484017+485017+486017+487017+488017+489017	WD	SWR	ROK	SWR
701018	480018+481018+482018+483018+484018+485018+486018+487018+488018+489018	WD	SWR	ROK	SWR
701019	480019+481019+482019+483019+484019+485019+486019+487019+488019+489019	WD	SWR	ROK	SWR
701020	480020+481020+482020+483020+484020+485020+486020+487020+488020+489020	WD	SWR	ROK	SWR
701021	480021+481021+482021+483021+484021+485021+486021+487021+488021+489021	WD	SWR	ROK	SWR
701022	480022+481022+482022+483022+484022+485022+486022+487022+488022+489022	WD	SWR	ROK	SWR
701023	480023+481023+482023+483023+484023+485023+486023+487023+488023+489023	WD	SWR	ROK	SWR
701024	480024+481024+482024+483024+484024+485024+486024+487024+488024+489024	WD	SWR	ROK	SWR
701025	480025+481025+482025+483025+484025+485025+486025+487025+488025+489025	WD	SWR	ROK	SWR
701026	480026+481026+482026+483026+484026+485026+486026+487026+488026+489026	WD	SWR	ROK	SWR
701027	480027+481027+482027+483027+484027+485027+486027+487027+488027+489027	WD	SWR	ROK	SWR
701028	480028+481028+482028+483028+484028+485028+486028+487028+488028+489028	WD	SWR	ROK	SWR
701029	480029+481029+482029+483029+484029+485029+486029+487029+488029+489029	WD	SWR	ROK	SWR
701030	480030+481030+482030+483030+484030+485030+486030+487030+488030+489030	WD	SWR	ROK	SWR
701031	480031+481031+482031+483031+484031+485031+486031+487031+488031+489031	WD	SWR	ROK	SWR
701032	480032+481032+482032+483032+484032+485032+486032+487032+488032+489032	WD	SWR	ROK	SWR
701033	480033+481033+482033+483033+484033+485033+486033+487033+488033+489033	WD	SWR	ROK	SWR
701034	480034+481034+482034+483034+484034+485034+486034+487034+488034+489034	WD	SWR	ROK	SWR
701035	480035+481035+482035+483035+484035+485035+486035+487035+488035+489035	WD	SWR	ROK	SWR
701036	480036+481036+482036+483036+484036+485036+486036+487036+488036+489036	WD	SWR	ROK	SWR
701037	480037+481037+482037+483037+484037+485037+486037+487037+488037+489037	WD	SWR	ROK	SWR
701038	480038+481038+482038+483038+484038+485038+486038+487038+488038+489038	WD	SWR	ROK	SWR
701039	480039+481039+482039+483039+484039+485039+486039+487039+488039+489039	WD	SWR	ROK	SWR
701040	480040+481040+482040+483040+484040+485040+486040+487040+488040+489040	WD	SWR	ROK	SWR
701041	480041+481041+482041+483041+484041+485041+486041+487041+488041+489041	WD	SWR	ROK	SWR
701042	480042+481042+482042+483042+484042+485042+486042+487042+488042+489042	WD	SWR	ROK	SWR
701043	480043+481043+482043+483043+484043+485043+486043+487043+488043+489043	WD	SWR	ROK	SWR
701044	480044+481044+482044+483044+484044+485044+486044+487044+488044+489044	WD	SWR	ROK	SWR
701045	480045+481045+482045+483045+484045+485045+486045+487045+488045+489045	WD	SWR	ROK	SWR
701046	480046+481046+482046+483046+484046+485046+486046+487046+488046+489046	WD	SWR	ROK	SWR
701047	480047+481047+482047+483047+484047+485047+486047+487047+488047+489047	WD	SWR	ROK	SWR
701048	480048+481048+482048+483048+484048+485048+486048+487048+488048+489048	WD	SWR	ROK	SWR
701049	480049+481049+482049+483049+484049+485049+486049+487049+488049+489049	WD	SWR	ROK	SWR
701050	480050+481050+482050+483050+484050+485050+486050+487050+488050+489050	WD	SWR	ROK	SWR
701051	480041+481051+482051+483051+484051+485051+486051+487051+488051+489051	WD	SWR	ROK	SWR
701052	480052+481052+482052+483052+484052+485052+486052+487052+488052+489052	WD	SWR	ROK	SWR
701053	480053+481053+482053+483053+484053+485053+486053+487053+488053+489053	WD	SWR	ROK	SWR
701054	480054+481054+482054+483054+484054+485054+486054+487054+488054+489054	WD	SWR	ROK	SWR
701055	480055+481055+482055+483055+484055+485055+486055+487055+488055+489055	WD	SWR	ROK	SWR
701056	480056+481056+482056+483056+484056+485056+486056+487056+488056+489056	WD	SWR	ROK	SWR
701057	480057+481057+482057+483057+484057+485057+486057+487057+488057+489057	WD	SWR	ROK	SWR
701058	480058+481058+482058+483058+484058+485058+486058+487058+488058+489058	WD	SWR	ROK	SWR
701059	480059+481059+482059+483059+484059+485059+486059+487059+488059+489059	WD	SWR	ROK	SWR
701060	480060+481060+482060+483060+484060+485060+486060+487060+488060+489060	WD	SWR	ROK	SWR
701061	480061+481061+482061+483061+484061+485061+486061+487061+488061+489061	WD	SWR	ROK	SWR
701060	480062+481062+482062+483062+484062+485062+486062+487062+488062+489062	WD	SWR	ROK	SWR

701/5 Formation: 5-car DMS+MS+TS+MS+DMS

701501	480101+481101+482101+483101+489101	WD	SWR	ROK	SWR
701502	480102+481102+482102+483102+489102	WD	SWR	ROK	SWR
701503	480103+481103+482103+483103+489103	WD	SWR	ROK	SWR
701504	480104+481104+482104+483104+489104	WD	SWR	ROK	SWR
701505	480105+481105+482105+483105+489105	WD	SWR	ROK	SWR
701506	480106+481106+482106+483106+489106	WD	SWR	ROK	SWR
701507	480107+481107+482107+483107+489107	WD	SWR	ROK	SWR
701508	480108+481108+482108+483108+489108	WD	SWR	ROK	SWR
701509	480109+481109+482109+483109+489109	WD	SWR	ROK	SWR
701510	480110+481110+482110+483110+489110	WD	SWR	ROK	SWR
701511	480111+481111+482111+483111+489111	WD	SWR	ROK	SWR
701512	480112+481112+482112+483112+489112	WD	SWR	ROK	SWR
701513	480113+481113+482113+483113+489113	WD	SWR	ROK	SWR
701514	480114+481114+482114+483114+489114	WD	SWR	ROK	SWR
701515	480115+481115+482115+483115+489115	WD	SWR	ROK	SWR
701516	480116+481116+482116+483116+489116	WD	SWR	ROK	SWR
701517	480117+481117+482117+483117+489117	WD	SWR	ROK	SWR
701518	480118+481118+482118+483118+489118	WD	SWR	ROK	SWR
701519	480119+481119+482119+483119+489119	WD	SWR	ROK	SWR
701520	480120+481120+482120+483120+489120	WD	SWR	ROK	SWR
701521	480121+481121+482121+483121+489121	WD	SWR	ROK	SWR
701522	480122+481122+482122+483122+489122	WD	SWR	ROK	SWR
701523	480123+481123+482123+483123+489123	WD	SWR	ROK	SWR
701524	480124+481124+482124+483124+489124	WD	SWR	ROK	SWR
701525	480125+481125+482125+483125+489125	WD	SWR	ROK	SWR
701526	480126+481126+482126+483126+489126	WD	SWR	ROK	SWR
701527	480127+481127+482127+483127+489127	WD	SWR	ROK	SWR
701528	480128+481128+482128+483128+489128	WD	SWR	ROK	SWR
701529	480129+481129+482129+483129+489129	WD	SWR	ROK	SWR
701530	480130+481130+482130+483130+489130	WD	SWR	ROK	SWR

Class 707
Siemens 5-car EMU Suburban 'Desiro City'

Built: 2014-2018
Vehicle length: Driving 67ft 4in (20.52m)
Intermediate 66ft 2in (20.16m)
Height: 12ft 1in (3.70m)
Width: 9ft 2in (2.80m)
Power: 750V dc third rail
Horsepower: 1,075hp (800kW)
Transmission: Electric

Formation: DMS+TS+TS+TS+DMS

707001	421001+422001+423001+424001+425001	SG	SET	ANG	SET
707002	421002+422002+423002+424002+425002	SG	SET	ANG	SET
707003	421003+422003+423003+424003+425003	SG	SET	ANG	SET
707004	421004+422004+423004+424004+425004	SG	SET	ANG	SET
707005	421005+422005+423005+424005+425005	SG	SET	ANG	SET
	Remembering Rt Hon James Brokenshire MP Old Bexley and Sidcup				
707006	421006+422006+423006+424006+425006	SG	SET	ANG	SET
707007	421007+422007+423007+424007+425007	SG	SET	ANG	SET
707008	421008+422008+423008+424008+425008	SG	SET	ANG	SET
707009	421009+422009+423009+424009+425009	SG	SET	ANG	SET
707010	421010+422010+423010+424010+425011	SG	SET	ANG	SET
707011	421011+422011+423011+424011+425011	SG	SET	ANG	SET
707012	421012+422012+423012+424012+425012	SG	SET	ANG	SET
707013	421013+422013+423013+424013+425013	SG	SET	ANG	SET
707014	421014+422014+423014+424014+425014	WD	SWS	ANG	SWR
707015	421015+422015+423015+424015+425015	WD	SWS	ANG	SWR
707016	421016+422016+423016+424016+425016	WD	SWS	ANG	SWR
707017	421017+422017+423017+424017+425017	WD	SWS	ANG	SWR
707018	421018+422018+423018+424018+425018	WD	SWS	ANG	SWR
707019	421019+422019+423019+424019+425019	WD	SWS	ANG	SWR
707020	421020+422020+423020+424020+425020	WD	SWS	ANG	SWR
707021	421021+422021+423021+424021+425021	WD	SWS	ANG	SWR
707022	421022+422022+423022+424022+425022	WD	SWS	ANG	SWR
707023	421023+422023+423023+424023+425023	WD	SWS	ANG	SWR
707024	421024+422024+423024+424024+425024	WD	SWS	ANG	SWR
707025	421025+422025+423025+424025+425025	SG	SET	ANG	SET
707026	421026+422026+423026+424026+425026	SG	SET	ANG	SET
707027	421027+422027+423027+424027+425027	SG	SET	ANG	SET
707028	421028+422028+423028+424028+425028	SG	SET	ANG	SET
707029	421029+422029+423029+424029+425029	SG	SET	ANG	SET
707030	421030+422030+423030+424030+425030	WD	SWS	ANG	SWR

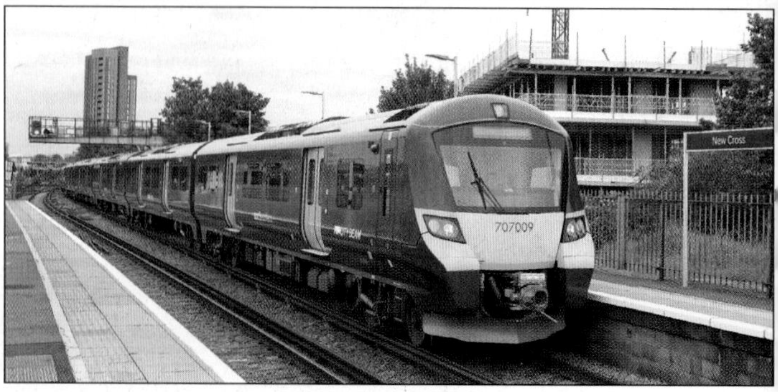

By Autumn 2022 all Class 707s will be operating for SouthEastern, an agreement was struck in January 2022 for 12 Class 707s to remain with SWR until August to cover shortages due to late delivery of Class 701s. No. 707009, leads a 10-car formation into New Cross on 30 September 2021 with a Cannon Street to Cannon Street via Dartford service. **CJM**

Class 710
Alstom 4 and 5-car EMU Suburban 'Aventra'

Built: 2018-2020
Vehicle length: Driving 77ft 5in (23.62m)
Intermediate 73ft 8in (22.50m)
Height: 12ft 4in (3.87m)
Width: 9ft 1in (2.78m)
Power: 710/1 25kV ac overhead
710/2, 710/3 25kV ac overhead and 750V dc third rail
Horsepower: 4-car 2,843hp (2120kW)
5-car 3,554hp (2650kW)
Transmission: Electric

710/1	Formation: DMS+MS+PMS+DMS				
710101	431101+431201+431301+431501	WN	LON	RFL	LOG
710102	431102+431202+431302+431502	WN	LON	RFL	LOG
710103	431103+431203+431303+431503	WN	LON	RFL	LOG
710104	431104+431204+431304+431504	WN	LON	RFL	LOG
710105	431105+431205+431305+431505	WN	LON	RFL	LOG
710106	431106+431206+431306+431506	WN	LON	RFL	LOG
710107	431107+431207+431307+431507	WN	LON	RFL	LOG
710108	431108+431208+431308+431508	WN	LON	RFL	LOG
710109	431109+431209+431309+431509	WN	LON	RFL	LOG
710110	431110+431210+431310+431510	WN	LON	RFL	LOG
710111	431111+431211+431311+431511	WN	LON	RFL	LOG
710112	431112+431212+431312+431512	WN	LON	RFL	LOG
710113	431113+431213+431313+431513	WN	LON	RFL	LOG
710114	431114+431214+431314+431514	WN	LON	RFL	LOG
710115	431115+431215+431315+431515	WN	LON	RFL	LOG
710116	431116+431216+431316+431516	WN	LON	RFL	LOG
710117	431117+431217+431317+431517	WN	LON	RFL	LOG
710118	431118+431218+431318+431518	WN	LON	RFL	LOG
710119	431119+431219+431319+431519	WN	LON	RFL	LOG
710120	431120+431220+431320+431520	WN	LON	RFL	LOG
710121	431121+431221+431321+431521	WN	LON	RFL	LOG
710122	431122+431222+431322+431522	WN	LON	RFL	LOG
710123	431123+431223+431323+431523	WN	LON	RFL	LOG
710124	431124+431224+431324+431524	WN	LON	RFL	(S)
710125	431125+431225+431325+431525	WN	LON	RFL	LOG
710126	431126+431226+431326+431526	WN	LON	RFL	LOG
710127	431127+431227+431327+431527	WN	LON	RFL	LOG
710128	431128+431228+431328+431528	WN	LON	RFL	LOG
710129	431129+431229+431329+431529	WN	LON	RFL	LOG
710130	431130+431230+431330+431530	WN	LON	RFL	LOG

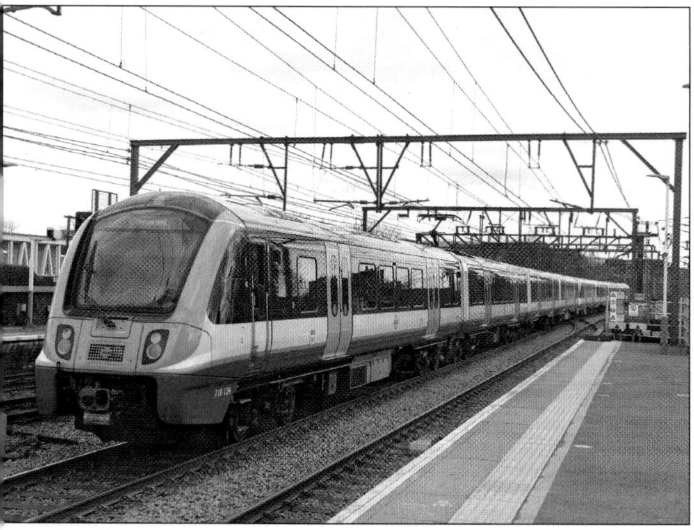

The first fleet of Bombardier 'Aventra' units to enter service were the Class 710s for London Overground. Class 710/1 No. 710129 is seen departing from Hackney Downs with a service for Liverpool Street. The Class 710/1s are ac power supply only. **CJM**

710/2	Formation: DMS+MS+PMS+DMS				
710256	432156+432256+432356+432556	WN	LON	RFL	LOG
710257	432157+432257+432357+432557	WN	LON	RFL	LOG
710258	432158+432258+432358+432558	WN	LON	RFL	LOG
710259	432159+432259+432359+432559	WN	LON	RFL	LOG
710260	432160+432260+432360+432560	WN	LON	RFL	LOG
710261	432161+432261+432361+432561	WN	LON	RFL	LOG
710262	432162+432262+432362+432562	WN	LON	RFL	LOG
710263	432163+432263+432363+432563	WN	LON	RFL	LOG
710264	432164+432264+432364+432564	WN	LON	RFL	LOG
710265	432165+432265+432365+432565	WN	LON	RFL	LOG
710266	432166+432266+432366+432566	WN	LON	RFL	LOG
710267	432167+432267+432367+432567	WN	LON	RFL	LOG
710268	432168+432268+432368+432568	WN	LON	RFL	LOG
710269	432169+432269+432369+432569	WN	LON	RFL	LOG
710270	432170+432270+432370+432570	WN	LON	RFL	LOG
710271	432171+432271+432371+432571	WN	LON	RFL	LOG
710272	432172+432272+432372+432572	WN	LON	RFL	LOG
710273	432173+432273+432373+432573	WN	LON	RFL	LOG

710/3	Formation: DMS+MS+PMS+MS+DMS				
710374 (710274)	432174+432274+432374+432474+432574	WN	LON	RFL	LOG
710375 (710275)	432175+432275+432375+432475+432575	WN	LON	RFL	LOG
710376 (710276)	432176+432276+432376+432476+432576	WN	LON	RFL	LOG
710377 (710277)	432177+432277+432377+432477+432577	WN	LON	RFL	LOG
710378 (710278)	432178+432278+432378+432478+432578	WN	LON	RFL	LOG
710379 (710279)	432179+432279+432379+432479+432579	WN	LON	RFL	LOG

Class 717
Siemens 6-car EMU Suburban 'Desiro City'

Built: 2014-2018
Vehicle length: Driving 67ft 4in (20.52m)
Intermediate 66ft 2in (20.16m)
Height: 12ft 1in (3.70m)
Width: 9ft 2in (2.80m)
Power: 25kV ac overhead and 750V dc third rail
Horsepower: 1,609hp (1,200kW)
Transmission: Electric

	Formation: DMS+TS+TS+MS+PMS+DMS				
717001	451001+452001+453001+454001+455001+456001	HE	TLK	ROK	GTR
717002	451002+452002+453002+454002+455002+456002	HE	TLK	ROK	GTR
717003	451003+452003+453003+454003+455003+456003	HE	TLK	ROK	GTR
717004	451004+452004+453004+454004+455004+456004	HE	TLK	ROK	GTR
717005	451005+452005+453005+454005+455005+456005	HE	TLK	ROK	GTR
717006	451006+452006+453006+454006+455006+456006	HE	TLK	ROK	GTR
717007	451007+452007+453007+454007+455007+456007	HE	TLK	ROK	GTR
717008	451008+452008+453008+454008+455008+456008	HE	TLK	ROK	GTR
717009	451009+452009+453009+454009+455009+456009	HE	TLK	ROK	GTR
717010	451010+452010+453010+454010+455010+456010	HE	TLK	ROK	GTR
717011	451011+452011+453011+454011+455011+456011	HE	TLK§	ROK	GTR
717012	451012+452012+453012+454012+455012+456012	HE	TLK	ROK	GTR
717013	451013+452013+453013+454013+455013+456013	HE	TLK	ROK	GTR
717014	451014+452014+453014+454014+455014+456014	HE	TLK	ROK	GTR
717015	451015+452015+453015+454015+455015+456015	HE	TLK	ROK	GTR
717016	451016+452016+453016+454016+455016+456016	HE	TLK	ROK	GTR
717017	451017+452017+453017+454017+455017+456017	HE	TLK	ROK	GTR
717018	451018+452018+453018+454018+455018+456018	HE	TLK	ROK	GTR
717019	451019+452019+453019+454019+455019+456019	HE	TLK	ROK	GTR
717020	451020+452020+453020+454020+455020+456020	HE	TLK	ROK	GTR
717021	451021+452021+453021+454021+455021+456021	HE	TLK	ROK	GTR
717022	451022+452022+453022+454022+455022+456022	HE	TLK	ROK	GTR
717023	451023+452023+453023+454023+455023+456023	HE	TLK	ROK	GTR
717024	451024+452024+453024+454024+455024+456024	HE	TLK	ROK	GTR
717025	451025+452025+453025+454025+455025+456025	HE	TLK	ROK	GTR

§ Carries NHS/Key Workers branding

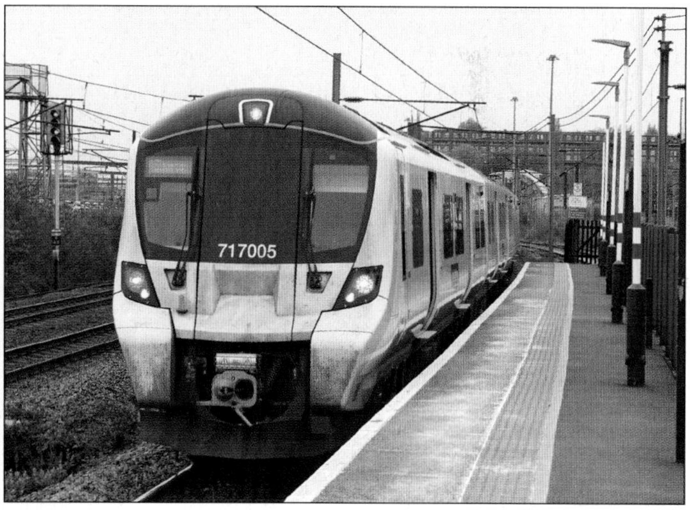

A fleet of 25 six-car Siemens 'Desiro City' sets are operated by GTR Great Northern on the Moorgate suburban route to Stevenage. These are a unique design, incorporating a fold down door in the front end to allow tunnel evacuation, seeing a rather unusual design of front end, which does not have a yellow high-visability panel. Set No. 717005 is shown. **CJM**

Class 720
Bombardier 5-car EMU Main Line 'Aventra'

Built: 2019-2021
Vehicle length: Driving 80ft 1in (24.47m)
Intermediate 79ft 5in (24.21m)
Height: 12ft 4in (3.87m)
Width: 9ft 1in (2.78m)
Power: 25kV ac overhead
Horsepower: 2,842hp (2,120kW)
Transmission: Electric

720/1	Formation: DMS+PMS+MS+MS+DTS				
720101	450101+451101+452101+453101+454101	IL	GAR	ANG	GAR
720102	450102+451102+452102+453102+454102	IL	GAR	ANG	GAR
720103	450103+451103+452103+453103+454103	IL	GAR	ANG	GAR
720104	450104+451104+452104+453104+459104	IL	GAR	ANG	GAR
720105	450105+451105+452105+453105+454105	IL	GAR	ANG	GAR
720106	450106+451106+452106+453106+454106	IL	GAR	ANG	GAR
720107	450107+451107+452107+453107+454107	IL	GAR	ANG	GAR
720108	450108+451108+452108+453108+454108	IL	GAR	ANG	GAR
720109	450109+451109+452109+453109+454109	IL	GAR	ANG	GAR
720110	450110+451110+452110+453110+454110	IL	GAR	ANG	GAR
720111	450111+451111+452111+453111+454111	IL	GAR	ANG	GAR
720112	450112+451112+452112+453112+454112	IL	GAR	ANG	GAR
720113	450113+451113+452113+453113+454113	IL	GAR	ANG	GAR
720114	450114+451114+452114+453114+454114	IL	GAR	ANG	GAR
720115	450115+451115+452115+453115+454115	IL	GAR	ANG	GAR
720116	450116+451116+452116+453116+454116	IL	GAR	ANG	GAR
720117	450117+451117+452117+453117+454117	IL	GAR	ANG	GAR
720118	450118+451118+452118+453118+454118	IL	GAR	ANG	GAR
720119	450119+451119+452119+453119+454119	IL	GAR	ANG	GAR
720120	450120+451120+452120+453120+454120	IL	GAR	ANG	GAR
720121	450121+451121+452121+453121+454121	IL	GAR	ANG	GAR
720122	450122+451122+452122+453122+454122	IL	GAR	ANG	GAR

720123	450123+451123+452123+453123+454123	IL	GAR	ANG	GAR
720124	450124+451124+452124+453124+454124	IL	GAR	ANG	GAR
720125	450125+451125+452125+453125+454125	IL	GAR	ANG	GAR
720126	450126+451126+452126+453126+454126	IL	GAR	ANG	GAR
720127	450127+451127+452127+453127+454127	IL	GAR	ANG	GAR
720128	450128+451128+452128+453128+454128	IL	GAR	ANG	GAR
720129	450129+451129+452129+453129+454129	IL	GAR	ANG	GAR
720130	450130+451130+452130+453130+454130	IL	GAR	ANG	GAR
720131	450131+451131+452131+453131+454131	IL	GAR	ANG	GAR
720132	450132+451132+452132+453132+454132	IL	GAR	ANG	GAR
720133	450133+451133+452133+453133+454133	IL	GAR	ANG	GAR
720134	450134+451134+452134+453134+454134	IL	GAR	ANG	GAR
720135	450135+451135+452135+453135+454135	IL	GAR	ANG	GAR
720136	450136+451136+452136+453136+454136	IL	GAR	ANG	GAR
720137	450137+451137+452137+453137+454137	IL	GAR	ANG	GAR
720138	450138+451138+452138+453138+454138	IL	GAR	ANG	GAR
720139	450139+451139+452139+453139+454139	IL	GAR	ANG	GAR
720140	450140+451140+452140+453140+454140	IL	GAR	ANG	GAR
720141	450141+451141+452141+453141+454141	IL	GAR	ANG	GAR
720142	450142+451142+452142+453142+454142	IL	GAR	ANG	GAR
720143	450143+451143+452143+453143+454143	IL	GAR	ANG	GAR
720144	450144+451144+452144+453144+454144	IL	GAR	ANG	GAR

720/5 Formation: DMS+PMS+MS+MS+DTS

720501	450501+451501+452501+453501+459501	IL	GAR	ANG	GAR
720502	450502+451502+452502+453502+459502	IL	GAR	ANG	GAR
720503	450503+451503+452503+453503+459503	IL	GAR	ANG	GAR
720504	450504+451504+452504+453504+459504	IL	GAR	ANG	GAR
720505	450505+451505+452505+453505+459505	IL	GAR	ANG	GAR
720506	450506+451506+452506+453506+459506	IL	GAR	ANG	GAR
720507	450507+451507+452507+453507+459507	IL	GAR	ANG	GAR
720508	450508+451508+452508+453508+459508	IL	GAR	ANG	GAR
720509	450509+451509+452509+453509+459509	IL	GAR	ANG	GAR
720510	450510+451510+452510+453510+459510	IL	GAR	ANG	GAR
720511	450511+451511+452511+453511+459511	IL	GAR	ANG	GAR
720512	450512+451512+452512+453512+459512	IL	GAR	ANG	GAR
720513	450513+451513+452513+453513+459513	IL	GAR	ANG	GAR
720514	450514+451514+452514+453514+459514	IL	GAR	ANG	GAR
720515	450515+451515+452515+453515+459515	IL	GAR	ANG	GAR
720516	450516+451516+452516+453516+459516	IL	GAR	ANG	GAR
720517	450517+451517+452517+453517+459517	IL	GAR	ANG	GAR
720518	450518+451518+452518+453518+459518	IL	GAR	ANG	GAR
720519	450519+451519+452519+453519+459519	IL	GAR	ANG	GAR
720520	450520+451520+452520+453520+459520	IL	GAR	ANG	GAR
720521	450521+451521+452521+453521+459521	IL	GAR	ANG	GAR
720522	450522+451522+452522+453522+459522	IL	GAR	ANG	GAR
720523	450523+451523+452523+453523+459523	IL	GAR	ANG	GAR
720524	450524+451524+452524+453524+459524	IL	GAR	ANG	GAR
720525	450525+451525+452525+453525+459525	IL	GAR	ANG	GAR
720526	450526+451526+452526+453526+459526	IL	GAR	ANG	GAR
720527	450527+451527+452527+453527+459527	IL	GAR	ANG	GAR
720528	450528+451528+452528+453528+459528	IL	GAR	ANG	GAR
720529	450529+451529+452529+453529+459529	IL	GAR	ANG	GAR
720530	450530+451530+452530+453530+459530	IL	GAR	ANG	GAR
720531	450531+451531+452531+453531+459531	IL	GAR	ANG	GAR
720532	450532+451532+452532+453532+459532	IL	GAR	ANG	GAR
720533	450533+451533+452533+453533+459533	IL	GAR	ANG	GAR
720534	450534+451534+452534+453534+459534	IL	GAR	ANG	GAR
720535	450535+451535+452535+453535+459535	IL	GAR	ANG	GAR
720536	450536+451536+452536+453536+459536	IL	GAR	ANG	GAR
720537	450537+451537+452537+453537+459537	IL	GAR	ANG	GAR
720538	450538+451538+452538+453538+459538	IL	GAR	ANG	GAR
720539	450539+451539+452539+453539+459539	IL	GAR	ANG	GAR
720540	450540+451540+452540+453540+459540	IL	GAR	ANG	GAR
720541	450541+451541+452541+453541+459541	IL	GAR	ANG	GAR
720542	450542+451542+452542+453542+459542	IL	GAR	ANG	GAR
720543	450543+451543+452543+453543+459543	IL	GAR	ANG	GAR
720544	450544+451544+452544+453544+459544	IL	GAR	ANG	GAR
720545	450545+451545+452545+453545+459545	IL	GAR	ANG	GAR
720546	450546+451546+452546+453546+459546	IL	GAR	ANG	GAR
720547	450547+451547+452547+453547+459547	IL	GAR	ANG	GAR
720548	450548+451548+452548+453548+459548	IL	GAR	ANG	GAR
720549	450549+451549+452549+453549+459549	IL	GAR	ANG	GAR
720550	450550+451550+452550+453550+459550	IL	GAR	ANG	GAR
720551	450551+451551+452551+453551+459551	IL	GAR	ANG	GAR
720552	450552+451552+452552+453552+459552	IL	GAR	ANG	GAR
720553	450553+451553+452553+453553+459553	IL	GAR	ANG	GAR
720554	450554+451554+452554+453554+459554	IL	GAR	ANG	GAR
720555	450555+451555+452555+453555+459555	IL	GAR	ANG	GAR
720556	450556+451556+452556+453556+459556	IL	GAR	ANG	GAR
720557	450557+451557+452557+453557+459557	IL	GAR	ANG	GAR
720558	450558+451558+452558+453558+459558	IL	GAR	ANG	GAR
720559	450559+451559+452559+453559+459559	IL	GAR	ANG	GAR
720560	450560+451560+452560+453560+459560	IL	GAR	ANG	GAR
720561	450561+451561+452561+453561+459561	IL	GAR	ANG	GAR
720562	450562+451562+452562+453562+459562	IL	GAR	ANG	GAR
720563	450563+451563+452563+453563+459563	IL	GAR	ANG	GAR
720564	450564+451564+452564+453564+459564	IL	GAR	ANG	GAR
720565	450565+451565+452565+453565+459565	IL	GAR	ANG	GAR
720566	450566+451566+452566+453566+459566	IL	GAR	ANG	GAR
720567	450567+451567+452567+453567+459567	IL	GAR	ANG	GAR
720568	450568+451568+452568+453568+459568	IL	GAR	ANG	GAR
720569	450569+451569+452569+453569+459569	IL	GAR	ANG	GAR
720570	450570+451570+452570+453570+459570	IL	GAR	ANG	GAR
720571	450571+451571+452571+453571+459571	IL	GAR	ANG	GAR
720572	450572+451572+452572+453572+459572	IL	GAR	ANG	GAR
720573	450573+451573+452573+453573+459573	IL	GAR	ANG	GAR
720574	450574+451574+452574+453574+459574	IL	GAR	ANG	GAR
720575	450575+451575+452575+453575+459575	IL	GAR	ANG	GAR
720576	450576+451576+452576+453576+459576	IL	GAR	ANG	GAR
720577	450577+451577+452577+453577+459577	IL	GAR	ANG	GAR
720578	450578+451578+452578+453578+459578	IL	GAR	ANG	GAR
720579	450579+451579+452579+453579+459579	IL	GAR	ANG	GAR
720580	450580+451580+452580+453580+459580	IL	GAR	ANG	GAR
720581	450581+451581+452581+453581+459581	IL	GAR	ANG	GAR
720582	450582+451582+452582+453582+459582	IL	GAR	ANG	GAR
720583	450583+451583+452583+453583+459583	IL	GAR	ANG	GAR
720584	450584+451584+452584+453584+459584	IL	GAR	ANG	GAR
720585	450585+451585+452585+453585+459585	IL	GAR	ANG	GAR
720586	450586+451586+452586+453586+459586	IL	GAR	ANG	GAR
720587	450587+451587+452587+453587+459587	IL	GAR	ANG	GAR
720588	450588+451588+452588+453588+459588	IL	GAR	ANG	GAR
720589	450589+451589+452589+453589+459589	IL	GAR	ANG	GAR

720/6 Formation: DMS+PMS+MS+MS+DTS

720601	450601+451601+452601+453601+459601	EM	c2c	PTR	c2c
720602	450602+451602+452602+453602+459602	EM	c2c	PTR	c2c
720603	450603+451603+452603+453603+459603	EM	c2c	PTR	c2c
720604	450604+451604+452604+453604+459604	EM	c2c	PTR	c2c
720605	450605+451605+452605+453605+459605	EM	c2c	PTR	c2c
720606	450606+451606+452606+453606+459606	EM	c2c	PTR	c2c
720607	450607+451607+452607+453607+459607	EM	c2c	PTR	c2c
720608	450608+451608+452608+453608+459608	EM	c2c	PTR	c2c
720609	450609+451609+452609+453609+459609	EM	c2c	PTR	c2c
720610	450610+451610+452610+453610+459610	EM	c2c	PTR	c2c
720611	450611+451611+452611+453611+459611	EM	c2c	PTR	c2c
720612	450612+451612+452612+453612+459612	EM	c2c	PTR	c2c

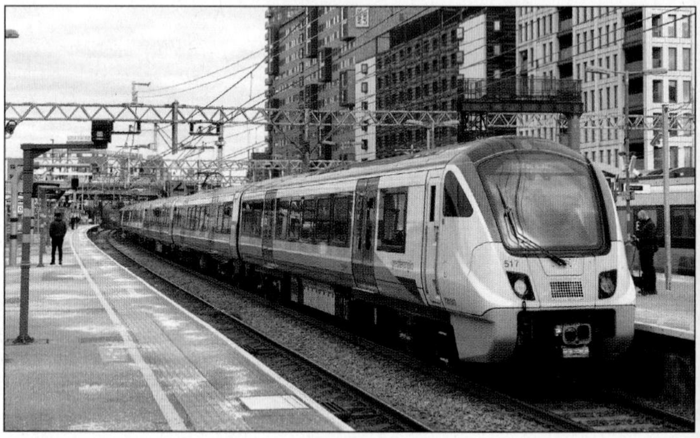

The slow delivery and commissioning of the Bombardier/Alstom Class 720 'Aventra' five-car sets for Greater Anglia is still ongoing in mid-2022, meaning a number of older classes have had to remain in service, such as the Class 317, 321, 322 and 379 fleets. By February 2022 deliveries were speeding up and dynamic testing of new sets was underway on the West Coast Main Line. Set No. 720517 is seen at Stratford on a Liverpool Street to Colchester North working. **CJM**

Class 730
Bombardier 3 and 5-car EMU Main Line 'Aventra'

Built: 2020-2021
Vehicle length: Driving 80ft 1in (24.47m)
Intermediate 79ft 5in (24.21m)
Height: 12ft 4in (3.87m)
Width: 9ft 1in (2.78m)
Power: 25kV ac overhead
Horsepower: 3-car 2,011hp (1,500kW)
5-car 3,352hp (2,500kW)
Transmission: Electric

730/0 Formation: DMS+PMS+DMS

730001	490001+492001+494001	WMR	COR	WMR
730002	490002+492002+494002	WMR	COR	WMR
730003	490003+492003+494003	WMR	COR	WMR
730004	490004+492004+494004	WMR	COR	WMR
730005	490005+492005+494005	WMR	COR	WMR
730006	490006+492006+494006	WMR	COR	WMR
730007	490007+492007+494007	WMR	COR	WMR
730008	490008+492008+494008	WMR	COR	WMR
730009	490009+492009+494009	WMR	COR	WMR
730010	490010+492010+494010	WMR	COR	WMR
730011	490011+492011+494011	WMR	COR	WMR
730012	490012+492012+494012	WMR	COR	WMR
730013	490013+492013+494013	WMR	COR	WMR
730014	490014+492014+494014	WMR	COR	WMR
730015	490015+492015+494015	WMR	COR	WMR
730016	490016+492016+494016	WMR	COR	WMR
730017	490017+492017+494017	WMR	COR	WMR
730018	490018+492018+494018	WMR	COR	WMR
730019	490019+492019+494019	WMR	COR	WMR
730020	490020+492020+494020	WMR	COR	WMR
730021	490021+492021+494021	WMR	COR	WMR
730022	490022+492022+494022	WMR	COR	WMR
730023	490023+492023+494023	WMR	COR	WMR
730024	490024+492024+494024	WMR	COR	WMR
730025	490025+492025+494025	WMR	COR	WMR
730026	490026+492026+494026	WMR	COR	WMR
730027	490027+492027+494027	WMR	COR	WMR
730028	490028+492028+494028	WMR	COR	WMR
730029	490029+492029+494029	WMR	COR	WMR

730030	490030+492030+494030	WMR	COR	WMR
730031	490031+492031+494031	WMR	COR	WMR
730032	490032+492032+494032	WMR	COR	WMR
730033	490033+492033+494033	WMR	COR	WMR
730034	490034+492034+494034	WMR	COR	WMR
730035	490035+492035+494035	WMR	COR	WMR
730036	490036+492036+494036	WMR	COR	WMR

730/1 Formation: DMC+MS+PMS+MS+DMS

730101	490101+491101+492101+493101+494101	LNW	COR	WMR
730102	490102+491102+492102+493102+494102	LNW	COR	WMR
730103	490103+491103+492103+493103+494103	LNW	COR	WMR
730104	490104+491104+492104+493104+494104	LNW	COR	WMR
730105	490105+491105+492105+493105+494105	LNW	COR	WMR
730106	490106+491106+492106+493106+494106	LNW	COR	WMR
730107	490107+491107+492107+493107+494107	LNW	COR	WMR
730108	490108+491108+492108+493108+494108	LNW	COR	WMR
730109	490109+491109+492109+493109+494109	LNW	COR	WMR
730110	490110+491110+492110+493110+494110	LNW	COR	WMR
730111	490111+491111+492111+493111+494111	LNW	COR	WMR
730112	490112+491112+492112+493112+494112	LNW	COR	WMR
730113	490113+491113+492113+493113+494113	LNW	COR	WMR
730114	490114+491114+492114+493114+494114	LNW	COR	WMR
730115	490115+491115+492115+493115+494115	LNW	COR	WMR
730116	490116+491116+492116+493116+494116	LNW	COR	WMR
730117	490117+491117+492117+493117+494117	LNW	COR	WMR
730118	490118+491118+492118+493119+494118	LNW	COR	WMR
730119	490119+491119+492119+493119+494119	LNW	COR	WMR
730120	490120+491120+492120+493120+494120	LNW	COR	WMR
730121	490121+491121+492121+493121+494121	LNW	COR	WMR
730122	490122+491122+492122+493122+494122	LNW	COR	WMR
730123	490123+491123+492123+493123+494123	LNW	COR	WMR
730124	490124+491124+492124+493124+494124	LNW	COR	WMR
730125	490125+491125+492125+493125+494125	LNW	COR	WMR
730126	490126+491126+492126+493126+494126	LNW	COR	WMR
730127	490127+491127+492127+493127+494127	LNW	COR	WMR
730128	490128+491128+492128+493128+494128	LNW	COR	WMR
730129	490129+491129+492129+493129+494129	LNW	COR	WMR

730/2 Formation: DMC+MS+PMS+MS+DMS

730201	490201+491201+492201+493201+494201	LNW	COR	WMR
730202	490202+491202+492202+493202+494202	LNW	COR	WMR
730203	490203+491203+492203+493203+494203	LNW	COR	WMR
730204	490204+491204+492204+493204+494204	LNW	COR	WMR
730205	490205+491205+492205+493205+494205	LNW	COR	WMR
730206	490206+491206+492206+493206+494206	LNW	COR	WMR
730207	490207+491207+492207+493207+494207	LNW	COR	WMR
730208	490208+491208+492208+493208+494208	LNW	COR	WMR
730209	490209+491209+492209+493209+494209	LNW	COR	WMR
730210	490210+491210+492210+493210+494210	LNW	COR	WMR
730211	490211+491211+492211+493211+494211	LNW	COR	WMR
730212	490212+491212+492212+493212+494212	LNW	COR	WMR
730213	490213+491213+492213+493213+494213	LNW	COR	WMR
730214	490214+491214+492214+493214+494214	LNW	COR	WMR
730215	490215+491215+492215+493215+494215	LNW	COR	WMR
730216	490216+491216+492216+493216+494216	LNW	COR	WMR

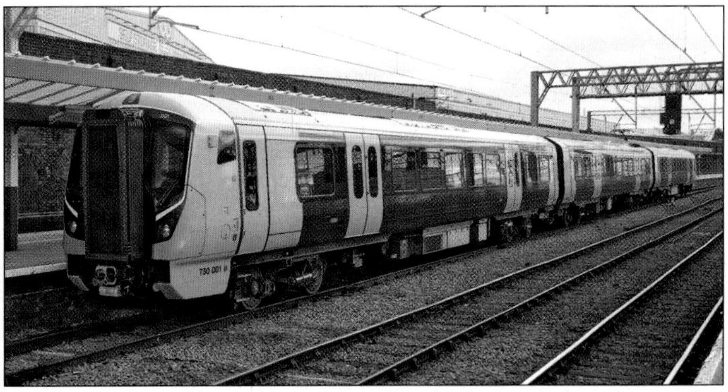

The Class 730 three and five car 'Aventra' sets for West Midlands are in the early stages of delivery and testing, which looks to be a long and drawn out affair. Three car gold and purple Class 730/0 No. 730001 is seen stabled at Crewe on 8 November 2021. **Antony Christie**

Class 745
Stadler 12-car EMU Main Line 'Flirt'

Built: 2019-2020
Train length: 776ft 4in (236.6m)
Height: 13ft 0in (3.95m)
Width: 8ft 11in (2.72m)
Power: 25kV ac overhead
Horsepower: 6,973hp (5,200kW)
Transmission: Electric

745/0 Formation: DMF+PTF+TS+TS+TS+MS+MS+TS+TS+TS+PTS+DMS - InterCity sets

745001	413001+426001+332001+343001+341001+301001+302001+342001+344001+346001+322001+312001	NC	GAR	ROK	GAR
745002	413002+426002+332002+334002+341002+301002+302002+342002+344002+346002+322002+312002	NC	GAR	ROK	GAR
745003	413003+426003+332003+343003+341003+301003+302003+342003+344003+346003+322003+312003	NC	GAR	ROK	GAR
745004	413004+426004+332004+343004+341004+301004+302004+342004+344004+346004+322004+312004	NC	GAR	ROK	GAR
745005	413005+426005+332005+343005+341005+301005+302005+342005+344005+346005+322005+312005	NC	GAR	ROK	GAR
745006	413006+426006+332006+343006+341006+301006+302006+342006+344006+346006+322006+312006	NC	GAR	ROK	GAR
745007	413007+426007+332007+343007+341007+301007+302007+342007+344007+346007+322007+312007	NC	GAR	ROK	GAR
745008	413008+426008+332008+343008+341008+301008+302008+342008+344008+346008+322008+312008	NC	GAR	ROK	GAR
745009	413009+426009+332009+343009+341009+301009+302009+342009+344009+346009+322009+312009	NC	GAR	ROK	GAR
745010	413010+426010+332010+343010+341010+301010+302010+342010+344010+346010+322010+312010	NC	GAR	ROK	GAR

The total route modernisation and complete replacement of trains on the Greater Anglia network saw two major fleets of 12-car Class 745 Stadler 'Flirt' units built. To operate the main line Liverpool Street to Norwich service, 12 high-quality Class 745/0 sets with first class seating were built. Usually the first class seating is located at the London end of the train. Set No. 745002 is shown heading south near Needham Market on 16 September 2021. **CJM**

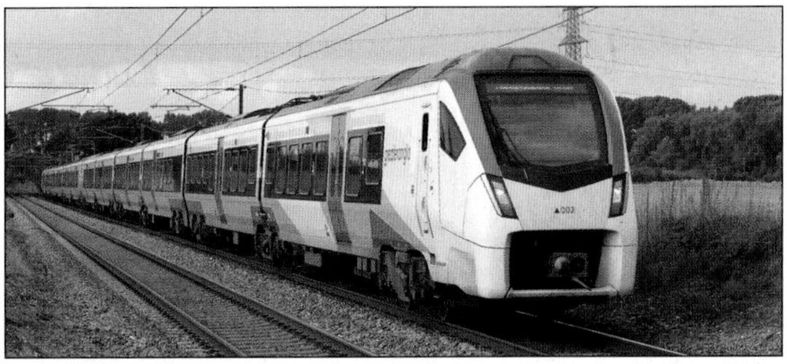

745/1 Formation: DMS+PTS+TS+TS+TS+MS+MS+TS+TS+TS+PTS+DMS - Stansted Express sets

745101	313001+326101+332101+343101+341101+301101+302101+342101+344101+346101+322101+312101	NC	GAR	ROK	GAR
745102	313002+326102+332102+343102+341102+301102+302102+342102+344102+346102+322102+312102	NC	GAR	ROK	GAR
745103	313003+326103+332103+343103+341103+301103+302103+342103+344103+346103+322103+312103	NC	GAR	ROK	GAR
745104	313004+326104+332104+343104+341104+301104+302104+342104+344104+346104+322104+312104	NC	GAR	ROK	GAR
745105	313005+326105+332105+343105+341105+301105+302105+342105+344105+346105+322105+312105	NC	GAR	ROK	GAR
745106	313006+326106+332106+343106+341106+301106+302106+342106+344106+346106+322106+312106	NC	GAR	ROK	GAR
745107	313007+326107+332107+343107+341107+301107+302107+342107+344107+346107+322107+312107	NC	GAR	ROK	GAR
745108	313008+326108+332108+343108+341108+301108+302108+342108+344108+346108+322108+312108	NC	GAR	ROK	GAR
745109	313009+326109+332109+343109+341109+301109+302109+342109+344109+346109+322109+312109	NC	GAR	ROK	GAR
745110	313010+326110+332110+343110+341110+301110+302110+342110+344110+346110+322110+312110	NC	GAR	ROK	GAR

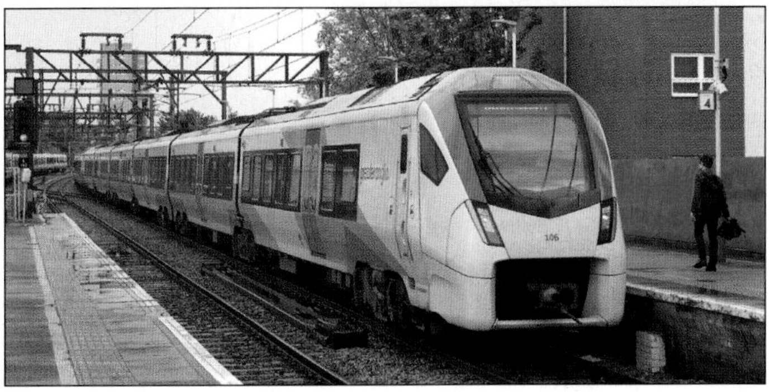

To operate the Stansted Express service between Liverpool Street and Stansted Airport, a fleet of 10 Class 745/1 sets were built, technically the same as the Class 745/0s but with all standard class seating and extra luggage stacks for airport passengers. A slightly different livery was applied. Sets of both sub-class are based at Norwich, seeing the Stansted sets used on some Norwich-London duties for stock balancing purposes. Set No. 745106 is seen passing Hackney Downs. **CJM**

Class 755
Stadler 3 and 4-car BMU Main Line 'Flirt'

Built: 2019-2020
Vehicle length: Driving 74ft 3in (20.81m)
Intermediate 50ft 0in (15.22m)
Power Pack 21ft 9in (6.69m)
Height: awaited
Width: 9ft 1in (2.78m)
Power: 25kV ac overhead or diesel
Horsepower: 3-car 1,287hp (960kW)
4-car 2,575hp (1,920kW)
Transmission: Electric

755/3 Formation: DMS+PP+PTSW+DMS

755325	911325+971325+981325+912325	NC	GAR	ROK	GAR
755326	911326+971326+981326+912326	NC	GAR	ROK	GAR
755327	911327+971327+981327+912327	NC	GAR	ROK	GAR
755328	911328+971328+981328+912328	NC	GAR	ROK	GAR
755329	911329+971329+981329+912329	NC	GAR	ROK	GAR
755330	911330+971330+981330+912330	NC	GAR	ROK	GAR
755331	911331+971331+981331+912331	NC	GAR	ROK	GAR
755332	911332+971332+981332+912332	NC	GAR	ROK	GAR
755333	911333+971333+981333+912333	NC	GAR	ROK	GAR
755334	911334+971334+981334+912334	NC	GAR	ROK	GAR
755335	911335+971335+981335+912335	NC	GAR	ROK	GAR
755336	911336+971336+981336+912336	NC	GAR	ROK	GAR
755337	911337+971337+981337+912337	NC	GAR	ROK	GAR
755338	911338+971338+981338+912338	NC	GAR	ROK	GAR

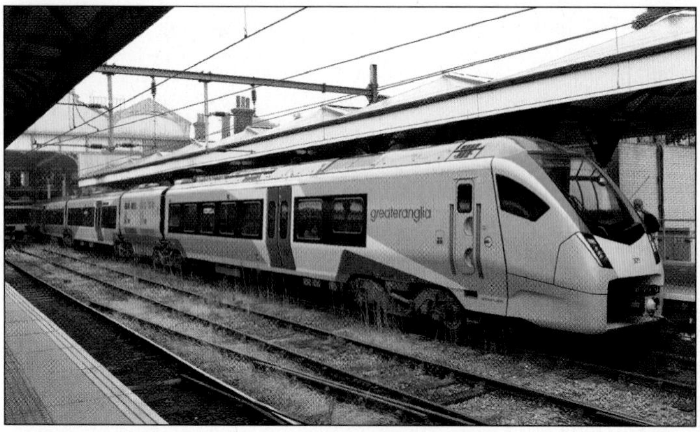

For regional operations Great Anglia operate two sub-classes of Class 755 Stadler 'Flirt'. The 14 three-car sets of Class 755/3 have two driving cars, one intermediate passenger coach and a power pack car. Set No. 755329 is seen at Norwich station with a service to Cromer. **CJM**

755/4 Formation: DMS+PTS+PP+PTSW+DMS

755401	911401+961401+971401+981401+912401	NC	GAR	ROK	GAR
755402	911402+961402+971402+981402+912402	NC	GAR	ROK	GAR
755403	911403+961403+971403+981403+912403	NC	GAR	ROK	GAR
755404	911404+961404+971404+981404+912404	NC	GAR	ROK	GAR
755405	911405+961405+971405+981405+912405	NC	GAR	ROK	GAR
755406	911406+961406+971406+981406+912406	NC	GAR	ROK	GAR
755407	911407+961407+971407+981407+912407	NC	GAR	ROK	GAR
755408	911408+961408+971408+981408+912408	NC	GAR	ROK	GAR
755409	911409+961409+971409+981409+912409	NC	GAR	ROK	GAR
755410	911410+961410+971410+981410+912410	NC	GAR	ROK	GAR
755411	911411+961411+971411+981411+912411	NC	GAR	ROK	GAR
755412	911412+961412+971412+981412+912412	NC	GAR	ROK	GAR
755413	911413+961413+971413+981413+912413	NC	GAR	ROK	GAR
755414	911414+961414+971414+981414+912414	NC	GAR	ROK	GAR
755415	911415+961415+971415+981415+912415	NC	GAR	ROK	GAR
755416	911416+961416+971416+981416+912416	NC	GAR	ROK	GAR
755417	911417+961417+971417+981417+912417	NC	GAR	ROK	GAR
755418	911418+961418+971418+981418+912418	NC	GAR	ROK	GAR
755419	911419+961419+971419+981419+912419	NC	GAR	ROK	GAR
755420	911420+961420+971420+981420+912420	NC	GAR	ROK	GAR
755421	911421+961421+971421+981421+912421	NC	GAR	ROK	GAR
755422	911422+961422+971422+981422+912422	NC	GAR	ROK	GAR
755423	911423+961423+971423+981423+912423	NC	GAR	ROK	GAR
755424	911424+961424+971424+981424+912424	NC	GAR	ROK	GAR

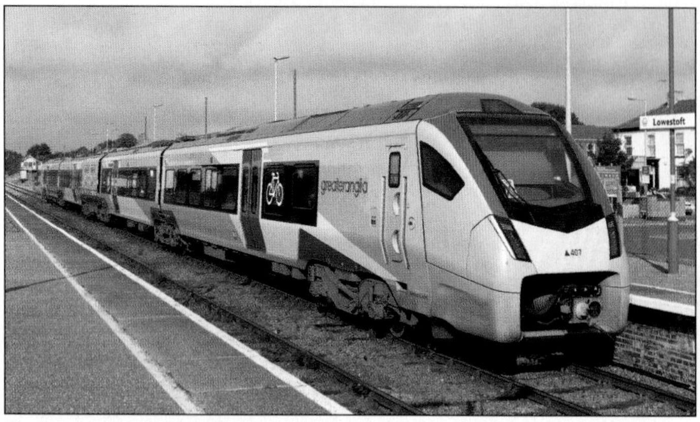

The four-car Class 755s of sub-class 755/4 have the power-pack vehicle in the middle, these vehicles are slightly wider than the passenger coaches. Set No. 755407 is seen departing from Lowestoft to Norwich on 17 September 2021. The cycle area on these sets is identified by a blue cant rail band and the disabled area by a green band. **CJM**

Class 756
Stadler 3 and 4-car TMU Main Line 'Flirt'

Built: 2021-2022
Vehicle length: Driving 74ft 3in (20.81m)
Intermediate 50ft 0in (15.22m)
Power Pack 21ft 9in (6.69m)
Height: awaited
Width: 9ft 1in (2.78m)
Power: 25kV ac overhead, diesel or battery
Horsepower: 3-car 1,287hp (960kW)
4-car 2,575hp (1,920kW)
Transmission: Electric

756/0 Formation: DMS+PP+PTS+DMS

756001	911001+971001+981001+912001	CV	TFW	SMB	TFW
756002	911002+971002+981002+912002	CV	TFW	SMB	TFW
756003	911003+971003+981003+912003	CV	TFW	SMB	TFW
756004	911004+971004+981004+912004	CV	TFW	SMB	TFW
756005	911005+971005+981005+912005	CV	TFW	SMB	TFW
756006	911006+971006+981006+912006	CV	TFW	SMB	TFW
756007	911007+971007+981007+912007	CV	TFW	SMB	TFW

756/1 Formation: DMS+PTS+PP+PTS+DMS

756101	911101+961101+971101+981101+912101	CV	TFW	SMB	TFW
756102	911102+961102+971102+981102+912102	CV	TFW	SMB	TFW
756103	911103+961103+971103+981103+912103	CV	TFW	SMB	TFW
756104	911104+961104+971104+981104+912104	CV	TFW	SMB	TFW
756105	911105+961105+971105+981105+912105	CV	TFW	SMB	TFW
756106	911106+961106+971106+981106+912106	CV	TFW	SMB	TFW
756107	911107+961107+971107+981107+912107	CV	TFW	SMB	TFW
756108	911108+961108+971108+981108+912108	CV	TFW	SMB	TFW
756109	911109+961109+971109+981109+912109	CV	TFW	SMB	TFW
756110	911110+961110+971110+981110+912110	CV	TFW	SMB	TFW
756111	911111+961111+971111+981111+912111	CV	TFW	SMB	TFW
756112	911112+961112+971112+981112+912112	CV	TFW	SMB	TFW
756113	911113+961113+971113+981113+912113	CV	TFW	SMB	TFW
756114	911114+961114+971114+981114+912114	CV	TFW	SMB	TFW
756115	911115+961115+971115+981115+912115	CV	TFW	SMB	TFW
756116	911116+961116+971116+981116+912116	CV	TFW	SMB	TFW
756117	911117+961117+971117+981117+912117	CV	TFW	SMB	TFW

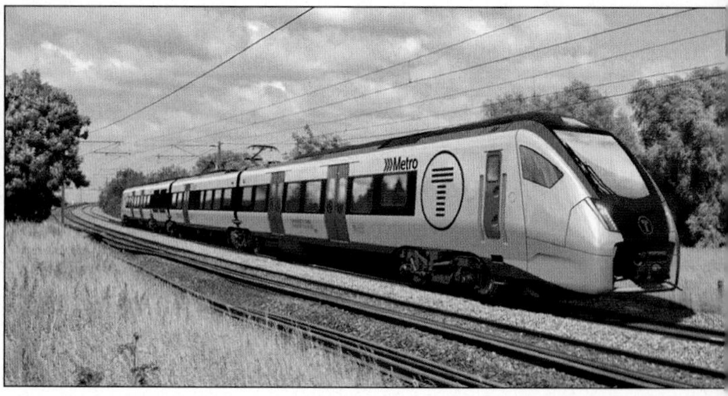

The first three and four passenger vehicle Class 756 sets for Transport for Wales are currently under construction in Switzerland. These are very much in line with the Class 755 Greater Anglia sets already in service and each will house a short wheelbase 'power pack' vehicle. From the Artist's impression, these sets will carry a TfW Metro livery. **TfW**

Class 768
Wabtec/Porterbrook 4-car BMU

Built: 2021-2022 (as 319s 1987-1990
Vehicle length: Driving - 65ft 0¾in (19.83m)
Intermediate - 65ft 4¼in (19.92m)
Height: 11ft 9in (3.58m)
Width: 9ft 3in (2.82m)
Power: 25kW ac overhead or diesel 2 x MAN D2876 LUE531 of 523hp (390kV)
Horsepower: 1,438hp (1,072kW)
Transmission: Electric

Formation: DTPMV+MPMV+TPMV+DTPMV

768001	(319010)	77309+62900+71781+77308	ZG	ORI	PTR	ROG
768002	(319011)	77311+62901+71782+77310	ZG	ORI	PTR	ROG
768003	(319009)	77307+62899+71780+77306	ZG	ORI	PTR	ROG

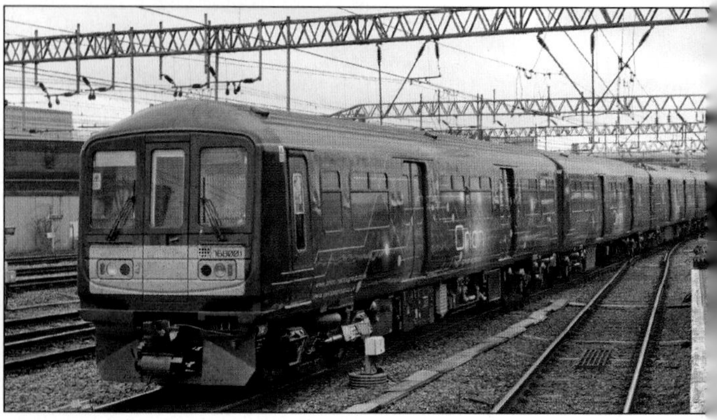

The Class 319 bi-mode conversions for the ROG Orion project have been reclassified as 768. These sets can operate from the 25kV ac overhead or diesel engines under both driving cars. Painted in orion livery, set No. 768001 is seen at Crewe, this set was modified from Class 319 No. 319010 **Spencer Conquest**

Class 769
Wabtec/Porterbrook 4-car BMU

Built: 2018-2020 (as 319s 1987-1990
Vehicle length: Driving - 65ft 0¾in (19.83m)
Intermediate - 65ft 4¼in (19.92m)
Height: 11ft 9in (3.58m)
Width: 9ft 3in (2.82m)

Power: 25kW ac overhead or diesel 2 x MAN D2876 LUE531 of 523hp (390kV), 769/9 also 750V dc
TfW sets diesel only
Horsepower: 1,438hp (1,072kW)
Transmission: Electric

769/0 Formation: DTS+MS+TS+DTS

769002	(319002)	77293+62892+71773+77292	CV	TFW	PTR	TFW
769003	(319003)	77295+62893+71774+77294	CV	TFW	PTR	TFW
769006	(319006)	77301+62896+71777+77300	CV	TFW	PTR	TFW
769007	(319007)	77303+62897+71778+77302	CV	TFW	PTR	TFW
769008	(319008)	77305+62898+71779+77304	CV	TFW	PTR	TFW

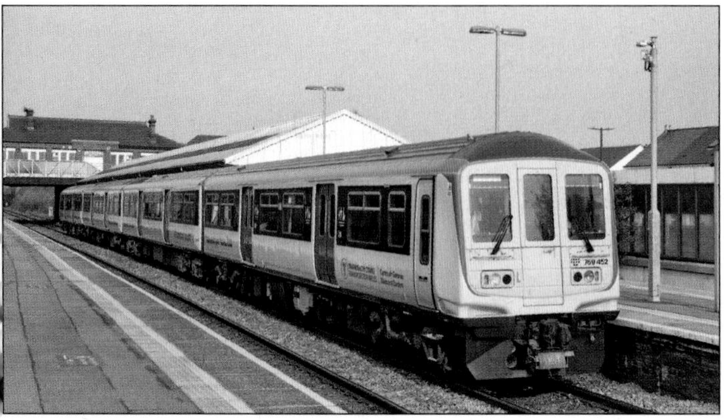

The Class 769 conversion project from Class 319 EMUs to dual power trains has been a major undertaking, with the technical work including the fitting of the diesel engine/alternator raft below the driving trailer vehicles undertaken at the Wabtec Loughborough (former Brush) site. Internal upgrade work has been undertaken at Wolverton Works. Transport for Wales was the first operator to introduce the stock. Set No. 769452 is seen in the above image at Caerphilly, below is detail of the engine/alternator below the driving car. Both: **CJM**

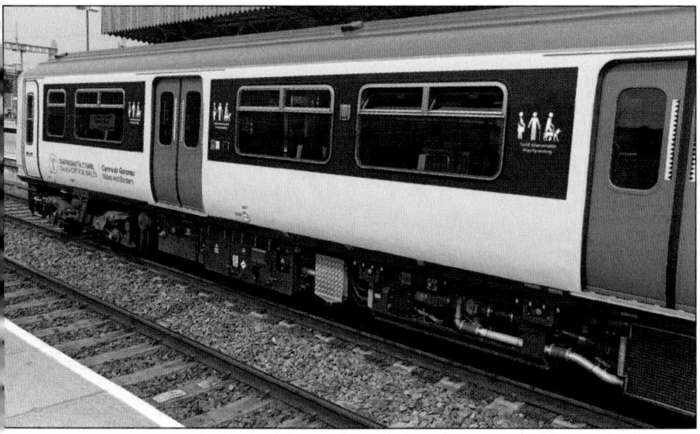

769/4 Formation: DTS+MS+TS+DTS

769421	(319421)	77331+62911+71792+77330	CV	TFW	PTR	TFW
769426	(319426)	77341+62916+71797+77340	CV	TFW	PTR	TFW
769424	(319424)	77337+62914+71795+77336	AN	NNR	PTR	NOR
769431	(319431)	77351+62921+71802+77350	AN	NNR	PTR	NOR
769434	(319434)	77357+62924+71805+77356	AN	NNR	PTR	NOR
769442	(319442)	77373+62932+71813+77372	AN	NNR	PTR	NOR
769445	(319445)	77379+62935+71816+77378	CV	TFW	PTR	TFW
769448	(319448)	77433+62962+71867+77432	AN	NNR	PTR	NOR
769450	(319450)	77437+62964+71869+77436	AN	NNR	PTR	NOR
769452	(319452)	77441+62966+71871+77440	CV	TFW	PTR	TFW
769456	(319456)	77449+62970+71875+77448	AN	NNR	PTR	NOR
769458	(319458)	77453+62972+71877+77452	AN	NNR	PTR	NOR

769/9 Formation: DTS+MS+TS+DTS

769922	(319422)	77333+62912+71793+77332	RG	GWG	PTR	GWR
769923	(319423)	77335+62913+71794+77334	RG	GWG	PTR	GWR
769925	(319425)	77339+62915+71796+77338	RG	GWG	PTR	GWR
769927	(319427)	77343+62917+71798+77342	RG	GWG	PTR	GWR
769928	(319428)	77345+62918+71799+77344	RG	GWG	PTR	GWR
769930	(319430)	77349+62920+71801+77348	RG	GWG	PTR	GWR
769932	(319432)	77353+62922+71803+77352	RG	GWG	PTR	GWR
769935	(319435)	77359+62925+71806+77358	RG	GWG	PTR	GWR
769936	(319436)	77361+62926+71807+77360	RG	GWG	PTR	GWR
769937	(319437)	77363+62927+71808+77362	RG	GWG	PTR	GWR
769938	(319438)	77365+62928+71809+77364	RG	GWG	PTR	GWR
769939	(319439)	77367+62929+71810+77366	RG	GWG	PTR	GWR
769940	(319440)	77369+62930+71811+77368	RG	GWG	PTR	GWR
769943	(319443)	77375+62933+71814+77374	RG	GWG	PTR	GWR
769944	(319444)	77377+62934+71815+77376	RG	GWG	PTR	GWR
769946	(319446)	77381+62936+71817+77380	RG	GWG	PTR	GWR
769947	(319447)	77431+62961+71866+77430	RG	GWG	PTR	GWR
769949	(319449)	77435+62963+71868+77434	RG	GWG	PTR	GWR
769959	(319459)	77455+62973+71878+77454	RG	GWG	PTR	GWR

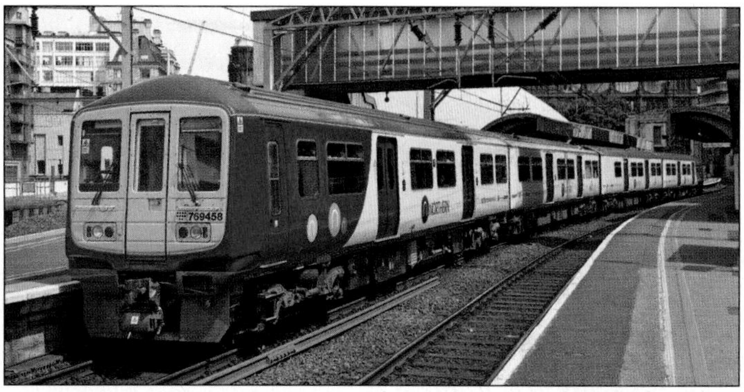

Northern operate a fleet of eight Class 769s, based at Allerton and used on Southport to Manchester services via Bolton, using both forms of power, diesel and electric. Set No. 769458 poses at Manchester Oxford Road. A restriction was imposed in May 2022 that Northern sets were to use diesel power only **CJM**

A fleet of 19 Class 769/9s are being delivered to Great Western at Reading for Thames Valley and Gatwick Airport services. These sets have received a heavier rebuilt and now sport first class seating, the ability to operate on either dc or ac power supply and incorporate a high-level marker light on the front end. Set No. 769959 (the original 319459 is seen under test at Didcot. **Spencer Conquest**

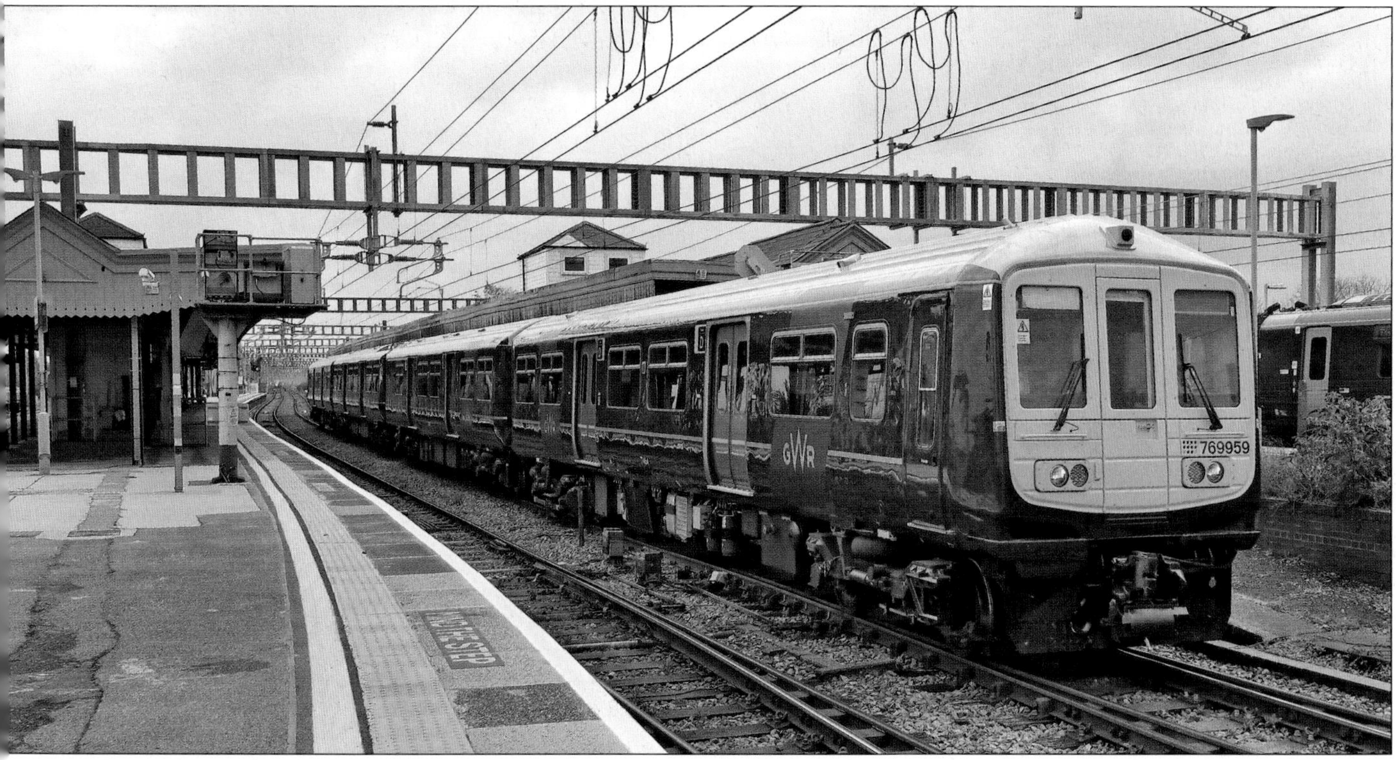

Class 777
Stadler 4-car EMU Metro

Built: 2020-2021
Vehicle length: Driving - 62ft 3in (19.0m)
Intermediate - 44ft 7in (13.6m)
Height: 12ft 6in (3.82m)
Width: 9ft 3in (2.82m)
Power: 750V dc third rail
Horsepower: 2,820hp (2,100kW)
Transmission: Electric

	Formation: DMS+MS+MS+DMS				
777001	427001+428001+429001+430001	KK	MEZ	LIV	MER
777002	427002+428002+429002+430002	KK	MEZ	LIV	MER
777003	427003+428003+429003+430003	KK	MEZ	LIV	MER
777004	427004+428004+429004+430004	KK	MEZ	LIV	MER
777005	427005+428005+429005+430005	KK	MEZ	LIV	MER
777006	427006+428006+429006+430006	KK	MEZ	LIV	MER
777007	427007+428007+429007+430007	KK	MEZ	LIV	MER
777008	427008+428008+429008+430008	KK	MEZ	LIV	MER
777009	427009+428009+429009+430009	KK	MEZ	LIV	MER
777010	427010+428010+429010+430010	KK	MEZ	LIV	MER
777011	427011+428011+429011+430011	KK	MEZ	LIV	MER
777012	427012+428012+429012+430012	KK	MEZ	LIV	MER
777013	427013+428013+429013+430013	KK	MEZ	LIV	MER
777014	427014+428014+429014+430014	KK	MEZ	LIV	MER
777015	427015+428015+429015+430015	KK	MEZ	LIV	MER
777016	427016+428016+429016+430016	KK	MEZ	LIV	MER
777017	427017+428017+429017+430017	KK	MEZ	LIV	MER
777018	427018+428018+429018+430018	KK	MEZ	LIV	MER
777019	427019+428019+429019+430019	KK	MEZ	LIV	MER
777020	427020+428020+429020+430020	KK	MEZ	LIV	MER
777021	427021+428021+429021+430021	KK	MEZ	LIV	MER
777022	427022+428022+429022+430022	KK	MEZ	LIV	MER
777023	427023+428023+429023+430023	KK	MEZ	LIV	MER
777024	427024+428024+429024+430024	KK	MEZ	LIV	MER
777025	427025+428025+429025+430025	KK	MEZ	LIV	MER
777026	427026+428026+429026+430026	KK	MEZ	LIV	MER
777027	427027+428027+429027+430027	KK	MEZ	LIV	MER
777028	427028+428028+429028+430028	KK	MEZ	LIV	MER
777029	427029+428029+429029+430029	KK	MEZ	LIV	MER
777030	427030+428030+429030+430030	KK	MEZ	LIV	MER
777031	427031+428031+429031+430031	KK	MEZ	LIV	MER
777032	427032+428032+429032+430032	KK	MEZ	LIV	MER
777033	427033+428033+429033+430033	KK	MEZ	LIV	MER
777034	427034+428034+429034+430034	KK	MEZ	LIV	MER
777035	427035+428035+429035+430035	KK	MEZ	LIV	MER
777036	427036+428036+429036+430036	KK	MEZ	LIV	MER
777037	427037+428037+429037+430037	KK	MEZ	LIV	MER
777038	427038+428038+429038+430038	KK	MEZ	LIV	MER
777039	427039+428039+429039+430039	KK	MEZ	LIV	MER
777040	427040+428040+429040+430040	KK	MEZ	LIV	MER
777041	427041+428041+429041+430041	KK	MEZ	LIV	MER
777042	427042+428042+429042+430042	KK	MEZ	LIV	MER
777043	427043+428043+429043+430043	KK	MEZ	LIV	MER
777044	427044+428044+429044+430044	KK	MEZ	LIV	MER
777045	427045+428045+429045+430045	KK	MEZ	LIV	MER
777046	427046+428046+429046+430046	KK	MEZ	LIV	MER
777047	427047+428047+429047+430047	KK	MEZ	LIV	MER
777048	427048+428048+429048+430048	KK	MEZ	LIV	MER
777049	427049+428049+429049+430049	KK	MEZ	LIV	MER
777050	427050+428050+429050+430050	KK	MEZ	LIV	MER
777051	427051+428051+429051+430051	KK	MEZ	LIV	MER
777052	427052+428052+429052+430052	KK	MEZ	LIV	MER
777053	427053+428053+429053+430053	KK	MEZ	LIV	MER

777040/042/044/046/048/050/053 to have traction batteries

Class 799
Porterbrook 4-car 'HydroFlex' development unit

Introduced: 2019-2021
Vehicle length: Driving - 65ft 0¾in (19.83m)
Intermediate - 65ft 4¼in (19.92m)
Height: 11ft 9in (3.58m)
Width: 9ft 3in (2.82m)
Power: Hydrogen Fuel Cell / 25kV ac overhead
Horsepower: 1,438hp (1,072kW)
Transmission: Electric

		Formation: DTSO(A)+PMSO+TSOL+DTSO(B)				
799001	(319001)	77291+62891+71772+77290 (disbanded)	LM	SPL	PTR	PTR
799201	(319382)	77975+63094+71980+77976	LM	SPL	PTR	PTR

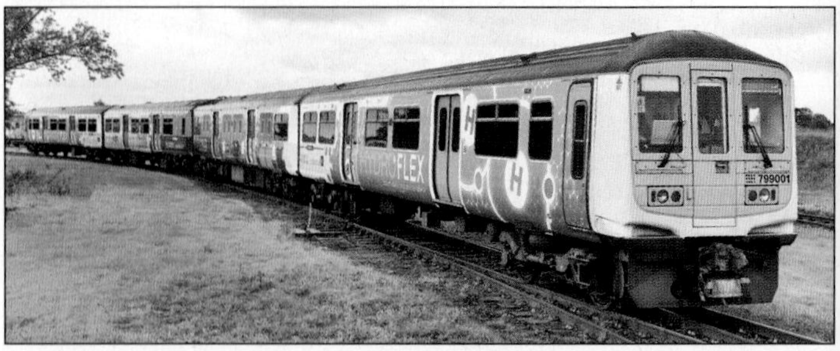

Porterbrook are one of the industry leaders in the development of hydrogen power technology. They originally converted ex Class 319 No. 319001 into a test bed, installing hydrogen fuel cell equipment inside the MSO. This set was renumbered as 799001 and is illustrated above It is now disbanded. In 2021 a second more advanced hydrogen test train was launched, 799201, rebuilt from Class 319 No. 319382, this had its hydrogen cell and storage tanks housed in the DTSO(A). In the below images, the set is seen from the hydrogen car in the upper image and the standard DTSO in the lower in Glasgow during demonstration runs at COP26 in November 2021. All: **CJM**

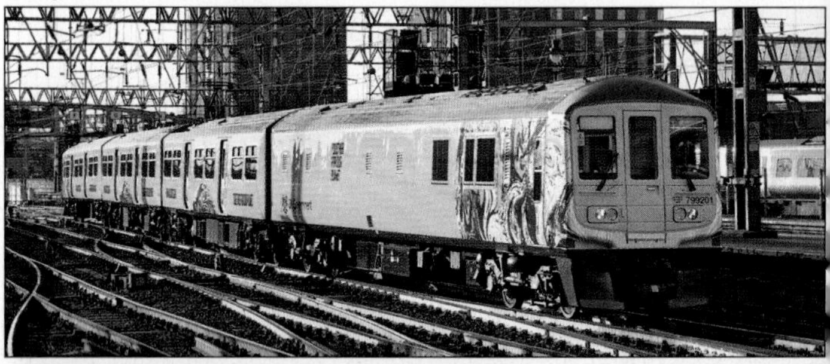

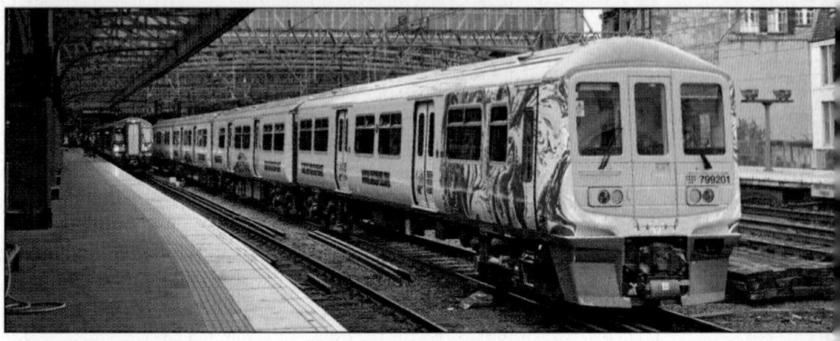

Stadler Class 777 four-car sets for Merseyrail are still under commissioning with only a handful of the 53 trains ordered so far delivered. Set No. 777014 is captured at Higgs Hill near Formby on 26 August 2021 with a test run rom Southport to Sandhills. **David Shore**

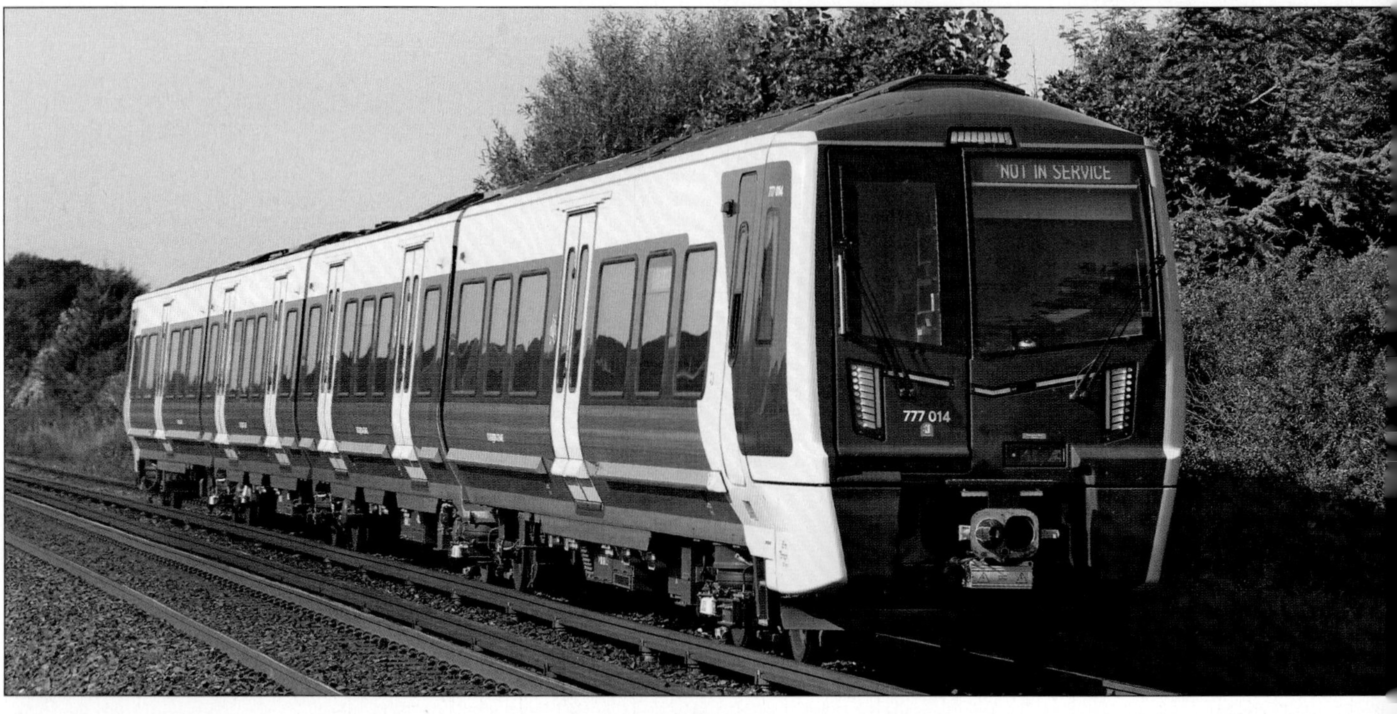

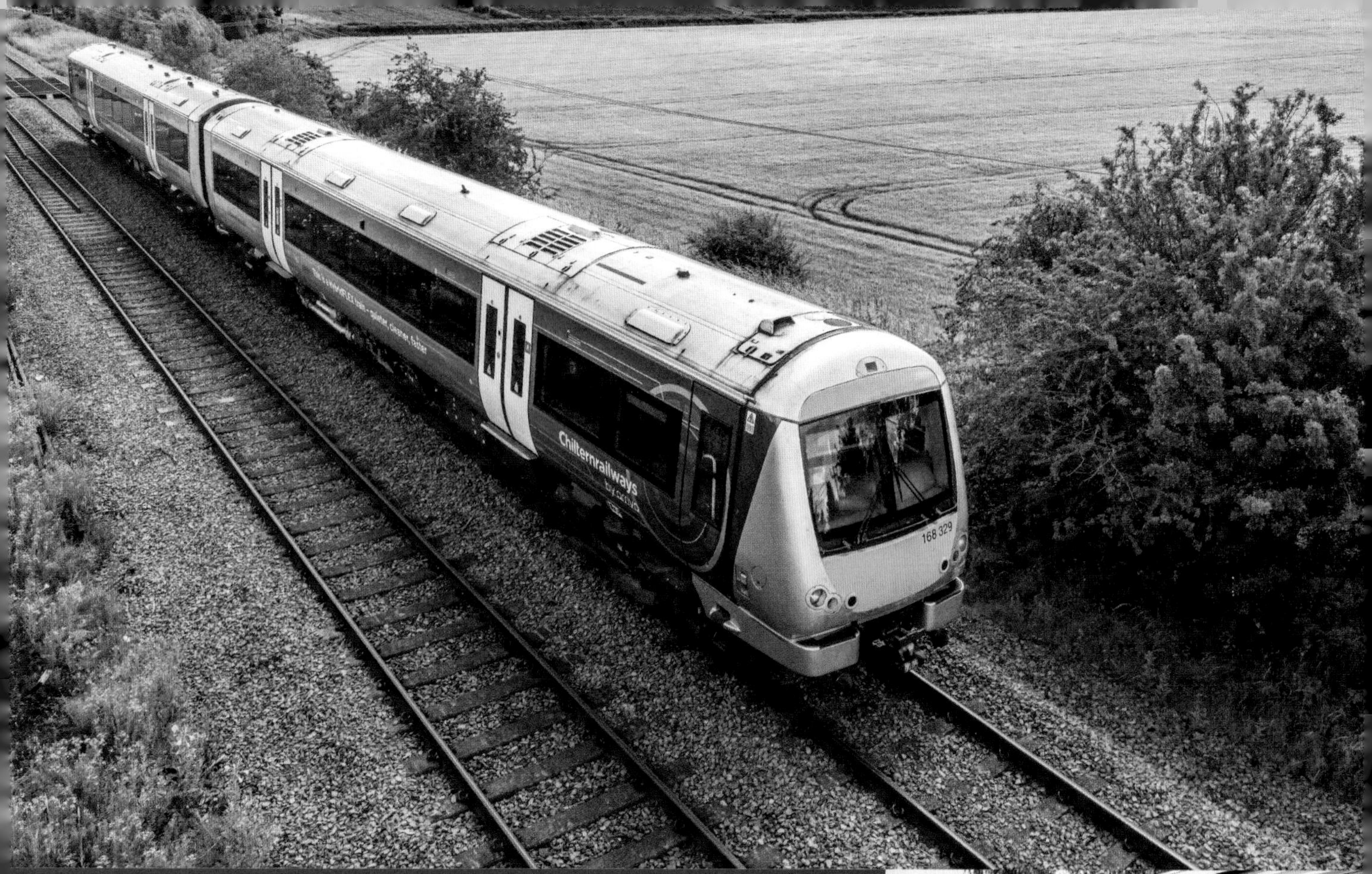
Chilternrailways
168 329

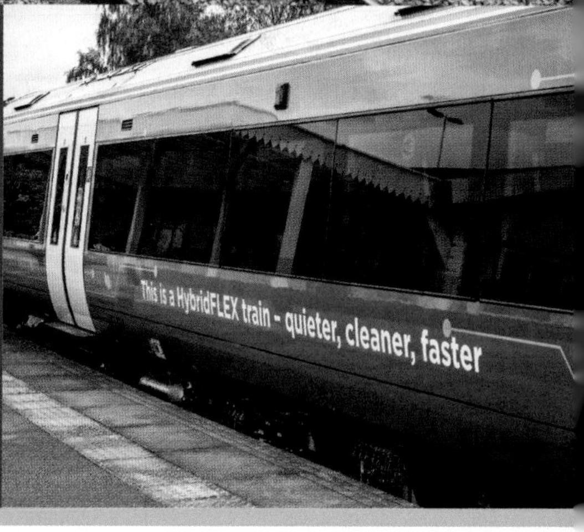
This is a HybridFLEX train - quieter, cleaner, faster

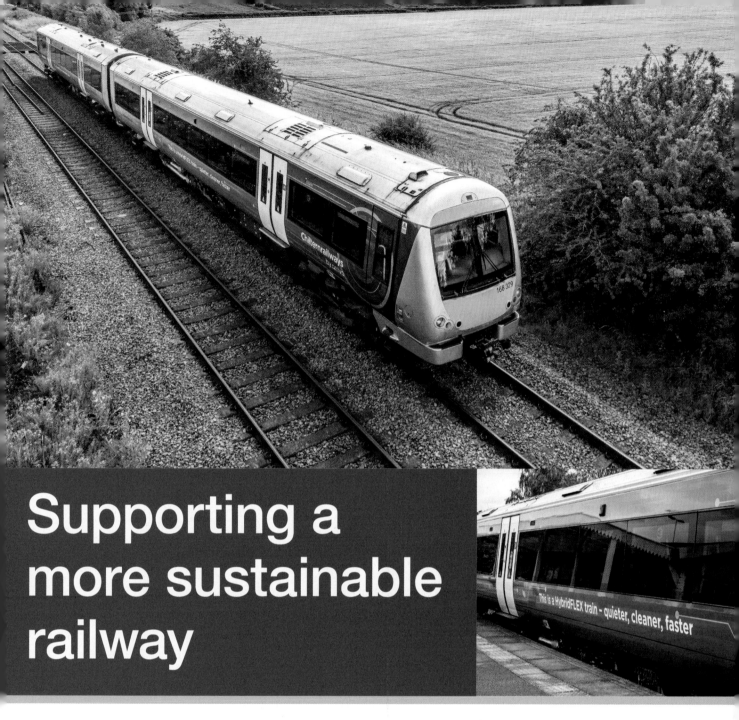

Class 800
Hitachi IET 5 or 9-car BMU Inter City (AT300)

Built: 2013-2020
Vehicle length: Driving 83ft 2in (25.35m)
Intermediate 82ft 0in (25.0m)
Height: 11ft 8in (3.62m)
Width: 8ft 10in (2.7m)

Power: 25kV ac overhead or MTU 1600R80L
Horsepower: 5-car 3,637hp (2,712kW)
9-car 6,062hp (4,520kW)
Transmission: Electric

800/0 Formation: PDTS+MS+MS+MC+PDTRF

800001	811001+812001+813001+814001+815001		NP	GWG	AGT	GWR
800002	811002+812002+813002+814002+815002		NP	GWG	AGT	GWR
800003	811003+812003+813003+814003+815003	*Queen Victoria/Queen Elizabeth II*	NP	GWG	AGT	GWR
800004	811004+812004+813004+814004+815004		NP	GWG	AGT	GWR
800005	811005+812005+813005+814005+815005		NP	GWG	AGT	GWR
800006	811006+812006+813006+814006+815006	*Tulbahadur Pun VC*	NP	GWG	AGT	GWR
800007	811007+812007+813007+814007+815007		NP	GWG	AGT	GWR
800008	811008+812008+813008+814008+815008	*Alan Turing*	NP	GWG	AGT	GWR
800009	811009+812009+813009+814009+815009	*Sir Gareth Edwards / John Charles*	NP	SPL	AGT	GWR
800010	811010+812010+813010+814010+815010	*Michael Bond / Paddington Bear*	NP	GWG	AGT	GWR
800011	811011+812011+813011+814011+815011		NP	GWG	AGT	GWR
800012	811012+812012+813012+814012+815012		NP	GWG	AGT	GWR
800013	811013+812013+813013+814013+815013		NP	GWG	AGT	GWR
800014	811014+812014+813014+814014+815014	*Edith New / Meghan Lloyd George*	NP	GWG	AGT	GWR
800015	811015+812015+813015+814015+815015		NP	GWG	AGT	GWR
800016	811016+812016+813016+814016+815016		NP	GWG	AGT	GWR
800017	811017+812017+813017+814017+815017		NP	GWG	AGT	GWR
800018	811018+812018+813018+814018+815018		NP	GWG	AGT	GWR
800019	811019+812019+813019+814019+815019	*Jonny Johnson MBE DFM / Joy Lofthouse*	NP	GWG	AGT	GWR
800020	811020+812020+813020+814020+815020	*Bob Woodward / Elizabeth Ralph*	NP	GWG	AGT	GWR
800021	811021+812021+813021+814021+815021		NP	GWG	AGT	GWR
800022	811022+812022+813022+814022+815022		NP	GWG	AGT	GWR
800023	811023+812023+813023+814023+815023	*Kathryn Osmond / Firefighter Fleur Lombard*	NP	GWG	AGT	GWR
800024	811024+812024+813024+814024+815024		NP	GWG	AGT	GWR
800025	811025+812025+813025+814025+815025	*Captain Sir Tom Moore*	NP	GWG	AGT	GWR
800026*	811026+812026+813026+814026+815026	*Don Cameron*	NP	GWG	AGT	GWR
800027	811027+812027+813027+814027+815027		NP	GWG	AGT	GWR
800028	811028+812028+813028+814028+815028		NP	GWG	AGT	GWR
800029	811029+812029+813029+814029+815029	*Christopher Dando / Evette Wakely*	NP	GWG	AGT	GWR
800030	811030+812030+813030+814030+815030	*Henry Cleary / Lincoln Callaghan*	NP	GWG	AGT	GWR
800031	811031+812031+813031+814031+815031	*Mazen Salmou / Charlotte Marsland*	NP	GWG	AGT	GWR
800032	811032+812032+813032+814032+815032	*Iain Bugler / Sarah Williams Martin*	NP	GWG	AGT	GWR
800033	811033+812033+813033+814033+815033		NP	GWG	AGT	GWR
800034	811034+812034+813034+814034+815034	*Tracy Devlin*	NP	GWG	AGT	GWR
800035	811035+812035+813035+814035+815035	*Liz Gallagher / Naomi Betts*	NP	GWG	AGT	GWR
800036	811036+812036+813036+814036+815036	*Dr Paul Stephenson OBE*	NP	GWG	AGT	GWR

** Long term out of use*

Agility Trains owned, Great Western five-car bi-mode Class 800/0 No. 800015 with its first class end leading is seen on the outskirts of Swindon heading to London on 20 July 2021. The 800/0s can be identified with white door surrounds and bogie brackets. **CJM**

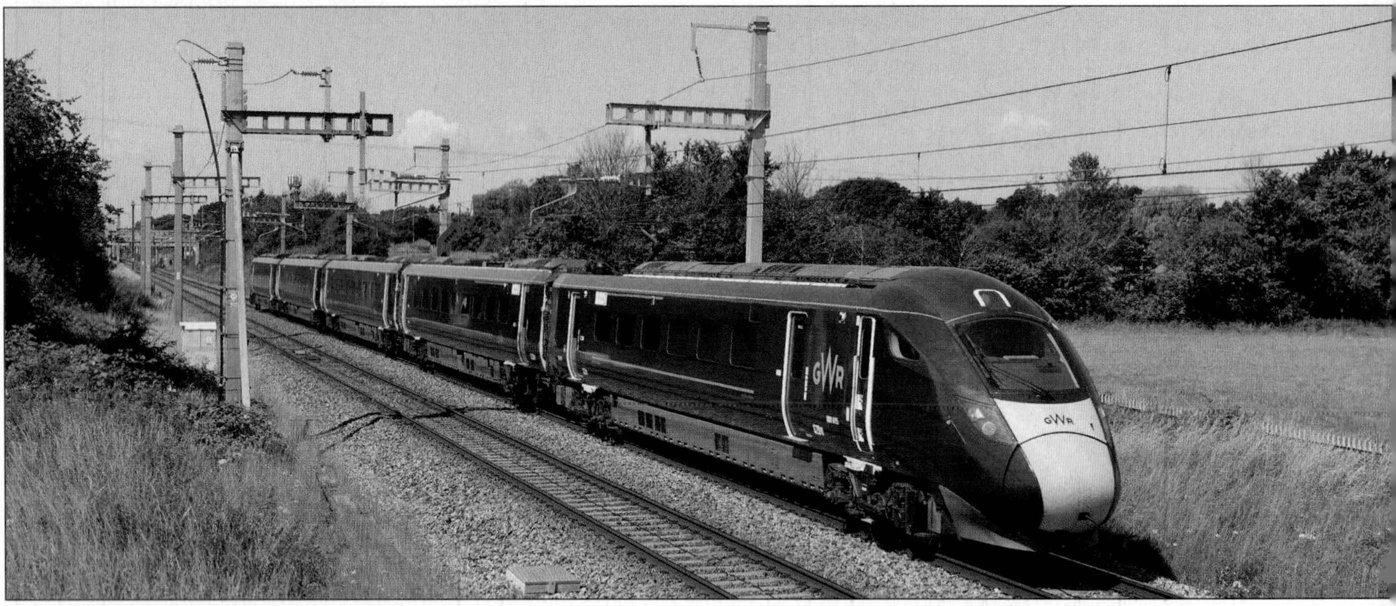

800/1 Formation: PDTS+MS+MS+TSB+MS+TS+MC+MF+PDTRF

800101	811101+812101+813101+814101+815101+816101+817101+818101+819101	DN	LNE	AGT	LNE
800102	811102+812102+813102+814102+815102+816102+817102+818102+819102	DN	LNE	AGT	LNE
800103	811103+812103+813103+814103+815103+816103+817103+818103+819103	DN	LNE	AGT	LNE
800104	811104+812104+813104+814104+815104+816104+817104+818104+819104	DN	SPL	AGT	LNE

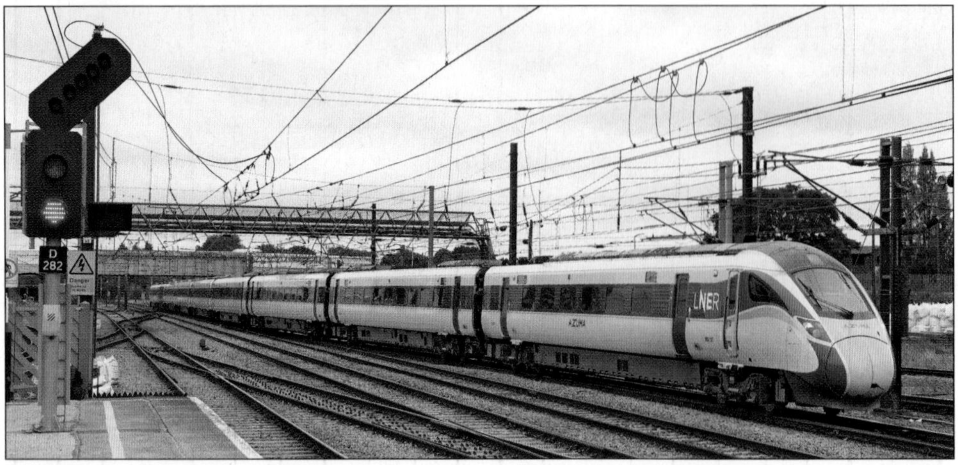

On LNER the Agility Trains-owned bi-mode nine car sets are classified as 800/1, with the 13 sets based at Doncaster. Set No. 800107 is seen on the approaches to Doncaster with its standard class driving car PDTS No. 811107 leading. **CJM**

800105	811105+812105+813105+814105+815105+816105+817105+818105+819105	DN	LNE	AGT	LNE
800106	811106+812106+813106+814106+815106+816106+817106+818106+819106	DN	LNE	AGT	LNE
800107	811107+812107+813107+814107+815107+816107+817107+818107+819107	DN	LNE	AGT	LNE
800108	811108+812108+813108+814108+815108+816108+817108+818108+819108	DN	LNE	AGT	LNE
800109	811109+812109+813109+814109+815109+816109+817109+818109+819109	DN	LNE	AGT	LNE
800110	811110+812110+813110+814110+815110+816110+817110+818110+819110	DN	LNE	AGT	LNE
800111	811111+812111+813111+814111+815111+816111+817111+818111+819111	DN	LNE	AGT	LNE
800112	811112+812112+813112+814112+815112+816112+817112+818112+819112	DN	LNE	AGT	LNE
800113	811113+812113+813113+814113+815113+816113+817113+818113+819113	DN	LNE	AGT	LNE

800/2	Formation: PDTS+MS+MS+MC+PDTRF				
800201	811201+812201+813201+814201+815201	DN	LNE	AGT	LNE
800202	811202+812202+813202+814202+815202	DN	LNE	AGT	LNE
800203	811203+812203+813203+814203+815203	DN	LNE	AGT	LNE
800204	811204+812204+813204+814204+815204	DN	LNE	AGT	LNE
800205	811205+812205+813205+814205+815205	DN	LNE	AGT	LNE
800206	811206+812206+813206+814206+815206	DN	LNE	AGT	LNE
800207	811207+812207+813207+814207+815207	DN	LNE	AGT	LNE
800208	811208+812208+813208+814208+815208	DN	LNE	AGT	LNE
800209	811209+812209+813209+814209+815209	DN	LNE	AGT	LNE
800210	811210+812210+813210+814210+815210	DN	LNE	AGT	LNE

Just 10 Class 800/2 five-car bi-mode sets are operated by LNER, again based at Doncaster. These sets either operate on their own or in multiple with another five car bi-mode or all-electric set. No. 800207 is seen at King's Cross from its standard class end. **Antony Christie**

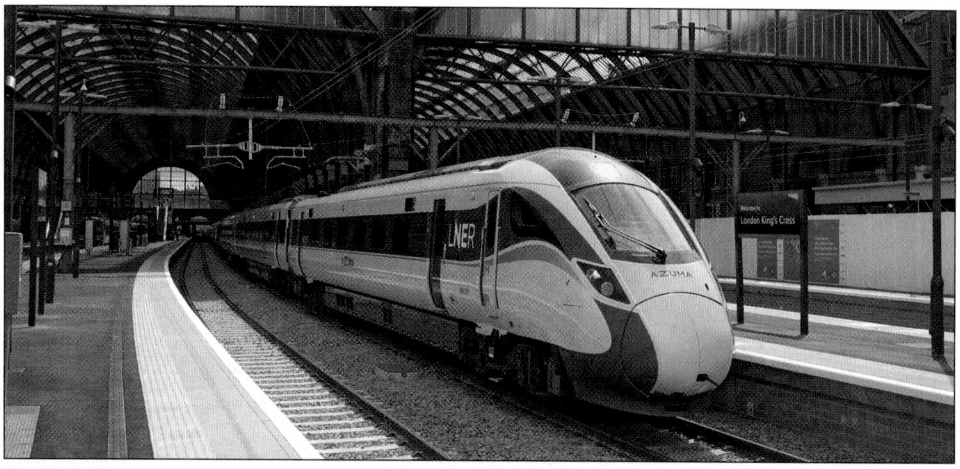

The Class 800/3 designation covers the Great Western nine-car Agility Trains owned sets, based at North Pole depot. The fleet consists of 21 sets, many of which now carry transfer applied nameplates on the cab side. Set No. 800320 passes Denchworth, between Didcot and Swindon on 9 June 2021 with the 09.02 Paddington to Bristol Temple Meads service. **CJM**

800/3	Formation: PDTS+MS+MS+TS+MS+TS+MS+MF+PDTRF					
800301	821001+822001+823001+824001+825001+826001+827001+828001+829001		NP	GWG	AGT	GWR
800302*	821002+822002+823002+824002+825002+826002+827002+828002+829002		NP	GWG	AGT	GWR
800303*	821003+822003+823003+824003+825003+826003+827003+828003+829003		NP	GWG	AGT	GWR
800304	821004+822004+823004+824004+825004+826004+827004+828004+829004		NP	GWG	AGT	GWR
800305	821005+822005+823005+824005+825005+826005+827005+828005+829005		NP	GWG	AGT	GWR
800306	821006+822006+823006+824006+825006+826006+827006+828006+829006	*Allan Leonard Lewis VC / Harold Day DSC*	NP	GWG	AGT	GWR
800307	821007+822007+823007+824007+825007+826007+827007+828007+829007		NP	GWG	AGT	GWR
800308	821008+822008+823008+824008+825008+826008+827008+828008+829008		NP	GWG	AGT	GWR
800309	821009+822009+823009+824009+825009+826009+827009+828009+829009		NP	GWG	AGT	GWR
800310	821010+822010+823010+824010+825010+826010+827010+828003+829010	*Wing Commander Ken Rees*	NP	GWG	AGT	GWR
800311	821011+822011+823011+824011+825011+826011+827011+828011+829011		NP	GWG	AGT	GWR
800312	821012+822012+823012+824012+825012+826012+827012+828012+829012		NP	GWG	AGT	GWR
800313	821013+822013+823013+824013+825013+826013+827013+828013+829013		NP	GWG	AGT	GWR
800314	821014+822014+823014+824014+825014+826014+827014+828014+829014	*Odette Hallowes GC MBE LdH VE 75 1945-2020*	NP	GWG	AGT	GWR
800315	821015+822015+823015+824015+825015+826015+827015+828015+829015		NP	GWG	AGT	GWR
800316	821016+822016+823016+824016+825016+826016+827016+828016+829016		NP	GWG	AGT	GWR
800317	821017+822017+823017+824017+825017+826017+827017+828017+829017	*Freya Bevan*	NP	GWG	AGT	GWR
800318	821018+822018+823018+824018+825018+826018+827018+828018+829018		NP	GWG	AGT	GWR
800319	821019+822019+823019+824019+825019+826019+827019+828019+829019		NP	GWG	AGT	GWR
800320	821020+822020+823020+824020+825020+826020+827020+828020+829020		NP	GWG	AGT	GWR
800321	821021+822021+823021+824021+825021+826021+827021+828021+829021		NP	GWG§	AGT	GWR

§ Carries facemask

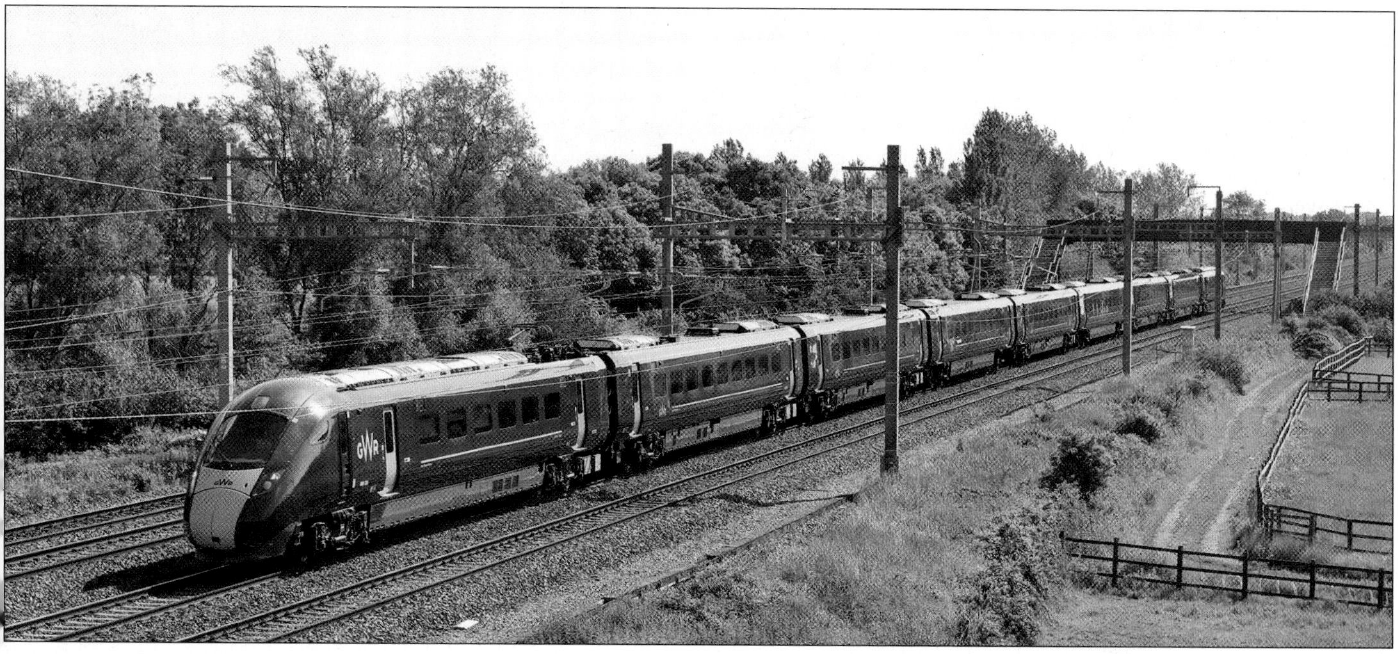

Class 801
Hitachi IET 5 or 9-car EMU Inter City (AT300)

Built: 2013-2020
Vehicle length: Driving 83ft 2in (25.35m)
Intermediate 82ft 0in (25.0m)
Height: 11ft 8in (3.62m)
Width: 8ft 10in (2.7m)

Power: 25kV ac overhead or MTU 1600R80L
Horsepower: 5-car 3,637hp (2,712kW)
9-car 6,062hp (4,520kW)
Transmission: Electric

801/1	Formation: PDTS+MSB+MS+MC+PDTRF				
801101	821101+822101+823101+824101+825101	DN	LNE	AGT	LNE
801102	821102+822102+823102+824102+825102	DN	LNE	AGT	LNE
801103	821103+822103+823103+824103+825103	DN	LNE	AGT	LNE
801104	821104+822104+823104+824104+825104	DN	LNE	AGT	LNE
801105	821105+822105+823105+824105+825105	DN	LNE	AGT	LNE
801106	821106+822106+823106+824106+825106	DN	LNE	AGT	LNE
801107	821107+822107+823107+824107+825107	DN	LNE	AGT	LNE
801108	821108+822108+823108+824108+825108	DN	LNE	AGT	LNE
801109	821109+822109+823109+824109+825109	DN	LNE	AGT	LNE
801110	821110+822110+823110+824110+825110	DN	LNE	AGT	LNE
801111	821111+822111+823111+824111+825111	DN	LNE	AGT	LNE
801112	821112+822112+823112+824112+825112	DN	LNE	AGT	LNE

The Class 801 classification ordered by Agility Trains covers the all-electric sets, all of which are operated by LNER. The sets are identical in terms of passenger accommodation to the 800 breed. On all-electric five-car sets one under-slung GU set (diesel/alternator) is located below the MSB vehicle, the second coach in this view of set No. 801101. **CJM**

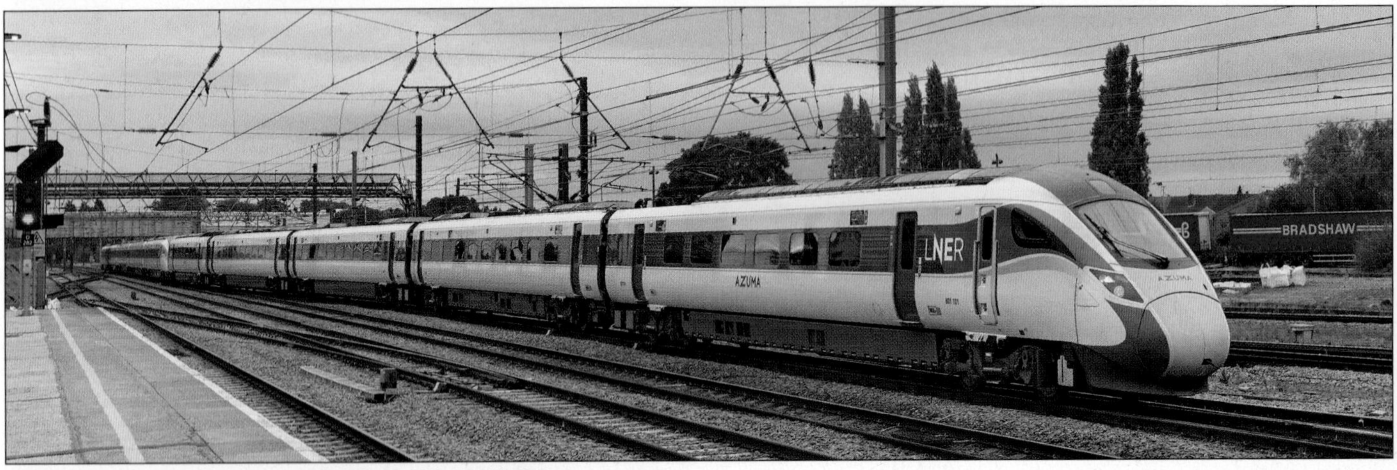

801/2	Formation: PDTS+MS+MS+TSB+MS+TS+MC+MF+PDTRF				
801201	821201+822201+823201+824201+825201+826201+827201+828201+829201	BN	LNE	AGT	LNE
801202	821202+822202+823202+824202+825202+826202+827202+828202+829202	BN	LNE	AGT	LNE
801203	821203+822203+823203+824203+825203+826203+827203+828203+829203	BN	LNE	AGT	LNE
801204	821204+822204+823204+824204+825204+826204+827204+828204+829204	BN	LNE	AGT	LNE
801205	821205+822205+823205+824205+825205+826205+827205+828205+829205	BN	LNE	AGT	LNE
801206	821206+822206+823206+824206+825206+826206+827206+828206+829206	BN	LNE	AGT	LNE
801207	821207+822207+823207+824207+825207+826207+827207+828207+829207	BN	LNE	AGT	LNE
801208	821208+822208+823208+824208+825208+826208+827208+828208+829208	BN	LNE	AGT	LNE
801209	821209+822209+823209+824209+825209+826209+827209+828209+829209	BN	LNE	AGT	LNE
801210	821210+822210+823210+824210+825210+826210+827210+828210+829210	BN	LNE	AGT	LNE
801211	821211+822211+823211+824211+825211+826211+827211+828211+829211	BN	LNE	AGT	LNE
801212	821212+822212+823212+824212+825212+826212+827212+828212+829212	BN	LNE	AGT	LNE
801213	821213+822213+823213+824213+825213+826213+827213+828213+829213	BN	LNE	AGT	LNE
801214	821214+822214+823214+824214+825214+826214+827214+828214+829214	BN	LNE	AGT	LNE
801215	821215+822215+823215+824215+825215+826215+827215+828215+829215	BN	LNE	AGT	LNE
801216	821216+822216+823216+824216+825216+826216+827216+828216+829216	BN	LNE	AGT	LNE
801217	821217+822217+823217+824217+825217+826217+827217+828217+829217	BN	LNE	AGT	LNE
801218	821218+822218+823218+824218+825218+826218+827218+828218+829218	BN	LNE	AGT	LNE
801219	821219+822219+823219+824219+825219+826219+827219+828219+829219	BN	LNE	AGT	LNE
801220	821220+822220+823220+824220+825220+826220+827220+828220+829220	BN	LNE	AGT	LNE
801221	821221+822221+823221+824221+825221+826221+827221+828221+829221	BN	LNE	AGT	LNE
801222	821222+822222+823222+824222+825222+826222+827222+828222+829222	BN	LNE	AGT	LNE
801223	821223+822223+823223+824223+825223+826223+827223+828223+829223	BN	LNE	AGT	LNE
801224	821224+822224+823224+824224+825224+826224+827224+828224+829224	BN	LNE	AGT	LNE
801225	821225+822225+823225+824225+825225+826225+827225+828225+829225	BN	LNE	AGT	LNE
801226	821226+822226+823226+824226+825226+826226+827226+828226+829226	BN	LNE	AGT	LNE
801227	821227+822227+823227+824227+825227+826227+827227+828227+829227	BN	LNE	AGT	LNE
801228	821228+822228+823228+824228+825228+826228+827228+828228+829228	BN	LNE	AGT	LNE
801229	821229+822229+823229+824229+825229+826229+827229+828229+829229	BN	LNE	AGT	LNE
801230	821230+822230+823230+824230+825230+826230+827230+828230+829230	BN	LNE	AGT	LNE

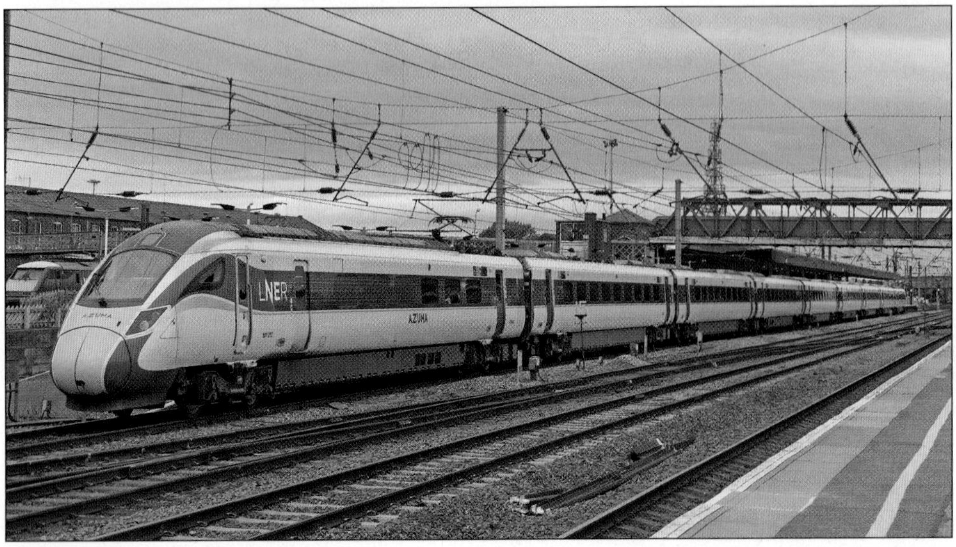

The nine-car all-electric sets are classified as 801/2 (the 801/1 classification would have been used on Great Western all-electric sets, but this order was changed). On these 30 sets, allocated to Bounds Green, one underslung GU is located below the MS coupled to the PDTS coach. Set No. 801212 is seen at Doncaster. **CJM**

Class 802
Hitachi IET 5 or 9-car BMU Inter City (AT300)

Built: 2013-2020
Vehicle length: Driving 83ft 2in (25.35m)
Intermediate 25m
Height: 11ft 8in (3.62m)
Width: 8ft 10in (2.7m)

Power: 25kV ac overhead or MTU 1600R80L
Horsepower: 5-car 3,637hp (2,712kW)
9-car 6,062hp (4,520kW)
Transmission: Electric

802/0	Formation: PDTS+MS+MS+MC+PDTRF					
802001	831001+832001+833001+834001+835001		NP	GWG	EVL	GWR
802002	832002+832002+833002+834002+835002	*Steve Whiteway*	NP	GWG	EVL	GWR
802003	833003+832003+833003+834003+835003		NP	GWG	EVL	GWR
802004	834004+832004+833004+834004+835004		NP	GWG	EVL	GWR
802005	835005+832005+833005+834005+835005		NP	GWG	EVL	GWR
802006	836006+832006+833006+834006+835006	*Donovan & Jenifer Gardner / Harry Billinge MBE, LdH*	NP	GWG	EVL	GWR
802007*	837007+832007+833007+834007+835007		NP	GWG	EVL	GWR
802008	838008+832008+833008+834008+835008	*RNLB Solomon Brown Penlee Lifeboat / Rick Rescorla*	NP	GWG	EVL	GWR
802009	839009+832009+833009+834009+835009		NP	GWG	EVL	GWR
802010	840010+832010+833010+834010+835010	*Kieron Griffin / Corporal George Sheard*	NP	GWG	EVL	GWR
802011	841011+832011+833011+834011+835011	*Sir Joshua Reynolds PRA / Capt. Robert Falcon Scott RN CVO*	NP	GWG	EVL	GWR
802012	842012+832012+833012+834012+835012		NP	GWG	EVL	GWR
802013	843013+832013+833013+834013+835013	*Michael Eavis*	NP	GWG	EVL	GWR
802014	844014+832014+833014+834014+835014		NP	GWG	EVL	GWR
802015	845015+832015+833015+834015+835015		NP	GWG	EVL	GWR
802016	846016+832016+833016+834016+835016		NP	GWG	EVL	GWR
802017	847017+832017+833017+834017+835017		NP	GWG	EVL	GWR
802018	848018+832018+833018+834018+835018	*Preston de Mendonca / Jeremy Doyle*	NP	GWG	EVL	GWR
802019	849019+832019+833019+834019+835019		NP	GWG§	EVL	GWR
802020	850020+832020+833020+834020+835020		NP	GWG	EVL	GWR
802021	851021+832021+833021+834021+835021		NP	GWG	EVL	GWR
802022	852022+832022+833022+834022+835022		NP	GWG	EVL	GWR

§ Carries NHS / Key Workers branding
* Long term out of use

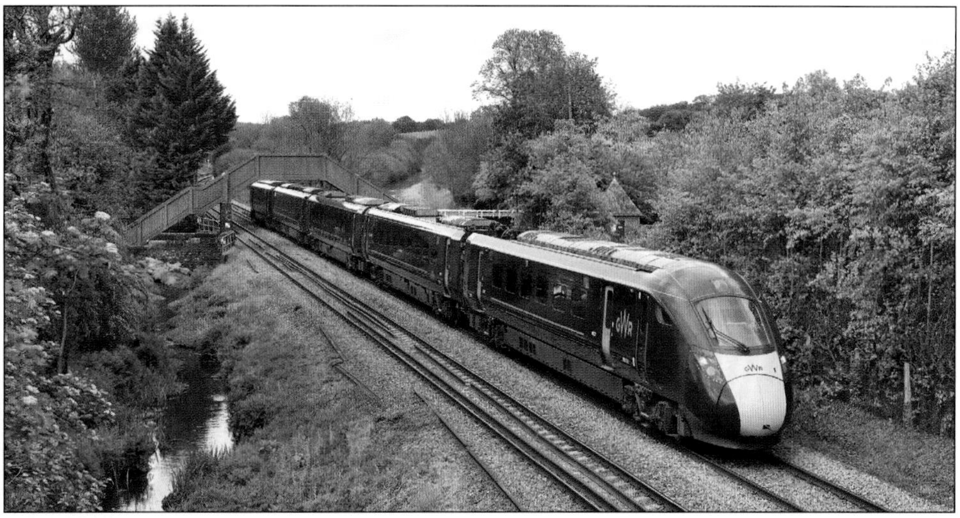

The Great Western upgrade saw Great Western Railway, through funding by Eversholt Leasing, procure 22 five car and 14 nine-car Class 802s for use on the West of England and Cotswold routes. These are identical in passenger accommodation to the Class 800s but have some minor technical differences. Five-car set No. 802021 passes Little Bedwyn on 26 May 2021 with the 14.37 Paddington to Plymouth. **CJM**

802/1	Formation: PDTS+MS+MS+TSB+MS+TS+MC+MF+PDTRF					
802101	831101+832101+833101+834101+835101+836101+837101+838101+839101	*Nancy Astor CH*	NP	GWG	EVL	GWR
802102	831102+832102+833102+834102+835102+836102+837102+838102+839102		NP	GWG	EVL	GWR
802103	831103+832103+833103+834103+835103+836103+837103+838103+839103		NP	GWG	EVL	GWR
802104	831104+832104+833104+834104+835104+836104+837104+838104+839104		NP	GWG	EVL	GWR
802105	831105+832105+833105+834105+835105+836105+837105+838105+839105		NP	GWG	EVL	GWR
802106	831106+832106+833106+834106+835106+836106+837106+838106+839106		NP	GWG	EVL	GWR
802107	831107+832107+833107+834107+835107+836107+837107+838107+839107		NP	GWG	EVL	GWR
802108	831108+832108+833108+834108+835108+836108+837108+838108+839108		NP	GWG	EVL	GWR
802109	831109+832109+833109+834109+835109+836109+837109+838109+839109		NP	GWG	EVL	GWR
802110	831110+832110+833110+834110+835110+836110+837110+838110+839110		NP	GWG	EVL	GWR
802111	831111+832111+833111+834111+835111+836111+837111+838111+839111		NP	GWG	EVL	GWR
802112	831112+832112+833112+834112+835112+836112+837112+838112+839112		NP	GWG	EVL	GWR
802113	831113+832113+833113+834113+835113+836113+837113+838113+839113		NP	GWG	EVL	GWR
802114	831114+832114+833114+834114+835114+836114+837114+838114+839114		NP	GWG	EVL	GWR

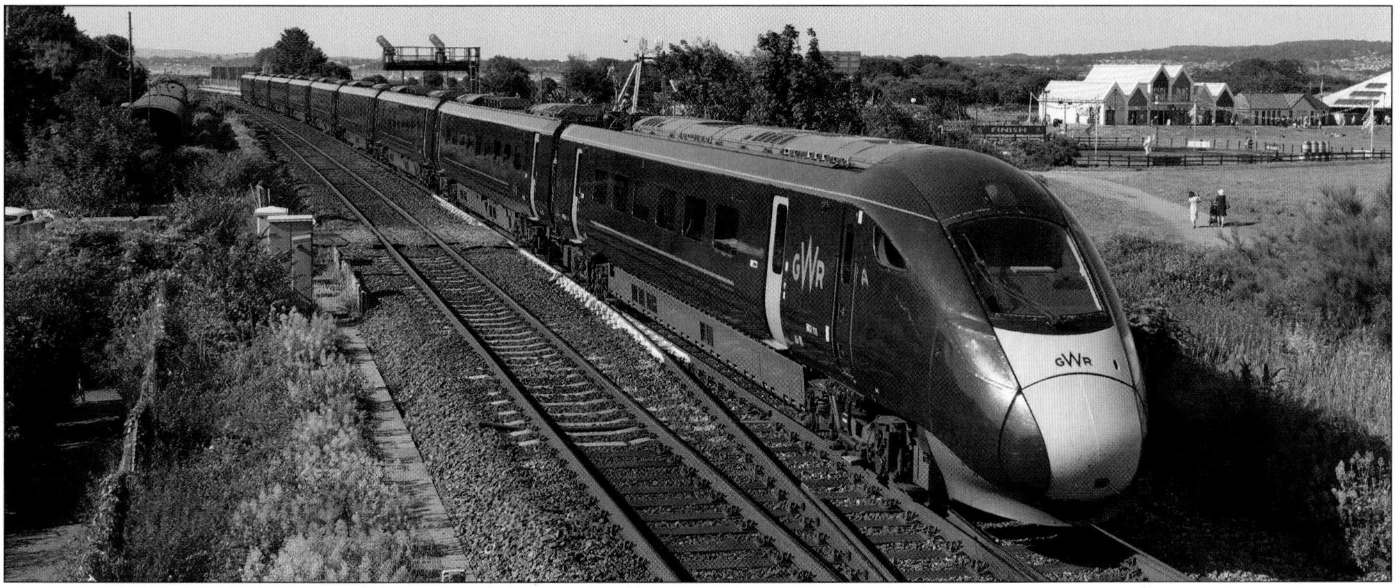

The 14 nine-car Class 802/1s are usually deployed on West of England services. On 18 July 2021, set No. 802111 passes Dawlish Warren on the middle road with the 15.03 Paddington to Plymouth. The set is formed in the booked way, with the standard class at the west end. **CJM**

802/2 Formation: PDTS+MS+MS+MS+PDTRF

802201	831201+832201+833201+834201+835201	EC	FTN	ANG	FTP
802202	831202+832202+833202+834202+835202	EC	FTN	ANG	FTP
802203	831203+832203+833203+834203+835203	EC	FTN	ANG	FTP
802204	831204+832204+833204+834204+835204	EC	FTN	ANG	FTP
802205	831205+832205+833205+834205+835205	EC	FTN	ANG	FTP
802206	831206+832206+833206+834206+835206	EC	FTN	ANG	FTP
802207	831207+832207+833207+834207+835207	EC	FTN	ANG	FTP
802208	831208+832208+833208+834208+835208	EC	FTN	ANG	FTP
802209	831209+832209+833209+834209+835209	EC	FTN	ANG	FTP
802210	831210+832210+833210+834210+835210	EC	FTN	ANG	FTP
802211	831211+832211+833211+834211+835211	EC	FTN	ANG	FTP
802212	831212+832212+833212+834212+835212	EC	FTN	ANG	FTP
802213	831213+832213+833213+834213+835213	EC	FTN	ANG	FTP
802214	831214+832214+833214+834214+835214	EC	FTN	ANG	FTP
802215	831215+832215+833215+834215+835215	EC	FTN	ANG	FTP
802216	831216+832216+833216+834216+835216	EC	FTN	ANG	FTP
802217	831217+832217+833217+834217+835217	EC	FTN	ANG	FTP
802218	831218+832218+833218+834218+835218	EC	FTN	ANG	FTP
802219	831219+832219+833219+834219+835219	EC	FTN	ANG	FTP

802/3 Formation: PDTS+MS+MS+MC+PDTRF

802301	831301+832301+833301+834001+835001	BN	FHT	ANG	FHT
802302	831302+832302+833302+834002+835002	BN	FHT	ANG	FHT
802303	831303+832303+833303+834003+835003	BN	FHT	ANG	FHT
802304	831304+832304+833304+834004+835004	BN	FHT	ANG	FHT
802305	831305+832305+833305+834005+835005	BN	SPL	ANG	FHT

First Hull Trains operate a fleet of five Class 802/3s on the Open Access King's Cross to Hull route, The sets are based at Bounds Green. The sets do not operate over any other route. They are branded as 'Paragon' sets and do not have a yellow warning end. Set No. 802303 is seen from its standard class end at Doncaster. **CJM**

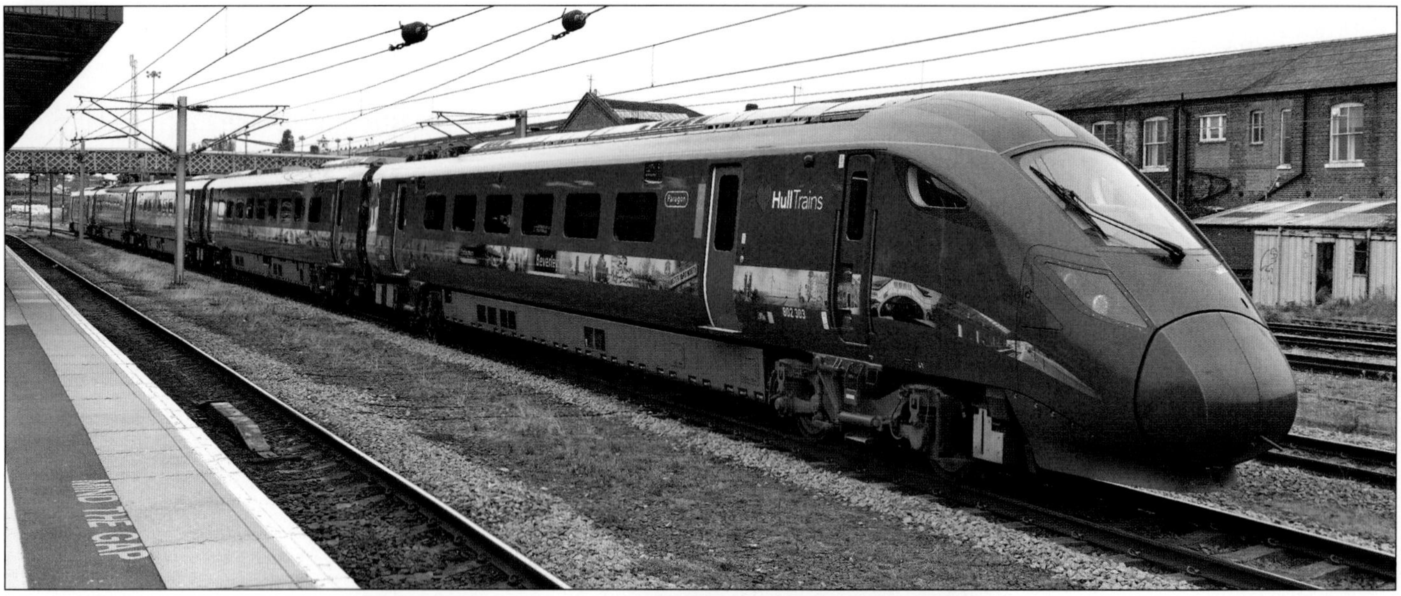

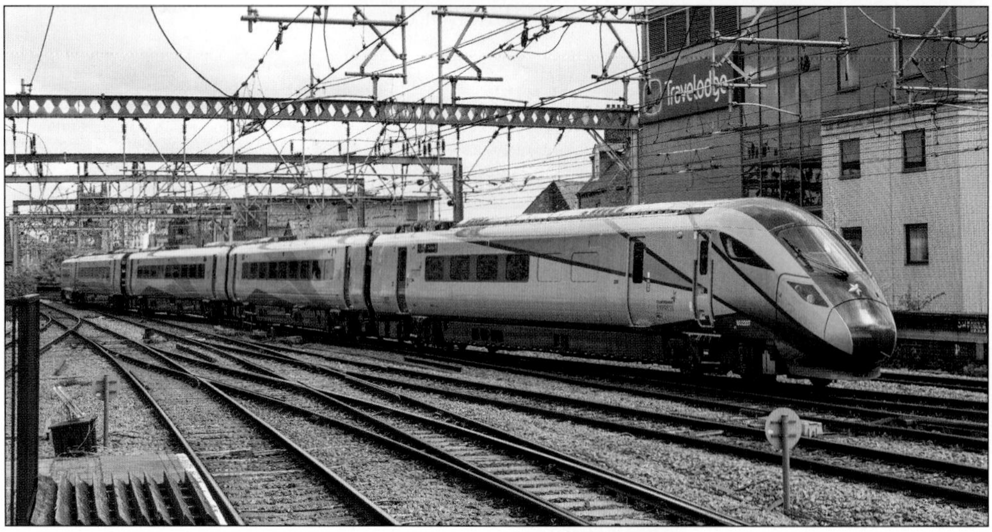

As part of route modernisation TransPennine Express, also part of First Group took on the lease of 19 five-car Class 802/2 from Angel Trains to operate Liverpool/Manchester to Newcastle/Edinburgh and from 2022 West Coast routed services. The sets, based at Edinburgh Craigentinny carry the TPE multi-coloured with no yellow warning end. First class accommodation is provided in one driving car, which also houses a kitchen. This is the nearest vehicle in this image of set No. 802207 at Leeds. **Antony Christie**

The most recent IET sets to enter service are the five Class 803s introduced in 2021 for First Group Open Access operator Lumo, who operate several trains each day on the King's Cross to Edinburgh corridor, offering one class low-cost travel. Seating is all 2+2 and an external catering service brings food to the train which has to be pre-ordered. The sets are maintained at Edinburgh Craigentinny. No. 803003 is seen passing south through Doncaster. **CJM**

Class 803 'Lumo'
Hitachi IET 5-car EMU Inter City (AT300)

Built: 2020-2021
Vehicle length: Driving 83ft 2in (25.35m)
Intermediate 82ft 0in (25.0m)
Height: 11ft 8in (3.62m)
Width: 8ft 10in (2.7m)
Power: 25kV ac overhead
Horsepower: 3,637hp (2,712kW)
Transmission: Electric

Formation: PDTS+MS+MS+MS+PDTS

803001	841001+842001+843001+844001+845001	EC	FEC	BEA	FEC
803002	841002+842002+843002+844002+845002	EC	FEC	BEA	FEC
803003	841003+842003+843003+844003+845003	EC	FEC	BEA	FEC
803004	841004+842004+843004+844004+845004	EC	FEC	BEA	FEC
803005	841005+842005+843005+844005+845005	EC	FEC	BEA	FEC

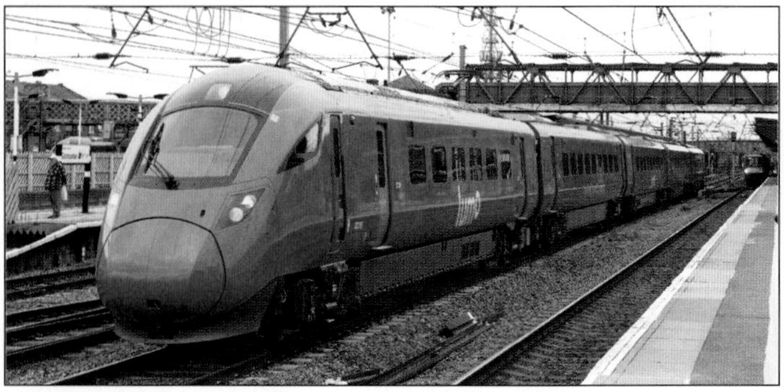

Class 805
Hitachi IET 5-car BMU Inter City (AT300)

Built: 2021-2022
Vehicle length: Driving 83ft 2in (25.35m)
Intermediate 82ft 0in (25.0m)
Height: 11ft 8in (3.62m)
Width: 8ft 10in (2.7m)
Power: 25kV ac overhead and diesel
Horsepower: 3,637hp (2,712kW)
Transmission: Electric

Formation: PDTS+MS+MS+MS+PDTF

805001	861001+862001+863001+864001+865001	OY	AWC	ROK	AWC
805002	861002+862002+863002+864002+865002	OY	AWC	ROK	AWC
805003	861003+862003+863003+864003+865003	OY	AWC	ROK	AWC
805004	861004+862004+863004+864004+865004	OY	AWC	ROK	AWC
805005	861005+862005+863005+864005+865005	OY	AWC	ROK	AWC
805006	861006+862006+863006+864006+865006	OY	AWC	ROK	AWC
805007	861007+862007+863007+864007+865007	OY	AWC	ROK	AWC
805008	861008+862008+863008+864008+865008	OY	AWC	ROK	AWC
805009	861009+862009+863009+864009+865009	OY	AWC	ROK	AWC
805010	861010+862010+863010+864010+865010	OY	AWC	ROK	AWC
805011	861011+862011+863011+864011+865011	OY	AWC	ROK	AWC
805012	861012+862012+863012+864012+865012	OY	AWC	ROK	AWC
805013	861013+862013+863013+864013+865013	OY	AWC	ROK	AWC

Class 807
Hitachi IET 7-car EMU Inter City (AT300)

Built: 2021-2022
Vehicle length: Driving 83ft 2in (25.35m)
Intermediate 82ft 0in (25.0m)
Height: 11ft 8in (3.62m)
Width: 8ft 10in (2.7m)
Power: 25kV ac overhead and diesel
Horsepower: 3,637hp (2,712kW)
Transmission: Electric

Formation: PDTS+MS+MS+MS+MS+MC+PDTF

807001	871001+872001+873001+874001+875001+876001+877001	OY	AWC	ROK	AWC
807002	871002+872002+873002+874002+875002+876002+877002	OY	AWC	ROK	AWC
807003	871003+872003+873003+874003+875003+876003+877003	OY	AWC	ROK	AWC
807004	871004+872004+873004+874004+875004+876004+877004	OY	AWC	ROK	AWC
807005	871005+872005+873005+874005+875005+876005+877005	OY	AWC	ROK	AWC
807006	871006+872006+873006+874006+875006+876006+877006	OY	AWC	ROK	AWC
807007	871007+872007+873007+874007+875007+876007+877007	OY	AWC	ROK	AWC
807008	871008+872008+873008+874008+875008+876008+877008	OY	AWC	ROK	AWC
807009	871009+872009+873009+874009+875009+876009+877009	OY	AWC	ROK	AWC
807010	871010+872010+873010+874010+875010+876010+877010	OY	AWC	ROK	AWC

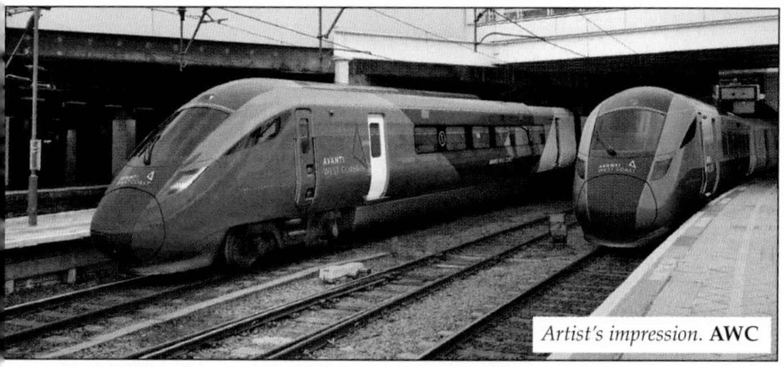

Artist's impression. **AWC**

Class 810 'Aurora'
Hitachi IET 5-car BMU Inter City (AT300)

Built: 2021-2022
Vehicle length: 78ft 8in (24m)
Height: 11ft 8in (3.62m)
Width: 8ft 10in (2.7m)
Power: 25kV ac overhead and diesel
Horsepower: 3,940hp (2,940kW)
Transmission: Electric

Formation: DMF+MC+TS+MS+DMS

810001	851001+852001+853001+854001+855001	DY	EMP	ROK	EMR
810002	851002+852002+853002+854002+855002	DY	EMP	ROK	EMR
810003	851003+852003+853003+854003+855003	DY	EMP	ROK	EMR
810004	851004+852004+853004+854004+855004	DY	EMP	ROK	EMR
810005	851005+852005+853005+854005+855005	DY	EMP	ROK	EMR
810006	851006+852006+853006+854006+855006	DY	EMP	ROK	EMR
810007	851007+852007+853007+854007+855007	DY	EMP	ROK	EMR
810008	851008+852008+853008+854008+855008	DY	EMP	ROK	EMR
810009	851009+852009+853009+854009+855009	DY	EMP	ROK	EMR
810010	851010+852010+853010+854010+855010	DY	EMP	ROK	EMR
810011	851011+852011+853011+854011+855011	DY	EMP	ROK	EMR
810012	851012+852012+853012+854012+855012	DY	EMP	ROK	EMR
810013	851013+852013+853013+854013+855013	DY	EMP	ROK	EMR
810014	851014+852014+853014+854014+855014	DY	EMP	ROK	EMR
810015	851015+852015+853015+854015+855015	DY	EMP	ROK	EMR
810016	851016+852016+853016+854016+855016	DY	EMP	ROK	EMR
810017	851017+852017+853017+854017+855017	DY	EMP	ROK	EMR
810018	851018+852018+853018+854018+855018	DY	EMP	ROK	EMR
810019	851019+852019+853019+854019+855019	DY	EMP	ROK	EMR
810020	851020+852020+853020+854020+855020	DY	EMP	ROK	EMR
810021	851021+852021+853021+854021+855021	DY	EMP	ROK	EMR
810022	851022+852022+853022+854022+855022	DY	EMP	ROK	EMR
810023	851023+852023+853023+854023+855023	DY	EMP	ROK	EMR
810024	851024+852024+853024+854024+855024	DY	EMP	ROK	EMR
810025	851025+852025+853025+854025+855025	DY	EMP	ROK	EMR
810026	851026+852026+853026+854026+855026	DY	EMP	ROK	EMR
810027	851027+852027+853027+854027+855027	DY	EMP	ROK	EMR
810028	851028+852028+853028+854028+855028	DY	EMP	ROK	EMR
810029	851029+852029+853029+854029+855029	DY	EMP	ROK	EMR
810030	851030+852030+853030+854030+855030	DY	EMP	ROK	EMR
810031	851031+852031+853031+854031+855031	DY	EMP	ROK	EMR
810032	851032+852032+853032+854032+855032	DY	EMP	ROK	EMR
810033	851033+852033+853033+854033+855033	DY	EMP	ROK	EMR

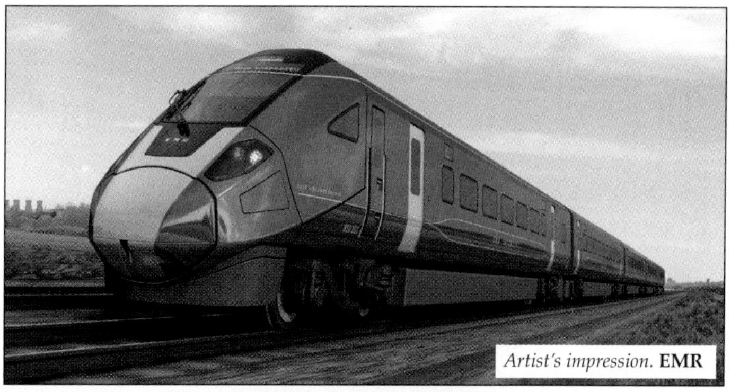

Artist's impression. **EMR**

Class 950
BREL 2-car DMU Track Inspection Train

Built: 1987
Vehicle length: 65ft 9¾in (20.06m)
Height: 12ft 4½in (3.77m)
Width: 9ft 3¼in (2.82m)
Engine: 1 x Cummins NT855R5 per car
Horsepower: 285hp (213kW) per car
Transmission: Hydraulic

Formation: DM+DM

950001	999600+999601	ZA	NRL	NRL	NRL

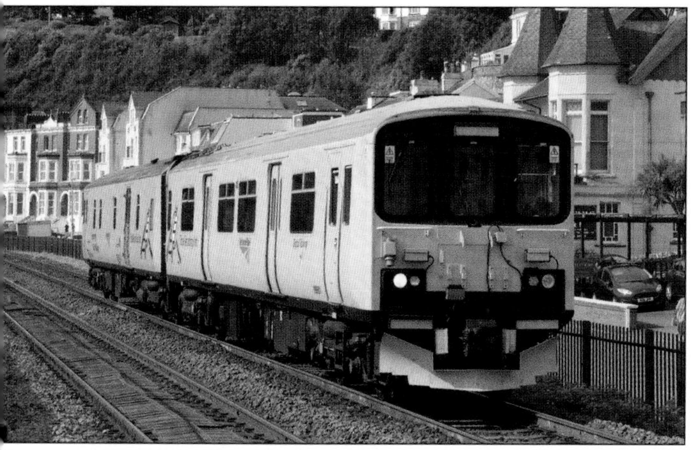

The two-car Network Rail Class 150 outline track testing train is classified 950 and numbered 950001. Based at Derby and currently operated by Loram, the sets operated over the entire rail network on a semi-timetabled basis. It is fitted with various different lights, cameras and recording equipment as required. The set is seen passing Dawlish. **CJM**

Unclassified
Very Light Weight Vehicle (VLR)

Built: 2021
Vehicle length: 18.5m
Height: 3.8m
Width: 2.8m
Engine: Cummins
Seating: 56
Transmission: Diesel-electric

Formation: DM

Un-numbered	Dudley

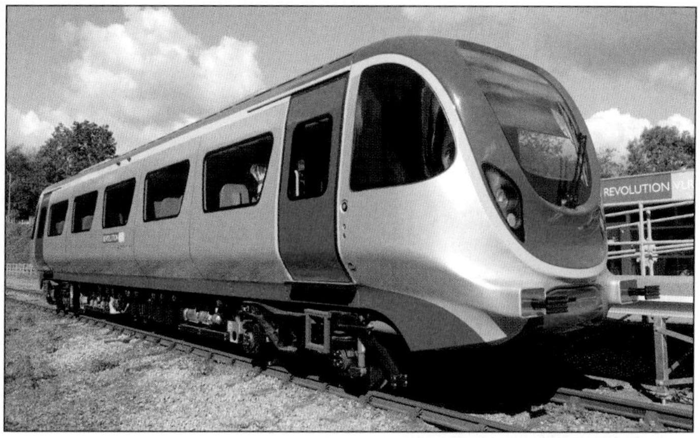

The Very Light Rail (VLR) vehicle is designed to demonstrate a new innovative, lightweight, energy-efficient vehicle that can operate on short routes where heavy rail/tram systems are not viable. The VLR was developed by a consortium of Transport Design International, Eversholt Rail, RSSB, the University of Warwick, Cummins and Transcal Engineering. The un-numbered vehicle is being tested in Warwickshire. **VLR**

At a Glance - Your Guide to UK Main Line Multiple Units 2022-2023

Class	Number Range	Builder	Year First Introduced	Operator
Diesel Units				
139	139001-139002	Parry	2007	WMR
150/0	150001-150002	BREL	1984	NOR
150/1	150101-150150	BREL	1985	NOR
150/2	150201-150285	BREL	1986	GWR, NOR, TFW
153	153301-153935	Hunslet Barclay	1991	ASR, TFW, OLS
155	155341-155347	Leyland	1987	NOR
158	158801-158959	BREL	1990	ASR, EMR, GWR, NOR, SWR, TFW
159/0	159001-159022	BREL	1992	SWR
159/1	159101-159108	BREL	2006	SWR
165/0	165001-165039	BREL/ABB	1990	CRW
165/1	165101-165137	BREL/ABB	1990	GWR
166	166201-166221	BREL/ABB	1992	GWR
168/0	168001-168005	Adtranz	1997	CRW
168/1	168106-168113	Bombardier	2000	CRW
168/2	168214-168219	Bombardier	2003	CRW
168/3	163321-168329	Bombardier	2000	CRW
170/1	170101-170117	Adtranz	1998	AXC
170/2	170201-170273	Adtranz	1999	TFW
170/3	170393-170398	Bombardier	2002	ASR, AXC
170/4	170401-170478	Adtranz	1999	ASR, EMR, NOR
170/5	170501-170535	Adtranz	1999	WMR
170/6	170623-170639	Adtranz	2000	AXC
171/2	171201-171202	Adtranz	2000	GTR
171/4	171401-171402	Adtranz	2000	GTR
171/7	171721-171730	Bombardier	2003	GTR
171/8	171801-171806	Bombardier	2004	GTR
172/0	172001-172008	Bombardier	2010	WMR
172/1	172101-172104	Bombardier	2011	WMR
172/2	172211-172222	Bombardier	2011	WMR
172/3	172331-172345	Bombardier	2011	WMR
175/0	175001-175011	Alstom	1999	TFW
175/1	175101-175116	Alstom	1999	TFW
180	180101-180114	Alstom	2000	GTL, EMR
185	185101-185154	Siemens	2005	FTP
195/0	195001-195025	CAF	2018	NOR
195/1	195101-195133	CAF	2018	NOR
196/0	196001-196012	CAF	2021	WMR
196/1	196101-196114	CAF	2020	WMR
197/0	197001-197051	CAF	2021	TFW
197/1	197101-197126	CAF	2021	TFW
220	220001-220034	Bombardier	2000	AXC
221	221101-221144	Bombardier	2001	AWC, AXC
222/0	222001-222023	Bombardier	2004	EMR
222/1	222101-222104	Bombardier	2005	EMR
230	230001-230010	Vivarail	2016	WMR, VIV, TFW
231	231001-231011	Stadler	2021	TFW
Electric Units, Hydrogen Units §, Bi-Mode Units *, Diesel Unit #				
313/1	313121	BREL	1976	NRL
313/2	313201-313220	BREL	1976	GTR
317/3	317337-317348	BREL	1981	GAR
317/5	317501-317515	BREL	1981	GAR
317/7	317708-317732	BREL	1981	OLS
317/8	317881-317886	BREL	1981	GAR
318	318250-318270	BREL	1985	ASR
319/0	319005-319013	BREL	1987	ROG, OLS
319/2	319214-319220	BREL	1987	OLS
319/3	319361-319386	BREL	1990	NOR, ROG, OLS
319/4	319429-319460	BREL	1988	OLS
320/3	320301-320322	BREL	1990	ASR
320/4	320403-320448	BREL	1989	ASR
321/3	321301-321343	BREL	1990	GAR, OLS
321/4	321403-321447	BREL	1989	GAR, OLS, EVL
321/9	321901-321903	BREL	1991	GAR
322	322401-322405	BREL	1990	GAR
323	323201-323243	Hunslet TPL	1992	WMR, NOR
325	325001-325016	Adtranz	1995	DBC
331/0	331001-331031	CAF	2018	NOR
331/1	331101-331112	CAF	2018	NOR
333	333001-333-016	CAF	2000	NOR
334	334001-334040	Alstom	1999	ASR
345	345001-345070	Bombardier	2017	CRO
350/1	350101-350130	Siemens	2004	WMR
350/2	350231-350267	Siemens	2008	WMR
350/3	350368-350377	Siemens	2014	WMR
350/4	350401-350410	Siemens	2014	WMR
357/0	357001-357046	Adtranz	1999	C2C
357/2	357201-357211	Bombardier	2001	C2C
357/3	357312-357328	Bombardier	2001	C2C
360/0	360101-360121	Siemens	2002	EMR
360/2	360201-360205	Siemens	2004	ROG
373/0	373007-373016	Alstom	1993	EUS

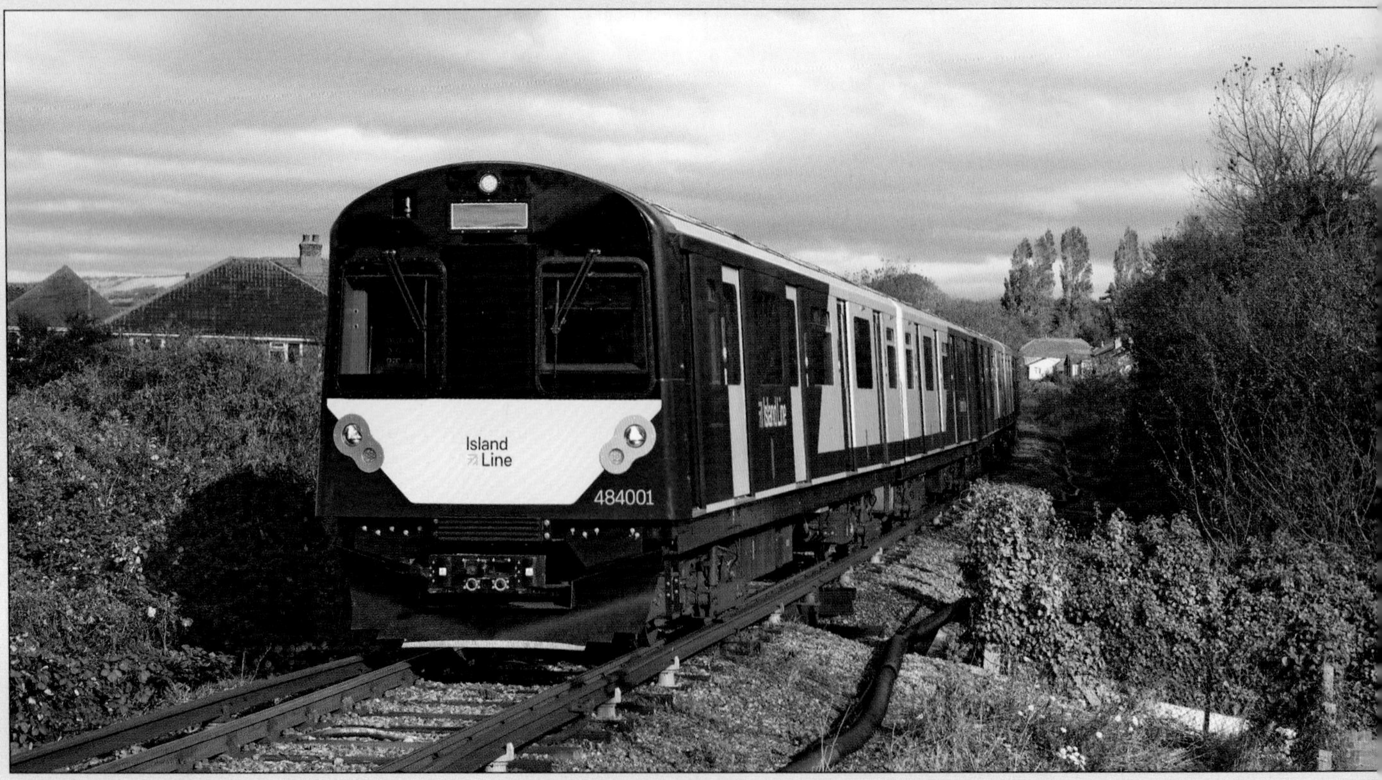

At the start of November 2021 South Western Railway Island Line successfully introduced Vivarail Class 484 stock on the Isle of Wight railway between Ryde Pier Head and Shanklin. During the first week of operation, set No. 484001 is recorded pulling into Lake station with a service from Ryde Pier Head to Shanklin. Five of the converted London Transport 'D' stock set are based at Ryde St Johns, with in the peak season two double unit trains in service and one set on maintenance. CJM

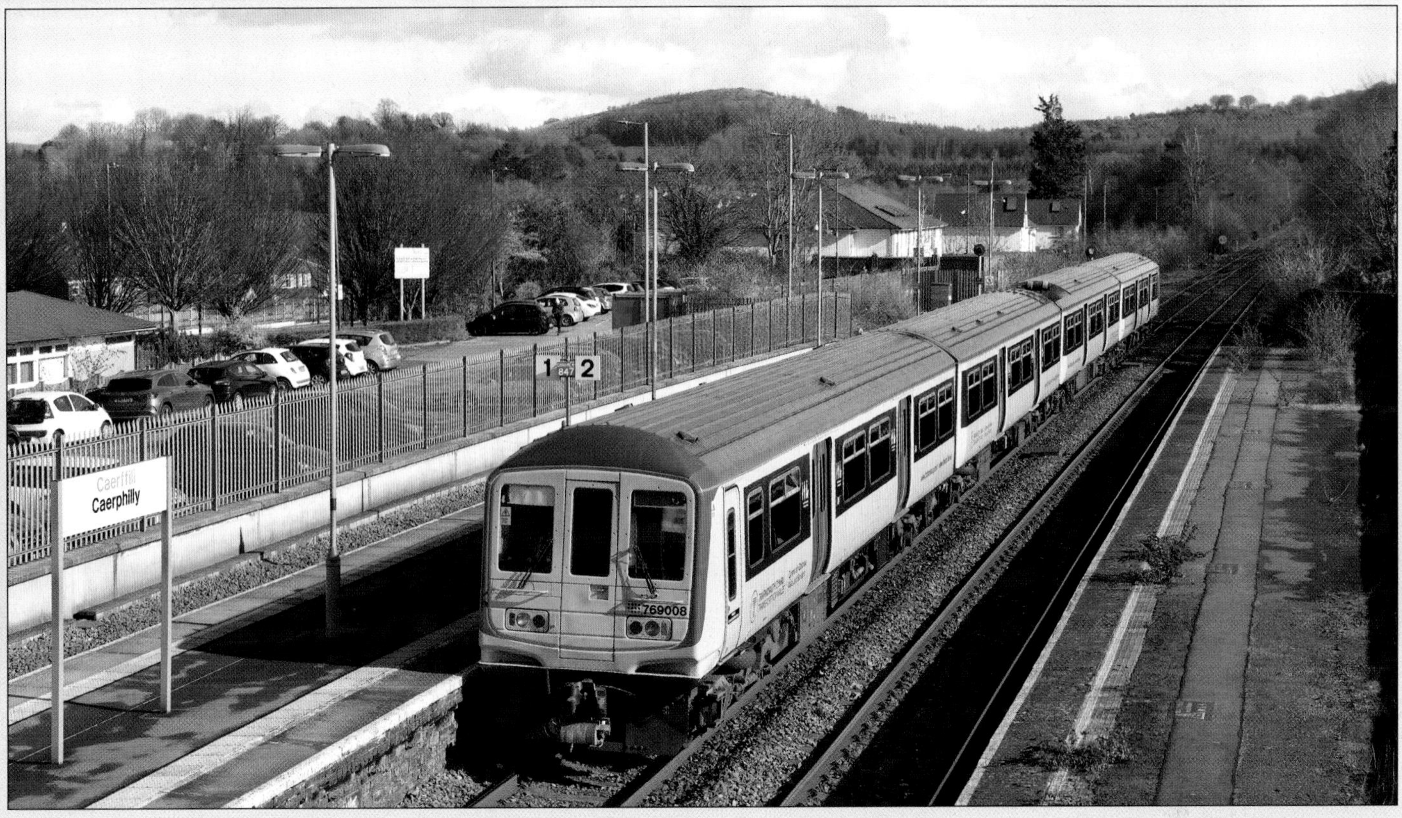

After a slow introduction and many technical and operational problems, the diesel-only version of the Class 769 operated by Transport for Wales on the Rhymney-Cardiff-Penarth route seem to have settled down well and operate the service alongside Class 150/153 DMUs. The '769s' being a little sluggish in acceleration on the graded sections of route. On 24 February 2022, set No. 769008 departs from Caerphilly with the 13.00 Bargoed to Penarth service. **CJM**

373/2	373205-373230	Alstom	1993	EUS
374	374001-374034	Siemens	2015	EUS
375/3	375301-375310	Bombardier	2001	SET
375/6	375601-375630	Adtranz	1999	SET
375/7	375701-375715	Bombardier	2001	SET
375/8	375801-375830	Bombardier	2003	SET
375/9	376901-376927	Bombardier	2003	SET
376	376001-376038	Bombardier	2004	SET
377/1	377101-377164	Bombardier	2002	GTR
377/2	377201-377215	Bombardier	2002	GTR
377/3	377301-377328	Bombardier	2001	GTR
377/4	377401-377475	Bombardier	2004	GTR
377/5	377501-377523	Bombardier	2008	SET
377/6	377601-377626	Bombardier	2013	GTR
377/7	377701-377708	Bombardier	2013	GTR
378/1	378135-378154	Bombardier	2009	LOG
378/2	378201-378257	Bombardier	2009	LOG
379	379001-379030	Bombardier	2010	OLS
380/0	380001-380022	Siemens	2010	ASR
380/1	380101-380116	Siemens	2010	ASR
385/0	385001-385046	Hitachi	2017	ASR
385/1	385101-385124	Hitachi	2017	ASR
387/0	387101-387174	Bombardier	2014	GTR, GWR, HEX
387/2	387201-387227	Bombardier	2016	GTR
387/3	387301-387306	Bombardier	2017	C2C
390/0	390001-390050	Alstom	2001	AWC
390/1	390103-390157	Alstom	2001	AWC
395	395001-395029	Hitachi	2007	SET
397	397001-397012	CAF	2018	TPE
398	398001-398036	Stadler	2021	TFW
399	399201-399207	Vossloh	2015	SST
444	444001-444045	Siemens	2003	SWR
450	450001-450127	Siemens	2002	SWR
455/7	455701-455743	BREL	1984	SWR
455/8	455801-455874	BREL	1982	OLS, SWR
455/9	455901-455920	BREL	1985	SWR
456	456001-456024	BREL	1990	OLS
458	458501-458536	Alstom	1999	SWR
465/0	465001-465050	BREL	1991	SET
465/1	465151-465197	ABB	1993	SET
465/2	465235-465250	Metro-Cammell	1991	OLS
465/9	465901-465934	Metro-Cammell	1991	SET
466	466001-466043	Metro-Cammell	1992	SET, OLS

484	484001-484005	Vivarail	2021	SWR
507	507001-507033	BREL	1978	MER
508	508103-508143	BREL	1979	MER
614§	614209	BREL	1979	-
700/0	700001-700060	Siemens	2015	GTR
700/1	700101-700155	Siemens	2015	GTR
701/0	701001-701062	Bombardier	2021	SWR
701/5	701501-701530	Bombardier	2021	SWR
707	707001-707030	Siemens	2015	SET, SWR
710/1	710101-710130	Bombardier	2018	LOG
710/2	710256-710273	Bombardier	2019	LOG
710/3	710374-710379	Bombardier	2020	LOG
717	717001-717025	Siemens	2018	GTR
720/1	720101-720144	Bombardier	2021	GAR
720/5	720501-720589	Bombardier	2020	GAR
730/0	730001-730036	Bombardier	2021	WMR
730/1	730101-730129	Bombardier	2021	WMR
730/2	730201-730216	Bombardier	2021	WMR
745/0	745001-745010	Stadler	2020	GAR
745/1	745101-745110	Stadler	2020	GAR
755/3*	755325-755338	Stadler	2019	GAR
755/4*	755401-755424	Stadler	2019	GAR
768*	768001-768003	Wabtec	2021	ROG
769/0#	769002-769008	Wabtec	2018	TFW
769/4*	769421-769458	Wabtec	2018	NOR, TFW
769/9*	769922-769959	Wabtec	2021	GWR
777	777001-777053	Stadler	2021	MER
799§	799001/799201	Porterbrook	2018	PTR
800/0*	800001-800036	Hitachi	2017	GWR
800/1*	800101-800113	Hitachi	2017	LNE
800/2*	800201-800210	Hitachi	2018	LNE
800/3*	800301-800321	Hitachi	2017	GWR
801/1	801101-801112	Hitachi	2017	LNE
801/2	801201-801230	Hitachi	2018	LNE
802/0*	802001-802022	Hitachi	2017	GWR
802/1*	802101-802114	Hitachi	2018	GWR
802/2*	802201-802219	Hitachi	2018	TPE
802/3*	802301-802305	Hitachi	2019	FHT
803	803001-803005	Hitachi	2021	FEC
805	805001-805013	Hitachi	2022	AWC
807	807001-807010	Hitachi	2022	AWC
810*	810001-810033	Hitachi	2022	EMR

Hauled Coaching Stock

Pullman Cars

Company Stock to Mk1 design

213 (99535)	*Minerva*	PFP	SL	PUL	BEL	BEL
232 (99970)	Car No. 79	PBT	NY	PUL	NYM	NYM
238	*Phyliss*	PFK	SL	PUL	BEL	BEL
239	*Agatha*	PFP	SL	PUL	BEL	BEL-S
243 (99541)	*Lucille*	PFP	SL	PUL	BEL	BEL
245 (99534)	*Ibis*	PFK	SL	PUL	BEL	BEL
254 (99536)	*Zena*	PFP	SL	PUL	BEL	BEL
255 (99539)	*Ione*	PFK	SL	PUL	BEL	BEL
264	*Ruth*	PCK	SL	PUL	BEL	BEL
280 (99537)	*Audrey*	PFK	SL	PUL	BEL	BEL
281 (99546)	*Gwen*	PFK	SL	PUL	BEL	BEL
283	*Mona*	PFK	SL	PUL	BEL	BEL-S
284 (99543)	*Vera*	PFK	SL	PUL	BEL	BEL
285	Car No. 85	PTP	SL	PUL	BEL	BEL-S
286	Car No. 86	PTP	SL	PUW	BEL	BEL-S
292 (99547)	Car No. 92	PTB	SL	PUL	BEL	BEL
293 (99548)	Car No. 93	PTB	SL	PUL	BEL	BEL
301 (99530)	*Perseus*	PFP	SL	PUL	BEL	BEL
302 (99531)	*Phoenix*	PFP	SL	PUL	BEL	BEL
307	*Carina*	PFK	SL	PUL	BEL	BEL-S
308 (99532)	*Cygnus*	PFP	SL	PUL	BEL	BEL
310	*Pegasus*	PBF	CL	PUL	LSL	LSL
325	*Amber*	PPF	CS	WCR	WCR	WCR
326 (95402)	*Emerald*	PPF	CS	PUL	WCR	WCR
328 (99974)	*Opal*	PPF	NY	PUL	NYM	NYM
335 (99362)	Car No. 335	PSK	TM	PUL	VTN	VTN
347 (99347)	*Diamond*	PPS	CS	PUL	WCR	WCR
348 (99348)	*Topaz*	PPS	CS	PUL	WCR	WCR
349 (99349)	Car No. 349	PPS	TM	PUL	VTN	VTN
350 (99350)	*Tanzanite*	PPS	CS	PUL	WCR	WCR
351 (99351)	*Sapphire*	PPS	CS	PUL	WCR	WCR
352 (99352)	*Amethyst*	PPS	CS	PUL	WCR	WCR
353 (99353)	Car No. 353	PPS	TM	PUL	VTN	VTN
354 (99354)	*The Hadrian Bar*	PBS	CS	PUL	WCR	WCR

Mk2 design

504 (99678)	*Ullswater*	PFK	CS	PUL	WCR	WCR
506 (99679)	*Windermere*	PFK	CS	PUL	WCR	WCR
546 (99670)	*City of Manchester*	PFP	CS	PUL	WCR	WCR
548 (99671)	*Grasmere*	PFP	CS	PUL	WCR	WCR
549 (99672)	*Bassenthwaite*	PFP	CS	PUL	WCR	WCR
550 (99673)	*Rydal Water*	PFP	CS	PUL	WCR	WCR
551 (99674)	*Buttermere*	PFP	CS	PUL	WCR	WCR
552 (99675)	*Ennerdale Water*	PFP	CS	PUL	WCR	WCR
553 (99676)	*Crummock Water*	PFP	CS	PUL	WCR	WCR
586 (99677)	*Derwentwater*	PFB	CS	PUL	WCR	WCR

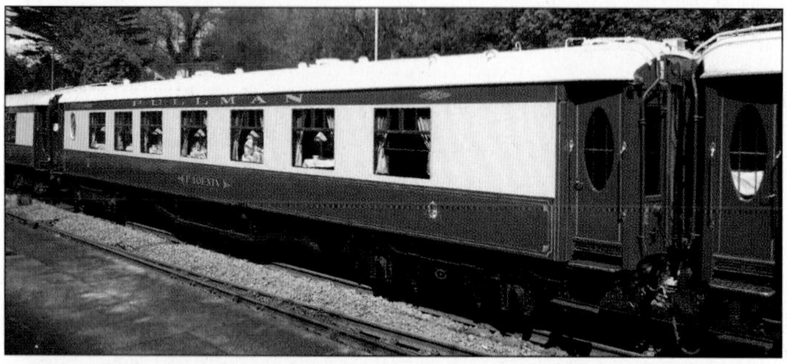

Pullman car Phoenix operating in the Belmond British Pullman was built in 1952 by Pullman at Preston Park, Brighton. Its number is 302 and its operational identity 99531. It is seen at St Austell in 2018. **Antony Christie**

1960s Mk2 BR Pullman. 586 Derwentwater *is operated by West Coast Railway, it is currently in umber and cream Pullman colours.* **Nathan Williamson**

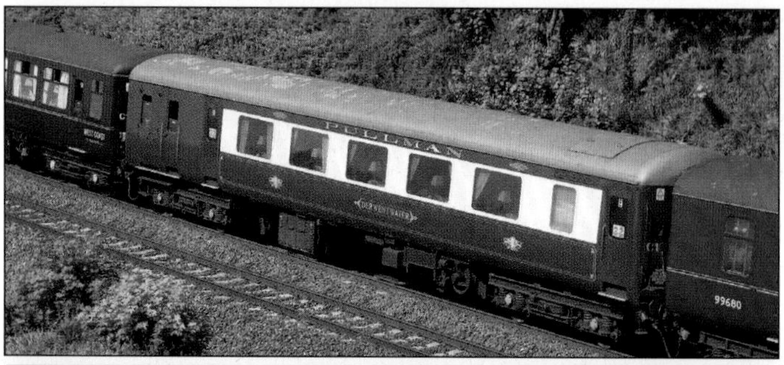

Pre-Nationalisation

41 (45018 / 99052)	LNWR Saloon	CS	MAR	WCR	WCR
159 (5159 / 99880)	LNWR Dining	CS	MAR	WCR	WCR
807 (4807 / 99881)	GNR First	CS	SPL	WCR	WCR
1999 (902260 / 99131)	LNER Saloon	CS	MAR	WCR	WCR
6320 (395707)	LMS GM Saloon	SK	MAR	MRC	MRC

Mk1, Mk2, Mk3, Mk4, Mk5

Mk1
Vehicle Length: 63ft 6in (20.11m)
Height: 12ft 9½in (3.89m)
Width: 9ft 3in (2.81m)

Mk2
Vehicle Length: 66ft 0in (19.35m)
Height: 12ft 9½in (3.89m)
Width: 9ft 3in (2.81m)

Mk 3
Vehicle Length: 75ft 0in (22.86m)
Height: 12ft 9in (3.88m)
Width: 8ft 11in (2.71m)

Mk 4
Vehicle Length: 75ft 0in (22.86m)
Height: 12ft 5in (3.78m)
Width: 8ft 11in (2.71m)

Mk 5
Vehicle Length: 72ft 10in (22.2m)
Height: 12ft 5in (3.78m)
Width: 9ft 0in (2.75m)

324	PFK	1	*Jos de Crau*	NY	PUL	NYM	NYM
325 (2907)	PFK	1	*Duart*	CS	PUL	WCR	WCR
1200 (3287, 6459)	FBO	2f		BU	BLG	RIV	RIV
1203 (3291)	FBO	2f		CL	CAR	LSL	LSL
1207 (3328, 6422)	FBO	2f		CS	VIR	WCR	WCR
1210 (3405, 6462)	FBO	2f		YM	FSR	ERS	ERS
1211 (3305)	FBO	2f	*Snaefell*	CL	PUL	LSL	LSL
1212 (3427, 6453)	FBO	2f		BU	BLG	RIV	RIV
1213 (3419)	FBO	2f		YM	FSR	ERS	ERS
1220 (3315, 6432)	FBO	2f		WO	FSR	ERS	ERS
1221 (3371)	FBO	2f		CS	ICS	WCR	WCR-S
1256 (3296)	RFO	2f	(PLPR3)	ZA	NRL	NRL	NRL
1566	RKR	1	*Caerdydd*	CS	NBL	WCR	WCR
1651	RBR	1		BU	CAR	RIV	RIV
1657	RBR	1		BU	BLG	RIV	RIV
1659	RBR	1		CL	CAR	LSL	LSL
1666	RBR	1		CS	MAR	RAM	WCR
1671	RBR	1		ZG	CHC	RIV	RIV
1683	RBR	1		BU	BLU	RIV	RIV
1691	RBR	1		BU	BLG	RIV	RIV
1692	RBR	1		YM	BLG	ERS	ERS
1694	RBR	1		YM	-	ERS	ERS
1730	RBR	1		BO	CAR	SRP	SRP
1813	RMB	1		BU	CHC	RIV	RIV
1823	RMB	1		NY	MAR	NYM	NYM
1832	RMB	1		ZG	CHC	RIV	RIV
1840	RMB	1		CS	MAR	WCR	WCR
1859	RMB	1		BO	MAR	SRP	SRP
1860	RMB	1		CS	MAR	WCR	WCR
1861	RMB	1		CS	MAR	WCR	WCR
1863	RMB	1		CL	CHC	LSL	LSL
1882 (99311)	RMB	1		CS	MAR	WCR	WCR
1953	RBR	1		CS	VIR	WCR	WCR-S
1961	RBR	1		CS	MAR	WCR	WCR
3045	FO	1		CL	CAR	LSL	LSL
3051	FO	1		YM	-	ERS	ERS
3058	FO	1	*Florence*	CS	MAR	WCR	WCR
3093	FO	1	*Florence*	CS	MAR	WCR	WCR
3096	FO	1		BO	MAR	SRP	SRP
3097	FO	1		BU	CHC	RIV	RIV
3098	FO	1		SH	CHC	RIV	RIV
3100	FO	1		CL	CAR	LSL	LSL
3105 (99121)	FO	1	*Julia*	CS	MAR	WCR	WCR
3106 (99122)	FO	1	*Alexandra*	CS	MAR	WCR	WCR
3110	FO	1		BU	CHC	RIV	RIV
3113 (99125)	FO	1	*Jessica*	CS	MAR	WCR	WCR
3115	FO	1		BO	MAR	SRP	SRP
3117 (99127)	FO	1	*Christina*	CS	MAR	WCR	WCR
3119	FO	1		BU	CHC	RIV	RIV
3120	FO	1		SH	CHC	RIV	RIV
3121	FO	1		BU	CHC	RIV	RIV
3122	FO	1		CL	CAR	LSL	LSL
3123	FO	1		BU	CHC	RIV	RIV
3125	FO	1		CL	CAR	LSL	LSL
3128 (99371)	FO	1	*Victoria*	CS	MAR	WCR	WCR
3130 (99128)	FO	1	*Pamela*	CS	MAR	WCR	WCR
3136	FO	1	*Diana*	CS	MAR	WCR	WCR
3141	FO	1		BU	CHC	RIV	RIV
3143	FO	1	*Patricia*	CS	MAR	WCR	WCR
3146	FO	1		BU	CHC	RIV	RIV
3147	FO	1		BU	CHC	RIV	RIV
3148	FO	1		CL	CAR	LSL	LSL
3149	FO	1		ZG	CHC	RIV	RIV
3150	FO	1		BO	CAR	SRP	SRP
3174	FO	2d	*Glamis*	CS	VIR	WCR	WCR
3182	FO	2d	*Warwick*	CS	VIR	WCR	WCR
3188	FO	2d	*Cadair Idris*	CL	PUL	LSL	LSL
3223	FO	2e	*Diamond*	CL	BLU	LSL	LSL
3229	FO	2e	*Snowdon*	CL	PUL	LSL	LSL
3231	FO	2e		CL	PUL	LSL	LSL
3232	FO	2e		CS	BLG	WCR	WCR
3240	FO	2e	*Sapphire*	CL	BLU	LSL	LSL
3247	FO	2e	*Chatsworth*	CS	NBL	WCR	WCR
3267	FO	2e	*Belvoir*	CS	NBL	WCR	WCR
3273	FO	2e	*Alnwick*	CS	NBL	WCR	WCR
3275	FO	2e	*Harlech*	CS	NBL	WCR	WCR
3278	FO	2f		BU	BLG	RIV	RIV
3304	FO	2f		BU	BLG	RIV	RIV
3312	FO	2f		CL	PUL	LSL	LSL
3313	FO	2f	*Helvellyn*	CS	MAR	WCR	WCR
3314	FO	2f		BU	BLG	RIV	RIV
3325	FO	2f		ZG	VIR	RIV	RIV
3326	FO	2f		CS	MAR	WCR	WCR

3330	FO	2f		CL	CAR	LSL	LSL
3333	FO	2f		BU	BLG	RIV	RIV
3340	FO	2f		BU	BLG	RIV	RIV
3344	FO	2f	*Ben Cruachan*	CL	PUL	LSL	LSL
3345	FO	2f		BU	BLG	RIV	RIV
3348	FO	2f	*Ingleborough*	CL	PUL	LSL	LSL
3350	FO	2f		CS	MAR	WCR	WCR
3352	FO	2f		CS	MAR	WCR	WCR
3356	FO	2f		BU	BLG	RIV	RIV
3359	FO	2f		CS	MAR	WCR	WCR
3360	FO	2f		CS	PUL	WCR	WCR
3362	FO	2f		CS	PUL	WCR	WCR
3364	FO	2f		BU	BLG	RIV	RIV
3384	FO	2f	*Pen-y-Ghent*	CL	PUL	LSL	LSL
3386	FO	2f		BU	BLG	RIV	RIV
3390	FO	2f		BU	BLG	RIV	RIV
3392	FO	2f		CS	MAR	WCR	WCR
3395	FO	2f		CS	MAR	WCR	WCR
3397	FO	2f		BU	BLG	RIV	RIV
3411	FO	2f		YM	BLU	ERS	ERS
3426	FO	2f	*Ben Nevis*	CL	PUL	LSL	LSL
3431	FO	2f		CS	MAR	WCR	WCR
3438	FO	2f	*Ben Lomond*	CL	PUL	LSL	LSL
3798	SO	1		NY	MAR	NYM	NYM
3801	SO	1		NY	CAR	NYM	NYM
3860	SO	1		NY	MAR	NYM	NYM
3872	SO	1		NY	BLG	NYM	NYM
3948	SO	1		NY	CAR	NYM	NYM
4198	SO	1		NY	CAR	NYM	NYM
4252	SO	1		NY	CAR	NYM	NYM
4286	SO	1		NY	CAR	NYM	NYM
4290	SO	1		NY	MAR	NYM	NYM
4455	SO	1		NY	CAR	NYM	NYM
4786	SO	1		NY	CHC	NYM	NYM
4817	SO	1		NY	MAR	NYM	NYM
4831	TSO	1		BO	MAR	SRP	SRP
4832	TSO	1		BO	MAR	SRP	SRP
4836	TSO	1		BO	MAR	SRP	SRP
4854	TSO	1		CS	MAR	WCR	WCR
4856	TSO	1		BO	MAR	SRP	SRP
4905	TSO	1		CS	MAR	WCR	WCR
4927	TSO	1		BU	CAR	RIV	RIV
4931 (99329)	TSO	1		CS	MAR	WCR	WCR
4940	TSO	1		CS	MAR	WCR	WCR
4946	TSO	1		BU	CHC	RIV	RIV
4949	TSO	1		BU	CHC	RIV	RIV
4951	TSO	1		CS	MAR	WCR	WCR
4954 (99326)	TSO	1		CS	MAR	WCR	WCR
4959	TSO	1		ZG	CHC	RIV	RIV
4960	TSO	1		CS	MAR	WCR	WCR
4973	TSO	1		CS	MAR	WCR	WCR
4984	TSO	1		CS	MAR	WCR	WCR
4990	TSO	1		NY	MAR	NYM	NYM
4991	TSO	1		BU	CHC	RIV	RIV
4994	TSO	1		CS	MAR	WCR	WCR
4998	TSO	1		BU	CHC	RIV	RIV
5000	TSO	1		NY	MAR	NYM	NYM
5009	TSO	1		BU	CHC	RIV	RIV
5028	TSO	1		BO	MAR	SRP	SRP
5029	TSO	1		NY	CHC	NYM	NYM
5032	TSO	1		CS	MAR	WCR	WCR
5033 (99328)	TSO	1		CS	MAR	WCR	WCR
5035	TSO	1		CS	MAR	WCR	WCR
5044 (99327)	TSO	1		CS	MAR	WCR	WCR
5157	TSO	2		TM	CHC	VTN	VTN
5171	TSO	2		CS	MAR	WCR	WCR
5177	TSO	2		TM	CHC	VTN	VTN
5191	TSO	2		TM	CHC	VTN	VTN
5198	TSO	2		TM	CHC	VTN	VTN
5200	TSO	2		CS	MAR	WCR	WCR
5212	TSO	2		TM	CHC	VTN	VTN
5216	TSO	2		CS	MAR	WCR	WCR
5222	TSO	2		CS	MAR	WCR	WCR
5229	TSO	2		CS	MAR	WCR	WCR
5236	TSO	2		CS	MAR	WCR	WCR
5237	TSO	2		CS	MAR	WCR	WCR
5239	TSO	2		CS	MAR	WCR	WCR
5249	TSO	2		CS	MAR	WCR	WCR
5278	TSO	2a		CS	MAR	WCR	WCR
5292	TSO	2a		BU	CAR	RIV	RIV
5366	TSO	2a		CL	CAR	LSL	LSL
5419	TSO	2a		CS	MAR	WCR	WCR
5482	TSO	2b		YM	BLG	ERS	ERS
5487	TSO	2b		CS	MAR	WCR	WCR
5626	TSO	2d		PM	BLU	GWR	GWR
5647	TSO	2d		YM	MAR	ERS	ERS
5787	TSO	2e		YM	BLU	ERS	ERS
5810	TSO	2e		CN	LOR	LSL	LOR
5842	TSO	2e		YM	MAR	ERS	ERS
5910	TSO	2f		BU	GRY	RIV	RIV
5912	TSO	2f		CL	PUL	LSL	LSL
5919	TSO	2f		CN	GRY	LSL	LOR
5921	TSO	2f		BU	ANG	RIV	RIV
5929	TSO	2f		BU	BLG	RIV	RIV
5937	TSO	2f		YM	BLU	ERS	ERS
5945	TSO	2f		BU	ASR	RIV	RIV
5950	TSO	2f		BU	ANG	RIV	RIV

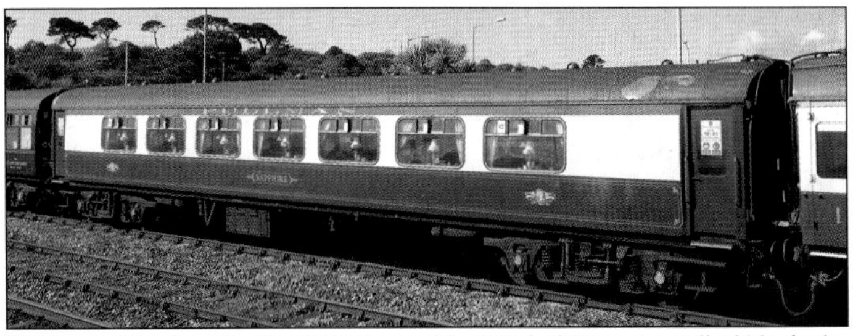

Pullman Car Sapphire, *No. 351 (99351) is one of the 1960s-built Metro-Cammell vehicles for the then Eastern Region. It is a Parlour Second and is now operated by West Coast Railway, based at Carnforth. It is seen at Penzance in September 2021.* **Antony Christie**

5955	TSO	2f		BU	ASR	RIV	RIV
5961	TSO	2f		BU	BLG	RIV	RIV
5964	TSO	2f		BU	ANG	RIV	RIV
5965	TSO	2f		BU	ASR	RIV	RIV
5971	TSO	2f		ZA	LOM	DRS	NRL
5976	TSO	2f		BU	ASR	RIV	RIV
5981	TSO	2f	(PLPR2)	ZA	NRL	NRL	NRL
5985	TSO	2f		BU	ASR	RIV	RIV
5987	TSO	2f		BU	ASR	RIV	RIV
5991	TSO	2f		CL	CAR	LSL	LSL
5995	TSO	2f		ZA	LOM	DRS	NRL
5998	TSO	2f		BU	BLG	RIV	RIV
6000	TSO	2f		CS	MAR	WCR	WCR
6001	TSO	2f		ZA	LOM	DRS	NRL
6006	TSO	2f		BU	ANG	RIV	RIV
6008	TSO	2f		ZA	LOM	DRS	NRL
6012	TSO	2f		CS	MAR	WCR	WCR
6021	TSO	2f		CS	PUL	WCR	WCR
6022	TSO	2f		CS	MAR	WCR	WCR
6024	TSO	2f		BU	BLG	RIV	RIV
6027	TSO	2f	Yorkshire Wolds Railway				
6042	TSO	2f		BU	ANG	RIV	RIV
6046	TSO	2f		CL	GRY	LSL	LSL
6051	TSO	2f		BU	BLG	RIV	RIV
6054	TSO	2f		BU	BLG	RIV	RIV
6064	TSO	2f		YM	BLU	ERS	ERS
6067	TSO	2f		BU	BLG	RIV	RIV
6103	TSO	2f		CS	MAR	WCR	WCR
6115	TSO	2f		CS	MAR	WCR	WCR
6117	TSO	2F		ZA	LOM	DRS	NRL
6122	TSO	2f		ZA	DRS	DRS	NRL
6137	TSO	2f		BU	ASR	RIV	RIV
6141	TSO	2f		BU	VIR	RIV	RIV
6158	TSO	2f		BU	BLG	RIV	RIV
6173	TSO	2f		YM	BLU	ERS	ERS
6176	TSO	2f		KM	DRS	DRS	DRS
6177	TSO	2f		BU	ASR	RIV	RIV
6183	TSO	2f		BU	ASR	RIV	RIV
6260 (92116)	GEN	1		ZA	NRL	NRL	NRL
6261 (92988)	GEN	1		ZA	NRL	NRL	NRL
6262 (92928)	GEN	1		ZA	NRL	NRL	NRL
6263 (92961)	GEN	1		ZA	NRL	NRL	NRL
6264 (92923)	GEN	1		ZA	NRL	NRL	NRL
6310 (81448)	GEN	1		ZG	CHC	RIV	RIV
6311 (92911)	GEN	1		CL	CAR	LSL	LSL
6312 (92925)	GEN	1		CS	MAR	WCR	WCR
6313 (92167)	GEN	1		SL	PUL	BEL	BEL
6330 (975629)	BAR	1		LR	ROG	ANG	ROG
6336 (92185)	BAR	1		LA	BLU	ANG	GWR
6338 (92180)	BAR	1		LR	BLU	ANG	ROG
6340 (975678)	BAR	1		LR	ROG	ANG	ROG
6344 (92080)	BAR	1		LR	ROG	ANG	ROG
6346 (9422)	BAR	1		LR	ROG	ANG	ROG
6348 (92963)	BAR	1		LA	BLU	ANG	GWR
6352 (19465)	BAR	1		HQ	HSB	EVL	OLS
6353 (19478)	BAR	1		NL	HSB	EVL	(S)
6376 (975973)	BAR	1		TO	PTR	DBC	GBR
6377 (975975)	BAR	1		TO	PTR	DBC	GBR
6378 (975971)	BAR	1		LR	PTR	ROG	ROG
6379 (975972)	BAR	1		LR	PTR	ROG	ROG
6392 (92183)	BFR	1		ZA	PTR	COL	COL
6393 (92196)	BAR	1		ZG	PTR	GBR	GBR
6394 (92906)	BAR	1		ZG	PTR	GBR	GBR
6397 (92190)	BFR	1		ZA	PTR	COL	COL

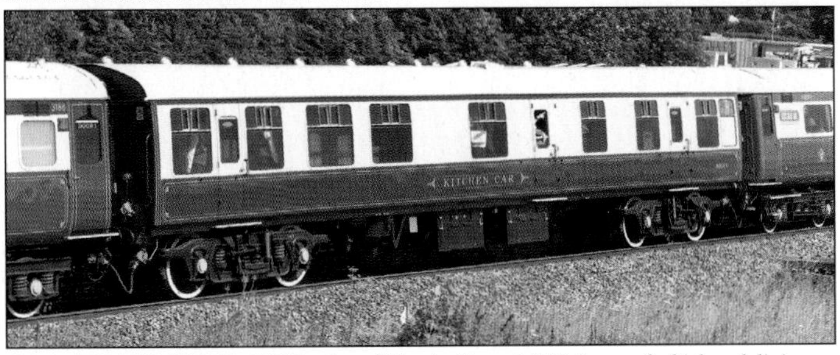

Original BR MK1 RBR No. 1680 has been fully rebuilt as a full kitchen car for high-end dining trains and renumbered as 80043. It is operated by Loco Services Ltd and painted in umber and cream Pullman colours. Is is seen working in 'The Statesman' train at Dawlish Warren in summer 2021. **CJM**

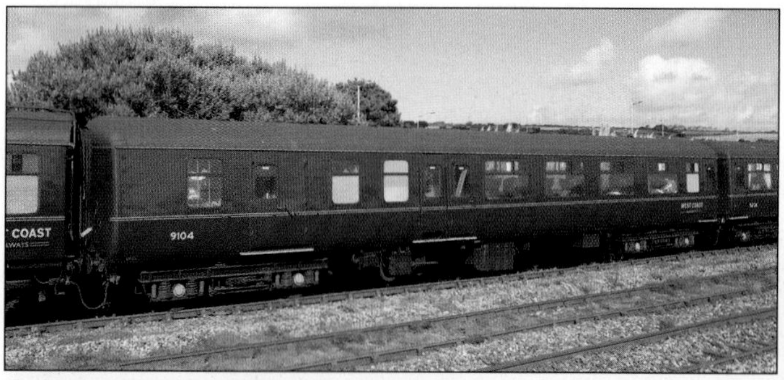

Displaying West Coast Railway lines maroon livery, Mk2 BSO No. 9104 is seen from its brake van end at Penzance in September 2021. The vehicle provides brake accommodation, 2+2 seating and a toilet at the non-brake end. **Antony Christie**

6398 (92126)	BAR	1		NL	EMR	PTR	EMR
6399 (92994)	BAR	1		NL	EMR	PTR	EMR
6410 (977390)	FO	2c		WO	GRN	ERS	ERS
6528 (5592)	TSOT	2c		CS	MAR	WCR	WCR
6700 (3347	RLO	2f		YM	CAL	ERS	ERS
6701 (3346)	RLO	2f		ZM	CAL	BRO	BRO
6702 (3421)	RLO	2f		YM	FSR	ERS	ERS
6703 (3308)	RLO	2f		WO	CAL	ERS	ERS
6704 (3341)	RLO	2f		YM	FSR	ERS	ERS
6705 (3310/6430)	OBS	2f	*Ardnamurchan*	CL	CAR	LSL	LSL
6706 (3283/6421)	RLO	2f	*Mount Mgahinga*	CL	CAR	LSL	LSL
6707 (3276/6418)	RLO	2f		YM	FSR	ERS	ERS
6708 (3370)	RLO	2f	*Mount Helicon*	CL	CAR	LSL	LSL
6723	RMBF	2d		CS	MAR	WCR	WCR
6724	RMBF	2d		CS	MAR	WCR	WCR
9101	BSOT	2		TM	CHC	VTN	VTN
9104	BSOT	2		CS	MAR	WCR	WCR
9225	BSO	1		NY	MAR	NYM	NYM
9274	BSO	1		NY	MAR	NYM	NYM
9391	BSOT	2		CS	MAR	WCR	WCR
9392	BSOT	2		CS	MAR	WCR	WCR
9419	ESC	2a		KM	DRS	DRS	DRS
9428	ESC	2a		KM	DRS	DRS	DRS
9448	BSO	2c		YM	MAR	ERS	ERS
9479	BSO	2d		CL	PUL	LSL	LSL
9481	BSO	2d	(support vehicle)	ZA	NRL	NRL	NRL
9488	BSO	2d		ML	ASR	DRS	DRS
9493	BSO	2d		CS	MAR	WCR	WCR
9497	BSO	2e		WO	CAL	ERS	ERS
9502	BSO	2e		SL	SPL	BEL	BEL
9504	BSO	2e		BU	BLG	RIV	RIV
9506	ESC	2e		KM	DRS	DRS	DRS
9507	BSO	2e		BU	BLG	RIV	RIV
9508	ESC	2e		KM	DRS	DRS	DRS
9509	BSO	2e		BU	ATW	RIV	RIV
9513	BSO	2f		WO	ICS	ERS	ERS
9516	BSO	2f	(Brake force runner)	ZA	NRL	NRL	NRL
9520	BSO	2f		BU	ANG	RIV	RIV
9521	BSO	2f		BU	DRS	RIV	RIV
9523	BSO	2f	(Brake force runner)	ZA	NRL	NRL	NRL
9525	BSO	2f		CN	GRY	LSL	LOM
9526	BSO	2f		BU	BLG	RIV	RIV
9527	BSO	2f		BU	ASR	RIV	RIV
9537	BSO	2f		BU	VIR	RIV	RIV
9539	BSO	2f		BU	ASR	RIV	RIV
9701 (9528)	DBSO	2f	(RTOV)	ZA	NRL	NRL	NRL
9702 (9510)	DBSO	2f	(RTOV)	ZA	NRL	NRL	NRL
9703 (9517)	DBSO	2f	(RTOV)	ZA	NRL	NRL	NRL
9704 (9512)	DBSO	2f		CL	BLU	LSL	LSL
9705 (9519)	DBSO	2f		BH	BLU	PRI	PRI
9707 (9511)	DBSO	2f		CL	DRS	LSL	LSL
9708 (9530)	DBSO	2f	(RTOV)	ZA	NRL	NRL	NRL
9709 (9515)	DBSO	2f		YM	BLU	ERS	ERS
9710 (9518)	DBSO	2f		YM	BLU	ERS	ERS
9714 (9536)	DBSO	2f	(RTOV)	ZA	NRL	NRL	NRL
9800 (5751)	BUO	2e		WO	CAL	ERS	ERS
9801 (5760)	BUO	2e	(Support vehicle)	ZA	CAL	ERS	NRL
9802 (5772)	BUO	2e		YM	CAL	ERS	ERS
9803 (5799)	BUO	2e	(Support vehicle)	ZA	CAL	ERS	NRL
9804 (5826)	BUO	2e		YM	CAL	ERS	ERS
9805 (5833)	BUO	2e		YM	CAL	ERS	ERS
9806 (5840)	BUO	2e	(Support vehicle)	WO	CAL	ERS	NRL
9807 (5851)	BUO	2e		YM	CAL	ERS	ERS
9808 (5871)	BUO	2e	(Support vehicle)	ZA	CAL	ERS	NRL
9809 (5890)	BUO	2e		YM	CAL	ERS	ERS
9810 (5892)	BUO	2e	(Support vehicle)	YM	CAL	ERS	NRL
10211	RFM	3a		TO	SPL	DBC	DBC
10212	RFM	3a		YM	GAR	ERS	ERS
10217	RFB	3a		PZ	GWG	PTR	GWR
10219	RFB	3a		PZ	GWG	PTR	GWR
10225	RFB	3a		PZ	GWG	PTR	GWR
10237	RFB	3a		RJ	BLU	DAS	DAS
10242	RFB	3a		BU	ICS	NEM	NEM
10249	RFM	3a		LR	TFW	ROG	ROG
10259	RFM	3a		LR	TFW	ROG	OLS
10271	RKF	3a		AL	CRW	ATR	CRW
10272	RKF	3a		AL	CRW	ATR	CRW
10273	RKF	3a		AL	CRW	ATR	CRW
10274	RKF	3a		AL	CRW	ATR	CRW

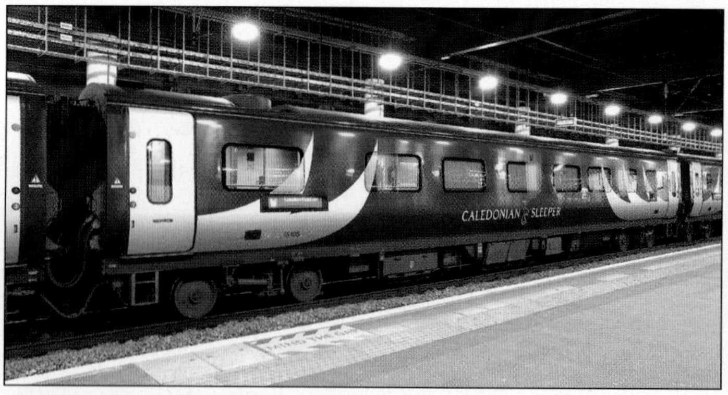

Caledonian Sleepers operate 10 CAF-built Lounge cars, in the 15101-15110 range. One of these is formed in each train section. No. 15105 (96 70 0015105-0) is seen at Euston in January 2022, from the staff access door end. All Caledonian Sleepers carry their full EVN identities. **Antony Christie**

10300	RSB	4	NL	LNE	EVL	LNE
10301	RSB	4	CV	BLK	TFW	TFW
10305	RSB	4	NL	LNE	EVL	LNE
10306	RSB	4	NL	LNE	EVL	LNE
10307	RSB	4	CV	LNE	TFW	TFW
10309	RSB	4	NL	LNE	EVL	LNE
10311	RSB	4	NL	LNE	EVL	LNE
10312	RSB	4	CV	TFW	TFW	TFW
10313	RSB	4	NL	LNE	EVL	LNE
10315	RSB	4	NL	LNE	EVL	LNE
10318	RSB	4	CV	BLK	TFW	TFW
10321	RSB	4	CV	BLK	TFW	TFW
10324	RSB	4	NL	LNE	EVL	LNE
10325	RSB	4	CV	TFW	TFW	TFW
10328	RSB	4	CV	TFW	TFL	TFW
10330	RSB	4	CV	BLK	TFL	OLS
10333	RSB	4	NL	LNE	EVL	LNE
10401	TSOB	3a	Mid Norfolk Railway			
10405	TSOB	3a	Mid Norfolk Railway			
10406	TSOB	3a	ETL at LR with ROG			
10411	TSOB	3a	CL	ICS	LSL	LSL
10413	TSOB	3a	YM	GAR	ERS	ERS
10414	TSOB	3a	Mid Norfolk Railway			
10415	TSOB	3a	CL	GAR	LSL	LSL
10416	TSOB	3a	CL	ICS	LSL	LSL
10417	TSOB	3a	The Auckland Project			
10501	SLEP	3	YM	FSR	ERS	ERS
10502	SLEP	3	YM	FSR	ERS	ERS
10504	SLEP	3	KR	FSR	LSL	LSL
10513	SLEP	3	KR	FSR	LSL	LSL
10519	SLEP	3	KR	FSR	LSL	LSL
10520	SLEP	3	KR	CAR	LSL	LSL
10532	SLEP	3	PZ	GWG	PTR	GWR
10534	SLEP	3	PZ	GWG	PTR	GWR
10541 (99968)	SLEP	3	CS	GSW	GSW	GSW
10546	SLEP	3	TO	SPL	DBC	DBC
10551	SLEP	3	PZ	GWG	PTR	GWR
10553	SLEP	3	PZ	GWG	PTR	GWR
10556 (99969)	SLEP	3	CS	GSW	GSW	GSW
10561	SLEP	3	Mid Norfolk Railway			
10563	SLEP	3	PZ	GWG	PTR	GWR
10584	SLEP	3	PZ	GWG	PTR	GWR
10589	SLEP	3	PZ	GWG	PTR	GWR
10590	SLEP	3	PZ	GWG	PTR	GWR
10594	SLEP	3	PZ	GWG	PTR	GWR
10596	SLEP	3	PZ	GWG	PTR	GWR
10598	SLEP	3	CS	FSR	WCR	WCR
10600	SLEP	3	YM	FSR	ERS	ERS
10601	SLEP	3	PZ	GWG	PTR	GWR
10610	SLEP	3	CS	FSR	WCR	WCR
10612	SLEP	3	PZ	GWG	PTR	GWR
10614	SLEP	3	CS	FSR	WCR	WCR
10616	SLEP	3	PZ	GWG	PTR	GWR
10648	SLE	3	KR	FSR	LSL	LSL
10650	SLE	3	KR	FSR	LSL	LSL
10675	SLE	3	KR	FSR	LSL	LSL
10683	SLE	3	KR	FSR	LSL	LSL
10688	SLE	3	CL	PUL	LSL	LSL
10699	SLE	3	YM	FSR	ERS	ERS
10703	SLE	3	CS	NBL	WCR	WCR
10706	SLE	3	WB	FSR	PTR	PTR
10714	SLE	3	CS	FSR	PRI	PRI
10718	SLE	3	CS	FSR	WCR	WCR
10719	SLE	3	CS	FSR	PRI	PRI
10729	SLE	3	CS	NBL	WCR	WCR
10734	SLE	3	CS	NBL	WCR	WCR
11018	FO	3	RJ	VIR	DAS	DAS
11039	FO	3	TO	SPL	DBC	DBC
11048	FO	3	RJ	VIR	DAS	DAS
11067	FO	3a	Mid Norfolk Railway			
11068	FO	3a	CL	ICS	LSL	LSL
11069	FO	3a	Mid Norfolk Railway			
11070	FO	3a	CL	ICS	LSL	LSL
11073	FO	3a	Mid Norfolk Railway			
11074	FO	3a	RJ	SPL	DAS	DAS
11075	FO	3a	CL	ICS	LSL	LSL
11076	FO	3a	CL	ICS	LSL	LSL

11077	FO	3a	CL	ICS	LSL	LSL
11078	FO	3a	HQ	GAR	ERS	ERS
11080	FO	3a	Mid Norfolk Railway			
11081	FO	3a	Mid Norfolk Railway			
11085	FO	3a	Mid Norfolk Railway			
11087	FO	3a	CL	ICS	LSL	LSL
11088	FO	3a	Richardson School, Smalley			
11090	FO	3a	RJ	GAR	DAS	DAS
11091	FO	3a	CL	ICS	LSL	LSL
11092	FO	3a	ETL at LR with ROG			
11093	FO	3a	Electric Traction Ltd at CD			
11095	FO	3a	YM	GAR	ERS	ERS
11098	FO	3a	CL	ICS	LSL	LSL
11099	FO	3a	ETL at LR with ROG			
11100	FO	3a	Mid Norfolk Railway			
11101	FO	3a	ETL at LR with ROG			
11229	FO	4	NL	LNE	EVL	LNE
11279	FO	4	NL	LNE	EVL	LNE
11284	FO	4	NL	LNE	EVL	LNE
11285	FO	4	NL	LNE	EVL	LNE
11286	FO	4	NL	LNE	EVL	LNE
11288	FO	4	NL	LNE	EVL	LNE
11295	FO	4	DN	LNE	EVL	LNE
11306	FOD	4	NL	LNE	EVL	LNE
11308	FOD	4	NL	LNE	EVL	LNE
11312	FOD	4	NL	LNE	EVL	LNE
11313	FOD	4	NL	LNE	EVL	LNE
11315	FOD	4	NL	LNE	EVL	LNE
11316	FOD	4	CV	LNE	TFW	TFW
11317	FOD	4	NL	LNE	EVL	LNE
11318	FOD	4	NL	LNE	EVL	LNE
11319	FOD	4	CV	BLK	TFW	TFW
11320	FOD	4	CV	BLK	TFW	TFW
11321	FOD	4	CV	BLK	TFW	TFW
11322	FOD	4	CV	BLK	TFW	TFW
11323	FOD	4	CV	TFW	TFW	TFW
11324	FOD	4	CV	TFW	TFW	TFW
11325	FOD	4	CV	TFW	TFW	TFW
11326	FOD	4	DN	LNE	EVL	LNE
11406	FO	4	NL	LNE	EVL	LNE
11408	FO	4	NL	LNE	EVL	LNE
11412	FO	4	NL	LNE	EVL	LNE
11413	FO	4	NL	LNE	EVL	LNE
11415	FO	4	NL	LNE	EVL	LNE
11416	FO	4	NL	LNE	EVL	LNE
11417	FO	4	NL	LNE	EVL	LNE
11418	FO	4	NL	LNE	EVL	LNE
11501	FO	5a	MA	FTP	BEA	FTP
11502	FO	5a	MA	FTP	BEA	FTP
11503	FO	5a	MA	FTP	BEA	FTP
11504	FO	5a	MA	FTP	BEA	FTP
11505	FO	5a	MA	FTP	BEA	FTP
11506	FO	5a	MA	FTP	BEA	FTP
11507	FO	5a	MA	FTP	BEA	FTP
11508	FO	5a	MA	FTP	BEA	FTP
11509	FO	5a	MA	FTP	BEA	FTP
11510	FO	5a	MA	FTP	BEA	FTP
11511	FO	5a	MA	FTP	BEA	FTP
11512	FO	5a	MA	FTP	BEA	FTP
11513	FO	5a	MA	FTP	BEA	FTP
12015	TSO	3a	The Auckland Project			
12017	TSO	3a	YM	CRW	ERS	ERS
12021	TSO	3a	HQ	GAR	ERS	ERS
12030	TSO	3a	Mid Norfolk Railway			
12032	TSO	3a	Mid Norfolk Railway			
12034	TSO	3a	The Auckland Project			
12036	TSO	3a	YM	CRW	ERS	ERS
12043	TSO	3a	YM	CRW	ERS	ERS
12061	TSO	3a	BU	GAR	NEM	NEM
12064	TSO	3a	RJ	GAR	DAS	DAS
12078	TSO	3a	RJ	VIR	DAS	DAS
12079	TSO	3a	BU	GAR	NEM	NEM
12084	TSO	3a	The Auckland Project			
12087	TSO	3a	125 Group, Ruddington			
12090	TSO	3a	Churnet Valley Railway			
12091	TSO	3a	RJ	GAR	DAS	DAS
12092	TSO	3a	RJ	SPL	DAS	DAS
12094	TSO	3a	ERS at Bay Studios, Swansea			
12097	TSO	3a	RJ	GAR	DAS	DAS
12098	TSO	3a	HQ	GAR	ERS	ERS
12100	TSO	3a	PZ	GWG	PTR	GWR
12109	TSO	3a	YM	GAR	ERS	ERS
12108	TSO	3a	The Auckland Project			
12111	TSO	3a	CL	GAR	LSL	LSL
12116	TSO	3a	Battlefield Line			
12122	TSO	3a	RJ	VIR	DAS	DAS
12125	TSO	3a	ETL with ROG			
12126	TSO	3a	The Auckland Project			
12129	TSO	3a	Mid Norfolk Railway			
12130	TSO	3a	Mid Norfolk Railway			
12132	TSO	3a	Mid Norfolk Railway			
12133	TSO	3a	RJ	VIR	DAS	DAS
12137	TSO	3a	Churnet Valley Railway			
12138	TSO	3a	LR	VIR	DAS	DAS
12142	TSO	3a	PZ	GWG	PTR	GWR
12143	TSO	3a	RJ	VIR	DAS	DAS

12146	TSO	3a	BU	GAR	NEM	NEM
12147	TSO	3a	Mid Norfolk Railway			
12154	TSO	3a	ETL with ROG			
12161	TSO	3a	PZ	GWG	PTR	GWR
12164	TSO	3a	BU	GAR	NEM	NEM
12167	TSO	3a	BU	GAR	NEM	NEM
12171	TSO	3a	CL	ICS	LSL	LSL
12176 (11064)	TSO	3a	LR	TFW	ROG	ROG
12180 (11084)	TSO	3a	LR	TFW	ROG	ROG
12182 (11013)	TSO	3a	LR	TFW	ROG	ROG
12202	TSOE	4	NL	LNE	EVL	LNE
12205	TSOE	4	NL	LNE	EVL	LNE
12208	TSOE	4	NL	LNE	EVL	LNE
12210	TSOE	4	CV	BLK	TFW	TFW
12211	TSOE	4	CV	BLK	TFW	TFW
12212	TSOE	4	NL	LNE	EVL	LNE
12213	TSOE	4	NL	LNE	EVL	LNE
12214	TSOE	4	NL	LNE	EVL	LNE
12215	TSOE	4	CV	LNE	TFW	TFW
12217	TSOE	4	CV	TFW	TFW	TFW
12219	TSOE	4	CV	TFW	EVL	TFW
12222	TSOE	4	CV	BLK	TFW	TFW
12223	TSOE	4	NL	LNE	EVL	LNE
12224	TSOE	4	CV	BLK	TFW	TFW
12225	TSOE	4	CV	TFW	EVL	TFW
12226	TSOE	4	NL	LNE	EVL	LNE
12228	TSOE	4	NL	LNE	EVL	LNE
12229	TSOE	4	CV	LNE	TFW	TFW
12230	TSOE	4	Office at York ROC			
12303	TSOD	4	NL	LNE	EVL	LNE
12304	TSOD	4	CV	LNE	TFW	TFW
12305	TSOD	4	WS	LNE	EVL	OLS
12308	TSOD	4	CV	LNE	TFW	TFW
12309	TSOD	4	CV	LNE	TFW	TFW
12310	TSOD	4	CV	BLK	TFW	TFW
12311	TSOD	4	DN	LNE	EVL	LNE
12312	TSOD	4	NL	LNE	EVL	LNE
12313	TSOD	4	NL	LNE	EVL	LNE
12315	TSOD	4	CV	LNE	TFW	TFW
12316	TSOD	4	CV	BLK	TFW	TFW
12323	TSOD	4	CV	BLK	TFW	TFW
12324	TSOD	4	CV	LNE	TFW	TFW
12325	TSOD	4	DN	LNE	EVL	LNE
12326	TSOD	4	CV	BLK	TFW	TFW
12328	TSOD	4	NL	LNE	EVL	LNE
12330	TSOD	4	NL	LNE	EVL	LNE
12404	TSO	4	NL	LNE	EVL	LNE
12406	TSO	4	NL	LNE	EVL	LNE
12407	TSO	4	NL	LNE	EVL	LNE
12409	TSO	4	NL	LNE	EVL	LNE
12410	TSO	4	NL	LNE	EVL	LNE
12415	TSO	4	Fire Service School, Moreton-in Marsh			
12417	TSO	4	Fire Service School, Moreton-in Marsh			
12420	TSO	4	NL	LNE	EVL	LNE
12422	TSO	4	NL	LNE	EVL	LNE
12424	TSO	4	NL	LNE	EVL	LNE
12426	TSO	4	NL	LNE	EVL	LNE
12427	TSO	4	NL	LNE	EVL	LNE
12428	TSO	4	NL	LNE	EVL	LNE
12429	TSO	4	DN	LNE	EVL	LNE
12430	TSO	4	NL	LNE	EVL	LNE
12431	TSO	4	NL	LNE	EVL	LNE
12432	TSO	4	NL	LNE	EVL	LNE
12433	TSO	4	NL	LNE	EVL	LNE
12434	TSO	4	CV	BLK	TFW	TFW
12442	TSO	4	NL	LNE	EVL	LNE
12443	TSO	4	Fire Service School, Moreton-in Marsh			
12444	TSO	4	NL	LNE	EVL	LNE
12446	TSO	4	CV	BLK	TRW	TFW
12447	TSO	4	CV	TFW	TFW	TFW
12452	TSO	4	CV	BLK	TFW	TFW
12454	TSO	4	CV	TFW	EVL	TFW
12461	TSO	4	CV	BLK	TFW	TFW
12464	TSO	4	CV	TFW	EVL	TFW
12465	TSO	4	DN	LNE	EVL	LNE
12467	TSO	4	NL	LNE	EVL	LNE
12468	TSO	4	Office at York ROC			
12469	TSO	4	NL	LNE	EVL	LNE
12474	TSO	4	DN	LNE	EVL	LNE
12477	TSO	4	CV	BLK	TFW	TFW
12480	TSO	4	NL	LNE	EVL	LNE
12481	TSO	4	NL	LNE	EVL	LNE
12485	TSO	4	NL	LNE	EVL	LNE
12486	TSO	4	WS	LNE	EVL	OLS
12515	TSO	4	NL	LNE	EVL	LNE
12526	TSO	4	CV	LNE	TFW	TFW
12602 (12072)	TSO	3a	AL	CRW	ATR	CRW
12603 (12053)	TSO	3a	AL	CRW	ATR	CRW
12604 (12131)	TSO	3a	AL	CRW	ATR	CRW
12605 (11040)	TSO	3a	AL	CRW	ATR	CRW
12606 (12048)	TSO	3a	AL	CRW	ATR	CRW
12607 (12038)	TSO	3a	AL	CRW	ATR	CRW
12608 (12069)	TSO	3a	AL	CRW	ATR	CRW
12609 (12014)	TSO	3a	AL	CRW	ATR	CRW
12610 (12117)	TSO	3a	AL	CRW	ATR	CRW
12613 (12173)	TSO	3a	AL	CRW	ATR	CRW

12614 (12145)	TSO	3a		AL	CRW	ATR	CRW
12615 (12059)	TSO	3a		AL	CRW	ATR	CRW
12616 (12127)	TSO	3a		AL	CRW	ATR	CRW
12617 (12174)	TSO	3a		AL	CRW	ATR	CRW
12618 (12169)	TSO	3a		AL	CRW	ATR	CRW
12619 (12175)	TSO	3a		AL	CRW	ATR	CRW
12620 (12124)	TSO	3a		AL	CRW	ATR	CRW
12621 (11046)	TSO	3a		AL	CRW	ATR	CRW
12623 (11019)	TSO	3a		AL	CRW	ATR	CRW
12625 (11030)	TSO	3a		AL	CRW	ATR	CRW
12627 (11054)	TSO	3a		AL	CRW	ATR	CRW
12701	TSO	5a		MA	FTP	BEA	FTP
12702	TSO	5a		MA	FTP	BEA	FTP
12703	TSO	5a		MA	FTP	BEA	FTP
12704	TSO	5a		MA	FTP	BEA	FTP
12705	TSO	5a		MA	FTP	BEA	FTP
12706	TSO	5a		MA	FTP	BEA	FTP
12707	TSO	5a		MA	FTP	BEA	FTP
12708	TSO	5a		MA	FTP	BEA	FTP
12709	TSO	5a		MA	FTP	BEA	FTP
12710	TSO	5a		MA	FTP	BEA	FTP
12711	TSO	5a		MA	FTP	BEA	FTP
12712	TSO	5a		MA	FTP	BEA	FTP
12713	TSO	5a		MA	FTP	BEA	FTP
12714	TSO	5a		MA	FTP	BEA	FTP
12715	TSO	5a		MA	FTP	BEA	FTP
12716	TSO	5a		MA	FTP	BEA	FTP
12717	TSO	5a		MA	FTP	BEA	FTP
12718	TSO	5a		MA	FTP	BEA	FTP
12719	TSO	5a		MA	FTP	BEA	FTP
12720	TSO	5a		MA	FTP	BEA	FTP
12721	TSO	5a		MA	FTP	BEA	FTP
12722	TSO	5a		MA	FTP	BEA	FTP
12723	TSO	5a		MA	FTP	BEA	FTP
12724	TSO	5a		MA	FTP	BEA	FTP
12725	TSO	5a		MA	FTP	BEA	FTP
12726	TSO	5a		MA	FTP	BEA	FTP
12727	TSO	5a		MA	FTP	BEA	FTP
12728	TSO	5a		MA	FTP	BEA	FTP
12729	TSO	5a		MA	FTP	BEA	FTP
12730	TSO	5a		MA	FTP	BEA	FTP
12731	TSO	5a		MA	FTP	BEA	FTP
12732	TSO	5a		MA	FTP	BEA	FTP
12733	TSO	5a		MA	FTP	BEA	FTP
12734	TSO	5a		MA	FTP	BEA	FTP
12735	TSO	5a		MA	FTP	BEA	FTP
12736	TSO	5a		MA	FTP	BEA	FTP
12737	TSO	5a		MA	FTP	BEA	FTP
12738	TSO	5a		MA	FTP	BEA	FTP
12739	TSO	5a		MA	FTP	BEA	FTP
12801	DSO	5a		MA	FTP	BEA	FTP
12802	DSO	5a		MA	FTP	BEA	FTP
12803	DSO	5a		MA	FTP	BEA	FTP
12804	DSO	5a		MA	FTP	BEA	FTP
12805	DSO	5a		MA	FTP	BEA	FTP
12806	DSO	5a		MA	FTP	BE A	FTP
12807	DSO	5a		MA	FTP	BEA	FTP
12808	DSO	5a		MA	FTP	BEA	FTP
12809	DSO	5a		MA	FTP	BEA	FTP
12810	DSO	5a		MA	FTP	BEA	FTP
12811	DSO	5a		MA	FTP	BEA	FTP
12812	DSO	5a		MA	FTP	BEA	FTP
12813	DSO	5a		MA	FTP	BEA	FTP
12814	DSO	5a		MA	FTP	BEA	FTP
13227	FK	1		CL	CAR	LSL	LSL
13229	FK	1		BO	MAR	SRP	SRP
13230	FK	1		BO	MAR	SRP	SRP
13306	FK	1	*Joana*	CS	MAR	WCR	WCR
13320	FO	1	*Ana*	CS	MAR	WCR	WCR
13440	FK	2a		CS	MAR	WCR	WCR
13573	FK	2d		WO	?	ERS	ERS
14007 (17007)	BFK	1	Support coach 61624	NY	MAR	NYM	NYM
14060 (17060)	BFK	2a	Support coach 45596	TM	MAR	VTN	VTN
15001	SSB	5		PO	SCS	LOM	SCS
15002	SSB	5		PO	SCS	LOM	SCS
15003	SSB	5		PO	SCS	LOM	SCS
15004	SSB	5		PO	SCS	LOM	SCS
15005	SSB	5		PO	SCS	LOM	SCS
15006	SSB	5		PO	SCS	LOM	SCS
15007	SSB	5		PO	SCS	LOM	SCS
15008	SSB	5		PO	SCS	LOM	SCS
15009	SSB	5		PO	SCS	LOM	SCS
15010	SSB	5		PO	SCS	LOM	SCS
15011	SSB	5		PO	SCS	LOM	SCS
15101	SL	5		PO	SCS	LOM	SCS
15102	SL	5		PO	SCS	LOM	SCS
15103	SL	5		PO	SCS	LOM	SCS
15104	SL	5		PO	SCS	LOM	SCS
15105	SL	5		PO	SCS	LOM	SCS
15106	SL	5		PO	SCS	LOM	SCS
15107	SL	5		PO	SCS	LOM	SCS
15108	SL	5		PO	SCS	LOM	SCS
15109	SL	5		PO	SCS	LOM	SCS
15110	SL	5		PO	SCS	LOM	SCS
15201	SLA	5		PO	SCS	LOM	SCS
15202	SLA	5		PO	SCS	LOM	SCS
15203	SLA	5		PO	SCS	LOM	SCS

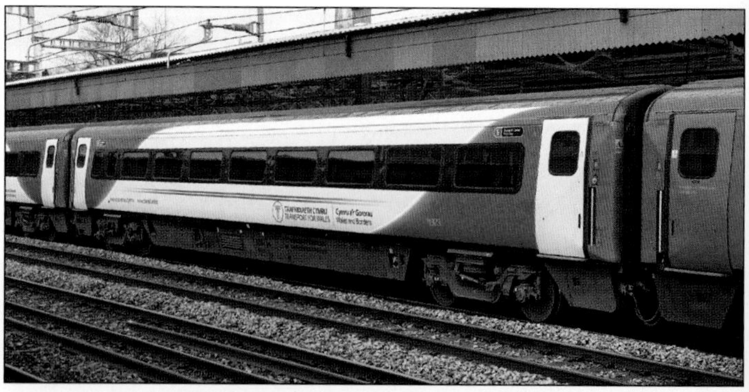

After displacement from LNER services by IET stock, a number of Mk4 vehicles became spare, some were broken up, while other transferred to Transport for Wales, replacing their Mk3s on long distance loco-hauled services. Further coaches will enter traffic in late 2022. FOD No. 11323 is shown at Newport in LNER colours with TfW branding. Note the bi-lingual branding on the vehicle side. **CJM**

15204	SLA	5		PO	SCS	LOM	SCS
15205	SLA	5		PO	SCS	LOM	SCS
15206	SLA	5		PO	SCS	LOM	SCS
15207	SLA	5		PO	SCS	LOM	SCS
15208	SLA	5		PO	SCS	LOM	SCS
15209	SLA	5		PO	SCS	LOM	SCS
15210	SLA	5		PO	SCS	LOM	SCS
15211	SLA	5		PO	SCS	LOM	SCS
15212	SLA	5		PO	SCS	LOM	SCS
15213	SLA	5		PO	SCS	LOM	SCS
15214	SLA	5		PO	SCS	LOM	SCS
15301	SLE	5		PO	SCS	LOM	SCS
15302	SLE	5		PO	SCS	LOM	SCS
15303	SLE	5		PO	SCS	LOM	SCS
15304	SLE	5		PO	SCS	LOM	SCS
15305	SLE	5		PO	SCS	LOM	SCS
15306	SLE	5		PO	SCS	LOM	SCS
15307	SLE	5		PO	SCS	LOM	SCS
15308	SLE	5		PO	SCS	LOM	SCS
15309	SLE	5		PO	SCS	LOM	SCS
15310	SLE	5		PO	SCS	LOM	SCS
15311	SLE	5		PO	SCS	LOM	SCS
15312	SLE	5		PO	SCS	LOM	SCS
15313	SLE	5		PO	SCS	LOM	SCS
15314	SLE	5		PO	SCS	LOM	SCS
15315	SLE	5		PO	SCS	LOM	SCS
15316	SLE	5		PO	SCS	LOM	SCS
15317	SLE	5		PO	SCS	LOM	SCS
15318	SLE	5		PO	SCS	LOM	SCS
15319	SLE	5		PO	SCS	LOM	SCS
15320	SLE	5		PO	SCS	LOM	SCS
15321	SLE	5		PO	SCS	LOM	SCS
15322	SLE	5		PO	SCS	LOM	SCS
15323	SLE	5		PO	SCS	LOM	SCS
15324	SLE	5		PO	SCS	LOM	SCS
15325	SLE	5		PO	SCS	LOM	SCS
15326	SLE	5		PO	SCS	LOM	SCS
15327	SLE	5		PO	SCS	LOM	SCS
15328	SLE	5		PO	SCS	LOM	SCS
15329	SLE	5		PO	SCS	LOM	SCS
15330	SLE	5		PO	SCS	LOM	SCS
15331	SLE	5		PO	SCS	LOM	SCS
15332	SLE	5		PO	SCS	LOM	SCS
15333	SLE	5		PO	SCS	LOM	SCS
15334	SLE	5		PO	SCS	LOM	SCS
15335	SLE	5		PO	SCS	LOM	SCS
15336	SLE	5		PO	SCS	LOM	SCS
15337	SLE	5		PO	SCS	LOM	SCS
15338	SLE	5		PO	SCS	LOM	SCS
15339	SLE	5		PO	SCS	LOM	SCS
15340	SLE	5		PO	SCS	LOM	SCS
15745	CK	1		NY	MAR	NYM	NYM
16156	CK	1		NY	CAR	NYM	NYM
17015	BFK	1	Support coach 71000	TM	CAR	BR8	VTN
17018 (14018)	BFK	1	*Botaurus*	TM	CHC	VTN	VTN
17025 (14025)	BFK	1	Support coach	CS	MAR	WCR	WCR
17041 (14041)	VFK	1	Support coach	TM	CAR	BR8	-
17056 (14056)	BFK	2a		CL	CAR	LSL	LSL
17080 (14080)	BFK	2a		CL	PUL	LSL	LSL
17090 (14090)	BFK	2a		TM	CHC	VTN	VTN
17096 (14096)	BFK	2a	Support coach 35028	SL	PUL	-	-
17102 (14102, 99680)	BFK	2a		CS	MAR	WCR	WCR
17105 (14105, 2905)	BFK	2b		BU	BLG	RIV	RIV
17159 (14159)	BFK	2d		CL	CAR	LSL	LSL
17167 (14167)	BFK	2d	*Mow Cop*	CS	NBL	WCR	WCR
17173	BUO	3b		PZ	GWG	PTR	GWR
17174	BUO	3b		PZ	GWG	PTR	GWR
17175	BUO	3b		PZ	GWG	PTR	GWR
18756 (25756)	CK	1		SH	MAR	WCR	WCR
21096	BCK	1	Support coach 60007	NY	MAR	NYM	NYM
21100	BCK	1		NY	CAR	NYM	NYM
21232 (99040)	BCK	1	Support coach 46201	SK	MAR	MRC	NYM
21241	BCK	1		BO	MAR	SRP	SRP

21249	BCK	1	Support coach 60163	SL	MAR	A1T	-
21256 (99304)	BCK	1		CS	MAR	WCR	WCR
21266	BCK	1		CS	MAR	WCR	WCR
21269	BCK	1		ZG	CAR	RIV	RIV
35089	BSK	1		NY	CAR	NYM	NYM
35185	BSK	1		BO	MAR	SRP	SRP
35317	BSK	1	Support coach LSL	CL	CAR	LSL	LSL
35322 (99035)	BSK	1	Support coach WCR	CS	MAR	WCR	WCR
35451	BSK	1	Support coach LSL	CL	CAR	LSL	LSL
35459 (99723)	BSK	1		CS	MAR	WCR	WCR
35461	BSK	1	Support coach 5029	CL	CHC	LSL	LSL
35463 (99312)	BSK	1	Support coach WCR	CS	MAR	WCR	WCR
35465	BSK	1		CL	CAR	LSL	LSL
35468 (99953)	BSK	1	Support coach NRM	YK	MAR	NRM	NRM
35469	BSK	1		BU	CHC	RIV	RIV
35470	BSK	1	Support coach Tyseley	TM	CHC	TYL	-
35476 (99041)	BSK	1	Support coach 46223	SK	MAR	MRC	-
35479	BSK	1	Support coach 61306	SH	MAR	WCR	WCR
35486 (99405)	BSK	1	Support coach	SH	MAR	WCR	-
35508 (14128)	BFK	2c	Support coach ELR	BQ	MAR	ELR	-
35511 (14130)	BPK	2c		CL	SPL	LSL	LSL
35517 (14088)	BFK	2a	Support coach ELR	BQ	MAR	ELR	-
35518	BFK	2a	Support coach 34067	CS	GRN		WCR
62287	MBS/CIG		(UTU2)	ZA	NRL	NRL	NRL
62384	MBS/CIG		(UTU1)	ZA	NRL	NRL	NRL
64664	DMO/508		(Barrier)	ZG	ARL	ARL	AFS
Livet Angel of Inventions							
64707	DMO/508		(Barrier)	ZG	ARL	ARL	AFS
Labezerin Angel of Success							
68501 (61281)	DMBS/489		(Barrier)	LR	AFG	AFG	AFS
68504 (61286)	DMBS/489		(Barrier)	LR	AFG	AFG	AFS
72612 (6156)	TSO	2f	(Brake force runner)	ZA	NRL	NRL	NRL
72616 (6007)	TSO	2f	(Brake force runner)	ZA	NRL	NRL	NRL
72630 (6094)	TSO	2f	(SGT1)	ZA	NRL	NRL	NRL
72631 (6096)	TSO	2f	(PLPR1)	ZA	NRL	NRL	NRL
72639 (6070)	TSO	2f	(PLPR4)	ZA	NRL	NRL	NRL
80041 (1690)	RBR	1		ZG	MAR	RIV	RIV
80042 (1646)	RBR	1		BU	CHC	RIV	RIV
80043 (1680)	RBR	1		CL	PUL	LSL	LSL
80044 (1659)	RBR	1		CL	CAR	LSL	LSL
80204	BCV	1		CS	MAR	WCR	WCR
80217	BCV	1		CS	MAR	WCR	WCR
80220	BCV	1	Support coach 62005	NY	MAR	NYM	-
80225	BCV	1		South Devon Railway			
82111	DVT	3		LM	NRL	NRL	OLS
82114	DVT	3		Northampton & Lamport Rly			
82115	DVT	3		RJ	BLU	DAS	DAS
82118	DVT	3		Crewe Heritage Centre			
82124	DVT	3		LM	NRL	NRL	OLS
82127	DVT	3		CL	ICS	LSL	LSL
82129	DVT	3		LM	NRL	NRL	OLS
82136	DVT	3		RJ	GAR	DAS	DAS
82138	DVT	3		RJ	VIR	DAS	DAS
82139	DVT	3		CL	ICS	LSL	LSL
82145	DVT	3		LM	NRL	NRL	OLS
82146	DVT	3		TO	SPL	DBC	DBC
82200	DVT	4		CV	BLK	TFW	TFW
82201	DVT	4		WS	BLK	EVL	OLS
82204	DVT	4		CV	LNR	TFW	TFW
82205	DVT	4		NL	LNR	EVL	(S)
82206	DVT	4		CV	LNR	TFW	TFW
82208	DVT	4		NL	LNR	EVL	LNR
82210	DVT	4		WS	LNR	EVL	OLS
82211	DVT	4		NL	LNR	EVL	LNR
82212	DVT	4		NL	LNR	EVL	LNR
82213	DVT	4		NL	LNR	EVL	LNR
82214	DVT	4		NL	LNR	EVL	LNR
82215	DVT	4		NL	LNR	EVL	LNR
82216	DVT	4		CV	SPL	TFW	TFW
82220	DVT	4		NL	LNR	EVL	LNR
82223	DVT	4		NL	LNR	EVL	LNR
82225	DVT	4		NL	LNR	EVL	LNR
82226	DVT	4		CV	SPL	TFW	TFW
82227	DVT	4		CV	BLK	TFW	TFW
82229	DVT	4		CV	SPL	TFW	TFW
82230	DVT	4		CV	BLK	TFW	TFW
82301 (82117)	DVT	3		AL	CRW	ATR	CRW
82302 (82151)	DVT	3		AL	CRW	ATR	CRW
82303 (82135)	DVT	3		AL	CRW	ATR	CRW
82304 (82130)	DVT	3		AL	CRW	ATR	CRW
82305 (82134)	DVT	3		AL	CRW	ATR	CRW
82306 (82144)	DVT	3		RJ	TFW	DAS	DAS
82309 (82104)	DVT	3		AL	CRW	ATR	CRW
92114 (81443) (S)	BG	1		ZA	NRL	NRL	NRL
92904 (99554)	GUV	1		CS	NBL	WCR	WCR
92939 (92039)	BG	1		ZA	SPL	NRL	NRL
94225 (93849)	BG	1		CS	MAR	WCR	WCR
96100 (93734)	GUV	1		TM	SPL	VTN	VTN
96175 (93628)	WCR	1		CS	MAR	WCR	WCR
96371 (10545)	GEN	3		YM	GRY	ERS	ERS
96372 (10564)	GEN	3		YM	GRY	ERS	ERS
96373 (10568)	GEN	3		YM	GRY	DRS	DRS
96374 (10585)	GEN	3		YM	ICS	ERS	ERS
96375 (10587)	GEN	3		YM	GRY	ERS	ERS
96380 (86386)	BAR	1		TI	BLU	EUS	EUS
96381 (86187)	BAR	1		TI	BLU	EUS	EUS
96383 (86664)	BAR	1		TI	BLU	EUS	EUS

96384 (86955)	BAR	1		TI	BLU	EUS	EUS
96602 (96150)	UBV	1	*Henry*	ZA	MGR	MGR	MGR
97 70 GB-MGRL 0096602							
96603 (96155)	UBV	1	*Oliver*	ZA	MGR	MGR	MGR
97 70 GB-MGRL 0096603							
96604 (96156)	NVA	1		RU	YEL	COL	COL
96605 (96157)	UBV	1	*Ernest*	ZA	MGR	MGR	MGR
97 70 GB-MGRL 0096605							
96606 (96213)	NVA	1		RU	YEL	COL	COL
96607 (96215)	UBV	1	*Philip*	ZA	MGR	MGR	MGR
97 70 GB-MGRL 0096607							
96608 (96216)	NVA	1		RU	YEL	COL	COL
96609 (96217)	NVA	1		RU	YEL	COL	COL
99316 (13321)	KIT	1		CS	MAR	WCR	WCR
99318 (4912)	BUF	1		CS	MAR	WCR	WCR
99337 (337)	PUL	1	State Spa Car	HN	GSW	GSW	GSW
99666 (3250)	FO	2e	(SGT1 barrier)	ZA	NRL	NRL	NRL
99712 (18893)	KIT	1		CS	MAR	WCR	WCR
99722 (18806)	TSO	1		CS	MAR	WCR	WCR
99545 (80207)	BCV	1	Support coach	SL	PUL	BEL	BEL
99960 (321)	PUL	1	Dining Car No. 2	HN	ROS	BEL	ROS
99961 (324)	PUL	1	State Car No. 1	HN	ROS	BEL	ROS
99662 (329)	PUL	1	State Car No. 2	HN	ROS	BEL	ROS
99663 (331)	PUL	1	State Car No. 3	HN	ROS	BEL	ROS
99664 (313)	PUL	1	State car No. 4	HN	ROS	BEL	ROS
99665 (319)	PUL	1	Observation Car	HN	ROS	BEL	ROS
99667 (317)	PUL	1	Dining Car No. 1	HN	ROS	BEL	ROS
99884 (19208)	SK	1	Support	YM	-	ERS	ERS
99886 (35407)	BSK	1	Service car	CS	MAR	WCR	WCR
99968 (10541)	SLE	3	State Car No. 5	HN	ROS	BEL	ROS
99969 (10556)	SLE	3	Service Car	HN	ROS	BEL	ROS
99993 (5067)	TSO	1	Club Car	CL	CAR	LSL	LSL
999506	OBS	1	Inspection saloon	CS	MAR	WCR	WCR

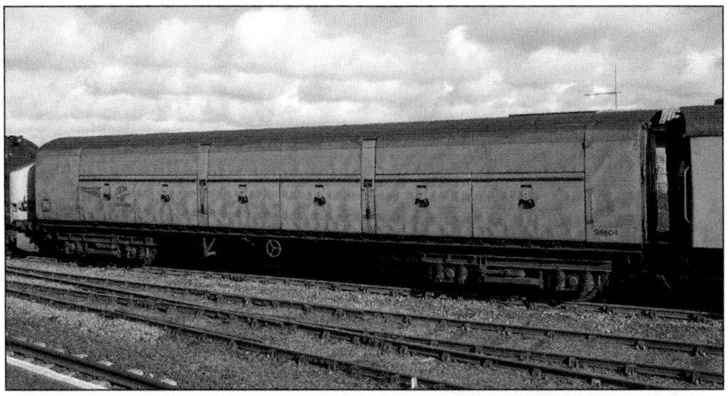

Modified for Colas/Network Rail use from a former side loading Great Western Motorail van, No. 96604 is one of four vehicles of this type frequently seen formed in Network Rail test trains as a make up vehicle. It is seen at Penzance. **Antony Christie**

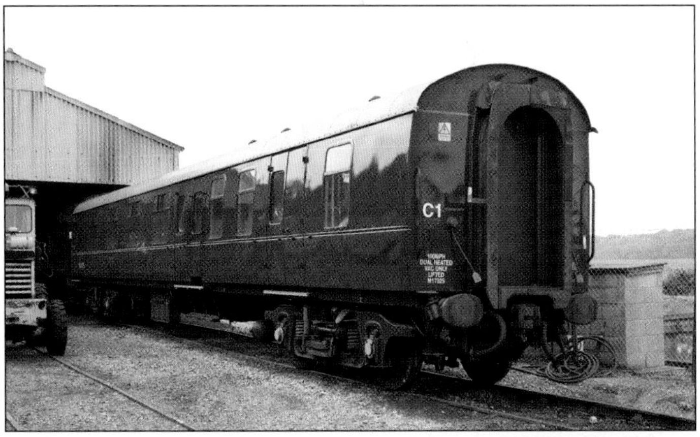

Former Mk 1 BFK No. 17025 is a steam loco support coach, operated by West Coast Railway Co. It is seen at Bishops Lydeard on the West Somerset Railway in September 2021 from its brake stores end. **Antony Christie**

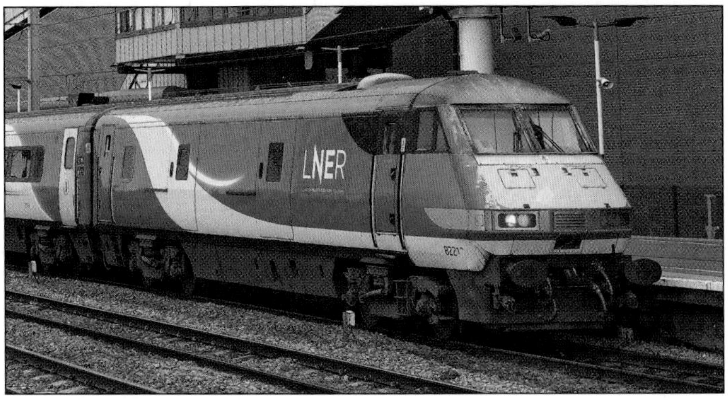

A small number of Mk4/Class 91 formations are still operating on LNER services, with Mk4 DVTs providing the remote cab No. 82213 is shown at Doncaster. **CJM**

Departmental

971001 (94150)	NKA	1	(Tool van)	SP	NRL	NRL	NRL
971002 (94190)	NKA	1	(Tool van)	SP	NRL	NRL	NRL
971003 (94191)	NKA	1	(Tool van)	BS	NRL	NRL	NRL
971004 (94168)	NKA	1	(Tool van)	SP	NRL	NRL	NRL
975025 (60755) *Caroline*	6B Buffet		(Inspection saloon)	ZA	GRN	NRL	NRL
975087	BSK	1	(Recovery train)	SP	NRL	NRL	NRL
975091 (34615)	BSK	1	(Test car *Mentor*)	ZA	NRL	NRL	NRL
975464 (35171)	BSK	1	(Snow train *Ptarmigan*)	SP	NRL	NRL	NRL
975477 (35108)	BSK	1	(Recovery train)	SP	NRL	NRL	NRL
975486 (34100)	BSK	1	(Snow train *Polar Bear*)	SP	NRL	NRL	NRL
975814 (41000)	TF	3	(NMT Conference Coach)	ZA	NRL	NRL	NRL
975864 (3849)	TRN	1	(Translator)	BU	HSB	EVL	-
975867 (1006)	TRN	1	(Translator)	BU	HSB	EVL	-
975875 (34643)	TRN	1	(Translator)	LR	SPL	EVL	ROG
975974 (1030) *Paschar*	RF	1	(Translator)	ZG	GRN	ANG	AFS
975978 (1025) *Perpetiel*	RF	1	(Barrier)	ZG	GRN	ANG	AFS
975984 (40000)	TRUB	3	(NMT Lecture Coach)	ZA	NRL	NRL	NRL
977087 (34971)	TRN	1	(Translator)	LR	SPL	EVL	ROG
977868 (5846)	TSO	2e	(Radio Survey coach)	ZA	NRL	NRL	NRL
977869 (5858)	TSO	2e	(Radio Survey coach)	ZA	NRL	NRL	NRL
977969 (14112)	BFK	2	(Staff coach)	ZA	NRL	NRL	NRL
977974 (5854)	TSO	2e	(TIC 1)	ZA	NRL	NRL	NRL
977983 (72503)	FO	2f	(EMV)	ZA	NRL	NRL	NRL
977984 (40501)	TRFK	3	(Staff Coach)	ZA	NRL	NRL	NRL
977985 (72715)	TSO	2f	(SGT2)	ZA	NRL	NRL	NRL
977986 (3189)	FO	2d	(SGT2 barrier)	ZA	NRL	NRL	NRL
977993 (44053)	TGS	3	(OH line test coach)	ZA	NRL	NRL	NRL
977994 (44087)	TGS	3	(NMT Recording coach)	ZA	NRL	NRL	NRL
977995 (40719)	TRFM	3	(NMT Generator coach)	ZA	NRL	NRL	NRL
977997 (72613)	TSO	2f	(Radio Survey)	ZA	NRL	NRL	NRL
999550 -	SPL	2f	(HSTRC)	ZA	NRL	NRL	NRL
999602 (62483)	Mk1/REP		(UTU3)	ZA	NRL	NRL	NRL
999605 (62482)	Mk1/REP		(UTU)	ZA	NRL	NRL	NRL
999606 (62356)	Mk1/CIG		(UTU4)	ZA	NRL	NRL	NRL

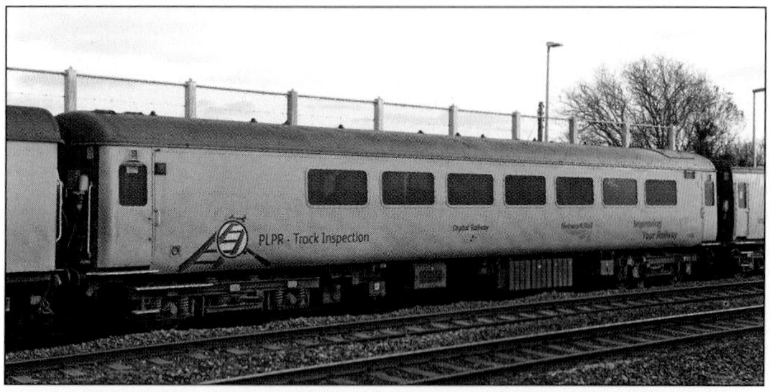

Plain Line Pattern Recognition (PLPR) track inspection coach 72631 is operated by Network Rail and based at the RTC Derby. It is rebuilt for departmental use from a Gatwick Express vehicle was previously Mk2f 6096. Although in Departmental use it has not been renumbered in the 977xxx series. **CJM**

Royal Train

2903 (11001)	HM The Queen's Saloon	ZN	ROY	ROY	DBC
2904 (12001)	HRH Special Saloon	ZN	ROY	ROY	DBC
2915 (10735)	Royal Household Sleeping Coach	ZN	ROY	ROY	DBC
2916 (40512)	HRH The Prince of Wales's Dining Coach	ZN	ROY	ROY	DBC
2917 (40514)	Kitchen Car & Royal Household Coach	ZN	ROY	ROY	DBC
2918 (40515)	Royal Household Coach	ZN	ROY	ROY	DBC
2919 (40518)	Royal Household Coach	ZN	ROY	ROY	DBC
2920 (17109)	Generator Coach & Household Coach	ZN	ROY	ROY	DBC
2921 (17107)	Brake, Coffin & Household Coach	ZN	ROY	ROY	DBC
2922	HRH The Prince of Wales's Sleeper	ZN	ROY	ROY	DBC
2923	HRH The Prince of Wales's Saloon	ZN	ROY	ROY	DBC

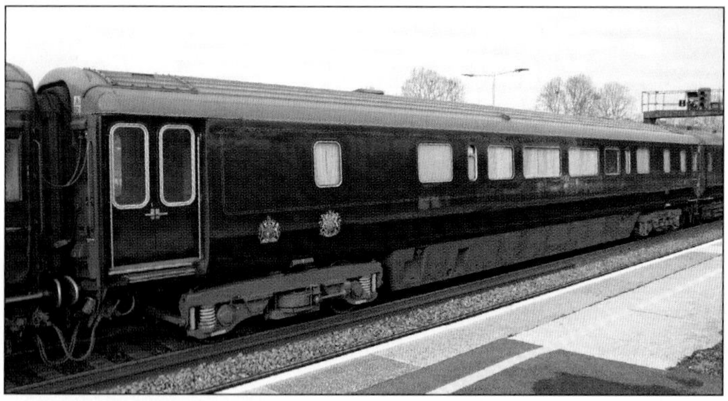

One of the most impressive trains on the UK national network is the Royal Train formed of up to nine vehicles. When not is use it is stabled at Wolverton. Purpose-built Mk3 No. 2922 The Prince of Wales's sleeper/lounge car is seen at Newton Abbot in 2021. **Nathan Williamson**

HST Vehicles

Buffet/Refreshment/Kitchen

40106 (42162)	TGB	CL	GWG	LSL	LSL
40204 (40004, 40404)	TFB	EL	EMR	ANG	OLS
40205 (40005, 40405)	TFB	EL	EMR	ANG	OLS
40221 (40021, 40421)	TFB	EL	EMR	ANG	OLS
40402 (40002)	TFB	ERS at Bay Studios, Swansea			
40601 (41032)	TGFB	IS	IC7	ANG	ASR
40602 (41038)	TGFB	IS	IC7	ANG	ASR
40603 (41006)	TGFB	IS	IC7	ANG	ASR
40604 (41024)	TGFB	IS	IC7	ANG	ASR
40605 (41094)	TGFB	IS	IC7	ANG	ASR
40606 (41104)	TGFB	IS	IC7	ANG	ASR
40607 (41136)	TGFB	IS	IC7	ANG	ASR
40608 (41122)	TGFB	IS	IC7	ANG	ASR
40609 (41020)	TGFB	IS	IC7	ANG	ASR
40610 (41103)	TGFB	IS	IC7	ANG	ASR
40611 (41130)	TGFB	IS	IC7	ANG	ASR
40612 (41134)	TGFB	IS	IC7	ANG	ASR
40613 (41135)	TGFB	IS	IC7	ANG	ASR
40614 (41010)	TGFB	IS	IC7	ANG	ASR
40615 (41022)	TGFB	IS	IC7	ANG	ASR
40616 (41142)	TGFB	IS	IC7	ANG	ASR
40617 (41144)	TGFB	IS	IC7	ANG	ASR
40618 (41016)	TGFB	IS	IC7	ANG	ASR
40619 (41124)	TGFB	IS	IC7	ANG	ASR
40620 (41158)	TGFB	IS	IC7	ANG	ASR
40621 (41146)	TGFB	IS	IC7	ANG	ASR
40624 (40511, 41180)	TGFB	IS	IC7	ANG	ASR
40624 (41116)	TGFB	IS	IC7	ANG	ASR
40625 (41137)	TGFB	IS	IC7	ANG	ASR
40626 (41012)	TGFB	IS	IC7	ANG	ASR
40701 (40301)	TRFK	Citzen Songwriters			
40702 (40302)	TRFK	Wensledale Railway			
40704 (40304)	TRFK	GCR at Leicester			
40706 (40306)	TRFK	Colne Valley Railway			
40711 (40311)	TRFK	Private in Northumbria			
40713 (40313)	TRFK	Lincolnshire Wolds Railway			
40715 (40315)	TRUK	EL	GWR	ANG	(S)
40720 (40320)	TRUK	EL	LNE	ANG	(S)
40728 (40328)	TRFK	LR	EMR	PTR	DAS
40730 (40330)	TRFK	125 Group, Midland Railway			
40732 (40332)	TRFK	Preserved-NRM, Shildon			
40734 (40334)	TRUK	EL	GWR	ANG	(S)
40741 (40341)	TRFK	125 Group, Midland Railway			
40750 (40350)	TRFK	EL	EMR	ANG	(S)
40751 (40351)	TRFK	Cambrian Heritage Railway			
40755 (40355)	TRFK	ZG	GWR	LSL	LSL
40801 (40027, 40427)	BAR	CL	BLP	LSL	LSL
40802 (40012, 40412)	TRK	CL	BLP	LSL	LSL
40804 (40032, 40432)	TFKB	CL	RCG	LSL	LSL
40807 (40035, 40435)	TRFK	The Wee Choo-Choo, Pitlochry (Thai Restaurant)			
40808 (40015, 40415)	TFKB	CL	GWB	LSL	LSL
40900 (40022, 40422)	TRB	LM	GWR	FGP	(S)
40902 (40023, 40423)	TRB	LM	GWR	FGP	(S)
40904 (40001, 40401)	TRB	Northumbria Rail			

Trailer First

41026	FO	LA	AXC	ANG	AXC
41035	FO	LA	AXC	ANG	AXC
41057	FO	125 Group, Midland Railway			
41059	FO	CL	BLP	LSL	LSL
41061	FO	GW	EMR	PTR	OLS
41063	FO	CL	EMR	LSL	LSL
41067	FO	125 Group, Midland Railway			
41087	FO	EL	LNE	ANG	(S)
41088	FO	Colne Valley Railway			
41091	FO	EL	LNE	ANG	(S)
41095	FO	Private in Northumbria			
41100	FO	EL	EMR	ANG	(S)
41106	FO	ZG	GWR	PTR	(S)
41108	FO	CL	BLP	LSL	LSL
41117	FO	CL	EMR	LSL	LSL
41118	FO	EL	LNE	ANG	(S)

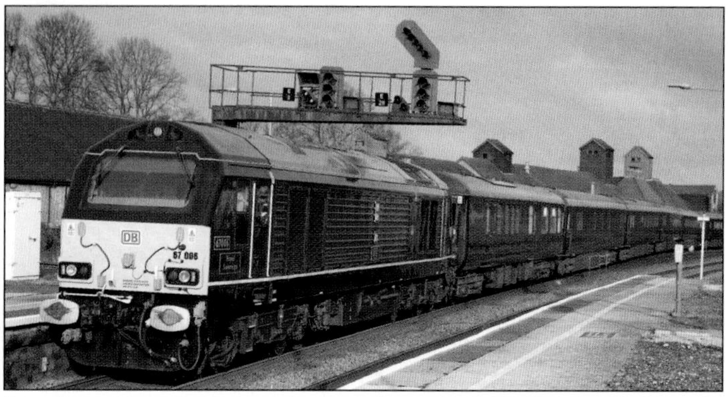

When the Royal Train is used, it is normally formed of between 7 and nine vehicle depending on use. It is usually powered by the two DB Royal-liveried Class 67s, Nos. 67005 and 67006. No. 67006 is seen hauling the train off the Heathfield line at Newton Abbot on 16 December 2021. **Nathan Williamson**

41149	FO	CL	?	LSL	LSL
41160	FO	CL	RCG	LSL	LSL
41161	FO	The Wee Choo-Choo, Pitlochry (Thai Restaurant)			
41162	FO	CL	BLP	LSL	LSL
41165	FO	Upside School, Essex			
41166	FO	CL	RCG	LSL	LSL
41167	FO	CL	GWG	LSL	LSL
41169	FO	CL	BLP	LSL	LSL
41170 (41001)	FO	EL	LNE	ANG	(S)
41176 (42142, 42352)	FO	CL	BLP	LSL	LSL
41182 (42278)	FO	CL	BLP	LSL	LSL
41183 (42274)	FO	CL	BLP	LSL	LSL
41187 (42311)	FO	CL	RCG	LSL	LSL
41189 (42298)	FO	International Metel Recycling Co, Long Marston			
41193 (11060)	FO	LA	AXC	PTR	AXC
41194 (11016)	FO	LA	AXC	PTR	AXC
41195 (11020)	FO	LA	AXC	PTR	AXC
41204 (11023)	FO	EL	EMR	ANG	OLS
41205 (11036)	FO	EL	EMR	ANG	OLS
41206 (11055)	FO	Privately preserved near Ely			
41207 (12033, 42403)	FO	Stannington Station			
41208 (12112, 42406)	FO	EL	EMR	ANG	OLS
41209 (12088, 42409)	FO	Privately preserved near Ely			

Trailer Standard

42002	TSO	IS	IC7	ANG	ASR
42004	TSO	IS	IC7	ANG	ASR
42009	TSO	IS	IC7	ANG	ASR
42010	TSO	IS	IC7	ANG	ASR
42012	TSO	IS	IC7	ANG	ASR
42013	TSO	IS	IC7	ANG	ASR
42014	TSO	IS	IC7	ANG	ASR
42019	TSO	IS	IC7	ANG	ASR
42021	TSO	IS	IC7	ANG	ASR
42023	TSO	IS	IC7	ANG	ASR
42024	TSO	EL	GWR	ANG	(S)
42026	TSO	EL	GWR	ANG	(S)
42029	TSO	IS	ASR	ANG	ASR
42030	TSO	IS	IC7	ANG	ASR
42032	TSO	IS	ASR	ANG	ASR
42033	TSO	IS	IC7	ANG	ASR
42034	TSO	IS	IC7	ANG	ASR

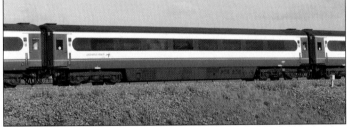

Former East Midlands Railway-operated HST TSO No. 42100 is now operated by Loco Services Limited and branded 'Locomotive InterCity Ltd'. The coach is part of the LSL hire and charter fleet. **CJM**

42035	TSO	IS	ASR	ANG	ASR
42036	TSO	LA	AXC	ANG	AXC
42037	TSO	LA	AXC	ANG	AXC
42038	TSO	LA	AXC	ANG	AXC
42045	TSO	IS	IC7	ANG	ASR
42046	TSO	IS	IC7	ANG	ASR
42047	TSO	IS	IC7	ANG	ASR
42051	TSO	LA	AXC	ANG	AXC
42052	TSO	LA	AXC	ANG	AXC
42053	TSO	LA	AXC	ANG	AXC
42054	TSO	IS	ASR	ANG	ASR
42055	TSO	IS	IC7	ANG	ASR
42056	TSO	IS	ASR	ANG	ASR
42072	TSO	IS	IC7	ANG	ASR
42075	TSO	IS	IC7	ANG	ASR
42077	TSO	IS	IC7	ANG	ASR
42078	TSO	IS	IC7	ANG	ASR
42094	TSO	LA	GWR	FGP	(S)
42095	TSO	LA	GWR	FGP	(S)
42096	TSO	IS	ASR	ANG	ASR
42097	TSO	LA	ACX	ANG	AXC
42100	TSO	CL	EMR	LSL	LSL
42107	TSO	IS	IC7	ANG	ASR
42109	TSO	Waltham Abbey School			
42110	TSO	Nemesis Rail, Burton			
42111	TSO	125 Group, Midland Railway			
42119	TSO	125 Group, Midland Railway			
42120	TSO	125 Group, Midland Railway			
42129	TSO	IS	IC7	ANG	ASR
42143	TSO	IS	IC7	ANG	ASR
42144	TSO	IS	IC7	ANG	ASR
42173	TSO	FGP at Wabtec Doncaster			
42175	TSO	LA	GWR	FGP	(S)
42176	TSO	LM	GWR	PTR	(S)
42179	TSO	EL	LNE	ANG	(S)
42183	TSO	IS	IC7	ANG	ASR
42184	TSO	IS	IC7	ANG	ASR
42185	TSO	IS	IC7	ANG	ASR
42195	TSO	FGP at Wabtec Doncaster			
42200	TSO	IS	IC7	ANG	ASR
42205	TSO	Fire training at Camberslang			
42206	TSO	IS	IC7	ANG	ASR
42207	TSO	IS	IC7	ANG	ASR
42208	TSO	IS	IC7	ANG	ASR
42209	TSO	IS	IC7	ANG	ASR
42210	TSO	Fire training at Aberdeen			
42213	TSO	IS	ASR	ANG	ASR
42217	TSO	FG at Wabtec Doncaster			
42220	TSO	CL	EMR	LSL	LSL
42234	TSO	LA	AXC	PTR	AXC
42242	TSO	EL	LNE	ANG	(S)
42243	TSO	EL	LNE	ANG	(S)
42245	TSO	IS	IC7	ANG	ASR
42250	TSO	IS	IC7	ANG	ASR
42252	TSO	IS	ASR	ANG	ASR
42253	TSO	IS	ASR	ANG	ASR
42255	TSO	IS	ASR	ANG	ASR
42256	TSO	IS	ASR	ANG	ASR
42257	TSO	IS	ASR	ANG	ASR
42259	TSO	IS	ASR	ANG	ASR
42265	TSO	IS	ASR	ANG	ASR
42267	TSO	IS	ASR	ANG	ASR
42268	TSO	IS	ASR	ANG	ASR
42269	TSO	IS	ASR	ANG	ASR
42275	TSO	IS	ASR	ANG	ASR
42276	TSO	IS	ASR	ANG	ASR
42277	TSO	IS	ASR	ANG	ASR
42279	TSO	IS	ASR	ANG	ASR
42280	TSO	IS	ASR	ANG	ASR
42281	TSO	IS	ASR	ANG	ASR
42288	TSO	IS	ASR	ANG	ASR
42290	TSO	LA	AXC	PTR	AXC
42291	TSO	IS	ASR	ANG	ASR
42292	TSO	IS	ASR	ANG	ASR
42293	TSO	IS	ASR	ANG	ASR
42295	TSO	IS	ASR	ANG	ASR
42296	TSO	IS	ASR	ANG	ASR
42297	TSO	IS	ASR	ANG	ASR
42299	TSO	IS	ASR	ANG	ASR
42300	TSO	IS	ASR	ANG	ASR
42301	TSO	IS	ASR	ANG	ASR

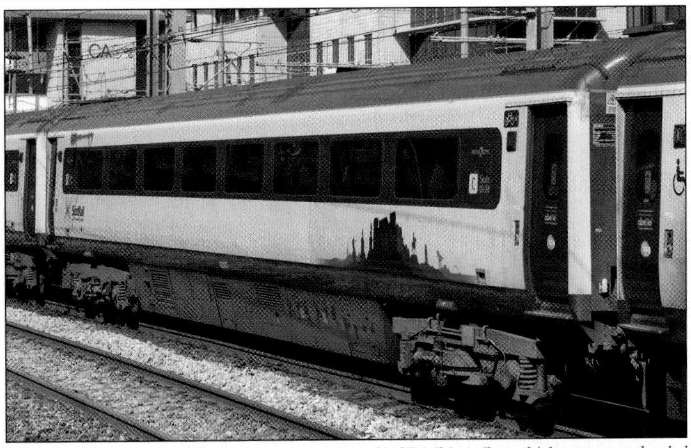

After finishing work on Great Western a number of HST Mk3 trailer vehicles were overhauled by Wabtec, fitted with sliding doors and transferred to Scotland for use on their I7C services. TSO No. 42107 is shown in I7C livery at Haymarket in June 2021. **CJM**

42310	TSO	FGP at Wabtec Doncaster			
42319	TSO	CL	?	LSL	LSL
42325	TSO	IS	ASR	ANG	ASR
42333	TSO	IS	ASR	ANG	ASR
42337	TSO	125 Group, Midland Railway			
42342 (44082)	TSO	LA	AXC	ANG	AXC
42343 (44095)	TSO	IS	IC7	ANG	ASR
42345 (44096)	TSO	IS	IC7	ANG	ASR
42347 (41054)	TSO	EL	GWR	ANG	(S)
42350 (41047)	TSO	IS	IC7	ANG	ASR
42351 (41048)	TSO	IS	ASR	ANG	ASR
42353 (42001, 41171)	TSO	Northumbria Rail			
42355 (42000, 41172)	TSO	EL	LNE	ANG	(S)
42356 (42002, 41173)	TSO	Northumbria Rail			
42357 (41002, 41174)	TSO	EL	LNE	ANG	(S)
42360 (44084, 45084)	TSO	IS	IC7	ANG	ASR
42363 (41082)	TSO	EL	LNE	ANG	(S)
42366 (12007)	TSO	LA	AXC	PTR	AXC
42367 (12025)	TSO	LA	AXC	PTR	AXC
42368 (12028)	TSO	LA	AXC	PTR	AXC
42369 (12050)	TSO	LA	AXC	PTR	AXC
42370 (12086)	TSO	LA	AXC	PTR	AXC
42371 (12052)	TSO	LA	AXC	PTR	AXC
42372 (12055)	TSO	LA	AXC	PTR	AXC
42373 (12071)	TSO	LA	AXC	PTR	AXC
42374 (12075)	TSO	LA	AXC	PTR	AXC
42375 (12113)	TSO	LA	AXC	PTR	AXC
42376 (12085)	TSO	LA	AXC	PTR	AXC
42377 (12102)	TSO	LA	AXC	PTR	AXC
42378 (12123)	TSO	LA	AXC	PTR	AXC
42379 (41036)	TSO	LA	AXC	ANG	AXC

42380 (41025)	TSO	LA	AXC	ANG	AXC
42401 (12149)	TSO	EL	EMR	ANG	OLS
42402 (12155)	TSO	EL	EMR	ANG	OLS
42404 (12152)	TSO	EL	EMR	ANG	OLS
42405 (12136)	TSO	EL	EMR	ANG	OLS
42408 (12121)	TSO	EL	EMR	ANG	OLS
42504 (40714)	TSO	Appleby-Frodingham RPS			
42502 (40731)	TSO	Wabtec owned by Wabtec			
42511 (40709)	TSO	Appleby-Frodingham RPS			
42551 (41003)	TSO	IS	IC7	ANG	ASR
42553 (41009)	TSO	IS	IC7	ANG	ASR
42555 (41015)	TSO	IS	IC7	ANG	ASR
42555 (41017)	TSO	IS	IC7	ANG	ASR
42557 (41019)	TSO	IS	IC7	ANG	ASR
42558 (41021)	TSO	IS	IC7	ANG	ASR
42559 (41023)	TSO	IS	IC7	ANG	ASR
42561 (41031)	TSO	IS	IC7	ANG	ASR
42562 (41037)	TSO	IS	IC7	ANG	ASR
42566 (41086)	TSO	PZ	GWB	FGP	(S)
42567 (41093)	TSO	IS	IC7	ANG	ASR
42568 (41101)	TSO	IS	ASR	ANG	ASR
42569 (41105)	TSO	EL	GWR	ANG	(S)
42571 (41121)	TSO	IS	IC7	ANG	ASR
42574 (41129)	TSO	IS	IC7	ANG	ASR
42575 (41131)	TSO	IS	IC7	ANG	ASR
42576 (41133)	TSO	IS	IC7	ANG	ASR
42577 (41141)	TSO	IS	IC7	ANG	ASR
42578 (41143)	TSO	IS	IC7	ANG	ASR
42579 (41145)	TSO	IS	IC7	ANG	ASR
42581 (41157)	TSO	IS	IC7	ANG	ASR
42583 (41153, 42385)	TSO	CL	GWG	LSL	LSL
42584 (11045, 41201)	TSO	EL	EMR	ANG	OLS
42585 (11017, 42203)	TSO	EL	EMR	ANG	OLS
48101 (42093, 48111)	TSO	LA	GWG	FGP	GWR
48102 (42218, 48113)	TSO	LA	GWG	FGP	GWR
48103 (42168, 48101)	TSO	LA	GWG	FGP	GWR
48104 (42365)	TSO	LA	GWG	FGP	GWR
48105 (42266)	TSO	LA	GWG	FGP	GWR
48106 (42258)	TSO	LA	GWG	FGP	GWR
48107 (42101)	TSO	LA	GWG	FGP	GWR
48108 (42174)	TSO	LA	GWG	FGP	GWR
48109 (42085)	TSO	LA	GWG	FGP	GWR
48110 (42315)	TSO	LA	GWG	FGP	GWR
48111 (42224)	TSO	LA	GWG	FGP	GWR
48112 (42222)	TSO	LA	GWG	FGP	GWR
48113 (42177, 48102)	TSO	LA	GWG	FGP	GWR
48114 (42317)	TSO	LA	GWG	FGP	GWR
48115 (42285)	TSO	LA	GWG	ANG	GWR
48116 (42273)	TSO	LA	GWG	ANG	GWR
48117 (42271)	TSO	LA	GWG	ANG	GWR
48118 (42073)	TSO	LA	GWG	ANG	GWR
48119 (42204)	TSO	LA	GWG	ANG	GWR
48120 (42201)	TSO	LA	GWG	ANG	GWR
48121 (42027)	TSO	LA	GWG	ANG	GWR
48122 (42214)	TSO	LA	GWG	ANG	GWR
48123 (42211)	TSO	LA	GWG	ANG	GWR
48124 (42212)	TSO	LA	GWG	ANG	GWR
48125 (42203)	TSO	LA	GWG	ANG	GWR
48126 (42138)	TSO	LA	GWG	ANG	GWR
48127 (41074, 42349)	TSO	LA	GWG	ANG	GWR
48128 (42044)	TSO	LA	GWG	ANG	GWR
48129 (42008)	TSO	LA	GWG	ANG	GWR
48130 (42102, 48131)	TSO	LA	GWG	FGP	GWR
48131 (42042)	TSO	LA	GWG	ANG	GWR
48132 (42202)	TSO	LA	GWG	ANG	GWR
48133 (42003)	TSO	LA	GWG	ANG	GWR
48134 (42264)	TSO	LA	GWG	ANG	GWR
48135 (42251)	TSO	LA	GWG	ANG	GWR
48136 (42570, 41114)	TSO	LA	GWG	FGP	GWR
48137 (42582, 41163)	TSO	LA	GWG	FGP	GWR
48140 (42005)	TSO	LA	GWG	ANG	GWR
48141 (42015)	TSO	LA	GWG	ANG	GWR
48142 (42016)	TSO	LA	GWG	ANG	GWR
48143 (42050)	TSO	LA	GWG	ANG	GWR
48144 (42066)	TSO	LA	GWG	ANG	GWR
48145 (42048)	TSO	LA	GWG	ANG	GWR
48146 (42074)	TSO	LA	GWG	ANG	GWR
48147 (42081)	TSO	LA	GWG	ANG	GWR
48148 (42071)	TSO	LA	GWG	ANG	GWR
48149 (42087)	TSO	LA	GWG	ANG	GWR
48150 (42580)	TSO	LA	GWG	ANG	GWR

Trailer Guards Standard (*First)

44000	TGS	125 Group, Midland Railway			
44004	TGS	Wabtec owned at Wabtec			
44012	TGS	LA	AXC	ANG	AXC
44015	TGS	ERS at Bay Studios, Swansea			
44017	TGS	LA	AXC	ANG	AXC
44020	TGS	Wabtec owned at Wabtec			
44021	TGS	LA	AXC	PTR	AXC
44024	TGS	Wabtec owned at Wabtec			
44034	TGS	EL	GWR	ANG	(S)
44035	TGS	Wabtec owned at Wabtec			
44040	TGS	Wabtec owned at Wabtec			
44047	TGS	CL	EMR	LSL	LSL
44052	TGS	LA	AXC	PTR	AXC
44058	TGS	Colne Valley Railway			
44059	TGS	Appleby-Frodingham RPS			
44061	TGS	EL	EMR	ANG	(S)
44063	TGS	EL	EMR	ANG	(S)
44066	TGS	Wabtec owned at Wabtec			
44071	TGS	NL	EMR	PTR	EMR
44072	TGS	LA	AXC	PTR	AXC
44078*	TGF	CL	BLP	LSL	LSL
44081	TGS	CL	RCG	LSL	LSL
44086	TGS	Wabtec owned at Wabtec			
44094	TGS	EL	EMR	ANG	(S)
44098	TGS	EL	LNE	ANG	(S)
44100	TGS	PZ	GWB	PTR	(S)

Trailer Composite Kitchen

45001 (12004)	TCK	LA	AXC	PTR	AXC
45002 (12106)	TCK	LA	AXC	PTR	AXC
45003 (12076)	TCK	LA	AXC	PTR	AXC
45004 (12077)	TCK	LA	AXC	PTR	AXC
45005 (12080)	TCK	LA	AXC	PTR	AXC

Trailer Composite

46006 (41081)	TC	CL	GWG	LSL	LSL
46012 (41147)	TC	CL	GWG	LSL	LSL
46014 (41168)	TC	CL	CAR	LSL	LSL

Trailer Guards Standard

49101 (44055)	TGS	LA	GWG	FGP	GWR
49102 (44083)	TGS	LA	GWG	FGP	GWR
49103 (44097)	TGS	LA	GWG	FGP	GWR
49104 (44101)	TGS	LA	GWG	FGP	GWR
49105 (44090)	TGS	LA	GWG	FGP	GWR
49106 (44033)	TGS	LA	GWG	ANG	GWR
49107 (44064)	TGS	LA	GWG	ANG	GWR
49108 (44067)	TGS	LA	GWG	ANG	GWR
49109 (44003)	TGS	LA	GWG	ANG	GWR
49110 (44014)	TGS	LA	GWG	ANG	GWR
49111 (44036)	TGS	LA	GWG	ANG	GWR
49112 (44079)	TGS	LA	GWG	FGP	GWR
49113 (44008)	TGS	LA	GWG	ANG	GWR
49114 (44005)	TGS	LA	GWG	ANG	GWR
49115 (44016)	TGS	LA	GWG	ANG	GWR
49116 (44002)	TGS	LA	GWG	ANG	GWR
49117 (44042)	TGS	LA	GWG	ANG	GWR

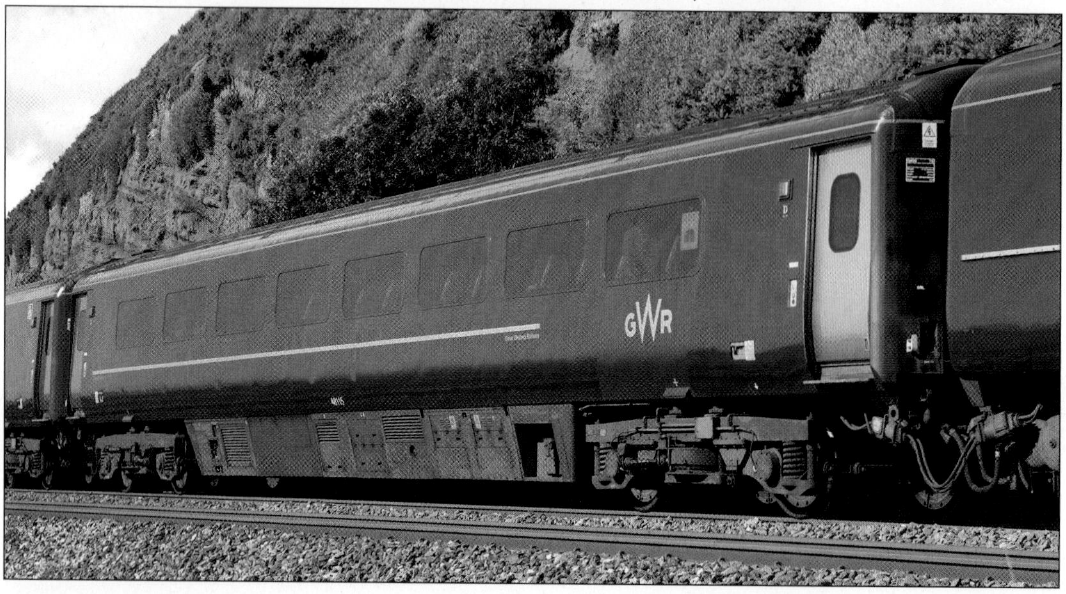

To operate in the Great Western 2+4 'Castle' sets, a number of 'new' TSO vehicles were rebuilt from both standard and first class vehicles at Wabtec, Doncaster and fitted with sliding passenger doors and high-density, mainly aircraft style interiors. The TSOs were renumbered in a new 481xx series and TGS coaches in a new 491xx range. Vehicle 48115 is illustrated, rebuilt from TSO 42285. **CJM**

Coaching Stock Semi-fixed Formations

Chiltern Railway Mk3 Sets

Set No.	Formation DVT+RFK+TSO+TSO+TSO+TSO+TSO+(loco)
AL01	82302+10272+12610+12621+12609+12606+12604
AL02	82301+10271+12605+12608+12607+12615+12616
AL03	82309+10274+12602+12613+12617+12623+12627
AL04	82304+10273+12603+12614+12618+12625+12619

These formations are constantly changing

CrossCountry

Set No.	Formation (DM)+TF+TBF+TS+TS+TS+TS+TGS+(DM)
XC01	41193+45001+42342+42097+42377+42374+44021
XC02	41194+45002+42234+42037+42367+42371+44072
XC03	41195+45003+42370+42378+42036+42376+44052
XC04	41026+45004+42375+42369+42051+42366+44012
XC05	41035+45005+42052+42038+42053+42379+44017

LNER 'Mk4 Sets'

Set No.	Formation DVT+FO+FO+FO+RSB+TS+TS+TS+TS+TSE+Loco
NL06	82208+11406+11306+11279+10309+12313+12422+12420+12406+12208
NL08	82211+11408+11308+11229+10300+12328+12407+12485+12481+12205
NL12	82212+11412+11312+11284+10333+12330+12426+12404+12431+12212
NL13	82213+11413+11313+11285+10313+12311+12424+12430+12469+12228
NL15	82214+11415+11315+11286+10306+12309+12515+12409+12442+12226
NL16	82222+11416+11318+11418+10315+12312+12467+12433+12428+11213
NL17	82225+11417+11317+11288+10324+12303+12432+12427+12444+12223
NL26	82223+11426+11326+11295+10311+12325+12429+12465+12474+12220

Great Western 'Castle Sets'

Set No.	Formation (DM)+TS+TS+TS+TGS+(DM)	Owner
GW01	48103+48102+48101+49101	FGP
GW02	48106+48105+48104+49102	FGP
GW03	48109+48108+48107+49103	FGP
GW04	48112+48111+48110+49104	FGP
GW05	48115+48114+48113+49105	FGP
GW06	48118+48117+48116+49106	ANG
GW07	48121+48120+48119+49107	ANG
GW08	48124+48123+48122+49108	ANG
GW09	48127+48126+48125+49109	ANG
GW10	48130+48129+48128+49110	ANG
GW11	48131+48132+48133+49111	ANG
GW12	48137+48134+48136+49112	FGP
GW13	48150+48135+48149+49113	FGP
GW14	48140+48141+48142+49114	ANG
GW15	48143+48144+48145+49115	ANG
GW16	48146+48147+48148+49116	ANG

Scotrail 'Inter7City Sets' 2+4 and 2+5 sets

Set No.	Formation (DM)+TFB+TS+TS+TS+TS+(DM)
HA01	40601+42004+42561+42046
HA02	40602+42292+42562+42045
HA03	40603+42021+42557+42143
HA04	40604+42183+42559+42343
HA05	40605+42345+42034+42184+42029
HA06	40606+42206+42208+42581+42033
HA07	40607+42207+42574+42288
HA08	40608+42055+42571+42019
HA09	40609+42253+42107+42257
HA10	40610+42360+42551+42252+42351
HA11	40611+42267+42325+42301+42023
HA12	40612+42275+42576+42276+42574
HA13	40613+42279+42280+42296
HA14	40614+42012+42013+42245
HA15	40615+42010+42030+42579
HA16	40616+42291+42577+42075
HA17	40617+42295+42558+42250
HA18	46018+42297+42555+42014
HA19	40619+42255+42568+42256+42029
HA20	40620+42129+42200+42575
HA21	40621+42299+42300+42277
HA22	46022+42007+42564+42145 (collision damage)
HA23	40623+42268+42567+42269
HA24	40624+42265+42553+42293
HA25	40625+42259+42578+42333
HA26	40626+42281+42072+42350

The following TSOs are due to be inserted into 2+4 sets to make 2+5 formations. Set numbers are to be advised
42009, 42032, 42033, 42035, 42047, 42054, 42056, 42077, 42078, 42096, 42144, 42185, 42209 and 42213

Transport for Wales 'Mk4 Sets'

Set No.	Formation DVT+FO+RSB+TSO+TSO+TSOE+(loco)
HD01	82226+11323+10325+12454+12225
HD02	82229+11324+10328+12447+12219
HD03	82216+11325+10312+12446+12217
GC01	82201+11319+10318+12310+12434+12211
GC02	82200+11320+10321+12326+12477+12224
GC03	82227+11321+10330+12323+12461+12222
GC04	82230+11322+10301+12316+12452+12210

Trans Pennine Express 'Mk5 Sets'

Set No.	Formation DTS+T2(TS)+T3-1(TS)+T3-2(TS)+T1(TF)+Loco
TP01	12801+12703+12702+12701+11501
TP02	12812+12706+12705+12704+11502
TP03	12803+12709+12708+12707+11503
TP04	12804+12712+12711+12710+11504
TP05	12805+12715+12714+12713+11505
TP06	12806+12718+12717+12716+11506
TP07	12807+12721+12720+12719+11507
TP08	12808+12724+12723+12722+11508
TP09	12809+12727+12726+12725+11509
TP10	12810+12730+12729+12728+11510
TP11	12811+12733+12732+12731+11511
TP12	12812+12736+12735+12734+11512
TP13	12813+12739+12738+12737+11513
TP14	12802 Spare vehicle

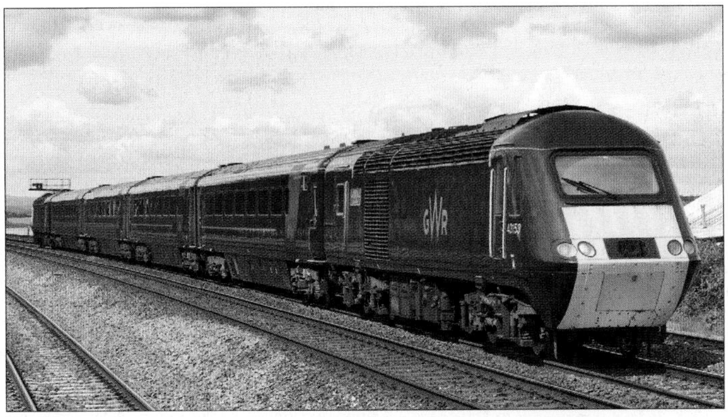

The GW 2+4 'Castle' sets should operate in fixed formations, identified by set numbers, but mixed formations are common 43153 with set GW16 formed of vehicles 49116, 48146, 48147 and 48148 with power car No. 43171 on the rear are seen passing Dawlish Warren in May 2021. **CJM**

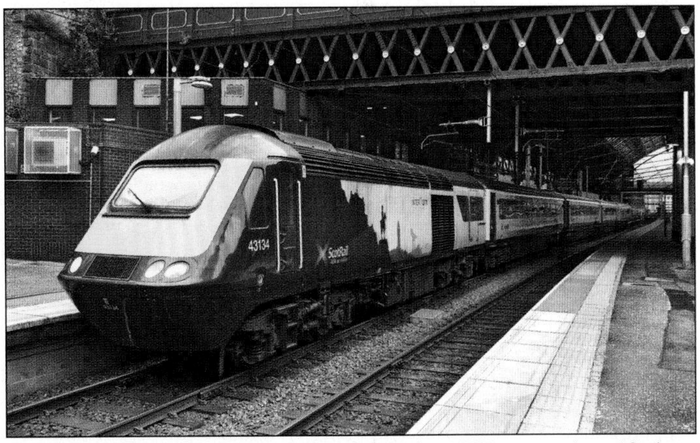

The Edinburgh Haymarket allocated Inter7City (I7C) 2+4 and 2+5 HST sets operate in semi-fixed formations of passenger stock, using what power cars are available. Formations of this fleet are known to be fluid. A 2+4 set is seen at Glasgow Queen Street led by power car No. 43134. **CJM**

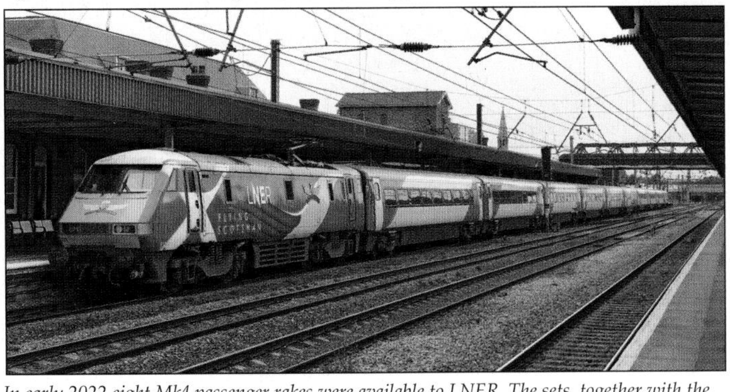

In early 2022 eight Mk4 passenger rakes were available to LNER. The sets, together with the Class 91s are based at Leeds Neville Hill. No. 91101 in Flying Scotsman branding is seen at Doncaster with a 10 vehicle Mk4 rake. **CJM**

Network Rail Track Machines and Equipment

No.	Name	Type	Op'r
DR72211		P&T DTS-62-N – Dynamic Stabiliser	BAL
DR72213		P&T DTS-62-N – Dynamic Stabiliser	BAL
DR73109		P&T 09-3X – Tamper/Liner	SBR
DR73111		P&T 09-3X-D-RT – Tamper/Liner	SBR
DR73113	*Dai Evans*	P&T 09-3X-D-RT – Tamper/Liner	NRL
DR73114	*Ron Henderson*	P&T 09-3X-D-RT – Tamper/Liner	NRL
DR73115		P&T 09-3X-D-RT – Tamper/Liner	NRL
DR73116		P&T 09-3X-D-RT – Tamper/Liner	NRL
DR73117		P&T 09-3X-D-RT – Tamper/Liner	NRL
DR73118		P&T 09-3X-D-RT – Tamper/Liner	NRL
DR73120 (99 70 9123 120-6)		P&T 09-2x – Dynamic Tamper/Liner	NRL
DR73121 (99 70 9123 121-4)		P&T 09-2x – Dynamic Tamper/Liner	NRL
DR73122 (99 70 9123 122-2)		P&T 09-2x – Dynamic Tamper/Liner	NRL
DR73803	*Alexander Graham Bell*	P&T 08-32U RT – Plain Line Tamper	SBR
DR73806	*Karine*	P&T 08-16(32)U RT – Plain Line Tamper	COL
DR73904	*Thomas Telford*	P&T 08-4x4/4S - RT – S&C Tamper	SBR
DR73905		P&T 08-4x4/4S - RT – S&C Tamper	COL
DR73906	*Panther*	P&T 08-4x4/4S - RT – S&C Tamper	COL
DR73907		P&T 08-4x4/4S - RT – S&C Tamper	COL
DR73908		P&T 08-4x4/4S - RT – S&C Tamper	COL
DR73909	*Saturn*	P&T 08-4x4/4S - RT – S&C Tamper	COL
DR73910	*Jupiter*	P&T 08-4x4/4S - RT – S&C Tamper	COL
DR73913		P&T 08-16/4x4 C/RT – S&C Tamper	COL
DR73914	*Robert McAlpine*	P&T 08-4x4S - RT – S&C Tamperr	SBR
DR73915	*William Arrol*	P&T 08-16/4x4C - RT – S&C Tamper	SBR
DR73916	*First Engineering*	P&T 08-16/4x4C - RT – S&C Tamper	SBR
DR73917		P&T 08-4x4S - RT – S&C Tamper	BAL
DR73918		P&T 08-4x4S - RT – S&C Tamper	BAL
DR73919		P&T 08-16/4x4 C100 - RT – Tamper+trailer	COL
DR73920		P&T 08-16/4x4C80 - RT – Tamper	COL
DR73921		P&T 08-16/4x4C80 - RT – Tamper	COL
DR73922	*John Snowdon*	P&T 08-16/4x4C80 - RT – Tamper	COL
DR73923		P&T 08-4x4S - RT – S&C Tamperr	COL
DR73924		P&T 08-16/4x4 C100 - RT – Tamper	COL
DR73925	*Europa*	P&T 08-16/4x4 C100 - RT – Tamper	COL
DR73926	*Stephen Keith Blanchard*	P&T 08-16/4x4 C100 - RT – Tamper	BAL
DR73927		P&T 08-16/4x4 C100 - RT – Tamper	BAL
DR73929		P&T 08-4x4S - RT – S&C Tamperr	COL
DR73930		P&T 08-4x4S - RT – S&C Tamperr	COL
DR73931		P&T 08-16/4x4C100 - RT – Tamper	COL
DR73932		P&T 08-4x4/4S - RT – S&C Tamper	SBR
DR73933		P&T 08-16/4x4C100 - RT – Tamper+trailer	SBR
DR73934		P&T 08-16/4x4C100 - RT – Tamper+trailer	SBR
DR73935		P&T 08-4x4/4S - RT – S&C Tamper	COL
DR73936		P&T 08-4x4/4S - RT – S&C Tamper	COL
DR73937		P&T 08-16/4x4 C100 - RT – Tamper	BAL
DR73938		P&T 08-16/4x4 C100 - RT – Tamper	BAL
DR73939	*Pat Best*	P&T 08-16/4x4 C100 - RT – Tamper	BAL
DR73940		P&T 08-4x4/4S - RT – S&C Tamper	SBR
DR73941		P&T 08-4x4/4S - RT – S&C Tamper	SBR
DR73942		P&T 08-4x4/4S - RT – S&C Tamper	COL
DR73943		P&T 08-16/4x4C100 - RT – Tamper	BAL
DR73944		P&T 08-16/4x4C100 - RT – Tamper	BAL
DR73945		P&T 08-16/4x4C100 - RT – Tamper	BAL
DR73946		P&T Euromat 08-4x4/4S	VRL
DR73947		P&T 08-4x4/4S - RT – S&C Tamper	COL
DR73948		P&T 08-4x4/4S - RT – S&C Tamper	COL
DR73949 (99 70 9123 016-6)		P&T 08-4x4/4S - RTv - S&C Tamper	BAL
DR73950 (99 70 9123 017-4)		P&T 08-4x4/4s - RTv - S&C Tamper	BAL
DR74002 (99 70 9128 002-1)		P&T 09-4x4/4s - Dynamic	SBR
DR75008 (99 70 9128 008-3)		P&T 09-4x4/4s - Dynamic	COL
DR75009 (99 70 9128 009-1)		P&T 09-4x4/4s - Dynamic	COL
DR75010 (99 70 9128 010-9)	*Roger Nicholas*	P&T 09-4x4/4s - Dynamic	COL
DR75011 (99 70 9128 011-7)	*Andrew Smith*	P&T 09-4x4/4s - Dynamic	COL
DR75012 (99 70 9128 012-5)		P&T 09-4x4/4s - Dynamic	SBR
DR75013 (99 70 9128 013-3)		P&T 09-4x4/4s - Dynamic	SBR
DR75301		Matisa B45UE Tamper	VRL
DR75302	*Gary Wright*	Matisa B45UE Tamper	VRL
DR75303		Matisa B45UE Tamper	VRL
DR75401		Matisa B41UE Tamper	VRL
DR75402		Matisa B41UE Tamper	VRL
DR75404		Matisa B41UE Tamper	VRL
DR75405		Matisa B41UE Tamper	VRL
DR75406	*Eric Machell*	Matisa B41UE Tamper	COL
DR75407	*Gerry Taylor*	Matisa B41UE Tamper	COL
DR75408		Matisa B41UE Tamper	BAL
DR75409		Matisa B41UE Tamper	BAL
DR75410		Matisa B41UE Tamper	BAL
DR75411		Matisa B41UE Tamper	BAL
DR75501		Matisa B66UC Tamper	BAL
DR75502		Matisa B66UC Tamper	BAL
DR75503		Matisa B66UC Tamper	VRL
DR75504		Matisa B66UC Tamper	VRL
DR76501		P&T RM900RT Ballast Cleaner (HOBC-1)	NRL
DR76502		P&T RM900RT Ballast Cleaner (HOBC-2)	NRL
DR76503		P&T RM900RT Ballast Cleaner (HOBC-3)	NRL
DR76504 (99 70 9314 504-0)		P&T RM900 Ballast Cleaner (HOBC-4)	NRL
DR76701 (S)		P&T VM80 (HOBC-3)	NRL
DR76703 (S)		P&T VM80 (HOBC-1)	NRL
DR76750		Matisa D75 Undercutter (HRTRT-2)	NRL
DR76751		Matisa D75 Undercutter (HRTRT-1)	NRL
DR76801		P&T 09-16 CM NR (HOBC-3)	NRL
DR76802 (99 70 9320 802-0)		P&T 09-16 CM NR (HOBC-4)	NRL
DR76901 (99 70 9131 001-8)	*Brunel*	Windhoff MPV - Electrification train	NRL
DR76903 (99 70 9131 003-4)		Windhoff MPV - Electrification train	NRL
DR76905 (99 70 9131 005-9)		Windhoff MPV - Electrification train	NRL
DR76906 (99 70 9131 006-7)		Windhoff MPV - Electrification train	NRL
DR76910 (99 70 9131 010-9)		Windhoff MPV - Electrification train	NRL
DR76911 (99 70 9131 011-7)		Windhoff MPV - Electrification train	NRL
DR76913 (99 70 9131 013-3)		Windhoff MPV - Electrification train	NRL
DR76914 (99 70 9131 014-1)		Windhoff MPV - Electrification train	NRL
DR76915 (99 70 9131 015-8)		Windhoff MPV - Electrification train	NRL
DR76918 (99 70 9131 018-2)		Windhoff MPV - Electrification train	NRL
DR76920 (99 70 9131 020-8)		Windhoff MPV - Electrification train	NRL
DR76921 (99 70 9131 021-6)		Windhoff MPV - Electrification train	NRL
DR76922 (99 70 9131 022-4)		Windhoff MPV - Electrification train	NRL
DR76923 (99 70 9131 023-2)	*Gavin Roberts*	Windhoff MPV - Electrification train	NRL
DR77001	*Anthony Lou Phillips*	P&T AFM 2000 RT – Finishing Machine	SBR
DR77002		P&T AFM 2000 RT – Finishing Machine	SBR
DR77010 (99 70 9125 010-7)		P&T USP 6000 – Ballast Regulator	NRL
DR77315(S)		P&T USP 5000C – Ballast Regulator	BAL
DR77316(S)		P&T USP 5000C – Ballast Regulator	BAL
DR77322(S)		P&T USP 5000C – Ballast Regulator	BAL
DR77327		P&T USP 5000C – Ballast Regulator	COL
DR77336(S)		P&T USP 5000C – Ballast Regulator	BAL
DR77801		Matisa R24S – Ballast Regulator	VRL
DR77802		Matisa R24S – Ballast Regulator	VRL
DR77901		P&T USP 5000RT – Ballast Regulator	COL
DR77903		P&T USP 5000RT – Ballast Regulator	SBR
DR77904		P&T USP 5000RT – Ballast Regulator	NRL
DR77905		P&T USP 5000RT – Ballast Regulator	NRL
DR77906		P&T USP 5000RT – Ballast Regulator	NRL
DR77907		P&T USP 5000RT – Ballast Regulator	NRL
DR77909 (99 70 9125 909-0)		P&T USP 5000RT – Ballast Regulator	NRL
DR78213		P&T Self-Propelled Twin Jib Crane	VRL
DR78215		P&T Self-Propelled Twin Jib Crane	BAB
DR78216(S)		P&T Self-Propelled Twin Jib Crane	BAL
DR78217		P&T Self-Propelled Twin Jib Crane	SBR
DR78218(S)		P&T Self-Propelled Twin Jib Crane	BAL
DR78219		P&T Self-Propelled Twin Jib Crane	BAB
DR78221(S)		P&T Self-Propelled Twin Jib Crane	BAL
DR78222(S)		P&T Self-Propelled Twin Jib Crane	BAL
DR78223(S)		P&T Self-Propelled Twin Jib Crane	BAL
DR78224(S)		P&T Self-Propelled Twin Jib Crane	BAL
DR78226		CS Self-Propelled Twin Jib Crane	COL
DR78229(S)		CS Self-Propelled Twin Jib Crane	NRL
DR78231(S)		CS Self-Propelled Twin Jib Crane	NRL
DR78234(S)		CS Self-Propelled Twin Jib Crane	NRL
DR78235		CS Self-Propelled Twin Jib Crane	COL
DR78237(S)		CS Self-Propelled Twin Jib Crane	COL
DR78701		HTL Track Construction Power Wagon	BAL
DR78702		HTL Track Construction Power Wagon	BAL
DR78801+DR78811+DR78821+DR78831		Matisa P95 Track Renewal Train	NRL
DR78802+DR78812+DR78822+DR78832		Matisa P95 Track Renewal Train	NRL
DR79101 (99 70 9427 063-1)		Linsinger MG31UK - Rail Milling Machine	CRO
DR79102		Linsinger SF06-UK - Rail Milling Machine	NRL
DR79103		Linsinger SF06-UK - Rail Milling Machine	NRL
DR79221+DR79222+DR79223+DR79224+DR79225+DR79226		Speno RPS-32 Grinder	Speno
DR79231+DR79232+DR79233+DR79234+DR79235+DR79236+DR79237		Loram C21 – Grinder Set 2101	NRL
DR79241+DR79242+DR79243+DR79244+DR79245+DR79246+DR79247	*Roger Smith*	Loram C21 – Grinder Set 2102	NRL
DR79251+DR79252+DR79253+DR79254+DR79255+DR79256+DR79257	*Martin Elwood*	Loram C21 – Grinder Set 2103	NRL
DR79261+DR79271		Harsco RGH-20C S&C Rail Grinder	NRL
DR79262+DR79272	*Chris Gibb*	Harsco RGH-20C S&C Rail Grinder	NRL
DR79263+DR79273		Harsco RGH-20C S&C Rail Grinder	NRL
DR79265+DR79274		Harsco RGH-20C S&C Rail Grinder	NRL
DR79267+DR79277	*Bridget Rosewell CBE*	Harsco RGH-20C S&C Rail Grinder	NRL
DR79301+DR79302+DR79303+DR79304 (99 70 9427 038 - 99 70 9427 041)		Loram C44 Rail Grinder Set C44-01	NRL
DR79401+DR79402+DR79403+DR79404 (99 70 9427 042 - 99 70 9427 045)		Loram C44 Rail Grinder Set C44-02	NRL

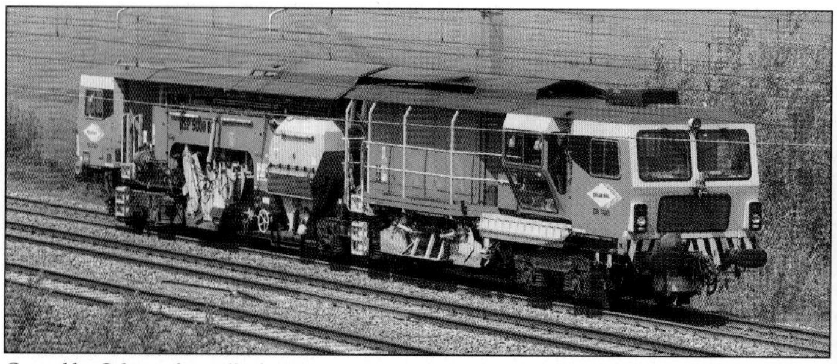

Owned by Colas and usually deployed on the Western Region, Plasser & Theurer USP5000RT ballast regulating machine is seen passing Denchworth, between Swindon and Didcot on 9 June 2021. **CJM**

DR79501+DR79502+DR79503+DR79504+DR79505+DR79506+DR79507 (99 70 9427 046 - 99 70 9427 052)	Loram C44 Grinder Set C44-03	NRL
DR79601	Schweerbau High Speed Milling Machine	SCH
DR79602	Schweerbau High Speed Milling Machine	SCH
DR79603	Schweerbau High Speed Milling Machine	SCH
DR79604	Schweerbau High Speed Milling Machine	SCH
DR80200	Pandrol Jackson – Stoneblower	HER
DR80201	Pandrol Jackson – Stoneblower	NRL
DR80202	Pandrol Jackson – Stoneblower	HER
DR80203	Pandrol Jackson – Stoneblower	HER
DR80205	Pandrol Jackson – Stoneblower	NRL
DR80206	Pandrol Jackson – Stoneblower	NRL
DR80207	Pandrol Jackson – Stoneblower (working in Sweden)	-
DR80208	Pandrol Jackson – Stoneblower	NRL
DR80209	Pandrol Jackson – Stoneblower	NRL
DR80210	Pandrol Jackson – Stoneblower	NRL
DR80211	Pandrol Jackson – Stoneblower	NRL
DR80213	HTL – Stoneblower	NRL
DR80214	HTL – Stoneblower	NRL
DR80215	HTL – Stoneblower	NRL
DR80216	HTL – Stoneblower	NRL
DR80217	HTL – Stoneblower	NRL
DR80301 *Stephen Cornish*	HTL – GP-Stoneblower	NRL
DR80302	HTL – GP-Stoneblower	NRL
DR80303	HTL – GP-Stoneblower	NRL
DR81505	P&T DH Crane	BAL
DR81507(S)	P&T DH Crane	BAL
DR81508	P&T DH Crane	BAL
DR81511(S)P&T DH Crane	BAL	
DR81513	P&T DH Crane	BAL
DR81517	P&T DH Crane	BAL
DR81519(S)	P&T DH Crane	BAL
DR81522	P&T DH Crane	BAL
DR81525	P&T DH Crane	BAL
DR81532	P&T DH Crane	BAL
DRK81601 *Nigel Chester*	Kirow KRC810UK 100 tonne DH Crane	VRL
DRK81602	Kirow KRC810UK 100 tonne DH Crane	BAL
DRK81611 *Malcolm L Pearce*	Kirow KRC1200UK 125 tonne DH Crane	BAL
DRK81612	Kirow KRC1200UK 125 tonne DH Crane	COL
DRK81613	Kirow KRC1200UK 125 tonne DH Crane	VRL
DRK81621	Kirow KRC250UK 25 tonne DH Crane	VRL
DRK81622	Kirow KRC250UK 25 tonne DH Crane	VRL
DRK81623	Kirow KRC250UK 25 tonne DH Crane	SBR
DRK81624	Kirow KRC250UK 25 tonne DH Crane	SBR
DRK81625	Kirow KRC250UK 25 tonne DH Crane	SBR
DRK81626 (99 70 9319 012-9)	Kirow KRC250UK 25 tonne DH Crane	SBR
DRK81627 (99 70 9319-013-7)	Kirow KRC1200UK 125 tonne DH Crane	NRL
DR89005	Cowens Rail Train Power Machine	NRL
DR89007	Cowens Rail Train Power Machine	NRL
DR89008	Cowens Rail Train Power Machine	NRL
DR92201	Starfer Single Line SHST	NRL
DR92202	Starfer Single Line SHST	NRL
DR92203	Starfer Single Line SHST	NRL
DR92204	Starfer Single Line SHST	NRL
DR92205	Starfer Single Line SHST	NRL
DR92206	Starfer Single Line SHST	NRL
DR92207	Starfer Single Line SHST	NRL
DR92208	Starfer Single Line SHST	NRL
DR92209	Starfer Single Line SHST	NRL
DR92210	Starfer Single Line SHST	NRL
DR92211	Starfer Single Line SHST	NRL
DR92212	Starfer Single Line SHST	NRL
DR92213	Skako Ballast Distribution Train 'Octopus'	NRL
DR92214	Skako Ballast Distribution Train 'Octopus'	NRL
DR92215	Skako Ballast Distribution Train 'Octopus'	NRL
DR92216	Skako Ballast Distribution Train 'Octopus'	NRL
DR92217	Skako Ballast Distribution Train 'Octopus'	NRL
DR92218	Skako Ballast Distribution Train 'Octopus'	NRL
DR92219	Skako Ballast Distribution Train 'Octopus'	NRL
DR92220	Skako Ballast Distribution Train 'Octopus'	NRL
DR92221	Skako Ballast Distribution Train 'Octopus'	NRL
DR92222	Skako Ballast Distribution Train 'Octopus'	NRL
DR92223	P&T NFS-D Ballast Train Hopper	NRL
DR92224	P&T NFS-D Ballast Train Hopper	NRL
DR92225	P&T NFS-D Ballast Train Hopper	NRL
DR92226	P&T NFS-D Ballast Train Hopper	NRL
DR92227	P&T NFS-D Ballast Train Hopper	NRL
DR92228	P&T NFS-D Ballast Train Hopper	NRL
DR92229	P&T NFS-D Ballast Train Hopper	NRL
DR92230	P&T NFS-D Ballast Train Hopper	NRL
DR92231	P&T NFS-D Ballast Train Hopper	NRL
DR92232	P&T NFS-D Ballast Train Hopper	NRL
DR92233	P&T NFS-D Ballast Train Hopper	NRL
DR92234	P&T NFS-D Ballast Train Hopper	NRL
DR92235	P&T NFS-D Ballast Train Hopper	NRL
DR92236	P&T NFS-D Ballast Train Hopper	NRL
DR92237	P&T NFS-D Ballast Train Hopper	NRL
DR92238	P&T NFS-D Ballast Train Hopper	NRL
DR92239	P&T NFS-D Ballast Train Hopper	NRL
DR92240	P&T NFS-D Ballast Train Hopper	NRL
DR92241	P&T MFS-D Ballast Train Hopper	NRL
DR92242	P&T MFS-D Ballast Train Hopper	NRL
DR92243	P&T MFS-D Ballast Train Hopper	NRL
DR92244	P&T MFS-D Ballast Train Hopper	NRL
DR92245	P&T MFS-D Ballast Train Hopper	NRL
DR92246	P&T MFS-D Ballast Train Hopper	NRL
DR92247	P&T MFS-D Ballast Train Hopper	NRL

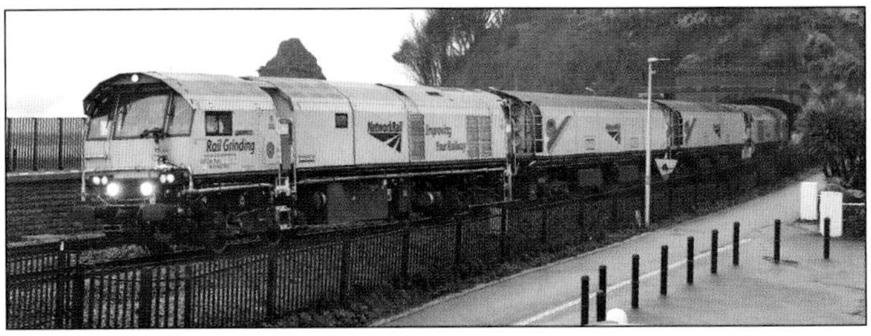

Rail grinding to keep the correct rail head profile is an important part of track maintenance. Several large grinding machines are in use. Here Network Rail owned, Loram-built C-44 Rail Grinder Nos DR79301-DR79304 is shown on a transit move. **CJM**

DR92248	P&T MFS-D Ballast Train Hopper	NRL
DR92249	P&T MFS-D Ballast Train Hopper	NRL
DR92250	P&T MFS-D Ballast Train Hopper	NRL
DR92251	P&T MFS-D Ballast Train Hopper	NRL
DR92252	P&T MFS-D Ballast Train Hopper	NRL
DR92253	P&T MFS-D Ballast Train Hopper	NRL
DR92254	P&T MFS-D Ballast Train Hopper	NRL
DR92259	P&T MFS-SB Swivel Conveyer Wagon	NRL
DR92260	P&T MFS-SB Swivel Conveyer Wagon	NRL
DR92261	P&T MFS-SB Swivel Conveyer Wagon	NRL
DR92262	P&T MFS-SB Swivel Conveyer Wagon	NRL
DR92263	P&T MFS-PW/NB/PW Power Wagon	NRL
DR92262	P&T MFS-PW/NB/PW Power Wagon	NRL
DR92265	P&T MFS-D Ballast Train Hopper	NRL
DR92266	P&T MFS-D Ballast Train Hopper	NRL
DR92267	P&T MFS-D Ballast Train Hopper	NRL
DR92268	P&T MFS-D Ballast Train Hopper	NRL
DR92269	P&T MFS-D Ballast Train Hopper	NRL
DR92270	P&T MFS-D Ballast Train Hopper	NRL
DR92271	P&T MFS-D Ballast Train Hopper	NRL
DR92272	P&T MFS-D Ballast Train Hopper	NRL
DR92273	P&T MFS-D Ballast Train Hopper	NRL
DR92274	P&T MFS-D Ballast Train Hopper	NRL
DR92275	P&T MFS-D Ballast Train Hopper	NRL
DR92276	P&T MFS-D Ballast Train Hopper	NRL
DR92277	P&T MFS-D Ballast Train Hopper	NRL
DR92278	P&T MFS-D Ballast Train Hopper	NRL
DR92279	P&T MFS-D Ballast Train Hopper	NRL
DR92280	P&T MFS-SB Swivel Conveyer Wagon	NRL
DR92281	P&T MFS-SB Swivel Conveyer Wagon	NRL
DR92282	P&T MFS-A Interfacer Wagon	NRL
DR92283	P&T MFS-A Interfacer Wagon	NRL
DR92285	P&T PW-RT Power Wagon	NRL
DR92286	P&T PW-RT Power Wagon	NRL
DR92287	P&T MFS-SB Swivel Conveyer Wagon	NRL
DR92288	P&T MFS-SB Swivel Conveyer Wagon	NRL
DR92289	P&T MFS-SB Swivel Conveyer Wagon	NRL
DR92290	P&T MFS-SB Swivel Conveyer Wagon	NRL
DR92291	P&T MFS-SB Swivel Conveyer Wagon	NRL
DR92292	P&T MFS-SB Swivel Conveyer Wagon	NRL
DR92293	P&T MFS-SB Swivel Conveyer Wagon	NRL
DR92294	P&T MFS-SB Swivel Conveyer Wagon	NRL
DR92295	P&T MFS-D Ballast Train Hopper	NRL
DR92296	P&T MFS-D Ballast Train Hopper	NRL
DR92297	P&T MFS-D Ballast Train Hopper	NRL
DR92298	P&T MFS-D Ballast Train Hopper	NRL
DR92299	P&T MFS-D Ballast Train Hopper	NRL
DR92300	P&T MFS-D Ballast Train Hopper	NRL
DR92301	P&T MFS-D Ballast Train Hopper	NRL
DR92302	P&T MFS-D Ballast Train Hopper	NRL
DR92303	P&T MFS-D Ballast Train Hopper	NRL
DR92304	P&T MFS-D Ballast Train Hopper	NRL
DR92305	P&T MFS-D Ballast Train Hopper	NRL
DR92306	P&T MFS-D Ballast Train Hopper	NRL
DR92307	P&T MFS-D Ballast Train Hopper	NRL
DR92308	P&T MFS-D Ballast Train Hopper	NRL
DR92309	P&T MFS-D Ballast Train Hopper	NRL
DR92310	P&T MFS-D Ballast Train Hopper	NRL
DR92311	P&T MFS-D Ballast Train Hopper	NRL
DR92312	P&T MFS-D Ballast Train Hopper	NRL
DR92313	P&T MFS-D Ballast Train Hopper	NRL
DR92314	P&T MFS-D Ballast Train Hopper	NRL
DR92315	P&T MFS-D Ballast Train Hopper	NRL
DR92316	P&T MFS-D Ballast Train Hopper	NRL
DR92317	P&T MFS-D Ballast Train Hopper	NRL
DR92318	P&T MFS-D Ballast Train Hopper	NRL
DR92319	P&T MFS-D Ballast Train Hopper	NRL
DR92320	P&T MFS-D Ballast Train Hopper	NRL
DR92321	P&T MFS-D Ballast Train Hopper	NRL
DR92322	P&T MFS-D Ballast Train Hopper	NRL
DR92323	P&T MFS-D Ballast Train Hopper	NRL
DR92324	P&T MFS-D Ballast Train Hopper	NRL
DR92325	P&T MFS-D Ballast Train Hopper	NRL
DR92326	P&T MFS-D Ballast Train Hopper	NRL
DR92327	P&T MFS-D Ballast Train Hopper	NRL
DR92328	P&T MFS-D Ballast Train Hopper	NRL
DR92329	P&T MFS-D Ballast Train Hopper	NRL
DR92330	P&T MFS-D Ballast Train Hopper	NRL
DR92331	P&T PW-RT Power Wagon	NRL
DR92332	P&T PW-RT Power Wagon	NRL
DR92333	P&T MFS-SB Swivel Conveyer Wagon	NRL
DR93334	P&T MFS-SB Swivel Conveyer Wagon	NRL

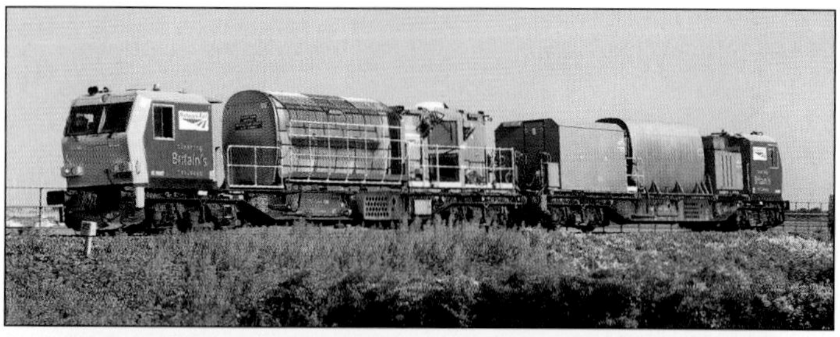

Network Rail operate a fleet of 32 twin-vehicle Windhoff-built Multi-Purpose Vehicles (MPVs) which can be used for a multitude of tasks, most frequently rail head cleaning and weed control. In Weed control use, Nos DR98907 and DR98957 are shown in June 2021. **CJM**

DR93335	P&T MFS-SB Swivel Conveyer Wagon	NRL
DR93336	P&T MFS-SB Swivel Conveyer Wagon	NRL
DR93337	P&T MFS-SB Swivel Conveyer Wagon	NRL
DR93338	P&T MFS-SB Swivel Conveyer Wagon	NRL
DR93339	P&T MFS-SB Swivel Conveyer Wagon	NRL
DR93340	P&T MFS-SB Swivel Conveyer Wagon	NRL
DR92341	P&T MFS-D Ballast Train Hopper	NRL
DR92342	P&T MFS-D Ballast Train Hopper	NRL
DR92343	P&T MFS-D Ballast Train Hopper	NRL
DR92344	P&T MFS-D Ballast Train Hopper	NRL
DR92345	P&T MFS-D Ballast Train Hopper	NRL
DR92346	P&T MFS-D Ballast Train Hopper	NRL
DR92347	P&T MFS-D Ballast Train Hopper	NRL
DR92348	P&T MFS-D Ballast Train Hopper	NRL
DR92349	P&T MFS-D Ballast Train Hopper	NRL
DR92350	P&T MFS-D Ballast Train Hopper	NRL
DR92351	P&T MFS-D Ballast Train Hopper	NRL
DR92352	P&T MFS-D Ballast Train Hopper	NRL
DR92353	P&T MFS-D Ballast Train Hopper	NRL
DR92354	P&T MFS-D Ballast Train Hopper	NRL
DR92355	P&T MFS-D Ballast Train Hopper	NRL
DR92356	P&T MFS-D Ballast Train Hopper	NRL
DR92357	P&T MFS-D Ballast Train Hopper	NRL
DR92358	P&T MFS-D Ballast Train Hopper	NRL
DR92359	P&T MFS-D Ballast Train Hopper	NRL
DR92360	P&T MFS-D Ballast Train Hopper	NRL
DR92361	P&T MFS-D Ballast Train Hopper	NRL
DR92362	P&T MFS-D Ballast Train Hopper	NRL
DR92363	P&T MFS-D Ballast Train Hopper	NRL
DR92364	P&T MFS-D Ballast Train Hopper	NRL
DR92365	P&T MFS-D Ballast Train Hopper	NRL
DR92366	P&T MFS-D Ballast Train Hopper	NRL
DR92367	P&T MFS-D Ballast Train Hopper	NRL
DR92368	P&T MFS-D Ballast Train Hopper	NRL
DR92369	P&T MFS-D Ballast Train Hopper	NRL
DR92370	P&T MFS-D Ballast Train Hopper	NRL
DR92371	P&T MFS-D Ballast Train Hopper	NRL
DR92372	P&T MFS-D Ballast Train Hopper	NRL
DR92373	P&T MFS-D Ballast Train Hopper	NRL
DR92374	P&T MFS-D Ballast Train Hopper	NRL
DR92375	P&T MFS-D Ballast Train Hopper	NRL
DR92376	P&T MFS-D Ballast Train Hopper	NRL
DR92377	P&T MFS-D Ballast Train Hopper	NRL
DR92400	P&T MFS-A Interfacer Wagon	COL
DR92431	P&T PW-RT Power Wagon	NRL
DR92432	P&T PW-RT Power Wagon	NRL
DR92133	P&T MFS-SB Swivel Conveyer Wagon	NRL
DR92434	P&T MFS-SB Swivel Conveyer Wagon	NRL
DR92435	P&T MFS-SB Swivel Conveyer Wagon	NRL
DR92436	P&T MFS-SB Swivel Conveyer Wagon	NRL
DR92437	P&T MFS-SB Swivel Conveyer Wagon	NRL
DR92438	P&T MFS-SB Swivel Conveyer Wagon	NRL
DR92439	P&T MFS-SB Swivel Conveyer Wagon	NRL
DR92440	P&T MFS-SB Swivel Conveyer Wagon	NRL
DR92441	P&T MFS-D Ballast Train Hopper	NRL
DR92442	P&T MFS-D Ballast Train Hopper	NRL
DR92443	P&T MFS-D Ballast Train Hopper	NRL
DR92444	P&T MFS-D Ballast Train Hopper	NRL
DR92445	P&T MFS-D Ballast Train Hopper	NRL
DR92446	P&T MFS-D Ballast Train Hopper	NRL
DR92447	P&T MFS-D Ballast Train Hopper	NRL
DR92448	P&T MFS-D Ballast Train Hopper	NRL
DR92449	P&T MFS-D Ballast Train Hopper	NRL
DR92450	P&T MFS-D Ballast Train Hopper	NRL
DR92451	P&T MFS-D Ballast Train Hopper	NRL
DR92452	P&T MFS-D Ballast Train Hopper	NRL
DR92453	P&T MFS-D Ballast Train Hopper	NRL
DR92454	P&T MFS-D Ballast Train Hopper	NRL
DR92455	P&T MFS-D Ballast Train Hopper	NRL
DR92456	P&T MFS-D Ballast Train Hopper	NRL
DR92457	P&T MFS-D Ballast Train Hopper	NRL
DR92458	P&T MFS-D Ballast Train Hopper	NRL
DR92459	P&T MFS-D Ballast Train Hopper	NRL
DR92460	P&T MFS-D Ballast Train Hopper	NRL
DR92461	P&T MFS-D Ballast Train Hopper	NRL
DR92462	P&T MFS-D Ballast Train Hopper	NRL
DR92463	P&T MFS-D Ballast Train Hopper	NRL
DR92464	P&T MFS-D Ballast Train Hopper	NRL
DR92465	P&T MFS-D Ballast Train Hopper	NRL
DR92466	P&T MFS-D Ballast Train Hopper	NRL
DR92467	P&T MFS-D Ballast Train Hopper	NRL

DR92468	P&T MFS-D Ballast Train Hopper	NRL
DR92469	P&T MFS-D Ballast Train Hopper	NRL
DR92470	P&T MFS-D Ballast Train Hopper	NRL
DR92471	P&T MFS-D Ballast Train Hopper	NRL
DR92472	P&T MFS-D Ballast Train Hopper	NRL
DR92473	P&T MFS-D Ballast Train Hopper	NRL
DR92474	P&T MFS-D Ballast Train Hopper	NRL
DR92475	P&T MFS-D Ballast Train Hopper	NRL
DR92476	P&T MFS-D Ballast Train Hopper	NRL
DR92477 (99 70 9310 477-3)	P&T PW-NPW Power Wagon	NRL
DR92478 (99 70 9310 478-1)	P&T PW-NPW Power Wagon	NRL
DR92944	Robel SPMMT intermediate	CRO
DR92945 (99 70 9550 005-1)	Robel SPMMT intermediate	CRO
DR92946 (99 70 9550-006-4)	Robel SPMMT intermediate	CRO
DR92601-DR92665	WH Davis Sleeper Wagons [65 vehicles]	NRL
DR92701	WH Davis Workshop / Barrier	NRL
DR92702	WH Davis Workshop / Barrier	NRL
DR92703	WH Davis Workshop / Barrier	NRL
DR92704	WH Davis Workshop / Barrier	NRL
DR92705	WH Davis Workshop / Barrier	NRL
DR92706	WH Davis Workshop / Barrier	NRL
DR969001-DR969050	International Sleeper Wagons [50 vehicles]	NRL
DR93325	SDL - Manipulator	NRL
DR93426	SDL - Manipulator	NRL
DR93427	SDL - Manipulator	NRL
DR93428	SDL - Manipulator	NRL
DR93429	SDL - Manipulator	NRL
DR93430	SDL - Manipulator	NRL
DR93431	SDL - Manipulator	NRL
DR93432	SDL - Manipulator	NRL
DR93433	SDL - Manipulator	NRL
DR93434	SDL - Manipulator	NRL
DR93435	SDL - Manipulator	NRL
ARDC96714 (S)	CS 75 tonne Hydraulic Recovery Crane	NRL
DR97001 (DU 94 B 001 URS)	Eiv de Brieve DU94BA – TRAMM	HS1
DR97011	Windhoff Overhead Line – MPV	HS1
DR97012 *Geoff Bell*	Windhoff Overhead Line – MPV	HS1
DR97013	Windhoff Overhead Line – MPV	HS1
DR97014	Windhoff Overhead Line – MPV	HS1
DR97501+DR97601+DR97801	Robel 69.70 Mobile Maintenance Train	NRL
DR97502+DR97602+DR97802	Robel 69.70 Mobile Maintenance Train	NRL
DR97503+DR97603+DR97803	Robel 69.70 Mobile Maintenance Train	NRL
DR97504+DR97604+DR97804	Robel 69.70 Mobile Maintenance Train	NRL
DR97505+DR97605+DR97805	Robel 69.70 Mobile Maintenance Train	NRL
DR97506+DR97606+DR97806	Robel 69.70 Mobile Maintenance Train	NRL
Andy King Works Delivery Manager MMT Romford 12th July 1962 - 7th April 2020		
DR97507+DR97607+DR97807	Robel 69.70 Mobile Maintenance Train	NRL
DR97508+DR97608+DR97808	Robel 69.70 Mobile Maintenance Train	NRL
DR97509 (99 70 6481 009-7)	Robel SPMMT	CRO
DR97510 (99 70 6481 010-5)	Robel SPMMT	CRO
DR97511 (99 70 6481 011-3)	Robel SPMMT	CRO
DR97512 (99 70 6481 012-1)	Robel SPMMT	CRO
DR98001	Windhoff Overhead Line – MPV	NRL
DR98002	Windhoff Overhead Line – MPV	NRL
DR98003 *Anthony Wrighton 1944-2011*	Windhoff Overhead Line – MPV	NRL
DR98004 *Philip Cattrell 1961-2011*	Windhoff Overhead Line – MPV	NRL
DR98005	Windhoff Overhead Line – MPV	NRL
DR98006 *Jason McDonnell 1970-2016*	Windhoff Overhead Line – MPV	NRL
DR98007	Windhoff Overhead Line – MPV	NRL
DR98008	Windhoff MPV Track Monitoring single car	NRL
DR98009 *Melvin Smith 1953-2011*	Windhoff Overhead Line – MPV	NRL
DR98010 *Benjamin Gautrey 1992-2011*	Windhoff Overhead Line – MPV	NRL
DR98011	Windhoff Overhead Line – MPV	NRL
DR98012 *Terence Hand 1962-2016*	Windhoff Overhead Line – MPV	NRL
DR98013 *David Wood 1951-2015*	Windhoff Overhead Line – MPV	NRL
DR98014 *Wayne Imlach 1955-2015*	Windhoff Overhead Line – MPV	NRL
DR98215 A+B	P&T GP-TRAMM	BAL
DR98216 A+B	P&T GP-TRAMM	BAL
DR98217 A+B	P&T GP-TRAMM	BAL
DR98218 A+B	P&T GP-TRAMM	BAL
DR98219 A+B	P&T GP-TRAMM	BAL
DR98220 A+B	P&T GP-TRAMM	BAL
DR98307 A	Geismar VMT860 PL / UM	COL
DR78307 B	Geismar trailer at Baglan Bay, propelling car	COL
DR98308 A+B	Geismar VMT860 PL / UM	COL
DR98901 + DR98951	Windhoff MPV	NRL
DR98902 + DR98952	Windhoff MPV	NRL
DR98903 + DR98953	Windhoff MPV	NRL
DR98904 + DR98954	Windhoff MPV	NRL
DR98905 + DR98955	Windhoff MPV	NRL
DR98906 + DR98956	Windhoff MPV	NRL
DR98907 + DR98957	Windhoff MPV	NRL
DR98908 + DR98958	Windhoff MPV	NRL
DR98909 + DR98959	Windhoff MPV	NRL
DR98910 + DR98960	Windhoff MPV	NRL
DR98911 + DR98961	Windhoff MPV	NRL
DR98912 + DR98962	Windhoff MPV	NRL
DR98913 + DR98963	Windhoff MPV	NRL
DR98914 + DR98964 *Dick Preston*	Windhoff MPV	NRL

DR98915 + DR98965	Windhoff MPV	NRL
Nigel Cummins		
DR98916 + DR98966	Windhoff MPV	NRL
DR98917 + DR98967	Windhoff MPV	NRL
DR98918 + DR98968	Windhoff MPV	NRL
DR98919 + DR98969	Windhoff MPV	NRL
DR98920 + DR98970	Windhoff MPV	NRL
DR98921 + DR98971	Windhoff MPV	NRL
DR98922 + DR98972	Windhoff MPV	NRL
DR98923 + DR98973	Windhoff MPV	NRL
Chris Lemon		
DR98924 + DR98974	Windhoff MPV	NRL
DR98925 + DR98975	Windhoff MPV	NRL
DR98926 + DR98976	Windhoff MPV	NRL
John Denyer		
DR98927 + DR98977	Windhoff MPV	NRL
DR98928 + DR98978	Windhoff MPV	NRL
DR98929 + DR98979	Windhoff MPV	NRL
DR98930 + DR98980	Windhoff MPV	NRL
DR98931 + DR98981	Windhoff MPV	NRL
DR98932 + DR98982	Windhoff MPV	NRL
DR979001-DR979134	Rail Wagon 'Perch' [134-vehicles]	NRL
DR979409-DR979415	Rail Clamp Wagon 'Perch' [3 vehicles]	NRL
DR979505-DR979515	Rail Train End Wagon 'Porpoise' [7 vehicles]	NRL
DR979500-DR979512	Rail Train Chute ' Porpoise' [8 vehicles]	NRL
DR979604-DR979614	Rail Train Gantry 'Perch' [7 Wagons]	NRL
642001	Rail Head Treatment Train	NRL
642002	Rail Head Treatment Train	NRL
642003	Rail Head Treatment Train	NRL
642004	Rail Head Treatment Train	NRL
642005	Rail Head Treatment Train	NRL
642006	Rail Head Treatment Train	NRL
642007	Rail Head Treatment Train	NRL
642008	Rail Head Treatment Train	NRL
642009	Rail Head Treatment Train	NRL
642010	Rail Head Treatment Train	NRL
642011	Rail Head Treatment Train	NRL
642012	Rail Head Treatment Train	NRL
642013	Rail Head Treatment Train	NRL
642014	Rail Head Treatment Train	NRL
642015	Rail Head Treatment Train	NRL
642016	Rail Head Treatment Train	NRL
642017	Rail Head Treatment Train	NRL
642018	Rail Head Treatment Train	NRL
642019	Rail Head Treatment Train	NRL
642020	Rail Head Treatment Train	NRL
642021	Rail Head Treatment Train	NRL
642022	Rail Head Treatment Train	NRL
642023	Rail Head Treatment Train	NRL
642024	Rail Head Treatment Train	NRL
642025	Rail Head Treatment Train	NRL
642026	Rail Head Treatment Train	NRL
642027	Rail Head Treatment Train	NRL
642028	Rail Head Treatment Train	NRL
642029	Rail Head Treatment Train	NRL
642030	Rail Head Treatment Train	NRL
642031	Rail Head Treatment Train	NRL
642032	Rail Head Treatment Train	NRL
642033	Rail Head Treatment Train	NRL
642034	Rail Head Treatment Train	NRL
642035	Rail Head Treatment Train	NRL
642036	Rail Head Treatment Train	NRL
642037	Rail Head Treatment Train	NRL
642038	Rail Head Treatment Train	NRL
642039	Rail Head Treatment Train	NRL
642040	Rail Head Treatment Train	NRL
642041	Rail Head Treatment Train	NRL
642042	Rail Head Treatment Train	NRL
642043	Rail Head Treatment Train	NRL
642044	Rail Head Treatment Train	NRL
642045	Rail Head Treatment Train	NRL
642046	Rail Head Treatment Train	NRL
642047	Rail Head Treatment Train	NRL
642048	Rail Head Treatment Train	NRL
642049	Rail Head Treatment Train	NRL
642050	Rail Head Treatment Train	NRL
99 70 9128 001-3	P&T Unimat 09-4x4/45 Tamper	BAB
99 70 9128 002-1	P&T Unimat 09-4x4/45 Tamper	BAB
99 70 9515 002-2	Railcare Railvac Machine, 16000-480UK	RAC
99 70 9515 003-0	Railcare Railvac Machine, 16000-480UK	RAC
99 70 9515 004-8	Railcare Railvac Machine, 16000-480UK	RAC
99 70 9515 005-5	Railcare Railvac Machine, 16000-480UK	RAC
99 70 9515 006-3	Railcare Railvac Machine, 16000-480UK	RAC

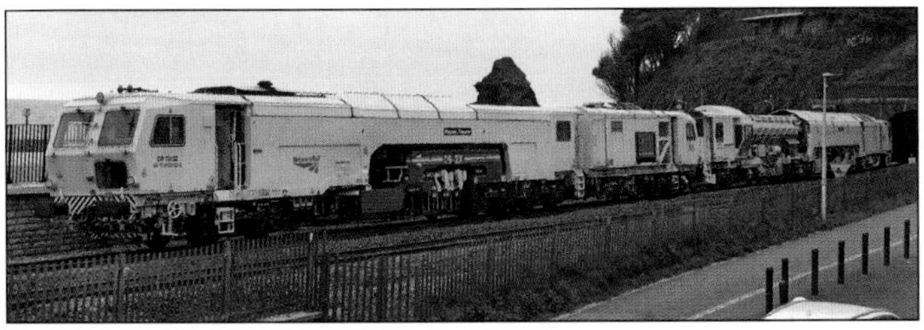

Often the larger Network Rail track machines operate between work sites in pairs. DR73122 nearest the camera is a Plasser & Theurer 09-2X Dynamic Tamper and Liner, while at the far end is DR77010 a Plasser & Theurer USP6000 Ballast Regulator **CJM**

99 70 9522 020-5	Railcare Ballast Feeder	RAC
99 70 9594 014-1	Winter Snow Patrol Train 'Perch'	NRL
DR 99 70 9231 001-7	Electrification Train - SVI RT250 Crane/platform vehicle	ABC
DR 99 70 9231 004-1	Electrification Train - SVI PT500 Wire/platform	ABC
DR 99 70 9231 005-8	Electrification Train - SVI RSM9 Platform	ABC
DR 99 70 9231 006-6	Electrification Train - SVI RSM9 Platform	ABC
DR 99 70 9231 007-4	Electrification Train - SVI APV250 Platform	ABC

Snowploughs and Snowblowers

Three-axle 'Drift' Ploughs

Number	Allocation	Number	Allocation
ADB965203	Carlisle	ADB965230	Inverness
ADB965206	York	ADB965231	Motherwell
ADB965208	Norwich	ADB965234	Inverness
ADB965209	Motherwell	ADB965235	Taunton
ADB965210	Tonbridge	ADB965236	Tonbridge
ADB965211	Tonbridge	ADB965237	Tonbridge
ADB965217	York	ADB965240	York
ADB965219	Norwich	ADB965241	York
ADB965223	Taunton	ADB965242	Carlisle
ADB965224	Inverness	ADB965243	Inverness

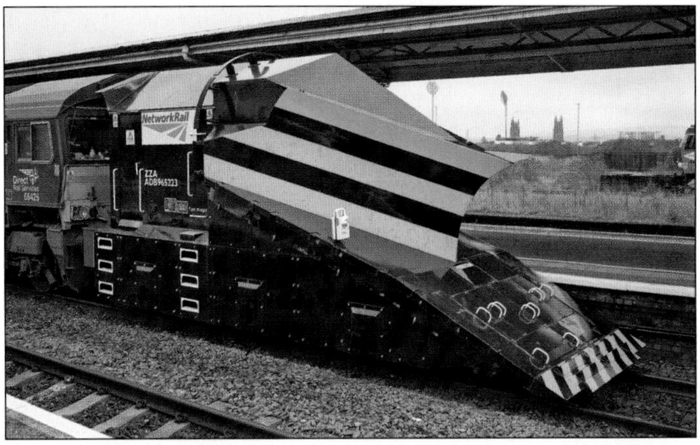

Network Rail still operate a fleet of heavy duty Drift Ploughs, which can be called to use after heavy snow. ZZA No. ADB965223 is one of a pair based at Taunton and is seen on its annual test run, operated by DRS. **Antony Christie**

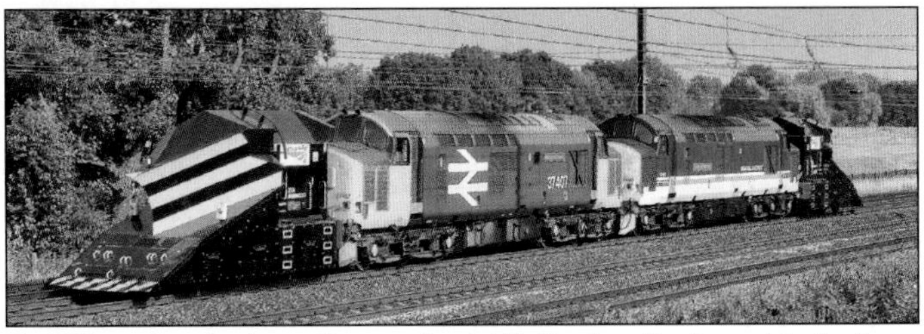

The NR heavy duty ploughs usually operate 'top & tail' of two locos. Two immaculate ploughs Nos. ADB965217 and 965240 operate a test run at Chaloners Whin, York on 7 September 2021, powered by DRS Class 37s Nos. 37407 and 37425. **Robin Patrick**

Beilhack 'Patrol' Ploughs

Number	Allocation
ADB965576	Doncaster (ex-Class 40 bogie)
ADB965577	Doncaster (ex-Class 40 bogie)
ADB965578	Carlisle (ex-Class 40 bogie)
ADB965579	Carlisle (ex-Class 40 bogie)
ADB965580	Wigan (ex-Class 40 bogie)
ADB965581	Wigan (ex-Class 40 bogie)
ADB966098	Doncaster (ex-Class 45 bogie)
ADB966099	Doncaster (ex-Class 40 bogie)

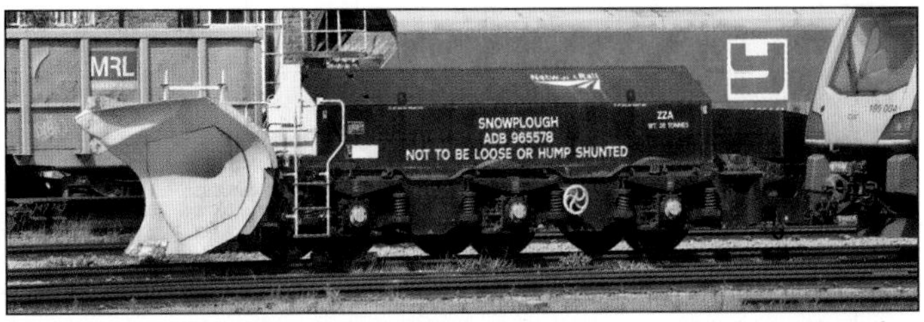

Four pairs of former bogie Beilhack patrol ploughs are operated by Network Rail, two pairs are kept at Doncaster, No. ADB965578 is shown. **Antony Christie**

Beilhack Snow Blowers

Number	Allocation	Number	Allocation
ADB968500	Rutherglen	ADB968501	Rutherglen

Eurotunnel

Shuttle Locomotives

Class 9/0, Brush Tri-Bo

Built: 1993-1999
Length: 72ft 2in (22.01m)
Height: 13ft 9in (4.20m)
Width: 9ft 9in (2.97m)
Power system: 25,000V ac overhead
Transmission: Electric
Horsepower: 7,725hp (5,760kW
Tractive effort: 69,500lb (310kN)

9005	*Jessye Norman*	A	CQ	EUR	EUR	EUR
9007	*Dame Joan Sutherland*	A	CQ	EUR	EUR	EUR
9011	*José Van Dam*	A	CQ	EUR	EUR	EUR
9013	*Maria Callas*	A	CQ	EUR	EUR	EUR
9015	*Lötschberg 1913*	A	CQ	EUR	EUR	EUR
9018	*Wilhelmena Fernandez*	A	CQ	EUR	EUR	EUR
9022	*Dame Janet Baker*	A	CQ	EUR	EUR	EUR
9024	*Gotthard 1882*	A	CQ	EUR	EUR	EUR
9026	*Furkatunnel 1982*	A	CQ	EUR	EUR	EUR
9029	*Thomas Allan*	A	CQ	EUR	EUR	EUR
9033	*Montserrat Caballé*	A	CQ	EUR	EUR	EUR
9036	*Alan Fondary*	A	CQ	EUR	EUR	EUR
9037	*Gabriel Bacquier*	A	CQ	EUR	EUR	EUR

Class 9/7, Brush Tri-Bo

Built: 2001
Length: 72ft 2in (22.01m)
Height: 13ft 9in (4.20m)
Width: 9ft 9in (2.97m)
Power system: 25,000V ac overhead
Transmission: Electric
Horsepower: 9,387hp (7,000kW
Tractive effort: 90,000lb (400kN)

9701	A	CQ	EUR	EUR	EUR
9702	A	CQ	EUR	EUR	EUR
9703	A	CQ	EUR	EUR	EUR
9704	A	CQ	EUR	EUR	EUR
9705	A	CQ	EUR	EUR	EUR
9706	A	CQ	EUR	EUR	EUR
9707	A	CQ	EUR	EUR	EUR
9711 (9101)	A	CQ	EUR	EUR	EUR
9712 (9102)	A	CQ	EUR	EUR	EUR
9713 (9103)	A	CQ	EUR	EUR	EUR
9714 (9104)	A	CQ	EUR	EUR	EUR
9715 (9105)	A	CQ	EUR	EUR	EUR
9716 (9106)	A	CQ	EUR	EUR	EUR
9717 (9107)	A	CQ	EUR	EUR	EUR
9718 (9108)	A	CQ	EUR	EUR	EUR
9719 (9109)	A	CQ	EUR	EUR	EUR
9720 (9110)	A	CQ	EUR	EUR	EUR
9721 (9111)	A	CQ	EUR	EUR	EUR
9722 (9112)	A	CQ	EUR	EUR	EUR
9723 (9113)	A	CQ	EUR	EUR	EUR

Class 9/8, Brush Tri-Bo

Built:1993-1994, rebuilt 2005-2010
Length: 72ft 2in (22.01m)
Height: 13ft 9in (4.20m)
Width: 9ft 9in (2.97m)
Power system: 25,000V ac overhead
Transmission: Electric
Horsepower: 9,387hp (7,000kW
Tractive effort: 90,000lb (400kN)

9801 (9001)	*Lesley Garrett*	A	CQ	EUR	EUR	EUR
9802 (9002)	*Stuart Burrows*	A	CQ	EUR	EUR	EUR
9803 (9003)	*Benjamin Luxon*	A	CQ	EUR	EUR	EUR
9804 (9004)		A	CQ	EUR	EUR	EUR
9806 (9006)	*Régine Crespin*	A	CQ	EUR	EUR	EUR
9808 (9008)	*Elisabeth Soderstrom*	A	CQ	EUR	EUR	EUR
9809 (9009)		A	CQ	EUR	EUR	EUR
9810 (9010)		A	CQ	EUR	EUR	EUR
9812 (9012)		A	CQ	EUR	EUR	EUR
9814 (9014)	*Lucia Popp*	A	CQ	EUR	EUR	EUR
9816 (9016)		A	CQ	EUR	EUR	EUR
9819 (9019)	*Maria Ewing*	A	CQ	EUR	EUR	EUR
9820 (9020)	*Nicolai Ghiaurov*	A	CQ	EUR	EUR	EUR
9821 (9021)		A	CQ	EUR	EUR	EUR
9823 (9023)	*Dame Elisabeth Legge-Schwarzkopf*	A	CQ	EUR	EUR	EUR
9825 (9025)		A	CQ	EUR	EUR	EUR
9827 (9027)	*Barbara Hendricks*	A	CQ	EUR	EUR	EUR
9828 (9028)		A	CQ	EUR	EUR	EUR
9831 (9031)		A	CQ	EUR	EUR	EUR
9832 (9032)	*Renata Tebaldi*	A	CQ	EUR	EUR	EUR
9834 (9034)	*Mirella Freni*	A	CQ	EUR	EUR	EUR
9835 (9035)	*Nicolai Gedda*	A	CQ	EUR	EUR	EUR
9838 (9036)	*Hildegard Behrens*	A	CQ	EUR	EUR	EUR
9840 (9040)		A	CQ	EUR	EUR	EUR

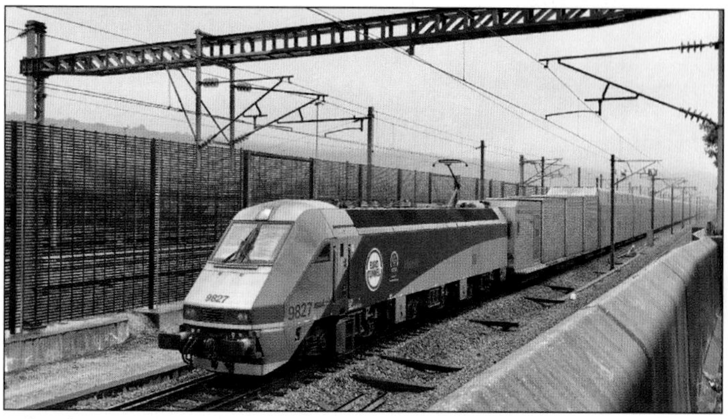

A fleet of 24 98xx 'Shuttle' locos, refurbished and upgraded from the original 90xx fleet are in regular use on EuroTunnel services. No. 9827 Barbara Hendricks *is seen arriving at the UK Cheriton terminal.* **Howard Lewsey**

Pilot / Rescue Locomotives

Krupp-MaK Bo-Bo

Built: 1991-1992
Length: 14.4m
Height: 3.89m
Width: 2.99m
Engine: MTU 12V396 TC13 of 1,275hp (960kW)
Transmission: Electric
Tractive effort: 68,600lb (305kN)
Fitted with TVM cab-signalling

Eurotunnel No.	TOPS No.				
0001	21901	A	GYL	EUR	EUR
0002	21902	A	GYL	EUR	EUR
0003	21903	A	GYL	EUR	EUR
0004	21904	A	GYL	EUR	EUR
0005	21905	A	GYL	EUR	EUR

Built: 1990-1991 to Eurotunnel 2011-2016
Length: 14.4m
Height: 3.89m
Width: 2.99m
Engine: MTU 12V396 TC13 of 1,580hp (1,180kW)
Transmission: Electric
Tractive effort: 31,500lb (140kN)

Eurotunnel No.	Ex DB-Cargo Netherlands No.				
0006	6456	A	GYL	EUR	EUR
0007	6457	A	GYL	EUR	EUR
0008	6450	A	GYL	EUR	EUR
0009	6451	A	GYL	EUR	EUR
0010	6447	A	GYL	EUR	EUR

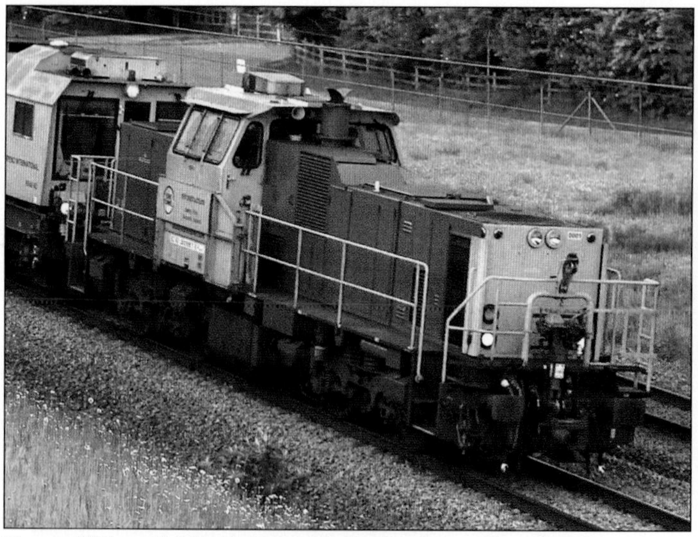

The powerful Krupp-Mak diesel locos operated y EuroTunnel are used for engineering trains as well as being available to rescue any train which becomes disabled in the Channel Tunnel. Loco No. 0001 (TOPS No. 21901) is seen working an engineering train on HS1. **Howard Lewsey**

Hunslet/Schöma 0-4-0

Built: 1989-1990 by Hunslet as 900mm gauge
Rebuilt 1993-1994 by Schöma as 1,438mm gauge
Length: 7.87m
Height: 3.79m
Width: 2.69m
Engine: Deutz F10L 413FW of 230hp (170kW)
Transmission: Mechanical
Tractive effort: 15,300lb (68kN)

0031	*Francis*	A	GYL	EUR	EUR
0032	*Elisabeth*	A	GYL	EUR	EUR
0033	*Silke*	A	GYL	EUR	EUR
0034	*Amanda*	A	GYL	EUR	EUR
0035	*Mary*	A	GYL	EUR	EUR
0036	*Laurence*	A	GYL	EUR	EUR
0037	*Lydie*	A	GYL	EUR	EUR
0038	*Jenny*	A	GYL	EUR	EUR
0039	*Pacita*	A	GYL	EUR	EUR
0040	*Jill*	A	GYL	EUR	EUR
0041	*Kim*	A	GYL	EUR	EUR
0042	*Nicole*	A	GYL	EUR	EUR

At the end of 2018, Eurotunnel announced an order for 19 two-axle 40 ton locos, to be built by Socofer. These will be battery powered, with a diesel engine for battery charging. Delivery is expected in 2023.

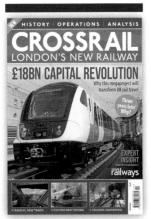

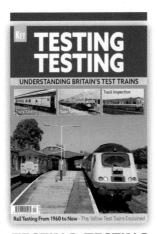

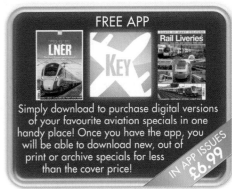

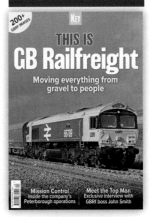

Metro & Light Rail

London Underground

1972 Tube Stock — BAKERLOO LINE

Builder: Metro-Cammell
Years built: 1972-1974
Formation: DM+T+T+M+UN+M+T+DM
Max speed: 45mph (72km/h)
Length: Driving - 52ft 8in (16.09m), Intermediate - 52ft 4in (15.98m)
Width: 8ft 6in (2.64m)
Height: 9ft 4in (2.87m)
Doors: Sliding bi-parting
Traction equipment: 4 x Brush LT115 of 71hp (53kW) on each power car

Four-car single-ended sets (formed at south end of train) DM+T+T+MM

3231+4231+4331+3331	3250+4250+4350+3350
3232+4232+4332+3332	3251+4251+4351+3351
3233+4233+4333+3333	3252+4252+4352+3352
3234+4234+4334+3334	3253+4253+4353+3353
3235+4235+4335+3335	3254+4254+4354+3354
3236+4236+4336+3336	3255+4255+4355+3355
3237+4237+4337+3337	3256+4256+4356+3356
3238+4238+4338+3338	3258+4258+4358+3358
3239+4239+4339+3339	3259+4259+4359+3359
3240+4240+4340+3340	3260+4260+4360+3360
3241+4241+4341+3341	3261+4261+4361+3361
3242+4242+4342+3342	3262+4262+4362+3362
3243+4243+4343+3343	3263+4263+4363+3363
3244+4244+4344+3344	3264+4264+4364+3364
3245+4245+4345+3345	3265+4265+4365+3365
3246+4246+4346+3346	3266+4266+4366+3366
3247+4247+4347+3347	3267+4267+4367+3367
3248+4248+4348+3348	3299+4299+4399+3399*

Three-car single-ended sets (formed at north end of train) UNDM+T+DM

3431+4531+3531	3450+4550+3550
3432+4532+3532	3451+4551+3551
3433+4533+3533	3452+4552+3552
3434+4534+3534	3453+4553+3553
3435+4535+3535	3454+4554+3554
3436+4536+3536	3455+4555+3555
3437+4537+3537	3456+4556+3556
3438+4538+3538	3457+4557+3557
3440+4540+3540	3458+4558+3558
3441+4541+3541	3459+4559+3559
3442+4542+3542	3460+4560+3560
3443+4543+3543	3461+4561+3561
3444+4544+3544	3462+4562+3562
3445+4545+3545	3463+4563+3563
3446+4546+3546	3464+4564+3564
3447+4547+3547	3465+4565+3565
3448+4548+3548	3466+4566+3566
3449+4549+3549	3467+4567+3567

Note: Nos. 4352-4363 fittted with de-icing equipment
* UNDM vehicle

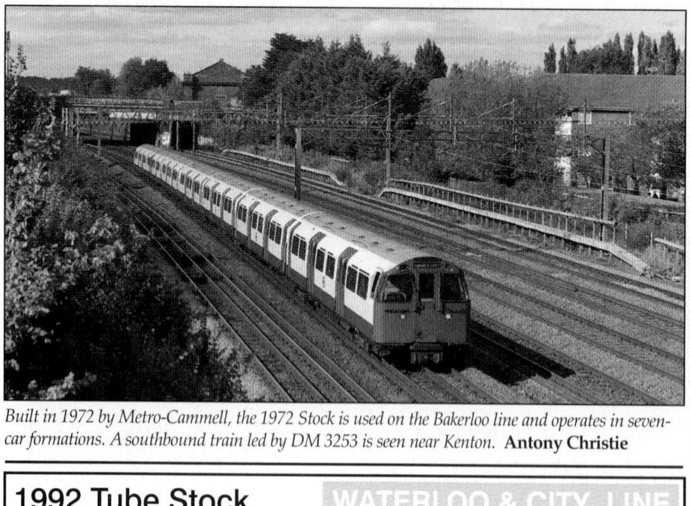

Built in 1972 by Metro-Cammell, the 1972 Stock is used on the Bakerloo line and operates in seven-car formations. A southbound train led by DM 3253 is seen near Kenton. **Antony Christie**

1992 Tube Stock — WATERLOO & CITY LINE

Builder: ADtranz
Years built: 1993
Formation: DM+M+M+DM
Max speed: 53mph (85km/h)
Length: 53ft 3in (16.25m)
Width: 8ft 5½in (2.62m)
Height: 9ft 4in (2.87m)
Doors: Sliding bi-parting
Traction equipment: 4 x Brush LT118 of 65hp (49kW) on each power car

Two-car single-ended sets DM+M (east end)

65501+67501	65507+67507
65503+67503	65509+67509
65505+67505	

Two-car single-ended sets M+DM (west end)

67502+65502	67508+65508
67504+65504	67510+65510
67506+65506	

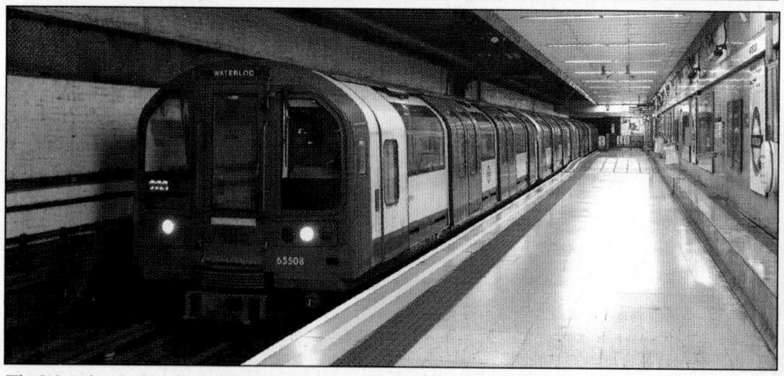

The Waterloo & City line, linking Waterloo with Bank was refurbished in 1993, when five four-car 1992 LU Central Line style sets were introduced. The then BR-operated line was then transferred to part of London Underground. Driving Motor car No. 65508 is seen at Waterloo in January 2022. **Antony Christie**

1992 Tube Stock — CENTRAL LINE

Builder: ADtranz
Years built: 1991-1994
Formation: DM+M+M+M+M+M+M+DM
Max speed: 53mph (85km/h)
Length: 53ft 3in (16.25m)
Width: 8ft 5½in (2.62m)
Height: 9ft 4in (2.87m)
Doors: Sliding bi-parting
Traction equipment: 4 x Brush LT118 of 65hp (49kW) on each power car

Two-car single-ended sets A+B - DM+NDM

91001+92001	91119+92119	91237+92237
91003+92003	91121+92121	91239+92239
91005+92005	91123+92123	91241+92241
91007+92007	91125+92125	91243+92243
91009+92009	91127+92127	91245+92245
91011+92011	91129+92129	91247+92247
91013+92013	91131+92131	91249+92249
91015+92015	91133+92133	91251+92251
91017+92017	91135+92135	91253+92253
91019+92019	91137+92137	91255+92255
91021+92021	91139+92139	91257+92257
91023+92023	91141+92141	91259+92259
91025+92025	91143+92143	91261+92261
91027+92027	91145+92145	91263+92263
91029+92029	91147+92147	91265+92265
91031+92031	91149+92149	91267+92267
91033+92033	91151+92151	91269+92269
91035+92035	91153+92153	91271+92271
91037+92037	91155+92155	91273+92273
91039+92039	91157+92157	91275+92275
91041+92041	91159+92159	91277+92277
91043+92043	91161+92161	91279+92279
91045+92045	91163+92163	91281+92281
91047+92047	91165+92165	91283+92283
91049+92049	91167+92167	91285+92285
91051+92051	91169+92169	91287+92287
91053+92053	91171+92171	91289+92289
91055+92055	91173+92173	91291+92291
91057+92057	91175+92175	91293+92293
91059+92059	91177+92177	91295+92295
91061+92061	91179+92179	91297+92297
91063+92063	91181+92181	91299+92299
91065+92065	91183+92183	91301+92301
91067+92067	91185+92185	91303+92303
91069+92069	91187+92187	91305+92305
91071+92071	91189+92189	91307+92307
91073+92073	91191+92191	91309+92309
91075+92075	91193+92193	91311+92311
91077+92077	91195+92195	91313+92313
91079+92079	91197+92197	91315+92315
91081+92081	91199+92199	91317+92317
91083+92083	91201+92201	91319+92319
91085+92085	91203+92203	91321+92321
91087+92087	91205+92205	91323+92323
91089+92089	91207+92207	91325+92325
91091+92091	91209+92209	91327+92327
91093+92093	91211+92211	91329+92329
91095+92095	91213+92213	91331+92331
91097+92097	91215+92215	91333+92333
91099+92099	91217+92217	91335+92335
91101+92101	91219+92219	91337+92337
91103+92103	91221+92221	91339+92339
91105+92105	91223+92223	91341+92341
91107+92107	91225+92225	91343+92343
91109+92109	91227+92227	91345+92345
91111+92111	91229+92229	91347+92347
91113+92113	91231+92231	91349+92349
91115+92115	91233+92233	
91117+92117	91235+92235	

Two-car non-driving sets B+C - NDM+NDM

92002+93002	92008+93008	92014+93014
92004+93004	92010+93010	92016+93016
92006+93006	92012+93012	92018+93018

92020+93020
92022+93022
92024+93024
92026+93026
92028+93028
92030+93030
92032+93032
92034+93034
92036+93036
92038+93038
92040+93040
92042+93042
92044+93044
92046+93046
92048+93048
92050+93050
92052+93052
92054+93054
92056+93056
92058+93058
92060+93060
92062+93062
92064+93064
92066+93066
92068+93068
92070+93070
92072+93072
92074+93074
92076+93076
92078+93078
92080+93080
92082+93082
92084+93084
92086+93086
92088+93088
92090+93090
92092+93092
92094+93094
92096+93096
92098+93098
92100+93100
92102+93102
92104+93104
92106+93106
92108+93108
92110+93110
92112+93112
92114+93114
92116+93116
92118+93118
92120+93120
92122+93122
92124+93124
92126+93126
92128+93128
92130+93130
92132+93132
92134+93134
92136+93136
92138+93138
92140+93140
92142+93142
92144+93144
92146+93146
92148+93148
92150+93150
92152+93152
92154+93154
92156+93156
92158+93158
92160+93160
92162+93162
92164+93164
92166+93166
92168+93168
92170+93170
92172+93172
92174+93174
92176+93176
92178+93178
92180+93180
92182+93182
92184+93184
92186+93186
92188+93188
92190+93190
92192+93192
92194+93194
92196+93196
92198+93198
92200+93200
92202+93202
92204+93204
92206+93206
92208+93208
92210+93210
92212+93212
92214+93214
92216+93216
92218+93218
92220+93220
92222+93222
92224+93224
92226+93226
92228+93228
92230+93230
92232+93232
92234+93234
92236+93236
92238+93238
92240+93240
92242+93242
92244+93244
92246+93246
92248+93248
92250+93250
92252+93252
92254+93254
92256+93256
92258+93258
92260+93260
92262+93262
92264+93264
92266+93266

Two-car non-driving sets B+D - NDM+NDM

92402+93402
92404+93404
92406+93406
92408+93408
92410+93410
92412+93412
92414+93414
92416+93416
92418+93418
92420+93420
92422+93422
92424+93424
92426+93426
92428+93428
92430+93430
92432+93432
92434+93434
92436+93436
92438+93438
92440+93440
92442+93442
92444+93444
92446+93446
92448+93448
92450+93450
92452+93452
92454+93454
92456+93456
92458+93458
92460+93460
92462+93462
92464+93464

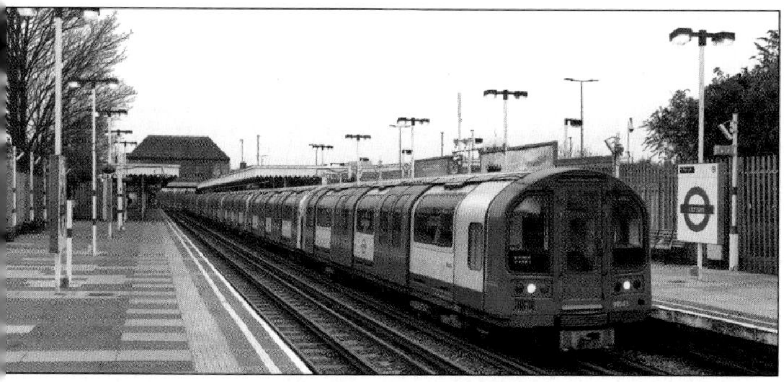

ADtranz-built 1992 stock on the Central Line are formed into eight-car trains. Led by DM No. 91043 a set is seen at Leyton in January 2022. **Antony Christie**

1973 Tube Stock

PICCADILLY LINE

Builder: Metro Cammell
Years built: 1974-1977
Formation: DM+T+UNDM+UNM+T+DM
or DM+T+UNDM+DM+T+DM
Max speed: 45mph (72km/h)
Length: Cab - 57ft 3in (17.47m)
Intermediate - 58ft 0in (17.68m)

Width: 8ft 5¾in (2.63m)
Height: 9ft 4in (2.88m)
Doors: Sliding bi-parting
Traction equipment: 4 x Brush LT118 of 65hp (49kW) on each power car

A fleet of 94 Siemens 'Inspiro' nine-car articulated sets, 2024 Stock are on order, to be built in Vienna (Austria) and Goole in the UK for delivery in 2024-2025

Three-car single-ended sets DM+T+UNDM

100+500+300
101+501+301
102+502+302
103+503+303
104+504+304
105+505+305
106+506+306
107+507+307
108+508+308
109+509+309
110+510+310
111+511+311
112+512+312
113+513+313
115+515+315
116+516+316
117+517+317
118+518+318
119+519+319
120+520+320
121+521+321
122+522+322
123+523+323
124+524+324
125+525+325
126+526+326
127+527+327
128+528+328
129+529+329
130+530+330
131+531+331
132+532+332
133+533+333
134+534+334
135+535+335
136+536+336
137+537+337
138+538+338
139+539+339
140+540+340
141+541+341
142+542+342
143+543+343
144+544+344
145+545+345
146+546+346
147+547+347
148+548+348
149+549+349
150+550+350
151+551+351
152+552+352
153+553+353
154+554+354
155+555+355
156+556+356
157+557+357
158+558+358
159+559+359
160+560+360
161+561+361
162+562+362
163+563+363
164+564+364
165+565+365
167+567+367
168+568+368
169+569+369
170+570+370
171+571+371
172+572+372
173+573+373
174+574+374
175+575+375
176+576+376
177+577+377
178+578+378
179+579+379
180+580+380
181+581+381
182+582+382
183+583+383
184+584+384
185+585+385
186+586+386
187+587+387
188+588+388
189+589+389
190+590+390
191+591+391
192+592+392
193+593+393
194+594+394
195+595+395
196+596+396
197+597+397
198+598+398
199+599+399
200+600+400
201+601+401
202+602+402
203+603+403
205+605+405
206+606+406
207+607+407
208+608+408
209+609+409
210+610+410
211+611+411
212+612+412
213+613+413
214+614+414
215+615+415
216+616+416
217+617+417
218+618+418
219+619+419
220+620+420
221+621+421
222+622+422
223+623+423
224+624+424
225+625+425
226+626+426
227+627+427
228+628+428
229+629+429
230+630+430
231+631+431
232+632+432
233+633+433
234+634+434
235+635+435
236+636+436
237+637+437
238+638+438
239+639+439
240+640+440
241+641+441
242+642+442
243+643+443
244+644+444
245+645+445
246+646+446
247+647+447
248+648+448
249+649+449
250+650+450
251+651+451
252+652+452
253+653+453

Three-car double-ended sets DM+T+DM

854+654+855
856+656+857
858+658+859
860+660+861
862+662+863
864+664+865
866+666+867
868+668+869■
870+670+871
872+672+873
874+674+875
876+676+877
878+678+879
880+680+881
882+682+883
884+684+885
886+686+887
890+690+891■
892+692+893
894+694+895
896+696+897

■ Sandite fitted

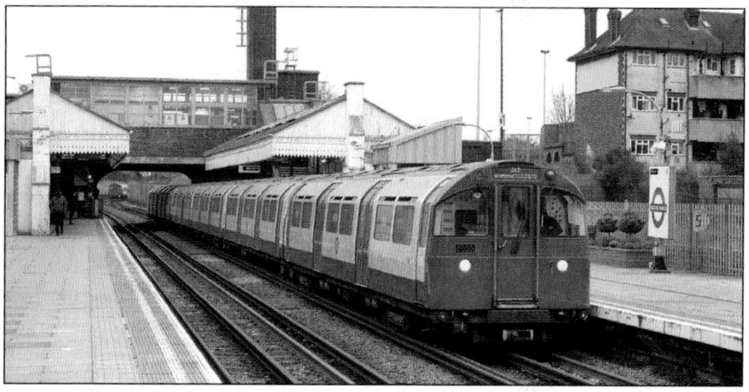

The Piccadilly Line sets, introduced in 1973 were built by Metro-Cammell and operate in six car formation. Led by Driving Motor 154, the train calls at Boston Manor on 26 January 2022 bound for Heathrow Airport. **Antony Christie**

1996 Tube Stock

JUBILEE LINE

Builder: GEC Alstom, CAF Spain●
Years built: 1996-1998, 2005●
Formation: DM+T+T+UNDM+UNDM+T+DM
Max speed: 62mph (100km/h)
Length: 58ft 2in (17.77m)

Width: 8ft 5¾in (2.63m)
Height: 9ft 4in (2.87m)
Doors: Sliding bi-parting
Traction equipment: 4 x GEC LT200 of 120hp (90kW) on each power car

Four-car single-ended sets. DM+T+T●+UNDM

96001+96201+96601+96401
96003+96203+96603+96403
96005+96205+96605+96405
96007+96207+96607+96407
96009+96209+96609+96409
96011+96211+96611+96411
96013+96213+96613+96413
96015+96215+96615+96415
96017+96217+96617+96417
96019+96219+96619+96419
96021+96221+96621+96421
96023+96223+96623+96423
96025+96225+96625+96425
96027+96227+96627+96427
96029+96229+96629+96429
96031+96231+96631+96431
96033+96233+96633+96433
96035+96235+96635+96435
96037+96237+96637+96437
96039+96239+96639+96439
96041+96241+96641+96441
96043+96243+96643+96443
96045+96245+96645+96445
96047+96247+96647+96447
96049+96249+96649+96449
96051+96251+96651+96451
96053+96253+96653+96453
96055+96255+96655+96455
96057+96257+96657+96457
96059+96259+96659+96459
96061+96261+96661+96461
96063+96263+96663+96463
96065+96265+96665+96465
96067+96267+96667+96467
96069+96269+96669+96469
96071+96271+96671+96471
96073+96273+96673+96473
96075+96275+96675+96475
96077+96277+96677+96477
96079+96279+96679+96479
96081+96281+96681+96481
96083+96283+96683+96483
96085+96285+96685+96485
96087+96287+96687+96487
96089+96289+96689+96489
96091+96291+96691+96491
96093+96293+96693+96493
96095+96295+96695+96495
96097+96297+96697+96497
96099+96299+96699+96499
96101+96301+96701+96501
96103+96303+96703+96503

96105+96305+96705+96505
96107+96307+96707+96507
96109+96309+96709+96509
96111+96311+96711+96511
96113+96313+96713+96513
96115+96315+96715+96515
96117+96317+96717+96517
96119+96319+96719+96519●
96121+96321+96721+96521●
96123+96323+96723+96523●
96125+96325+96725+96525●

Three-car single-ended sets. UNDM+T+DM

96402+96202+96002
96404+96204+96004
96406+96206+96006
96408+96208+96008
96410+96210+96010
96412+96212+96012
96414+96214+96014
96416+96216+96016
96418+96218+96018
96420+96220+96020
96422+96222+96022
96424+96224+96024
96426+96226+96026
96428+96228+96028
96430+96230+96030
96432+96232+96032
96434+96234+96034
96436+96236+96036
96438+96238+96038
96440+96240+96040
96442+96242+96042
96444+96244+96044
96446+96246+96046
96448+96248+96048
96450+96250+96050
96452+96252+96052
96454+96254+96054
96456+96256+96056
96458+96258+96058
96460+96260+96060
96462+96262+96062
96464+96264+96064
96466+96266+96066
96468+96268+96068
96470+96270+96070
96472+96272+96072
96474+96274+96074
96476+96276+96076
96478+96278+96078
96480+96280+96080
96482+96282+96082
96484+96284+96084
96486+96286+96086
96488+96288+96088
96490+96290+96090
96492+96292+96092
96494+96294+96094
96496+96296+96096
96498+96298+96098
96500+96300+96100
96502+96302+96102
96504+96304+96104
96506+96306+96106
96508+96308+96108
96510+96310+96110
96512+96312+96112
96514+96314+96114
96516+96316+96116
96518+96318+96118
96520+96320+96120●
96522+96322+96122●
96524+96324+96124●
96526+96326+96126●

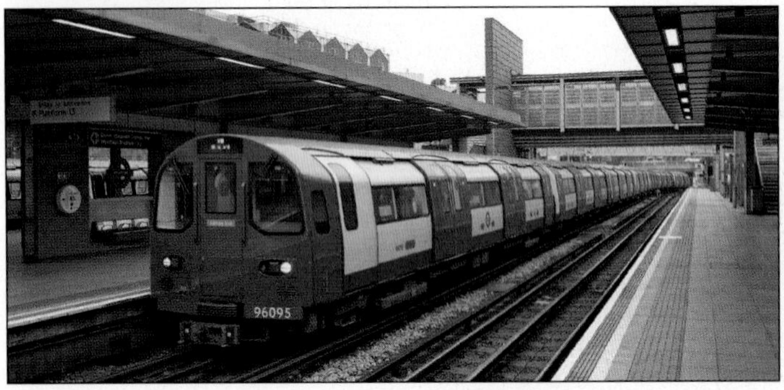

The Jubilee Line tube stock was built between 1996 and 1998 by GEC Alstom (previously Metro-Cammell) with extra trailers built by CAF in 2005. Trains operate in seven-car formation. DM No. 96095 leads a train at Stratford in January 2022. **Antony Christie**

1995 Tube Stock — NORTHERN LINE

Builder: GEC Alstom
Years built: 1996-2000
Formation: DM+T+UNDM+UNDM+T+DM
Max speed: 45mph (72km/h)
Length: 58ft 2in (17.77m)
Width: 8ft 5¾in (2.63m)
Height: 9ft 4in (2.87m)
Doors: Sliding bi-parting
Traction equipment: 4 x GEC G355AZ of 114hp (85kW) on each power car

Six-car double-ended sets DM+T+UNDM+UNDM+T+DM

51501+52501+53501+53701+52701+51701●
51502+52502+53502+53503+52503+51503
51504+52504+53504+53505+52505+51505
51506+52506+53506+53507+52507+51507
51508+52508+53508+53702+52702+51702●
51509+52509+53509+53510+52510+51510
51511+52511+53511+53512+52512+51512
51513+52513+53513+53514+52514+51514
51515+52515+53515+53703+52703+51703●
51516+52516+53516+53517+52517+51517
51518+52518+53518+53519+52519+51519
51520+52520+53520+53704+52704+51704●
51521+52521+53521+53522+52522+51522
51523+52523+53523+53524+52524+51524
51525+52525+53525+53705+52705+51705●
51526+52526+53526+53527+52527+51527
51528+52528+53528+53529+52529+51529
51530+52530+53530+53531+52531+51531
51532+52532+53532+53706+52706+51706●
51533+52533+53533+53534+52534+51534
51535+52535+53535+53536+52536+51536
51537+52537+53537+53538+52538+51538
51539+52539+53539+53707+52707+51707●
51540+52540+53540+53541+52541+51541
51542+52542+53542+53543+52543+51543
51544+52544+53544+53545+52545+51545
51546+52546+53546+53708+52708+51708●
51547+52547+53547+53548+52548+51548
51549+52549+53549+53550+52550+51550
51551+52551+53551+53711+52711+51711●
51553+52553+53553+53709+52709+51709
51554+52554+53554+53555+52555+51555
51556+52556+53556+53557+52557+51557
51558+52558+53558+53559+52559+51559
51560+52560+53560+53710+52710+51710●
51561+52561+53561+53562+52562+51562
51563+52563+53563+53564+52564+51564
51565+52565+53565+53566+52566+51566
51567+52567+53567+53552+52552+51552
51568+52568+53568+53569+52569+51569
51570+52570+53570+53571+52571+51571
51572+52572+53572+53573+52573+51573
51574+52574+53574+53712+52712+51712●
51575+52575+53575+53576+52576+51576
51577+52577+53577+53578+52578+51578
51579+52579+53579+53580+52580+51580
51581+52581+53581+53713+52713+51713●
51582+52582+53582+53583+52583+51583
51584+52584+53584+53585+52585+51585
51586+52586+53586+53587+52587+51587
51588+52588+53588+53714+52714+51714●
51589+52589+53589+53590+52590+51590
51591+52591+53591+53592+52592+51592
51593+52593+53593+53594+52594+51594
51595+52595+53595+53715+52715+51715●
51596+52596+53596+53597+52597+51597
51598+52598+53598+53599+52599+51599
51600+52600+53600+53601+52601+51601
51602+52602+53602+53716+52716+51716●
51603+52603+53603+53604+52604+51604
51605+52605+53605+53606+52606+51606
51607+52607+53607+53608+52608+51608
51609+52609+53609+53717+52717+51717●
51610+52610+53610+53611+52611+51611
51612+52612+53612+53613+52613+51613
51614+52614+53614+53615+52615+51615
51616+52616+53616+53718+52718+51718●
51617+52617+53617+53618+52618+51618
51619+52619+53619+53620+52620+51620
51621+52621+53621+53622+52622+51622
51623+52623+53623+53719+52719+51719●
51624+52624+53624+53625+52625+51625
51626+52626+53626+53627+52627+51627
51628+52628+53628+53629+52629+51629
51630+52630+53630+53720+52720+51720●
51631+52631+53631+53632+52632+51632
51633+52633+53633+53634+52634+51634
51635+52635+53635+53636+52636+51636
51637+52637+53637+53721+52721+51721●
51638+52638+53638+53639+52639+51639
51640+52640+53640+53641+52641+51641
51642+52642+53642+53643+52643+51643
51644+52644+53644+53722+52722+51722●
51645+52645+53645+53646+52646+51646
51647+52647+53647+53648+52648+51648
51649+52649+53649+53650+52650+51650
51651+52651+53651+53723+52723+51723●
51652+52652+53652+53653+52653+51653
51654+52654+53654+53655+52655+51655
51656+52656+53656+53657+52657+51657
51658+52658+53658+53724+52724+51724●
51659+52659+53659+53660+52660+51660
51661+52661+53661+53662+52662+51662
51663+52663+53663+53664+52664+51664
51665+52665+53665+53725+52725+51725●
51666+52666+53666+53667+52667+51667
51668+52668+53668+53669+52669+51669
51670+52670+53670+53671+52671+51671
51672+52672+53672+53726+52726+51726●
51673+52673+53673+53674+52674+51674
51675+52675+53675+53676+52676+51676
51677+52677+53677+53678+52678+51678
51679+52679+53679+53680+52680+51680
51681+52681+53681+53682+52682+51682
51683+52683+53683+53684+52684+51684
51685+52685+53685+53686+52686+51686

● Fitted with Sandite equipment

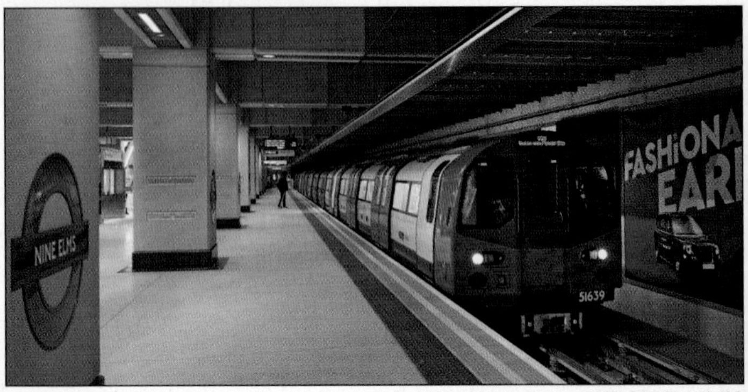

Six-car trains of GEC-Alstom built 1995 stock operate on the Northern Line. With DM No. 51639 a set is seen on the 2021 opened Battersey Power Station extension at Nine Elms. **CJM**

2009 Tube Stock — VICTORIA LINE

Builder: Bombardier, Derby
Years built: 2009-2011
Formation: DM+T+NDM+UNDM+UNDM+NDM+T+DM
Max speed: 50mph (80.5km/h)
Length: Driving - 54ft 4in (16.60m)
Intermediate - 53ft 6in (16.35m)
Width: 8ft 5½in (2.61m)
Height: 9ft 4⅜in (2.88m)
Doors: Sliding bi-parting
Traction equipment: 4 x Bombardier Mitrac of 100hp (75kW) each power car

Eight-car double-ended sets DM(south)+T+NDM+UNDM+UNDM+NDM+T+DM(north)

11001+12001+13001+14001+14002+13002+12002+11002
11003+12003+13003+14003+14004+13004+12004+11004
11005+12005+13005+14005+14006+13006+12006+11006
11007+12007+13007+14007+14008+13008+12008+11008
11009+12009+13009+14009+14010+13010+12010+11010
11011+12011+13011+14011+14012+13012+12012+11012
11013+12013+13013+14013+14014+13014+12014+11014
11015+12015+13015+14015+14016+13016+12016+11016
11017+12017+13017+14017+14018+13018+12018+11018
11019+12019+13019+14019+14020+13020+12020+11020
11021+12021+13021+14021+14022+13022+12022+11022
11023+12023+13023+14023+14024+13024+12024+11024
11025+12025+13025+14025+14026+13026+12026+11026
11027+12027+13027+14027+14028+13028+12028+11028
11029+12029+13029+14029+14030+13030+12030+11030
11031+12031+13031+14031+14032+13032+12032+11032
11033+12033+13033+14033+14034+13034+12034+11034
11035+12035+13035+14035+14036+13036+12036+11036
11037+12037+13037+14037+14038+13038+12038+11038
11039+12039+13039+14039+14040+13040+12040+11040
11041+12041+13041+14041+14042+13042+12042+11042
11043+12043+13043+14043+14044+13044+12044+11044
11045+12045+13045+14045+14046+13046+12046+11046
11047+12047+13047+14047+14048+13048+12048+11048
11049+12049+13049+14049+14050+13050+12050+11050
11051+12051+13051+14051+14052+13052+12052+11052
11053+12053+13053+14053+14054+13054+12054+11054
11055+12055+13055+14055+14056+13056+12056+11056
11057+12057+13057+14057+14058+13058+12058+11058
11059+12059+13059+14059+14060+13060+12060+11060
11061+12061+13061+14061+14062+13062+12062+11062
11063+12063+13063+14063+14064+13064+12064+11064
11065+12065+13065+14065+14066+13066+12066+11066
11067+12067+13067+14067+14068+13068+12068+11068
11069+12069+13069+14069+14070+13070+12070+11070
11071+12071+13071+14071+14072+13072+12072+11072
11073+12073+13073+14073+14074+13074+12074+11074
11075+12075+13075+14075+14076+13076+12076+11076
11077+12077+13077+14077+14078+13078+12078+11078
11079+12079+13079+14079+14080+13080+12080+11080
11081+12081+13081+14081+14082+13082+12082+11082
11083+12083+13083+14083+14084+13084+12084+11084
11085+12085+13085+14085+14086+13086+12086+11086
11087+12087+13087+14087+14088+13088+12088+11088
11089+12089+13089+14089+14090+13090+12090+11090
11091+12091+13091+14091+14092+13092+12092+11092
11093+12093+13093+14093+14094+13094+12094+11094

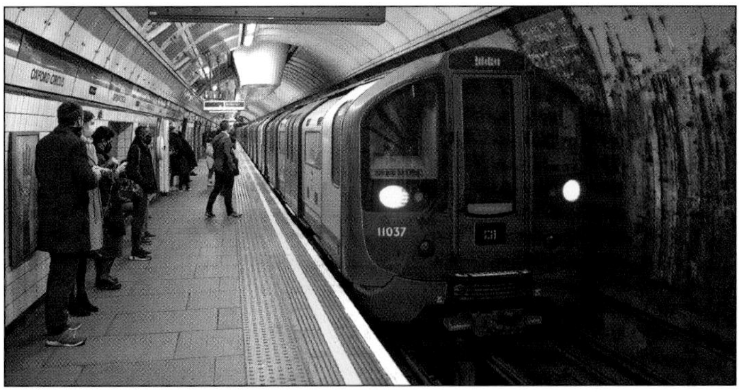

Currently the most modern tube stock are the 2009 Bombardier eight-car sets on the Victoria Line. DM No. 11037 leads a Brixton bound service at Oxford Circus in January 2022. **Antony Christie**

S7 Sub-Surface Stock

CIRCLE LINE

DISTRICT LINE

HAMMERSMITH & CITY LINE

Builder: Bombardier, Derby
Years built: 2011-2015
Formation: DM+M1+MS+MS+M2+M1+DM
Max speed: 62mph (100km/h)
Length: Driving - 57ft 2in (17.44m)
Intermediate - 50ft 6in (15.43m)
Width: 9ft 5in (2.92m)
Height: 12ft 0in (3.68m)
Doors: Sliding bi-parting
Traction equipment: 4 x Bombardier MJB20093 of 87hp (65kW) on each power car

Seven-car double-ended sets DM+M1+MS+MS+M2+M1+DM

21301+22301+24301+24302+25302+22302+21302
21303+22303+24303+24304+25304+22304+21304
21305+22305+24305+24306+25306+22306+21306
21307+22307+24307+24308+25308+22308+21308
21309+22309+24309+24310+25310+22310+21310
21311+22311+24311+24312+25312+22312+21312
21313+22313+24313+24314+25314+22314+21314
21315+22315+24315+24316+25316+22316+21316
21317+22317+24317+24318+25318+22318+21318
21319+22319+24319+24320+25320+22320+21320
21321+22321+24321+24322+25322+22322+21322
21325+22325+24325+24326+25326+22326+21326
21327+22327+24327+24328+25328+22328+21328
21329+22329+24329+24330+25330+22330+21330
21331+22331+24331+24332+25332+22332+21332
21333+22333+24333+24334+25334+22334+21334
21335+22335+24335+24336+25336+22336+21336
21337+22337+24337+24338+25338+22338+21338
21339+22339+24339+24340+25340+22340+21340
21341+22341+24341+24342+25342+22342+21342
21343+22343+24343+24344+25344+22344+21344
21345+22345+24345+24346+25346+22346+21346
21347+22347+24347+24348+25348+22348+21348
21349+22349+24349+24350+25350+22350+21350
21351+22351+24351+24352+25352+22352+21352
21353+22353+24353+24354+25354+22354+21354
21355+22355+24355+24356+25356+22356+21356
21357+22357+24357+24358+25358+22358+21358
21359+22359+24359+24360+25360+22360+21360
21361+22361+24361+24362+25362+22362+21362
21363+22363+24363+24364+25364+22364+21364
21365+22365+24365+24366+25366+22366+21366
21367+22367+24367+24368+25368+22368+21368
21369+22369+24369+24370+25370+22370+21370
21371+22371+24371+24372+25372+22372+21372
21373+22373+24373+24374+25374+22374+21374
21375+22375+24375+24376+25376+22376+21376
21377+22377+24377+24378+25378+22378+21378
21379+22379+24379+24380+25380+22380+21380
21381+22381+24381+24382+25382+22382+21382
21383+22383+24383+24384+25384+22384+21384
21385+22385+24385+24386+23386+22386+21386
21387+22387+24387+24388+23388+22388+21388
21389+22389+24389+24390+23390+22390+21390
21391+22391+24391+24392+23392+22392+21392
21393+22393+24393+24394+23394+22394+21394
21395+22395+24395+24396+23396+22396+21396
21397+22397+24397+24398+23398+22398+21398
21399+22399+24399+24400+23400+22400+21400
21401+22401+24401+24402+23402+22402+21402
21403+22403+24403+24404+23404+22404+21404
21405+22405+24405+24406+23406+22406+21406
21407+22407+24407+24408+23408+22408+21408
21409+22409+24409+24410+23410+22410+21410
21411+22411+24411+24412+23412+22412+21412
21413+22413+24413+24414+23414+22414+21414
21415+22415+24415+24416+23416+22416+21416
21417+22417+24417+24418+23418+22418+21418
21419+22419+24419+24420+23420+22420+21420
21421+22421+24421+24422+23422+22422+21422
21423+22423+24423+24424+23424+22424+21424
21425+22425+24425+24426+23426+22426+21426
21427+22427+24427+24428+23428+22428+21428
21429+22429+24429+24430+23430+22430+21430
21431+22431+24431+24432+23432+22432+21432
21433+22433+24433+24434+23434+22434+21434
21435+22435+24435+24436+23436+22436+21436
21437+22437+24437+24438+23438+22438+21438
21439+22439+24439+24440+23440+22440+21440
21441+22441+24441+24442+23442+22442+21442
21443+22443+24443+24444+23444+22444+21444
21445+22445+24445+24446+23446+22446+21446
21447+22447+24447+24448+23448+22448+21448
21449+22449+24449+24450+23450+22450+21450
21451+22451+24451+24452+23452+22452+21452
21453+22453+24453+24454+23454+22454+21454
21455+22455+24455+24456+23456+22456+21456
21457+22457+24457+24458+23458+22458+21458
21459+22459+24459+24460+23460+22460+21460
21461+22461+24461+24462+23462+22462+21462
21463+22463+24463+24464+23464+22464+21464
21465+22465+24465+24466+23466+22466+21466
21467+22467+24467+24468+23468+22468+21468
21469+22469+24469+24470+23470+22470+21470
21471+22471+24471+24472+23472+22472+21472
21473+22473+24473+24474+23474+22474+21474
21475+22475+24475+24476+23476+22476+21476
21477+22477+24477+24478+23478+22478+21478
21479+22479+24479+24480+23480+22480+21480
21481+22481+24481+24482+23482+22482+21482
21483+22483+24483+24484+23484+22484+21484
21485+22485+24485+24486+23486+22486+21486
21487+22487+24487+24488+23488+22488+21488
21489+22489+24489+24490+23490+22490+21490
21491+22491+24491+24492+23492+22492+21492
21493+22493+24493+24494+23494+22494+21494
21495+22495+24495+24496+23496+22496+21496
21497+22497+24497+24498+23498+22498+21498
21499+22499+24499+24500+23500+22500+21500
21501+22501+24501+24502+23502+22502+21502
21503+22503+24503+24504+23504+22504+21504
21505+22505+24505+24506+23506+22506+21506
21507+22507+24507+24508+23508+22508+21508
21509+22509+24509+24510+23510+22510+21510
21511+22511+24511+24512+23512+22512+21512
21513+22513+24513+24514+23514+22514+21514
21515+22515+24515+24516+23516+22516+21516
21517+22517+24517+24518+23518+22518+21518
21519+22519+24519+24520+23520+22520+21520
21521+22521+24521+24522+23522+22522+21522
21523+22523+24523+24524+23524+22524+21524
21525+22525+24525+24526+23526+22526+21526
21527+22527+24527+24528+23528+22528+21528
21529+22529+24529+24530+23530+22530+21530
21531+22531+24531+24532+23532+22532+21532
21533+22533+24533+24534+23534+22534+21534
21535+22535+24535+24536+23536+22536+21536
21537+22537+24537+24538+23538+22538+21538
21539+22539+24539+24540+23540+22540+21540
21541+22541+24541+24542+23542+22542+21542
21543+22543+24543+24544+23544+22544+21544
21545+22545+24545+24546+23546+22546+21546
21547+22547+24547+24548+23548+22548+21548
21549+22549+24549+24550+23550+22550+21550
21551+22551+24551+24552+23552+22552+21552
21553+22553+24553+24554+23554+22554+21554
21555+22555+24555+24556+23556+22556+21556
21557+22557+24557+24558+23558+22558+21558
21559+22559+24559+24560+23560+22560+21560
21561+22561+24561+24562+23562+22562+21562
21563+22563+24563+24564+23564+22564+21564
21565+22565+24565+24566+23566+22566+21566
21567+22567+24567+24568+23568+22568+21568

S7+1 Sub-Surface Stock

Eight-car double-ended sets DM+M1+M2+MS+MS+M2+M1+DM

21323+22323+25384+24323+24324+25324+22324+21324

Note
25xxx coaches classified as M2D and fitted with de-icing equipment

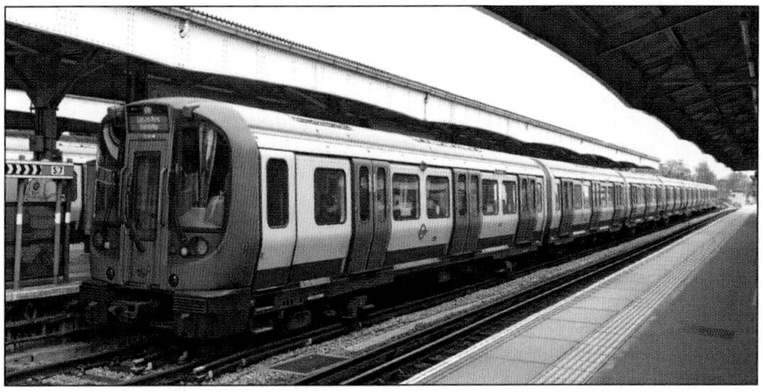

The S7 and S8 surface stock on London Underground look very similar, but the interiors are very different. S7 District/Circle and Hammersmith & City set with DM No. 21381 nearest the camera is seen at Wimbledon. **CJM**

S8 Sub-Surface Stock METROPOLITAN LINE

Builder: Bombardier, Derby
Years built: 2008-2012
Formation: DM+M1+M2+MS+MS+M2+M1+DM
Max speed: 62mph (100km/h)
Length: Driving - 57ft 2in (17.44m)
Intermediate - 50ft 6in (15.43m)
Width: 9ft 5in (2.92m)
Height: 12ft 0in (3.68m)
Doors: Sliding bi-parting
Traction equipment: 4 x Bombardier MJB20093 of 87hp (65kW) each power car

Eight-car double-ended sets DM+M1+M2+MS+MS+M2+M1+DM

21001+22001+23001+24001+24002+25002+22002+21002
21003+22003+23003+24003+24004+25004+22004+21004
21005+22005+23005+24005+24006+25006+22006+21006
21007+22007+23007+24007+24008+25008+22008+21008
21009+22009+23009+24009+24010+25010+22010+21010
21011+22011+23011+24011+24012+25012+22012+21012
21013+22013+23013+24013+24014+25014+22014+21014
21015+22015+23015+24015+24016+25016+22016+21016
21017+22017+23017+24017+24018+25018+22018+21018
21019+22019+23019+24019+24020+25020+22020+21020
21021+22021+23021+24021+24022+25022+22022+21022
21023+22023+23023+24023+24024+25024+22024+21024
21025+22025+23025+24025+24026+25026+22026+21026
21027+22027+23027+24027+24028+25028+22028+21028
21029+22029+23029+24029+24030+25030+22030+21030
21031+22031+23031+24031+24032+25032+22032+21032
21033+22033+23033+24033+24034+25034+22034+21034
21035+22035+23035+24035+24036+25036+22036+21036
21037+22037+23037+24037+24038+25038+22038+21038
21039+22039+23039+24039+24040+25040+22040+21040
21041+22041+23041+24041+24042+25042+22042+21042
21043+22043+23043+24043+24044+25044+22044+21044
21045+22045+23045+24045+24046+25046+22046+21046
21047+22047+23047+24047+24048+25048+22048+21048
21049+22049+23049+24049+24050+25050+22050+21050
21051+22051+23051+24051+24052+25052+22052+21052
21053+22053+23053+24053+24054+25054+22054+21054
21055+22055+23055+24055+24056+25056+22056+21056
21057+22057+23057+24057+24058+23058+22058+21058
21059+22059+23059+24059+24060+23060+22060+21060
21061+22061+23061+24061+24062+23062+22062+21062
21063+22063+23063+24063+24064+23064+22064+21064
21065+22065+23065+24065+24066+23066+22066+21066
21067+22067+23067+24067+24068+23068+22068+21068
21069+22069+23069+24069+24070+23070+22070+21070
21071+22071+23071+24071+24072+23072+22072+21072
21073+22073+23073+24073+24074+23074+22074+21074
21075+22075+23075+24075+24076+23076+22076+21076
21077+22077+23077+24077+24078+23078+22078+21078
21079+22079+23079+24079+24080+23080+22080+21080
21081+22081+23081+24081+24082+23082+22082+21082
21083+22083+23083+24083+24084+23084+22084+21084
21085+22085+23085+24085+24086+23086+22086+21086
21087+22087+23087+24087+24088+23088+22088+21088
21089+22089+23089+24089+24090+23090+22090+21090
21091+22091+23091+24091+24092+23092+22092+21092
21093+22093+23093+24093+24094+23094+22094+21094
21095+22095+23095+24095+24096+23096+22096+21096
21097+22097+23097+24097+24098+23098+22098+21098
21099+22099+23099+24099+24100+23100+22100+21100
21101+22101+23101+24101+24102+23102+22102+21102
21103+22103+23103+24103+24104+23104+22104+21104
21105+22105+23105+24105+24106+23106+22106+21106
21107+22107+23107+24107+24108+23108+22108+21108
21109+22109+23109+24109+24110+23110+22110+21110
21111+22111+23111+24111+24112+23112+22112+21112
21113+22113+23113+24113+24114+23114+22114+21114
21115+22115+23115+24115+24116+23116+22116+21116

Notes
25xxx coaches classified as M2D and fitted with de-icing equipment
Names applied 21100 *Tim O'Toole CBE*

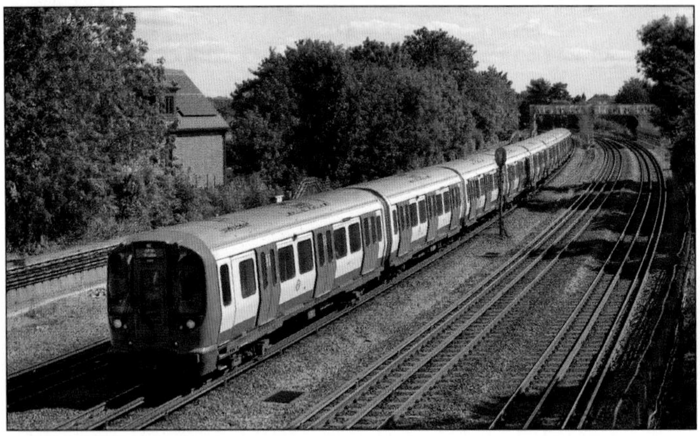

Eight-car 'S' stock (S8) works on the Metropolitan Line and has a more conventional seating layout with bench and group layout. With DM No. 21007 leading a service for Watford passes Northwood in late 2019. **Antony Christie**

Engineering and Service Stock

Rail Adhesion Train (RAT)

Former D78 stock
7010+8123+17010+8010+7123 | 7040+8107+17040+8040+7107

Track Recording Train

1960, 1967, 1972 and 1973 Tube stock
L132 (3901)+TRC666 (514)+L133 (3905)

Rail Adhesion (Sandite)

1956 and 1962 Stock
1406+2682+9125+1681+1682+9577+2406+1407
1570+9691+2440+9441+1441

Filming Train

1972 Stock
3229+4229+4329+3329 based at Aldwych

Locomotives

Built by Schoma/Clayton

1	*Britta Lotta*	DH	8	*Emma*	Battery/Electric
2	*Nikki*	Battery/Electric	9	*Debora*	DH
3	*Claire*	DH	10	*Clementine*	Battery/Electric
4	*Pam*	Battery/Electric	11	*Joan*	Battery/Electric
5	*Sophie*	Battery/Electric	12	*Melanie*	DH
6	*Denise*	Battery/Electric	13	*Michele*	Battery/Electric
7	*Annemarie*	Battery/Electric	14	*Carol*	Battery/Electric

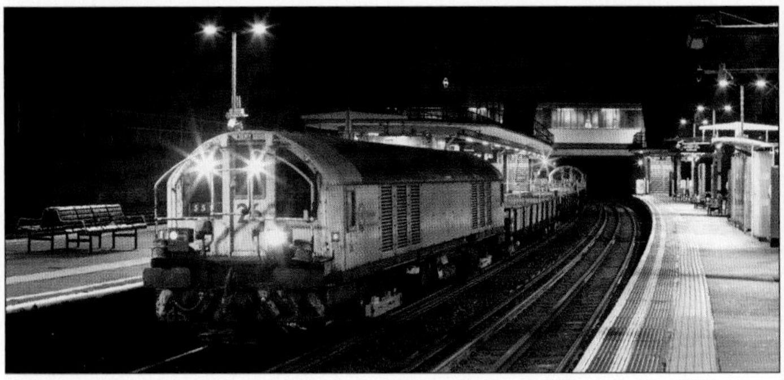

Refurbished battery/electric loco No. L26 in seen in the early hours of Christmas Day 2021 at South Ealing with a work train to Ruislip depot. **Jamie Squibbs**

Battery / Electric

L15	69015, 97015, 97715
L16●	69016, 97016 - Seltrac compliant
L17●	69017, 97017 - Seltrac compliant
L18●	69018. 97018 - Seltrac compliant
L19●	69019, 97019 - Seltrac compliant
L20	69020, 97020, 97720 - Seltrac compliant
L21	64021, 97021 - Seltrac compliant
L22●	64022, 97022, 97722
L23●	64023, 97023
L24●	64024, 97024
L25●	64025, 97025
L26●	64026, 97026
L27●	64027, 97027 - Victoria line ATP compliant
L28●	64028, 97028 - Victoria line ATP compliant
L29●	64029, 97029 - Victoria line ATP compliant
L30●	64030, 97030 - Victoria line ATP compliant
L31●	64031, 97031 - Victoria line ATP compliant
L32●	64032, 97032, 97732 - Victoria line ATP compliant
L44●	73044, 97044 - Seltrac compliant
L45●	73045, 97045 - Seltrac compliant
L46●	73046, 97046 - Seltrac compliant
L47	73047, 97047 - Seltrac compliant
L48	73048, 97048 - Seltrac compliant
L49●	73049, 97049 - Seltrac compliant
L50●	73050, 97050, 97750 - Seltrac compliant
L51●	73051, 97051, 97751 - Seltrac compliant
L52	73052, 97052, 97752 - Seltrac compliant
L53●	73053, 97053, 97753 - Seltrac compliant
L54	73054, 97054 - Seltrac compliant

● - Refurbished

Track Machines

C623	7.5t crane
C624	7.5t crane
C625	7.5t crane
C626	7.5t crane
TRM627	Track relaying crane
TRM628	Track relaying crane
TMM771	Plasser 07-16 Universal
TMM772	Plasser 07-16 Universal
TMM773	Plasser 07-16 Universal - *Alan Jenkins*
TMM774	Plasser 08-275
TMM775	Matisa B45UE (99 70 9128 003-9)
TMM776	Matisa B45UE (99 70 9128 004-7)

Preserved Stock

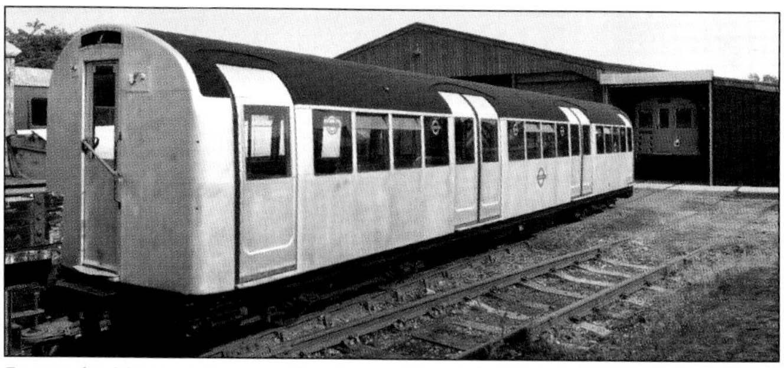

Preserved at Mangapps Farm near Burnham-on-Crouch, is 1959 tube stock trailer No. 2044, restored to silver livery. In the shed behind is CO/CP DM 54256. **CJM**

Locomotives

Number	Name	System	Type	Year	Preservation Site
)S75		Electric	Bo	1898	NRM, Shildon
)L82		Diesel	0-6-0	1967	Hardingham Station Norfolk
)L83		Diesel	0-6-0	1967	Nene Valley Railway
13		Electric	Bo	1890	London Transport Museum
5	*John Hampden*	Electric	Bo-Bo	1922	London Transport Museum
2	*Sarah Siddons*	Electric	Bo-Bo	1922	LU Ruislip Depot
.11		Electric	Bo-Bo	1964	Cravens Heritage, Epping
ESL107		Electric	Bo-2-2-Bo	1940	London Transport, Acton
.35		Batt/Elec	Bo-Bo	1938	London Transport, Acton

EMU Stock

Numbers	Design	Type	Railway	Preservation Site
MR4 → LPTB9486	1904 Stock	Trailer	Metropolitan Railway	London Transport Museum, Acton
)R644 → LPTB4148 → LT4248	Q23	DM	District Railway	London Transport Museum
)R662 → LPTB4184	Q23	DM	District Railway	London Transport Museum, Acton
.PTB2749 → LT ESL118B	T	DM	Metropolitan Railway	Buckingham Railway Centre
.PTB2758 → LT ESL118A	T	DM	Metropolitan Railway	Buckingham Railway Centre
.ER297 → LPTB3327	Std Stock	DM	London Electric Railway	London Transport Museum, Acton
.ER320 → LPTB3370 → L134	Std Stock	DM	London Electric Railway	London Transport Museum, Acton
.PTB3693 → L131	Std Stock	DM	London Electric Railway	London Transport Museum, Acton
.ER1789 → LPTB5279 → BR27	Std Stock	DT	London Electric Railway	London Transport Museum, Acton
.ER846 → LPTB7296 → BR49	Std Stock	DT	London Electric Railway	London Transport Museum, Acton
.PTB8063 → LT08063	Q35	T	London Passenger Transport Board	London Transport Museum, Acton
.PTB13028 → LT53028	CO/CP	DM	London Passenger Transport Board	Buckingham Railway Centre
.PTB013063 → LT013063	CO/CP	T	London Passenger Transport Board	Buckingham Railway Centre
.PTB14233 → LT54233	CO/CP	DM	London Passenger Transport Board	Buckingham Railway Centre
.PTB14256 → LT54256	CO/CP	DM	London Passenger Transport Board	Mangapps Farm Museum
.PTB4416 → LT L126	Q38	DM	London Passenger Transport Board	London Transport Museum, Acton
.PTB4417 → LT L127	Q38	DM	London Passenger Transport Board	London Transport Museum, Acton
.PTB10012 → LT10012	1938 Stock	DM	London Passenger Transport Board	London Transport Museum, Acton
.PTB11178 → LT11178(11012)	1938 Stock	DM	London Passenger Transport Board	London Transport Museum, Acton
.PTB11182 → LT11182	1938 Stock	DM	London Passenger Transport Board	London Transport Museum, Acton
.PTB92048 → LT92048(12048)	1938 Stock	M	London Passenger Transport Board	London Transport Museum, Acton
.PTB012229 → LT012229(4927)	1938 Stock	T	London Passenger Transport Board	Cravens Heritage Trains, Epping
.PTB012256 → LT012256	1938 Stock	T	London Passenger Transport Board	London Transport Museum, Acton
T22624	R38	DM	London Transport	Mangapps Railway Museum
.T21147	R49	DM	London Transport	Private in Beaconsfield
T22679	R49	DM	London Transport	London Transport Museum, Acton
T1018	1959	DM	London Transport	Mangapps Farm Museum
T1030	1959	DM	London Transport	Mangapps Railway Museum
T1044	1959	DM	London Transport	Alderney Railway
T1045	1959	DM	London Transport	Alderney Railway
T1085 (1031)	1959	DM	London Transport	Epping-Ongar Rly
T1304	1959	DM	London Transport	Old Cement works, Banbury
T1305	1959	DM	London Transport	Longstowe Station
T2018	1959	T	London Transport	Motcombe, Dorset
T2044	1959	T	London Transport	Mangapps Farm Museum
T2304	1959	T	London Transport	Old Cement works, Banbury
T9305	1959	M	London Transport	Old Cement works, Banbury
T3906	1960	DM	London Transport	Cravens Heritage Trains, Epping
T3907	1960	DM	London Transport	Cravens Heritage Trains, Epping
T5008 (5034)	A60	DM	London Transport	London Transport Museum, Acton
T1506	1962	DM	London Transport	Cravens Heritage Trains, Epping
T1507	1962	DM	London Transport	Cravens Heritage Trains, Epping
T2506	1962	T	London Transport	Cravens Heritage Trains, Epping
T9507	1962	M	London Transport	Cravens Heritage Trains, Epping
T3052	1967	DM	London Transport	London Transport Museum, Acton
T3186	1967	DM	London Transport	Walthamstowe Pumphouse Museum
T3530	1972	DM	London Transport	London Transport Museum, Acton
T4079	1972	T	London Transport	Private in Essex
T4179	1972	T	London Transport	Private in Essex
T5721	C77	DM	London Transport	London Transport Museum, Acton
T7012	D78	DM	London Transport	London Transport Museum, Acton
T7027	D78	DM	London Transport	Coopers Lane School, Grove Park
T3662	1983	DM	London Transport	Village Underground, Shoreditch
T3721	1983	DM	London Transport	Washington Fire Training base
T3733	1983	DM	London Transport	Village Underground, Shoreditch
T3734	1983	DM	London Transport	London Transport Museum, Acton
T4633	1983	T	London Transport	Village Underground, Shoreditch
T4662	1983	T	London Transport	Village Underground, Shoreditch
T16	1986	DM	London Transport	London Transport Museum, Acton

Hauled Stock

Numbers	Date	Detail	Preservation Site
)	1890	City & South London Railway 'Padded Cell'	London Transport Museum, Acton
5	1902	City & South London Railway (body only)	Private at Hope Farm, Sellindge, Kent
0	1884	Metropolitan Railway 4-wheel First	Kent & East Sussex Railway
3	1892	Metropolitan Railway 'Jubilee'	Kent & East Sussex Railway
	1896	Metropolitan Railway Milk Van	London Transport Museum, Acton
R368 → LPTB9702 → LT515	1898	C Metropolitan Railway 'Chesham'	Bluebell Railway
R387 → LPTB2671 → LT512	1900	DBT Metropolitan Railway 'Chesham'	Bluebell Railway
R394 → LPTB6702 → LT518	1900	DTT Metropolitan Railway 'Chesham'	Bluebell Railway
R400 → LPTB6703 → LT519	1900	DTT Metropolitan Railway	LT Museum, Covent Garden
R412 → LPTB9705 → LT516	1900	C Metropolitan Railway 'Chesham'	Bluebell Railway
R427	1910	T Metropolitan Railway 'Dreadnought'	Keighley & Worth Valley
R465	1919	T Metropolitan Railway 'Dreadnought'	Keighley & Worth Valley
R509	1923	F Metropolitan Railway 'Dreadnought'	Keighley & Worth Valley

Key		
3R - British Rail	ESL - Electric Sleet Loco	LT - London Transport
)R - District Railway	LER - London Electric Railway	MR - Metropolitan Railway
	LPTB - London Passenger Transport Board	

Transport for London

Croydon Tramlink

Bombardier *Flexity Swift* CR4000

Tram Length: 98ft 9in (30.1m)	*Horsepower: 643hp (480kW)*
Seating: 70	*Power Supply: 750V dc overhead*
Width: 8ft 7in (2.65m)	*Electrical Equipment: Bombardier*

2530	2536	2542	2548
2531	2537	2543	2549
2532	2538	2544	2550
2533	2539	2545	2552
2534	2540	2546	2553
2535	2541	2547	

Name - 2535 *Stephen Parascandolo 1980-2007*

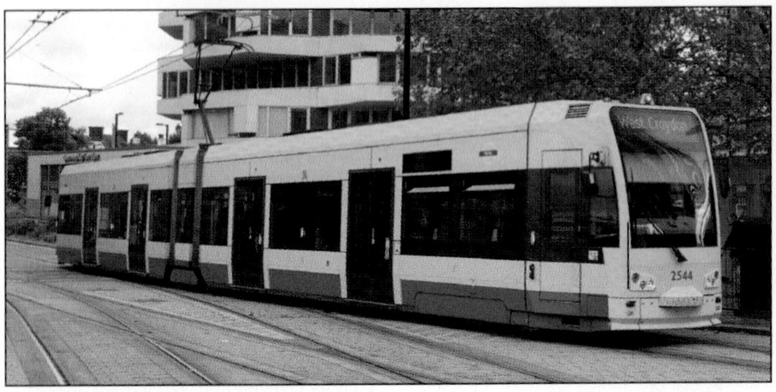

Bombardier Flexity Swift *three-section tram No. 2544 is seen in standard 'Tramlink' livery at East Croydon.* **CJM**

Stadler *Variobahn*

Train Length: 106ft 2½in (32.37m)	*Horsepower: 650hp (483kW)*
Seating: 70	*Power Supply: 750V dc overhead*
Width: 8ft 7in (2.65m)	*Electrical Equipment: Stadler*

2554	2557	2560	2563
2555	2558	2561	2564
2556	2559	2562	2565

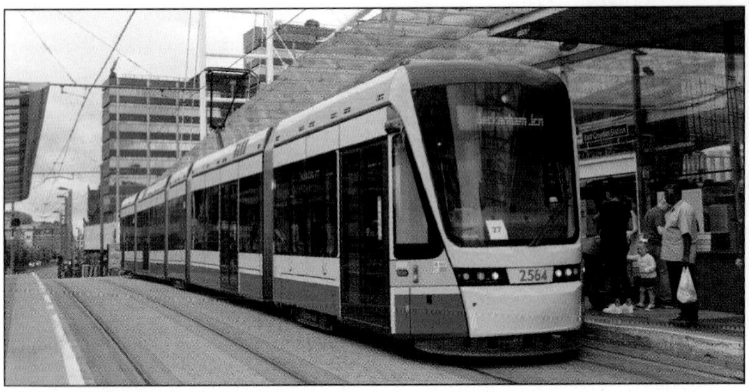

A fleet of 12Stadler Variobahn *five-section trams operate on the Croydon Tramlink system. No. 2564 is illustrate at East Croydon on a Beckenham Junction service.* **CJM**

Docklands Light Railway

Bombardier B90

Train Length: 94ft 5in (28.80m)	*Horsepower: 375hp (280kW)*
Seating: 52 + 4 tip-up	*Power Supply: 750V dc third rail*
Width: 8ft 7in (2.65m)	*Electrical Equipment: Brush*

22	26	30	34	38	42
23	27	31	35	39	43
24	28	32	36	40	44
25	29	33	37	41	

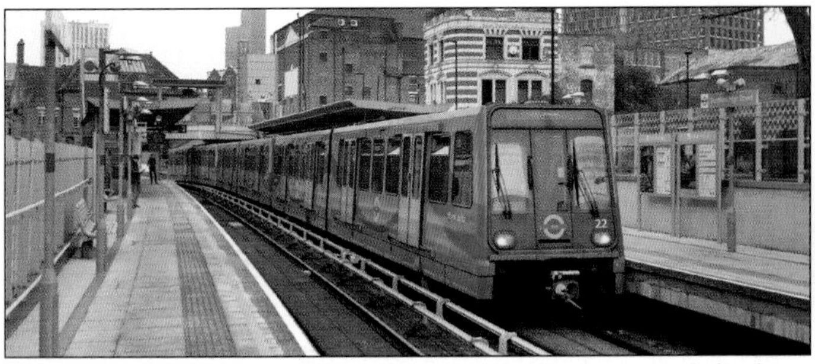

The Docklands Light Railway fleet operates as a common pool and any set types can be found on any duty. Soon a new fleet of CAF trains will start to arrive. B90 train No. 22 leads a three vehicle (6-car) formation at Stratford High Street. **Antony Christie**

Bombardier B92

Train Length: 94ft 5in (28.80m)	*Horsepower: 375hp (280kW)*
Seating: 54 + 4 tip-up	*Power Supply: 750V dc third rail*
Width: 8ft 7in (2.65m)	*Electrical Equipment: Brush*

45	53	61	69	77	85
46	54	62	70	78	86
47	55	63	71	79	87
48	56	64	72	80	88
49	57	65	73	81	89
50	58	66	74	82	90
51	59	67	75	83	91
52	60	68	76	84	

Bombardier B2K

Train Length: 94ft 5in (28.80m)	*Horsepower: 375hp (280kW)*
Seating: 52 + 4 tip-up	*Power Supply: 750V dc third rail*
Width: 8ft 7in (2.65m)	*Electrical Equipment: Brush*

01	05	09	13	92	96
02	06	10	14	93	97
03	07	11	15	94	98
04	08	12	16	95	99

Bombardier B07

Train Length: 94ft 5in (28.80m)	*Horsepower: 375hp (280kW)*
Seating: 52 + 4 tip-up	*Power Supply: 750V dc third rail*
Width: 8ft 7in (2.65m)	*Electrical Equipment: Bombardier*

101	111	121	131	141	151
102	112	122	132	142	152
103	113	123	133	143	153
104	114	124	134	144	154
105	115	125	135	145	155
106	116	126	136	146	
107	117	127	137	147	
108	118	128	138	148	
109	119	129	139	149	
110	120	130	140	150	

A new fleet of 54 trains for DLR have been ordered from CAF, these will be to a new five-car design and should enter service from 2023.

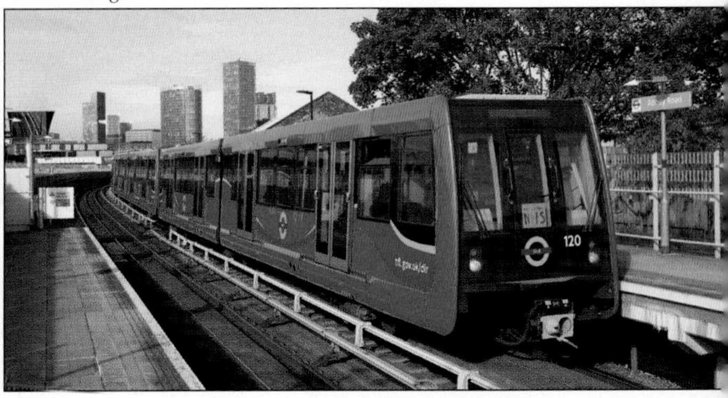

No. 120, one of the mid-2000s introduced sets calls at Abbey Road station on the Stratford International extension, located between West Ham and Stratford High Street. **Antony Christi**

Edinburgh Tramway

CAF *Urbos-3* 7-section vehicles

Train Length: 140ft 5in (42.8m)	*Horsepower: 1,287hp (960kW)*
Seating: 78 + 170 standing	*Power Supply: 750V dc overhead*
Width: 8ft 7in (2.65m)	*Electrical Equipment: CAF*

251	256	261	266	271	276
252	257	262	267	272	277
253	258	263	268	273	
254	259	264	269	274	
255	260	265	270	275	

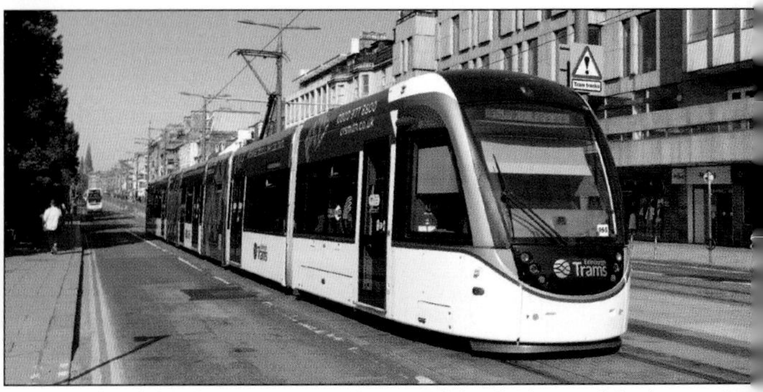

At present the Edinburgh Tramway operates between Edinburgh Airport and the city centre but soon an extension to Leith Docks will open. The network operates a fleet of CAF Urbos-3 seven section trams, No. 258 is seen in Princess Street in June 2021. **CJM**

Blackpool Trams

Bombardier *Flexity 2*

Train Length: 105ft 9in (32.23m)
Seating: 74 + 148 standing
Width: 8ft 8in (2.65m)
Horsepower: 4 x 160hp (120kW) three phase TMs
Power Supply: 600V dc overhead
Electrical Equipment: Bombardier

001	007 *Alan Whitbread*	013
002 *Alderman E E Wynne*	008	014
003	009	015
004	010	016
005	011	017
006	012	018

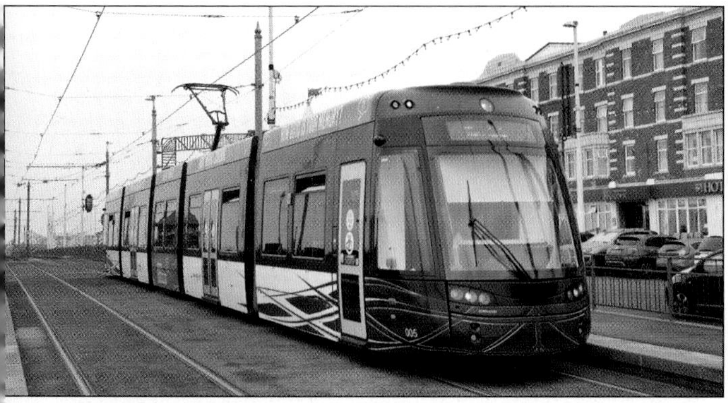

Blackpool operates a fleet of 18 Bombardier Flexity 2 five-section trams, which are based at Starr Gate depot. Vehicle carry a mix of white/purple and advertising liveries. No. 005 is seen at Cabin. **CJM**

Heritage Fleet

40	Fleetwood Box	711	Balloon
66	Bolton Tram	713	Balloon
147	Standard	715	Balloon
600	Boat	717	Balloon
621	Brush	718	Balloon
631	Brush *Reginald Dixon MBE*	719	Balloon
642	Centenary	723	Balloon
648	Centenary	733+734	Twin
680	Railcoach	736	Illuminated (Frigate)
700	Balloon	737	Illuminated (Boat)
701	Balloon	754	Diesel Works Car

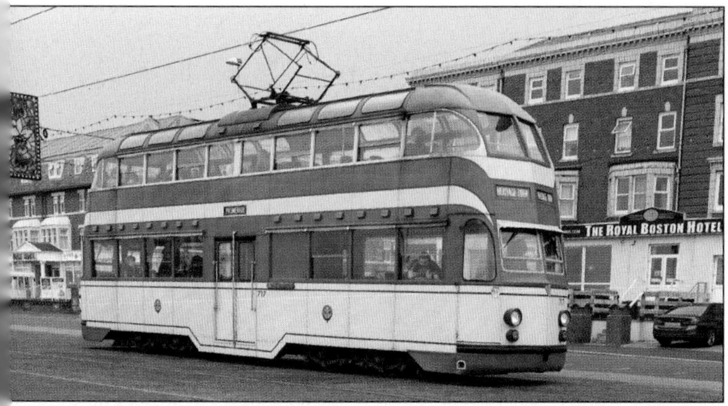

A superb collection of vintage Blackpool trams are based at Rigby Road depot and used on selected days during the summer, allowing tram enthusiasts and holiday visitors the chance to sample heritage tram travel. No. 717 a Balloon car is shown near Cabin in June 2021. **CJM**

Manchester Metrolink

Bombardier *Flexity Swift* M5000

Train Length: 93ft 1in (28.4m)
Seating: 52 + 8 tip-up
Width: 8ft 7in (2.65m)
Horsepower: 643hp (480kW)
Power Supply: 750V dc overhead
Electrical Equipment: Bombardier

3001	3018	3036
3002	3019	3037
3003	3020 *Lancashire Fusilier*	3038
3004	3021	3039
3005	3022 *Spirit of MCR*	3040
3006	3023	3041
3007	3024	3042
3008	3025	3043
3009 *50th Anniversary of*	3026	3044
Coronation Street 1960-2010	3027	3045
3010	3028	3046
3011	3029	3047
3012	3030	3048
3013	3031	3049
3014	3032	3050
3015	3033	3051
3016	3034	3052
3017	3035	3053

3054	3086	3118
3055	3087	3119
3056	3088	3120
3057	3089	3121
3058	3090	3122
3059	3091	3123
3060	3092	3124
3061	3093	3125
3062	3094	3126
3063	3095	3127
3064	3096	3128
3065	3097	3129
3066	3098 *Gracie Fields*	3130
3067	3099	3131
3068	3100	3132
3069	3101	3133
3070	3102	3134
3071	3103	3135
3072	3104	3136
3073	3105	3137
3074	3106	3138
3075	3107	3139
3076	3108	3140
3077	3109	3141
3078	3110	3142
3079	3111	3143
3080	3112	3144
3081	3113	3145
3082	3114	3136
3083	3115	3147
3084	3116	
3085	3117	

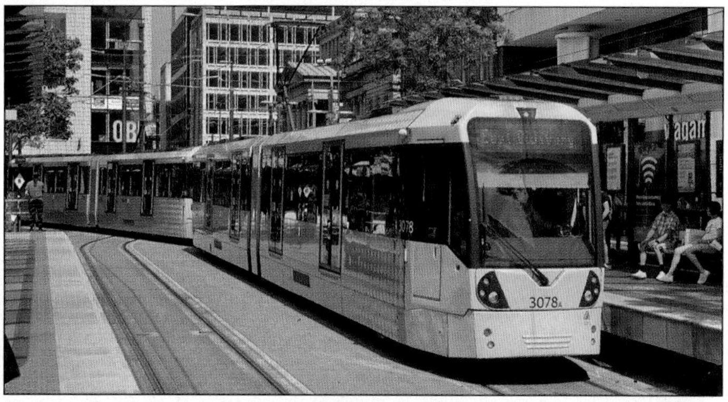

The largest fleet on single design trams in the UK are the 147 Bombardier Flexity Swift vehicles operated on the Manchester Metrolink system. No. 3078 is seen arriving at St Peter's Square with an East Didsbury service on 2 June 2021. **CJM**

West Midlands Metro

CAF *Urbos-3* 5-section vehicles

Train Length: 108ft 3in (29m)
Seating: 54 + 156 standing
Width: 8ft 8in (2.65m)
Horsepower: 1,320hp (960kW)
Power Supply: 750V dc overhead
Electrical Equipment: CAF

17	32	48*
18	33	49*
19	34	50*
20	35	51*
21	36	52*
22	37 *Ozzy Osbourne*	53*
23	38	54*
24	39	55*
25	40	56*
26	41	57*
27	42	58*
28 *Jasper Carrott*	43	* On delivery
29	44	
30	45	All fitted with traction
31 *Cyrille Regis MBE*	46*	batteries
1958-2018	47*	

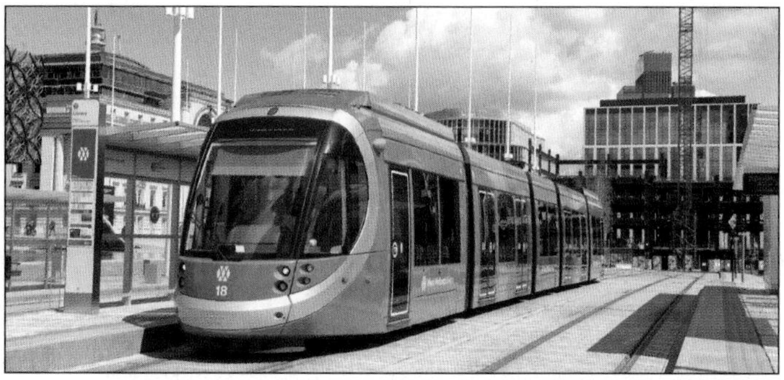

The West Midlands Metro operates a fleet of CAF Urbos-3 five-section vehicles. In late 2021 the line was closed due to cracks in the trams and slowly sets have been returned to traffic. Some of the additional order for trams arrived in late 2021. No. 18 is seen in the city centre at the Library stop, operating on battery power. **CJM**

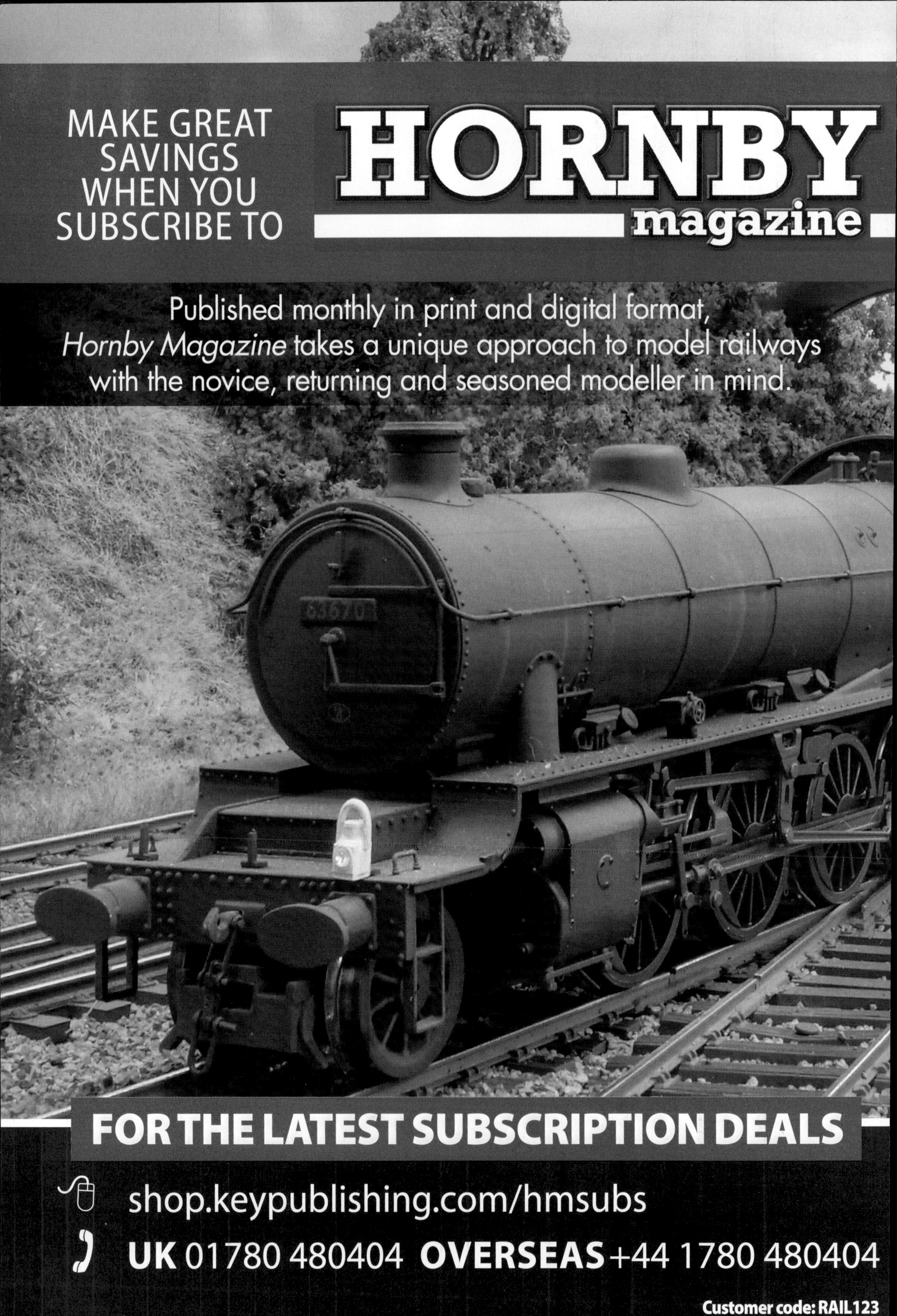
MAKE GREAT SAVINGS WHEN YOU SUBSCRIBE TO
HORNBY magazine
Published monthly in print and digital format, Hornby Magazine takes a unique approach to model railways with the novice, returning and seasoned modeller in mind.
FOR THE LATEST SUBSCRIPTION DEALS
shop.keypublishing.com/hmsubs
UK 01780 480404 OVERSEAS +44 1780 480404
Customer code: RAIL123

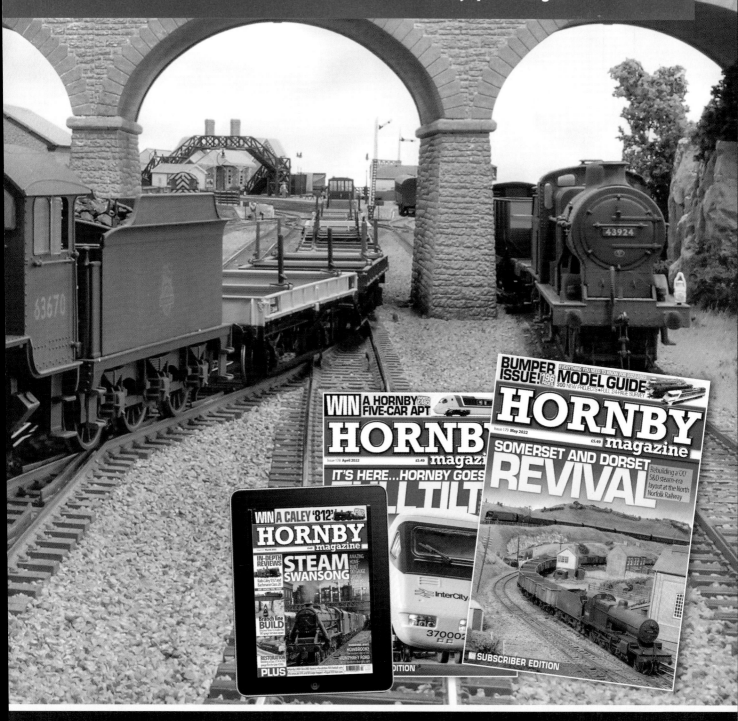

Nottingham Express Transit

Bombardier *Incento* AT6/5 5-section vehicles

Train Length: 108ft 3in (29m)
Seating: 54 + 4 tip-up
Width: 7ft 9in (2.4m)
Horsepower: 697hp (520kW)
Power Supply: 750V dc overhead
Electrical Equipment: Bombardier

201	*Torvill and Dean*	209	*Sidney Standard*
202	*DH Lawrence*	210	*Sir Jesse Boot*
203	*Bendigo Thompson*	211	*Robin Hood*
204	*Erica Beardsmore*	212	*William Booth*
205	*Lord Byron*	213	*Mary Potter*
206	*Angela Alcock*	214	*Dennis McCarthy MBE*
207	*Mavis Worthington*	215	*Brian Clough MBE*
208	*Dinah Minton*		

Alstom *Citadis 302* 5-section vehicles

Train Length: 104ft 11¾in (32m)
Seating: 58 + 6 tip-up
Width: 7ft 9in (2.4m)
Horsepower: 644hp (480kW)
Power Supply: 750V dc overhead
Builder: Alstom

216	*Dame Laura Knight*	227	*Sir Peter Mansfield*
217	*Carl Froch MBE*	228	*Local Armed Forces Heroes*
218	*Jim Taylor*	229	*Viv Anderson MBE*
219	*Alan Sillitoe*	230	*George Green*
220	*Sir Martyn Poliakoff*	231	*Rebecca Adlington OBE*
221	*Stephen Lowe*	232	*William Ivory*
222	*David S Stewart OBE*	233	*Ada Lovelace*
223	*Colin Slater MBE*	234	*George Africanus*
224	*Vicky McClure*	235	*David Clarke*
225	*Doug Scott CBE*	236	*Sat Bains*
226	*Jimmy Sirrel & Jack Wheeler*	237	*Stuart Broad MBE*

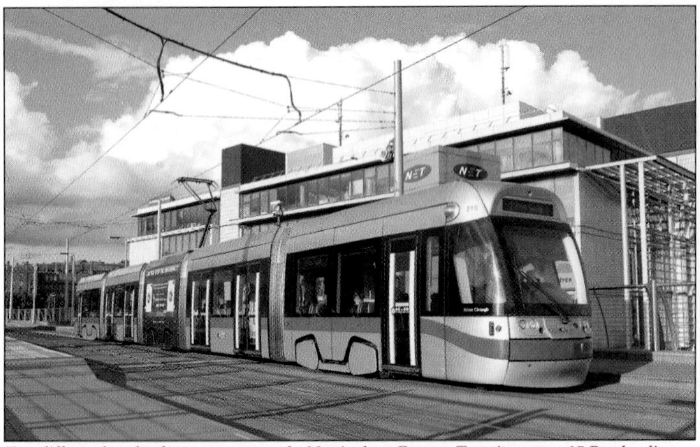

Two different breeds of tram operate on the Nottingham Express Transit system, 15 Bombardier Incento *vehicles and 22 Alstom* Citadis 302 *sets.* Incento *No. 215* Brian Clough MBE *is illustrated at Nottingham National Rail station.* **Nathan Williamson**

South Yorkshire Supertram

Siemens 3-section vehicles

Train Length: 113ft 6in (34.75m)
Seating: 88 + 6 tip-up
Width: 8ft 7in (2.65m)
Horsepower: 800hp (596kW)
Power Supply: 750V dc overhead
Electrical Equipment: Siemens

101	110	119
102	111	120
103	112	121
104	113	122
105	114	123 *Pete McKee*
106	115	124
107	116	125
108	117	
109	118	

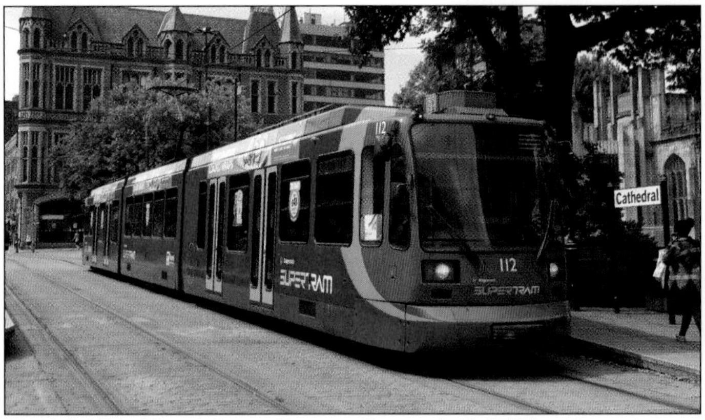

The original fleet of Siemens three-section trams still operate the Sheffield Super Tram system. Painted in standard Stagecoach colours, set No. 112 is seen at the Cathedral stop in Sheffield City centre. **CJM**

Tyne & Wear Metro, Network Rail Class 599

Metro-Cammell 6-axle 2-section vehicles

Train Length: 91ft 3in (27.80m)
Seating: 68
Width: 8ft 7in (2.65m)
Horsepower: 500hp (374kW)
Power Supply: 1500V dc overhead
Electrical Equipment: Siemens

4001 (599001)	4025 (599025)	4047 (599047)	4070 (599070)
4002 (599002)	4026 (599026)	4048 (599048)	4071 (599071)
4003 (599003)	4027 (599027)	4049 (599049)	4072 (599072)
4004 (599004)	4028 (599028)	4050 (599050)	4073 (599073)
4005 (599005)	4029 (599029)	4051 (599051)	4074 (599074)
4006 (599006)	4030 (599030)	4052 (599052)	4075 (599075)
4007 (599007)	4031 (599031)	4053 (599053)	4076 (599076)
4008 (599008)	4032 (599032)	4054 (599054)	4077 (599077)
4009 (599009)	4033 (599033)	4055 (599055)	4078 (599078)
4010 (599010)	4034 (599034)	4056 (599056)	4079 (599079)
4011 (599011)	4035 (599035)	4057 (599057)	4080 (599080)
4012 (599012)	4036 (599036)	4058 (599058)	4081 (599081)
4013 (599013)	4037 (599037)	4059 (599059)	4082 (599082)
4014 (599014)	4038 (599038)	4060 (599060)	4083 (599083)
4015 (599015)	4039 (599039)	4061 (599061)	4084 (599084)
4016 (599016)	4040 (599040)	4062 (599062)	4085 (599085)
4017 (599017)	4041 (599041)	4063 (599063)	4086 (599086)
4018 (599018)	*Harry Cowans*	4064 (599064)	4087 (599087)
4019 (599019)	4042 (599042)	4065 (599065)	4088 (599088)
4020 (599020)	4043 (599043)	4066 (599066)	4089 (599089)
4021 (599021)	4044 (599044)	4067 (599067)	4090 (599090)
4023 (599023)	4045 (599045)	4068 (599068)	
4024 (599024)	4046 (599046)	4069 (599069)	

A fleet of 46 new five-car sets are on order from Stadler Rail to replace the present fleet, units will be delivered from late 2022 to enter service in 2023, classified as Network Rail Class 555, Nos. 555001-555046.

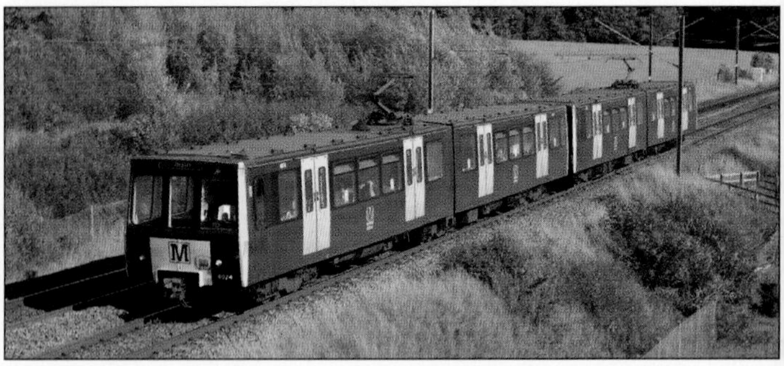

Soon to be replaced by new Stadler five-section trams, the Tyne & Wear Metro currently uses Metro-Cammell two-section trams. Painted in standard black and yellow livery, No. 4074 leads another set near Bolden bound for Newcastle Airport **Jamie Squibbs**

Glasgow Subway

Metro-Cammell Single Power Cars

Length: 42ft 2in (12.81m)
Seating: 36S
Width: 7ft 7in (2.34m)
Horsepower: 190hp (142.4kW)
Power Supply: 600V dc third rail
Electrical Equipment: GEC
Gauge: 4ft 0in (1219mm)

101	108	115	122(S)	129
102	109	116	123	130
103	110	117	124	131
104	111	118	125	132
105	112	119	126	133
106	113	120	127	
107	114	121	128	

Hunslet-Barclay Trailer Cars

Length: 41ft 6in (12.70m)
Seating: 40S
Width: 7ft 7in (2.34m)

201	203	205	207	208
202	204	206		

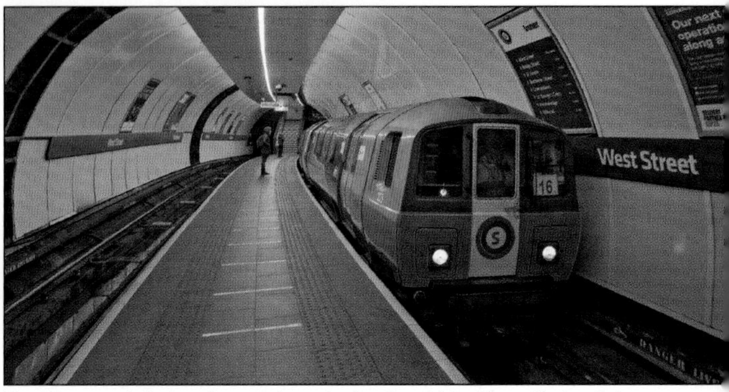

Providing commissioning of new stock goes to plan, these Metro-Cammell sets only have a very limited time remaining on the Glasgow Underground. Car No. 113 leads a train at West Street on the Inner Circle line on 9 November 2021. **Antony Christie**

Stadler 4-car Sets

Train Length: 128ft 9in (39.24m) | *Width: 7ft 7in (2.34m)*
Height: 8ft 8in (2.65m) | *Seating: 104S + 6 folding, standing for 199S*

301	305	309	313	317
302	306	310	314	
303	307	311	315	
304	308	312	316	

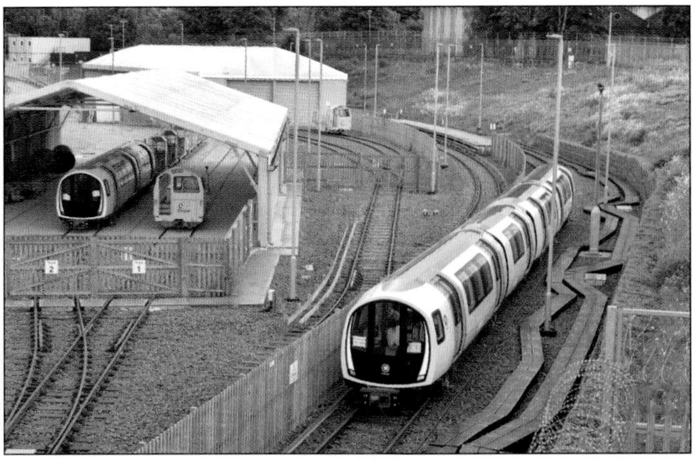

Two of the new four-car Stadler Glasgow Subway sets are seen under test at the new facility built at Broomloan depot. Which included a short test track for commissioning runs. **Robin Ralston**

Great Orme Tramway

Hurst Nelson Bogie Cars

Seating: 48 | *Power: Cable*
Introduced: 1902 | *Gauge: 3ft 6in (1067mm)*
Speed: 5mph (8km/h)

Lower section		Upper section	
4	*St Tudno*	6	*St Seiriol*
5	*St Silio*	7	*St Trillo*

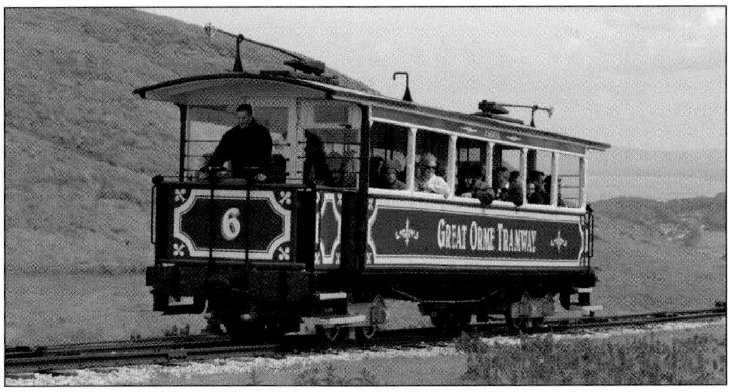

Upper section Great Orme Tramway car No. 6 approaches Great Orme station. **CJM**

Southend Pier Tramway

Severn Lamb Engineering 6-car sets

Seating: Train - 264S | *Power: Battery*
Introduced: 2022 | *Gauge: 3ft (914mm)*
Speed: 10mph (16km/h)

1 *David Amess*	2

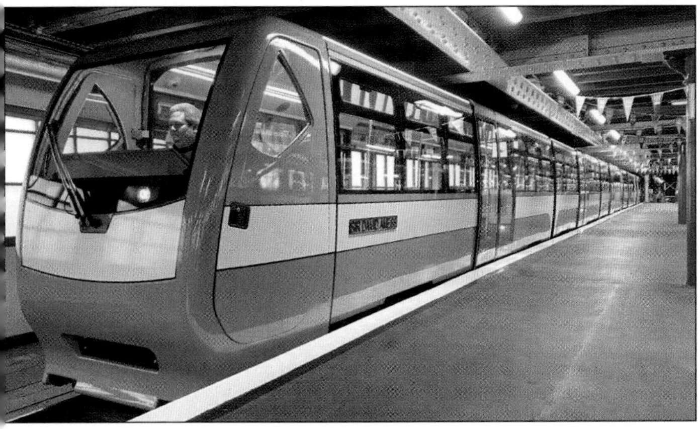

One of two new Severn Lamb Engineering Southend Pier trams which entered service for the pier's 2022 season. No. 1 was named David Amess after the MP for Southend West who was murdered in 2021. **SBC**

Volks Electric Railway

Open single cars

3	40 seat open of 1892	8	40 seat open of 1901
4	40 seat open of 1892	9	40 seat open of 1910
6	40 seat open of 1901	10	40 seat open of 1926
7	40 seat open of 1901	Gauge: 2ft 8½in (825mm)	

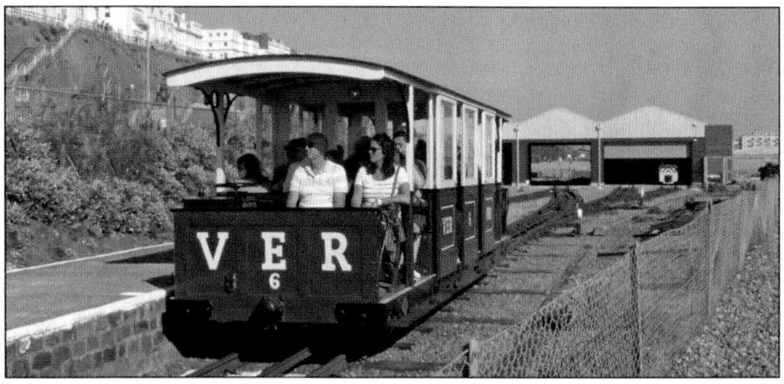

The unique Volks Electric Railway, which operates along the sea front in Brighton, is a great touriest attraction and is a facinating light railway. 1901 vintage car No. 6 is seen at Peter Pan's Playground station. **Adrian Paul**

Hythe Pier Tramway

Brush 4-wheel locos

Built By: Brush | *Speed: 10mph (16km/h)*
Seating: Nil | *Power: 250V dc third rail*
Introduced: 1917 as battery, now electric | *Gauge: 2ft (610mm)*

1	*Gerald Yorke*	Works No. 16302	2	Works No. 16307

Stock

Two bogie passenger carriages
Two bogie passenger carriages fitted with remote driving controls
One four-wheel freight wagon
One tank car

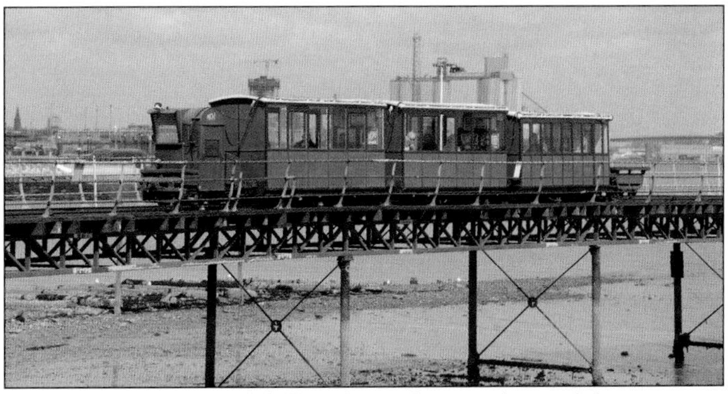

Powered by locomotive No. 1, a Hythe Pier train nears the town station, note the luggage wagon on the rear. **CJM**

Seaton Tramway

Various vehicles

02	1952 works vehicle
2	1964 replica, based on London Metropolitan Tramways Type A
4	1961 replica, based on Blackpool 'Boat' design
6	1954 replica, based on Bournemouth open top, previously single deck
7	1958 replica, based on Bournemouth open top
8	1968 replica, based on Bournemouth open top
9	2004 hybrid, based on Blackburn and Plymouth design
10	2006 hybrid, based on Blackburn and Plymouth design
11	2007 replica, based on Bournemouth open top
12	1966 replica, based on London Transport 'Feltham' tram
14	1904 original Metropolitan Tramways Type A car No. 94
15	1988 replica, based on Isle of Man design
16	1921 original Bournemouth open top car No. 106
19	1909 original Exeter Tram vehicle

Gauge: 2ft 9in (838mm)

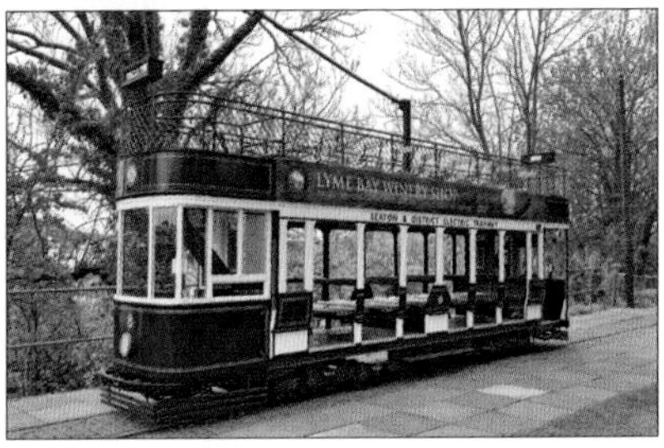

Seaton Tramway No. 8 is a replica built in 1968, based on a Bournemouth open top tram. **CJM**

Irish Railways

Northern Ireland Railways (NIR) / Translink

Locomotives

General Motors Class 111 (JT22CW)

Built: 1980-1984
Length: 57ft 0in (17.37m)
Height: 13ft 3in (4.04m)
Width: 9ft 5¾in (2.89m)
Engine: EMD 12-645E3B of 2,450hp (1,830kW)
Transmission: Electric
Tractive effort: 65,000lb (289kN)
Same as Irish Rail 071 class

8111	*Great Northern*
8112	*Northern Counties*
8113	*Belfast & County Down*

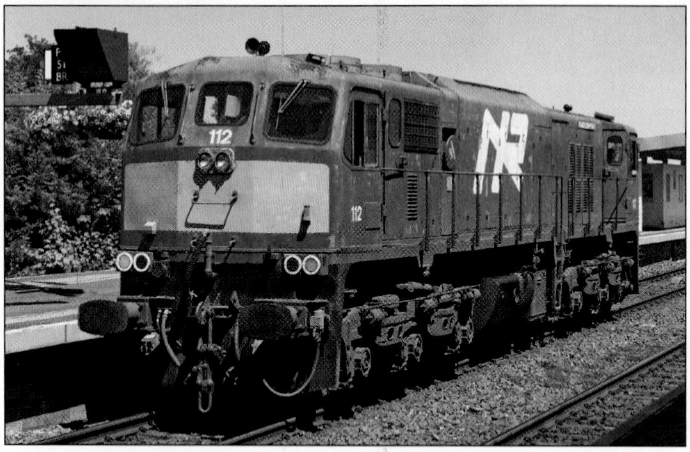

The Northern Ireland 111 class are the same as the Irish Rail 071 class. Built by General Motors in the 1980s as type JT22CW. The three locos are used on engineering trains and based at York Road. No. 112 Northern Counties is shown. **CJM**

General Motors Class 201 (JT42HCW)

Built: 1994
Length: 68ft 9in (20.95m)
Height: 13ft 2in (4.02m)
Width: 8ft 8in (2.64m)
Engine: EMD 12-710G3B of 3,200hp (2,400kW)
Transmission: Electric
Tractive effort: 43,700lb (194kN)

8208	*(River Lagan)*
8209	*(River Froyle)*

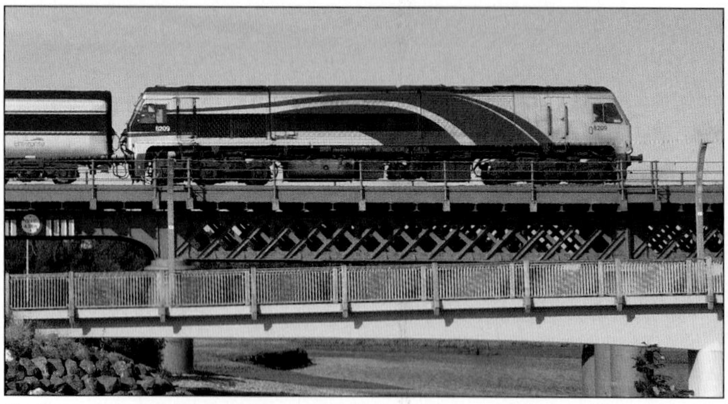

The 'Enterprise' service between Belfast and Dublin is jointly operated by NIR and IR. NIR 'own' two locos of the Class 201 fleet, the locos are of the General Motors JT42HCW platform. No. 8209 is shown crossing Laytown Viaduct on 23 August 2019 with the 08.35 Portadown to Dublin. **CJM**

Diesel Multiple Units

CAF Class 3000 - C3K

Built: 2004-2005
Vehicle length: Driving 23.74m
Intermediate 23.14m
Height: 3.62m
Width: 2.76m
Power: One MAN D2876 LUH03 per car
Horsepower: 453hp (338kW) per car
Transmission: Hydraulic
Sets 3001-3006 fitted with CAWS and able to operate on cross-border services on Irish Rail

Formation: DMSO+MSO+DMSO

3001	3301+3501+3401
3002	3302+3502+3402
3003	3303+3503+3403
3004	3304+3504+3404
3005	3305+3505+3405
3006	3306+3506+3406
3007	3307+3507+3407
3008	3308+3508+3408
3009	3309+3509+3409
3010	3310+3510+3410
3011	3311+3511+3411
3012	3312+3512+3412
3013	3313+3513+3413
3014	3314+3514+3414
3015	3315+3515+3415
3016	3316+3516+3416
3017	3317+3517+3417
3018	3318+3518+3418
3019	3319+3519+3419
3020	3320+3520+3420
3021	3321+3521+3421
3022	3322+3522+3422
3023	3323+3523+3423

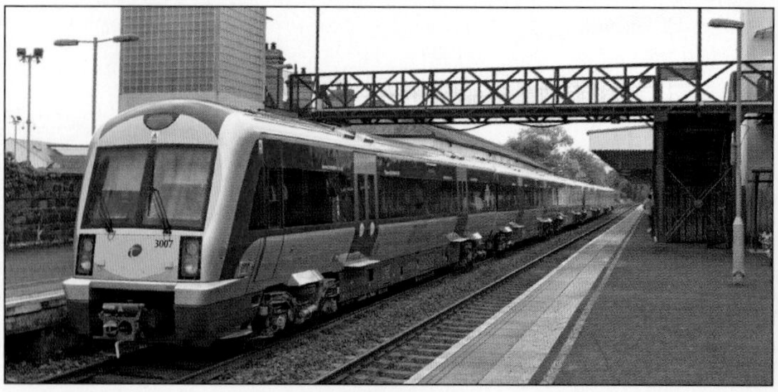

Local NIR services around Belfast are formed of DMU stock, a fleet of 23 CAF Class 3000 sets are in use. These work ether as three or six car sets, but can only operate in multiple with other class members and not with Class 4000 stock. No. 3007 is seen at Lisburn. **CJM**

CAF Class 4000 - C4K

Built: 2010-2011
Vehicle length: Driving 23.74m
Intermediate 23.14m
Height: 3.62m
Width: 2.76m
Power: One MTU 6H1800R84 per car
Horsepower: 520hp (390kW) per car
Transmission: Mechanical

Three-car sets

Formation: DMSO+MSO+DMSO

4001	4301+4501+4401
4002	4302+4502+4402
4003	4303+4503+4403
4004	4304+4504+4404
4005	4305+4505+4405
4006	4306+4506+4406
4007	4307+4507+4407
4008	4308+4508+4408
4009	4309+4509+4409
4010	4310+4510+4410
4011	4311+4511+4411
4012	4312+4512+4412
4013	4313+4513+4413

Six-car sets. 46xx, 47xx and 48xx MSOs added progressively in 2022, mix of three and six car sets currently in operation

Formation: DMSO+MSO+MSO+MSO+MSO+DMSO

4014	4314+4514+4614+4714+4814+4414
4015	4315+4515+4615+4715+4815+4415
4016	4316+4516+4616+4716+4816+4416
4017	4317+4517+4617+4717+4817+4417
4018	4318+4518+4618+4718+4818+4418
4019	4319+4519+4619+4719+4819+4419
4020	4320+4520+4620+4720+4820+4420

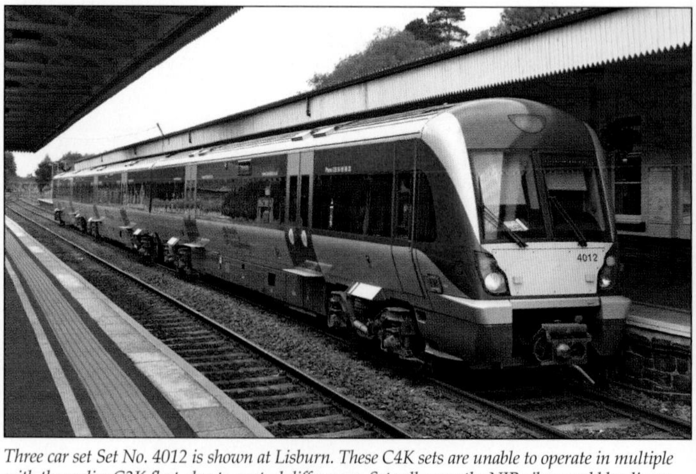

Three car set Set No. 4012 is shown at Lisburn. These C4K sets are unable to operate in multiple with the earlier C3K fleet, due to control differences. Sets all carry the NIR silver and blue livery, C4K sets have a rectangular yellow end, C3Ks had a rounded yellow end. **CJM**

Northern Ireland Railways (NIR) and Irish Rail (IR) 'Joint Stock' for *Enterprise* service

Built: 1996
Builder: De Dietrich, France
Length: 23.0m
Height: 4.02m
Width: 2.86m)

Driving Trailer Brake First (DTBF)

9001	9002	9003	9004

First Open (FO)

9101	9102	9103	9104

Standard Open (SO)

9201	9205	9209	9213
9202	9206	9210	9214
9203	9207	9211	9215
9204	9208	9212	9216

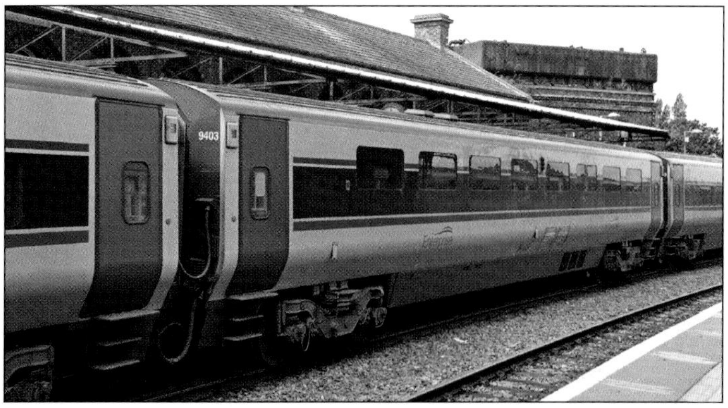

The joint 'Enterprise' service between Belfast and Dublin operated by NIR and IR uses a fleet of four French built De Dietrich sets. They are finished in a silver and black livery off-set by a red and purple stripe. Cafe car 9403 is illustrated. **CJM**

Trailer Cafe (RS)

9401	9402	9403	9404

Generator Car [Mk3]

Built: 1984-1988
Builder: BREL Derby/CIE Inchicore BR Mk3
Length: 23.0m
Height: 3.88m
Width: 2.74m

9602 (7601)	9604 (7605)	9605 (7608)	9608 (7613)

Service Stock

Class 80

A fleet of five former NIR Class 80 DMU vehicles are retained by NIR for autumn sandite and rail cleaning duties, based at York Road depot, Belfast.

8069 (DMBSO)	8097 (DMBSO)	8752 (DTSO)
8094 (DMBSO)	8749 (DTSO)	

Class 450

One former NIR Class 450 DMU is retained by NIR for autumn sandite and rail cleaning duties, based at York Road depot, Belfast.

005 8455+8795+8785 *Galgorm Castle* Stored at Ballymena

Irish Railways (IR)

Locomotives

General Motors Class 071 (JT22CW) Co-Co

Built: 1980-1984
Length: 57ft 0in (17.37m)
Height: 13ft 3in (4.04m)
Width: 9ft 5¾in (2.89m)
Engine: EMD 12-645E3B of 2,450hp (1,830kW)
Transmission: Electric
Tractive effort: 65,000lb (289kN)
Same as NIR 111 class

071 *Great Southern & Western*	081
072	082 *Cumann Na nInnealtoiri / The Institution Of Engineers Of Ireland*
073	083
074	084
075	085
076	086
077	087
078	088
079	
080	

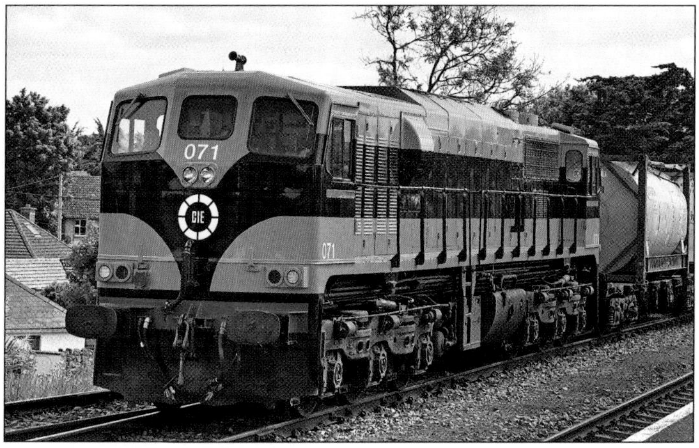

Most freight operated on Irish Rail is powered by a fleet of 18, 071 class Co-Co General Motors diesels. Most of the freight operations consists of container and log traffic. No. 071, named Great Southern & Western is seen passing Athlone with a container train for Ballina. **CJM**

General Motors Class 201 (JT42HCW) Co-Co

Built: 1994
Length: 68ft 9in (20.95m)
Height: 13ft 2in (4.02m)
Width: 8ft 8in (2.64m)
Engine: EMD 12-710G3B of 3,200hp (2,400kW)
Transmission: Electric
Tractive effort: 43,700lb (194kN)

201(S)	*River Shannon*	Note 1
202(S)	*Abhainn na Laoi / River Lee*	Note 1
203(S)	*Abhainn na Coiribe / River Corrib*	Note 1
204(S)	*Abhainn na Bearu / River Barrow*	Note 1
205(S)	*Abhainn na Feoire / River Nore*	Note 1
206		Note 3
207	*Abhainn na Bóinne / River Boyne*	Note 3
210(S)	*Abhainn na hEirne / River Erne*	Note 1
211(S)		Note 1
212(S)	*Abhainn na Slaine / River Slaney*	Note 1
213(S)	*Abhainn na Muaidhe / River Moy*	Note 1
214(S)	*Abhainn na Broshai / River Brosna*	Note 1
215	*An Abhainn Mhor / River Avonmore*	Note 2
216*	*Abhainn na Dothra / River Dodder*	Note 2
217	*Abhainn na Fleisce / River Flesk*	Note 2
218	*River Garavogue*	Note 2
219	*River Tolka*	Note 2
220	*An Abhainn Dhubh / River Blackwater*	Note 2
221	*Abhainn na Feilge / River Fealge*	Note 2
222	*River Dargle*	Note 2
223	*Abhainn na hAinnire / River Anner*	Note 2
224(S)	*Abhainn na Feile*	Note 2
225	*Abhainn na Daoile / River Deel*	Note 2
226	*Abhainn na Siuire*	Note 2
227	*River Laune*	Note 2
228		Note 3
229	*Abhainn na Mainge / River Maine*	Note 2
230(S)		Note 3
231	*Abhainn na Maighe*	Note 3
232	*River Cummeragh*	Note 2
233	*Abhainn na Chlair / River Clare*	Note 3
234		Note 2

Note 1: Fitted with fixed buffers and shackle couplings
Note 2: Fitted with push-pull control, retractable buffers, electronic fuel system, knuckle and shackle couplings
Note 3: As Note 2, but also have event recorders and cab equipment allowing operation on the NIR network

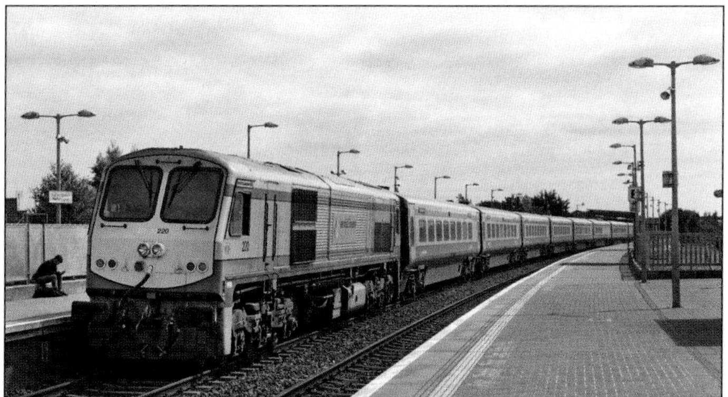

The most modern diesels in use on Irish Rail are the General Motors 201 class, introduced from 1994, although a large number are now stored out of use. No. 220 is one of the locos used to power the IR Intercity service between Dublin and Cork and is seen passing Portarlington with a Mk 4 set. **CJM**

Diesel Units

2600 Class Tokyu Car 2-car units 'Arrow'

Built: 1993
Vehicle length: Driving 20.26m
Height: 3.62m
Width: 2.90m
Power: One Cummins NTA-855-R1 per car
Horsepower: 350hp (260kW) per car
Transmission: Hydraulic

2601 + 2602	2607 + 2608
2603 + 2604	2610 + 2613
2605 + 2616	2611 + 2612
2606 + 2615	2614 + 2617

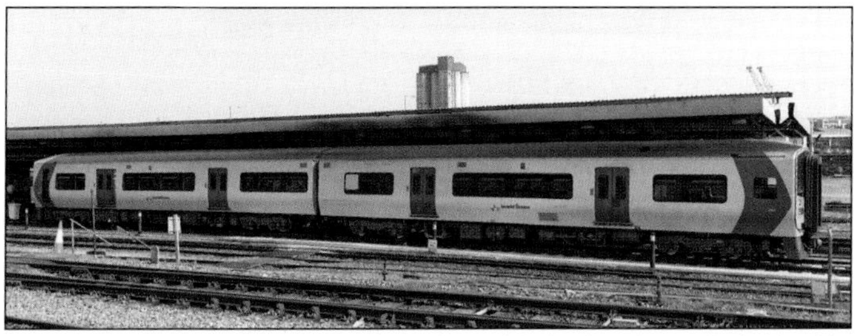

The eight two-car Class 2600 units are used in and around Cork and are also seen in the Limerick area. Vehicle Nos. 2601 and 2602 are seen on shed at Cork. **CJM**

2800 Class Tokyu Car 2-car units 'Arrow'

Built: 2000
Vehicle length: Driving 20.73m
Height: 3.62m
Width: 2.90m
Power: One Cummins NTA-855-R1 per car
Horsepower: 350hp (260kW) per car
Transmission: Hydraulic

2801 + 2802	2811 + 2812
2803 + 2804	2813 + 2814
2805 + 2806	2815 + 2816
2807 + 2808	2817 + 2818
2809 + 2810	2819 + 2820

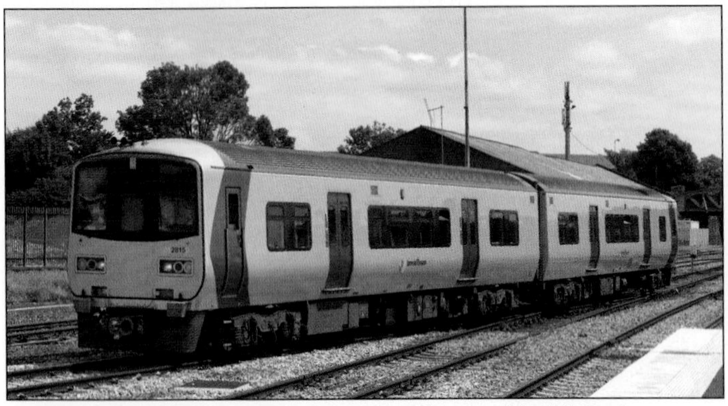

Introduced in 2000, these two-car 'Arrow' sets built by Tokyu Car, originally had end gangways, but following overhaul these have been removed. The fleet are used and based in the Limerick area, where nos. 2815 and 2816 are recorded. **CJM**

22000 Class Rotem 3-5-car units

Built: 2007-20011
Vehicle length: Driving 23.5m
intermediate 23.0m
Height: 3.62m
Width: 2.84m
Power: One MTU 6H1800 per car
Horsepower: 480hp (360kW) per car
Transmission: Hydraulic

Three-car Intercity/commuter units, authorised to operate into Northern Ireland

Formation: DMSO+MSO+DMSO

22001	22301+22401+22202	22004	22304+22404+22204
22002	22302+22402+22201	22005	22305+22405+22205
22003	22303+22403+22203	22006	22306+22406+22206

Three-car Intercity/commuter sets

Formation: DMSO+MSO+DMSO

22007	22307+22407+22207	22009	22309+22409+22209
22008	22308+22408+22208	22010	22310+22410+22210

Four-car Intercity/commuter sets

Formation: DMSO+MSO+MSO+DMSO

22011	22311+22411+22811 (22531)+22211
22012	22312+22412+22812 (22532)+22212
22013	22313+22413+22813 (22533)+22213
22014	22314+22414+22814 (22534)+22214
22015	22315+22415+22815 (22535)+22215
22016	22316+22416+22816 (22536)+22216
22017	22317+22417+22817 (22537)+22217
22018	22318+22418+22818 (22538)+22218
22019	22319+22419+22819 (22539)+22219
22020	22320+22420+22820 (22540)+22220
22021	22321+22421+22821 (22641)+22221
22022	22322+22422+22822 (22741)+22222
22023	22323+22423+22823 (22642)+22223
22024	22324+22424+22824 (22742)+22224
22025	22325+22425+22825 (22643)+22225
22026	22326+22426+22826 (22743)+22226
22027	22327+22427+22827 (22644)+22227
22028	22328+22428+22828 (22744)+22228
22029	22329+22429+22829 (22645)+22229
22030	22330+22430+22830 (22745)+22230

Five-car Intercity Premier sets

Formation: DMSO+MSO+MSO+MSO+DRBFO

22031	22331+22431+22631+22731+22131
22032	22332+22432+22632+22732+22132
22033	22333+22433+22633+22733+22133
22034	22334+22434+22634+22734+22134
22035	22335+22435+22635+22735+22135
22036	22336+22436+22636+22736+22136
22037	22337+22437+22637+22737+22137
22038	22338+22438+22638+22738+22138
22039	22339+22439+22639+22739+22139
22040	22340+22440+22640+22740+22140

Four-car commuter high-capacity sets

Formation: DMSO+MSO+MSO+DMSO

22041	22341+22441+22541+22241	22043	22343+22443+22543+22243
22042	22342+22442+22542+22242	22044	22344+22444+22544+22244
		22045	22345+22445+22545+22245

Three-car Intercity/commuter sets

Formation: DMSO+MSO+DMSO

22046	22346+22446+22246	22048	22348+22448+22248
22047	22347+22447+22247	22049	22349+22449+22249
		22050	22350+22450+22250

22051	22351+22451+22251	22058	22358+22458+22258
22052	22352+22452+22252	22059	22359+22459+22259
22053	22353+22453+22253	22060	22360+22460+22260
22054	22354+22454+22254	22061	22361+22461+22261
22055	22355+22455+22255	22062	22362+22462+22262
22056	22356+22456+22256	22063	22363+22463+22263
22057	22357+22457+22257		

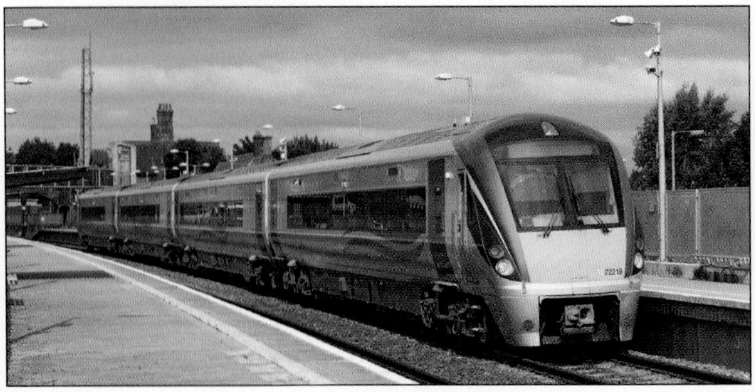

The most common main line unit class in Ireland are the Rotem-built 22000 class, which today are formed in 3, 4 or 5-car formations. Four-car Intercity and commuter set No. 19, with driving car 22219 leading is recorded at Portarlington, heading to Dublin. **CJM**

29000 Class CAF 4-car units

Built: 2002-2005
Vehicle length: Driving 20.4m
intermediate 20.2m
Height: 3.62m
Width: 2.90m
Power: One MAN D2876LUH per car
Horsepower: 394hp (294kW) per car
Transmission: Hydraulic

Formation: DMSO+MSO+MSO+DMSO

29001	29101+29201+29301+29401	29015	29115+29215+29315+29415
29002	29102+29202+29302+29402	29016	29116+29216+29316+29416
29003	29103+29203+29303+29403	29017	29117+29217+29317+29417
29004	29104+29204+29304+29404	29018	29118+29218+29318+29418
29005	29105+29205+29305+29405	29019	29119+29219+29319+29419
29006	29106+29206+29306+29406	29020	29120+29220+29320+29420
29007	29107+29207+29307+29407	29021	29121+29221+29321+29421
29008	29108+29208+29308+29408	29022	29122+29222+29322+29429
29009	29109+29209+29309+29409	29023	29123+29223+29323+29423
29010	29110+29210+29310+29410	29024	29124+29224+29324+29424
29011	29111+29211+29311+29411	29025	29125+29225+29325+29425
29012	29112+29212+29312+29412	29026	29126+29226+29326+29426
29013	29113+29213+29313+29413	29027	29127+29227+29327+29427
29014	29114+29214+29314+29414	29028	29128+29228+29328+29428
		29029	29129+29229+29329+29422

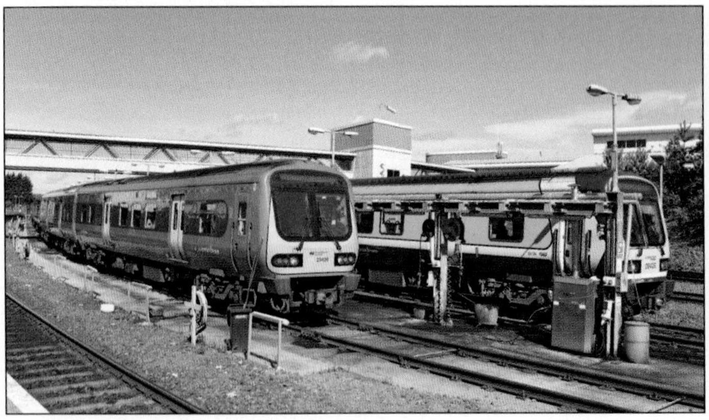

The 29 Class 29000 diesel units were introduced between 2002-2005 and were built by CAF in Spain. The sets sport two liveries, all-over mid green or the earlier light green and dark blue. Both liveries are shown in this view at Drogheda. **CJM**

Dublin Dart

8100 Class Linke-Hofmann-Busch 2-car units

Built: 1983
Vehicle length: Driving 21.0m
Height: 3.60m
Width: 2.9m
Power: Electric 1,500V dc overhead
Horsepower: 735hp (548kW) per DMSO car
Transmission: Electric

Formation DMSO+DTSO

	8114+8314	8128+8328
	8115+8315	8129+8329
8101+8301	8116+8316	8130+8330
8102+8302	8117+8317	8131+8331
8103+8303	8118+8318	8132+8332
8104+8304	8119+8319	8133+8333
8105+8305	8120+8320	8134+8334
8106+8306	8121+8321	8135+8335
8107+8307	8122+8322	8137+8337
8108+8308	8123+8323	8138+8338
8109+8309	8124+8324	8139+8339
8111+8311	8125+8325	8140+8340
8112+8312	8126+8326	
8113+8313	8127+8327	

8500 Tokyu Car 4-car units

Built: 2000
Vehicle length: Driving 20.73m
Intermediate 20.50m
Height: 3.60m
Width: 2.9m
Power: Electric 1,500V dc overhead
Horsepower: 735hp (548kW) per MSO car
Transmission: Electric

Formation DTSO+PMSO+PMSO+DTSO

8601+8501+8502+8602	8603+8503+8504+8604
	8605+8505+8506+8606
	8607+8507+8508+8608

8510 Tokyu Car 4-car units

Built: 2001
Vehicle length: Driving 20.73m
Intermediate 20.50m
Height: 3.60m
Width: 2.9m
Power: Electric 1,500V dc overhead
Horsepower: 735hp (548kW) per MSO car
Transmission: Electric

Formation DTSO+PMSO+PMSO+DTSO

8611+8511+8512+8612	8613+8513+8514+8614
	8615+8515+8516+8616

8520 Tokyu Car 4-car units

Built: 2003-2004
Vehicle length: Driving 20.73m
Intermediate 20.50m
Height: 3.60m
Width: 2.9m
Power: Electric 1,500V dc overhead
Horsepower: 735hp (548kW) per MSO car
Transmission: Electric

Formation DTSO+PMSO+PMSO+DTSO

8621+8521+8526+8626	8629+8529+8530+8630
8623+8523+8524+8624	8631+8531+8532+8632
8625+8525+8522+8622	8633+8533+8534+8634
8627+8527+8528+8628	8635+8535+8536+8636
	8637+8537+8538+8638
	8639+8539+8540+8640

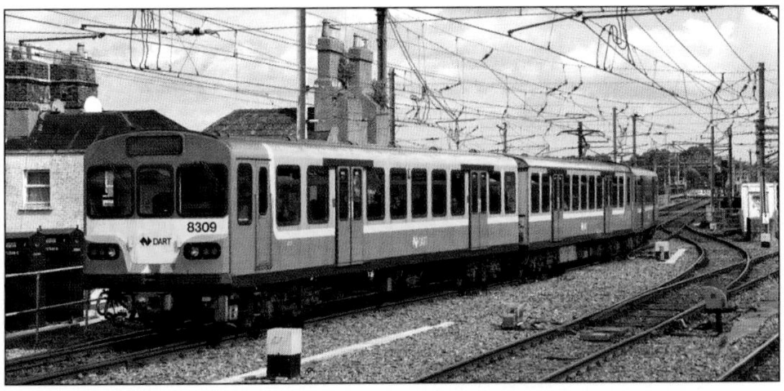

Local main line rail transport around the Dublin area is operated by the Dublin Area Rapid Transport (DART) system using four fleets of EMUs, 40 two-car 8100 class and 17 85xx class four-car sets. Two-car 8100 class No. 8309 is seen departing from Dublin Connolly. New trains are on the way for Dublin, in the form of 19 Alstom 5-car 'X-trapolis' sets, six all electric and 13 battery-electric, the first of which should arrive in 2025. **CJM/Alstom**

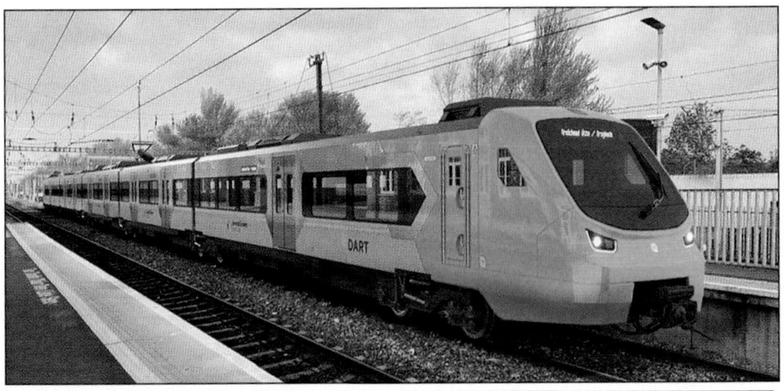

Mk 4 Inter-City stock

Built: 2004-2005
Builder: CAF
Vehicle length: Driving 23.81m
Intermediate 23.66 - 23.81m
Height: 3.62m
Width: 2.85m

Driving Brake Generator Van (DBGV)

4001	4003	4005	4007
4002	4004	4006	4008

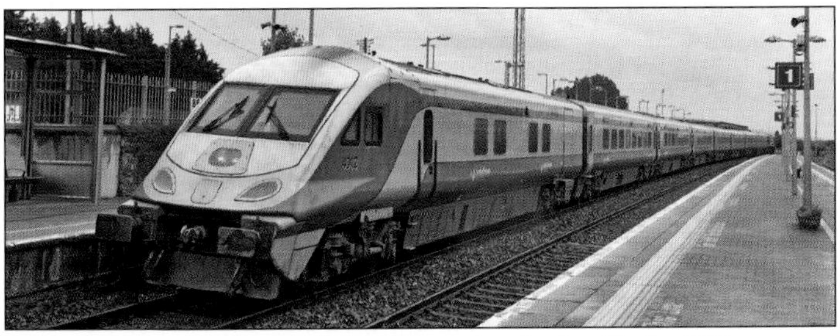
Driving Brake Generator Van (DBGV) No. 4002, seen departing from Thurles. **CJM**

Open Standard / Open Standard End (OS/OSE§)

4101	4112	4123	4134
4102	4113	4124	4135§
4103	4114	4125§	4136
4104	4115§	4126	4137
4105§	4116	4127	4138
4106	4117	4128	4139
4107	4118	4129	4140§
4108	4119	4130§	4141
4109	4120§	4131	4142
4110§	4121	4132	4143
4111	4122	4133	

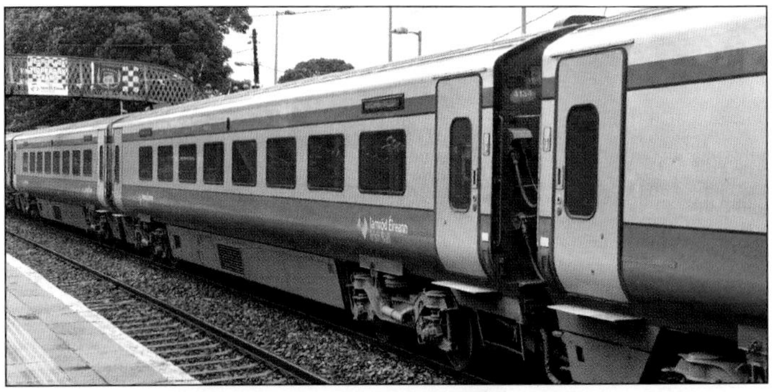
Standard class accommodation on the Irish Rail Intercity services is provided by a fleet of 42 open standard coaches, of which eight are end vehicles. No. 4134 is shown. **CJM**

Open First (OF)

4201	4203	4205	4207
4202	4204	4206	4208

Restaurant Buffet Standard (RBS)

4401	4403	4405	4407
4402	4404	4406	4408

Luas Trams - Dublin

Alstom 'Citadis' TGA301 5-section

Introduced: 2002-2003
Train Length: 40.80m
Seating: 72 + 8 tip-up
Width: 2.40m
Horsepower: 560kW
Power Supply: 750V dc overhead
Electrical Equipment: Alstom

3001	3004	3007	3010	3013	3016	3019	3022	3025
3002	3005	3008	3011	3014	3017	3020	3023	3026
3003	3006	3009	3012	3015	3018	3021	3024	

Alstom 'Citadis' TGA401 5-section

Introduced: 2002-2003
Train Length: 40.80m
Seating: 72 + 8 tip-up
Width: 2.40m
Horsepower: 560kW
Power Supply: 750V dc overhead
Electrical Equipment: Alstom

4001	4003	4005	4007	4009	4011	4012	4013	4014
4002	4004	4006	4008	4010				

Alstom 'Citadis' TGA402/502§ 9-section

Introduced: 2008-2009 as 7-section, extended 2010-20
Train Length: 43.5 - 54.7m
Seating: 70-92 + 8 tip-up
Width: 2.40m
Horsepower: 720kW
Power Supply: 750V dc overhead
Electrical Equipment: Alstom

5001	5006	5011	5016	5021	5026	5031§	5036§	5041§
5002	5007	5012	5017	5022	5027§	5032§	5037§	
5003	5008	5013	5018	5023	5028§	5033§	5038§	
5004	5009	5014	5019	5024	5029§	5034§	5039§	
5005	5010	5015	5020	5025	5030§	5035§	5040§	

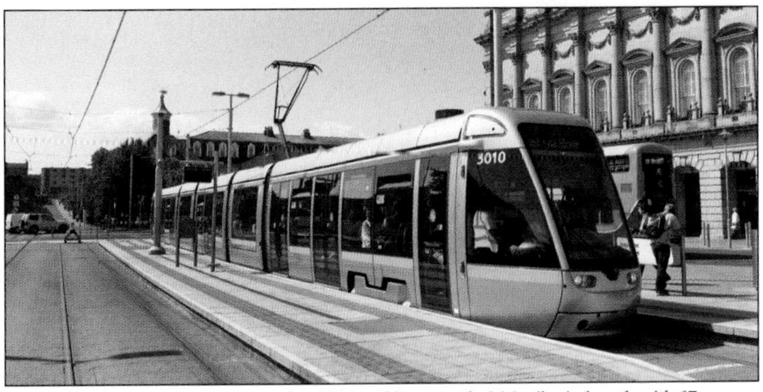

The Dublin Luas tram system opened in 2004 and is currently 26.2miles in length with 67 stations on two lines. Alstom Citadis TGA301 5-section tram No. 3010 is seen outside Dublin Heuston. **CJM**

Isle of Man Railways

Steam Railway

Locomotives

Steam

No.	Name	Builder/Year	Type	Notes
1	*Sutherland*	Beyer Peacock / 1873	2-4-0T	At Port Erin Museum
3	*Pender*	Beyer Peacock / 1873	2-4-0T	Manchester MSI
4	*Loch*	Beyer Peacock / 1874	2-4-0T	
5	*Mona*	Beyer Peacock / 1874	2-4-0T	
6	*Peveril*	Beyer Peacock / 1875	2-4-0T	At Port Erin Museum
8	*Fenella*	Beyer Peacock / 1894	2-4-0T	
9	*Douglas*	Beyer Peacock / 1896	2-4-0T	
10	*G. H. Wood*	Beyer Peacock / 1905	2-4-0T	
11	*Maitland*	Beyer Peacock / 1905	2-4-0T	
12	*Hutchinson*	Beyer Peacock / 1908	2-4-0T	
13	*Kissack*	Beyer Peacock / 1910	2-4-0T	
14	*Thornhill*	Beyer Peacock / 1880	2-4-0T	Private on Isle of Man
4	*Caledonia*	Dübs & Co / 1885	0-6-0T	Previously No. 15
16	*Mannin*	Beyer Peacock / 1926	2-4-0T	

Diesel

No.	Name	Builder / Year	Type	Notes
17	*Viking*	Schoema / 1958	0-4-0 DH	Stored
18	*Ailsa*	Hunslet / 1994	0-4-0 DE	
21		MPI / 2013	Bo-Bo DE	MP550-B1
22		D Wickham / 1956	4-wheel P	Ex Lochaber Railway
23		D Wickham / 1961	4-wheel P	Ex Lochaber Railway
24		Motorail / 1959	4-wheel DM	
25		Motorail / 1966	4-wheel DM	

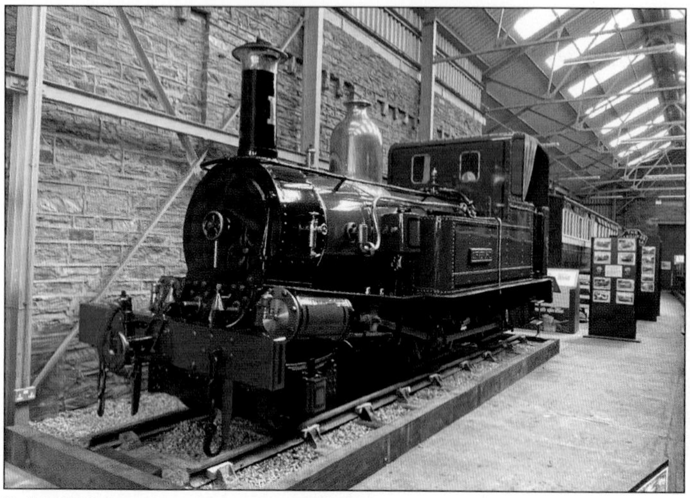

Built in 1879, Beyer Peacock 2-4-0T No. 1 Sutherland *is currently preserved a the Steam Railway museum at Port Erin, it carried green livery and was restored in 2021. The exhibits in the museum are part of the operational fleet and could be restored to full use.* **CJM**

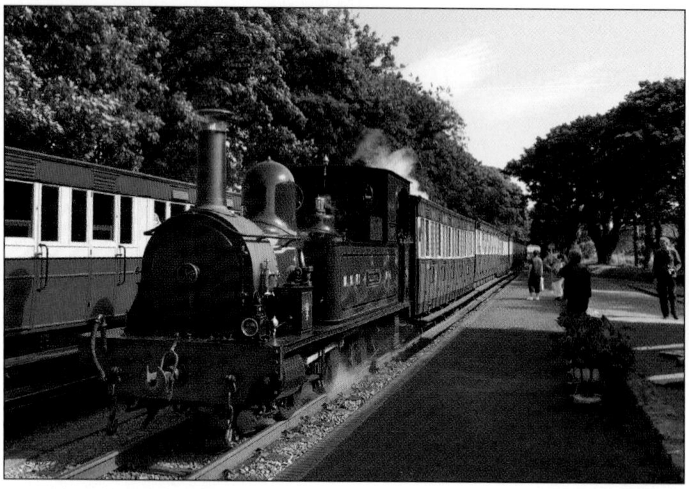

One of the prime locos operating Isle of Man steam services for the last few seasons is their largest loco, Dübs & Co 1885-built No. 4 Caledonia, *restored to Manx Northern Railway maroon. It is shown as Castletown with a train for Port Erin in August 2021.* **CJM**

Railcars

Number	Builder	Year built	Notes
19(S)	Walker	1949	Ex-County Donegal Railway - out of use
20(S)	Walker	1950	Ex-County Donegal Railway - out of use

Coaching Stock

No.	Builder / Year	Type	Notes
F9	Brown Marshalls / 1881	Bogie	
F10	Brown Marshalls / 1881	Bogie	
F11	Brown Marshalls / 1881	Bogie	
F15	Brown Marshalls / 1894	Bogie	
F18	Brown Marshalls / 1894	Bogie	
F21(S)	Metropolitan C&W / 1896	Bogie	
F25(S)	Metropolitan C&W / 1896	Bogie	
F26	Metropolitan C&W / 1896	Bogie	
F27	Metropolitan C&W / 1897	Bogie	Now Kitchen and Luggage
F28(S)	Metropolitan C&W / 1897	Bogie	Now Kitchen and Luggage
F29	Metropolitan C&W / 1905	Bogie	
F30	Metropolitan C&W / 1905	Bogie	
F31	Metropolitan C&W / 1905	Bogie	
F32	Metropolitan C&W / 1905	Bogie	
F35	Metropolitan C&W / 1905	Bogie	
F36§	Metropolitan C&W / 1905	Bogie	Port Erin Museum
F39	Oldbury C & W / 1887	Bogie	
F43	Metropolitan C&W / 1908	Bogie	
F45	Metropolitan C&W / 1913	Bogie	
F46	Metropolitan C&W / 1913	Bogie	
F47	Metropolitan C&W / 1923	Bogie	
F48	Metropolitan C&W / 1923	Bogie	
F49	Metropolitan C&W / 1926	Bogie	
F54	Metropolitan C&W / 1923	Bogie	
F62	Metropolitan C&W / 1926	Bogie	
F63(S)	Metropolitan C&W / 1920	Bogie	
F66(S)	Metropolitan C&W / 1920	Bogie	
F67(S)	Metropolitan C&W / 1920	Bogie	
F74(S)	Metropolitan C&W / 1921	Bogie	
F75§	Metropolitan C&W / 1926	Bogie	

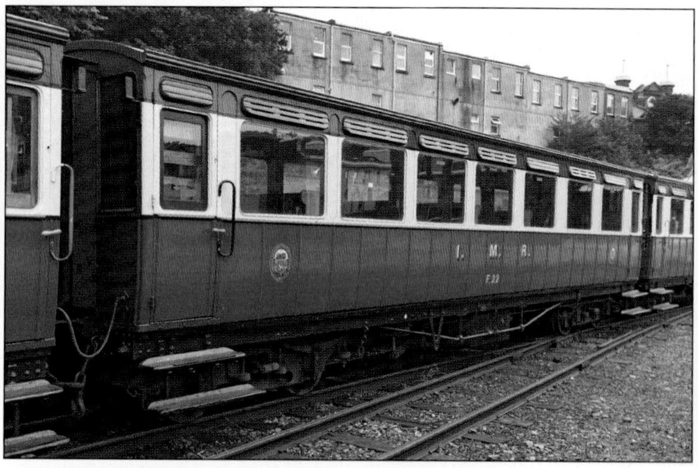

The Isle of Man Steam Railway operates a full catering service and for this a special set of coaches with side seating, a central corridor, a kitchen car and a bar car are maintained. Car F.32 a 1905-built vehicle from the catering train is seen stabled at Douglas station. **CJM**

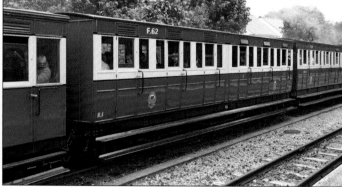

1926-built Metropolitan C&W Trailer Composite No. F.62 was restored for the 2021 season and is a credit to the railways engineering skills. It is seen from its second class end at Colby on 9 August 2021. **CJM**

Non Passenger Stock

No.	Type	Builder / Year	Notes
G1	Van (6-ton)	Metropolitan C&W / 1873	
W2	Well	IOM / 1998	
WW111	Well	IOM / 2014	
Gr12	Van 6-ton	Swansea Wagon / 1879	
G19	Van 6-ton	IOM / 1921	Port Erin Museum
F23	Flat	Metropolitan C&W / 1896	
F33	Flat	Metropolitan C&W / 1905	

F40	Flat	Metropolitan C&W / 1905	
F41	Flat	Metropolitan C&W / 1905	
F44	Flat	Metropolitan C&W / 1905	
F50	Flat	Metropolitan C&W / 1911	
F57	Flat	Metropolitan C&W / 1919	
F65	Hopper	Metropolitan C&W / 1910	Chassis only
F70	Hopper	Metropolitan C&W / 1922	
F71	Flat	Metropolitan C&W / 1911	
F73	Flat	Metropolitan C&W / 1920	
M69	2-plank wagon	Metropolitan C&W / 1926	Port Erin Museum
M78	2-plank wagon	Metropolitan C&W / 1926	Port Erin Museum
F430	Flat	Hudson / 1980	
RF274	Flat	Hudson / 1980	Fitted with Hiab crane

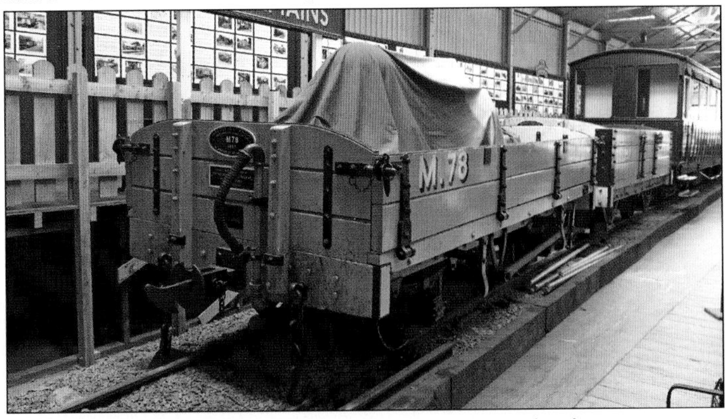

Although the IOM Steam Railway does not operate freight trains, a number of non passenger vehicles are on their books. Some, such as No. M.78 is preserved at the Port Erin Museum. This vehicle was built in 1926 for IOM use. **CJM**

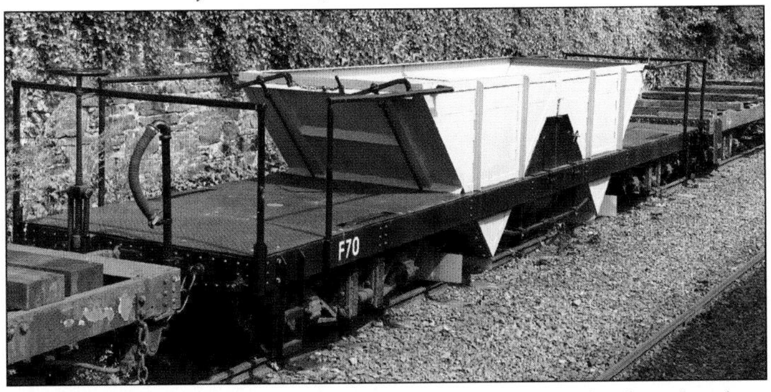

The only non-passenger trains operated by the IOM Steam Railway are engineering trains to keep the line in top condition. One such vehicle is F70 a local built ballast hopper. When not in use these vehicles are often stabled in the siding at Douglas station. **CJM**

Manx Electric Railway

Power Cars

No.	Type	Builder / Year	Notes
1	Un-vestibuled saloon	G F Milnes / 1893	
2	Un-vestibuled saloon	G F Milnes / 1893	
5	Vestibuled 'Tunnel car'	G F Milnes / 1894	
6	Vestibuled 'Tunnel car'	G F Milnes / 1894	
7	Vestibuled 'Tunnel car'	G F Milnes / 1894	
9	Vestibuled 'Tunnel car'	G F Milnes / 1894	

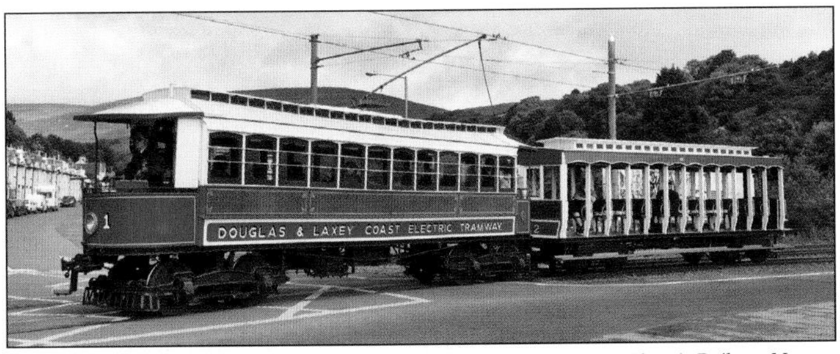

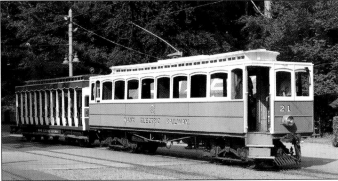

Considered as the oldest operational electric tram car in the World, Manx Electric Railway No. 1, painted in Douglas & Laxey Coast electric Tramway colours is seen arriving at Laxey from Ramsey, with trailer No. 42. **CJM**

14	Cross-bench open saloon	G F Milnes / 1898	
15	Cross-bench open saloon	G F Milnes / 1898	Stored
16	Cross-bench open saloon	G F Milnes / 1898	
17	Cross-bench open saloon	G F Milnes / 1898	Stored
18	Cross-bench open saloon	G F Milnes / 1898	Stored
19	Winter saloon	G F Milnes / 1899	
20	Winter saloon	G F Milnes / 1899	
21	Winter saloon	G F Milnes / 1899	
22	Winter saloon	McArds & MER / 1992*	New body
23	Locomotive	MER Co / 1900	Stored
25	Cross-bench open	G F Milnes / 1893	Stored
26	Cross-bench open	G F Milnes / 1893	Stored
27	Cross-bench open	G F Milnes / 1893	Stored
28	Cross-bench open	ER&T Ltd / 1904	Stored
29 (S)	Cross-bench open	ER&T Ltd / 1904	
30 (S)	Cross-bench open	ER&T Ltd / 1904	
31 (S)	Cross-bench open	ER&T Ltd / 1904	
32	Cross-bench 'Toastrack'	United Car / 1906	
33	Cross-bench 'Toastrack'	United Car / 1906	
34	Locomotive	IOM / 1996	

1899 Milnes built 'Winter Saloon' No. 21, one of four such trams in regular use, displays the short lived Manx Electric Railway green and white livery. It is seen at Laxey, with a trailer, heading towards Derby Castle, Douglas. **CJM**

Trailer Cars

Number	Type	Builder / Year	Notes
36	Cross-bench	G F Milnes / 1894	Under restoration
37	Cross-bench	G F Milnes /1894	
40	Cross-bench	English Electric / 1930	
41	Cross-bench	English Electric / 1930	
42	Cross-bench	G F Milnes / 1903	
43	Cross-bench	G F Milnes / 1903	
44	Cross-bench	English Electric / 1930	
46	Cross-bench	G F Milnes / 1899	
47	Cross-bench	G F Milnes / 1899	
48	Cross-bench	G F Milnes / 1899	
49	Cross-bench	G F Milnes / 1893	Stored
50	Cross-bench	G F Milnes / 1893	Under restoration
51	Cross-bench	G F Milnes / 1893	
53	Cross-bench	G F Milnes / 1893	Stored
54	Cross-bench	G F Milnes / 1893	Stored
55	Cross-bench	ER&T Ltd / 1904	Stored
56	Disabled persons	ER&T Ltd / 1904	Rebuilt in 1995
57	Enclosed saloon	ER&T Ltd / 1904	
58	Enclosed saloon	ER&T Ltd / 1904	
59	Special/Directors saloon	G F Milnes / 1895	
60	Cross-bench	G F Milnes / 1896	
61	Cross-bench	United Electric / 1906	
62	Cross-bench	United Electric / 1906	

In the above view one of the original 1893-built trailers No. 51, looking a little flimsy by more modern standards is seen at Laxey in 2019. Below, is slightly more modern, 1899-built trailer No. 48, showing the roller shutters, which can be lowered in poor weather, these offer some protection but no visibility from the coach. Both: **CJM**

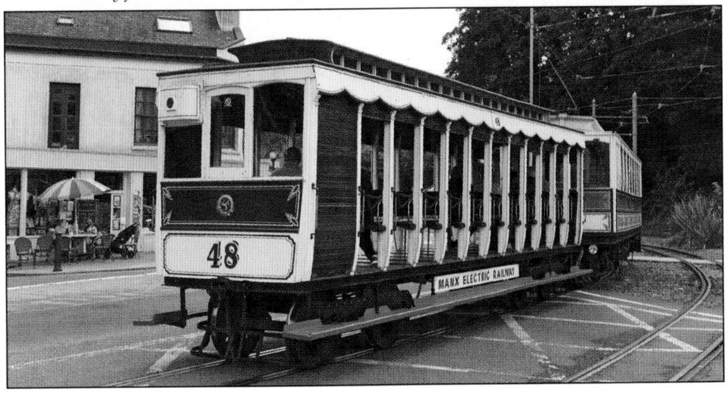

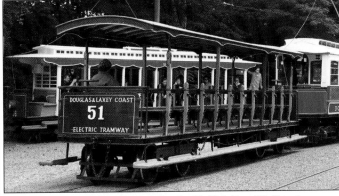

Non Passenger Stock

No.	Type	Builder / Year	Notes
1	Tower wagon	G F Milnes / 1894	
3	Van	G F Milnes / 1894	
4	Travelling Post Office	G F Milnes / 1894	
8	Open wagon	G F Milnes / 1897	
10	Open wagon	G F Milnes / 1897	
11	Van (6-ton)	G F Milnes / 1898	
12	Van (6-ton)	G F Milnes / 1899	
13	Van (5-ton)	G F Milnes / 1903	
14	Van (5-ton)	G F Milnes / 1904	
16	Mail van	MER / 1908	
21	Flat wagon	MER / 1926	
26	Freight trailer	G F Milnes / 1918	Previously Power Car 10
45	Flat wagon	G F Milnes / 1899	Previously Trailer 45
52	Flat with work lift	G F Milnes / 1893	Previously Trailer 52
RF308	Tipper wagon	Hudson / 1993	Ex-EuroTunnel
13/24-4	Tipper wagon	W G Allan / 1997	Stored
13/24-5	Tipper wagon	W G Allan / 1997	Stored
13/24-6	Tipper wagon	W G Allan / 1997	Stored
7442/2	Trailer	Wickham / 2014	

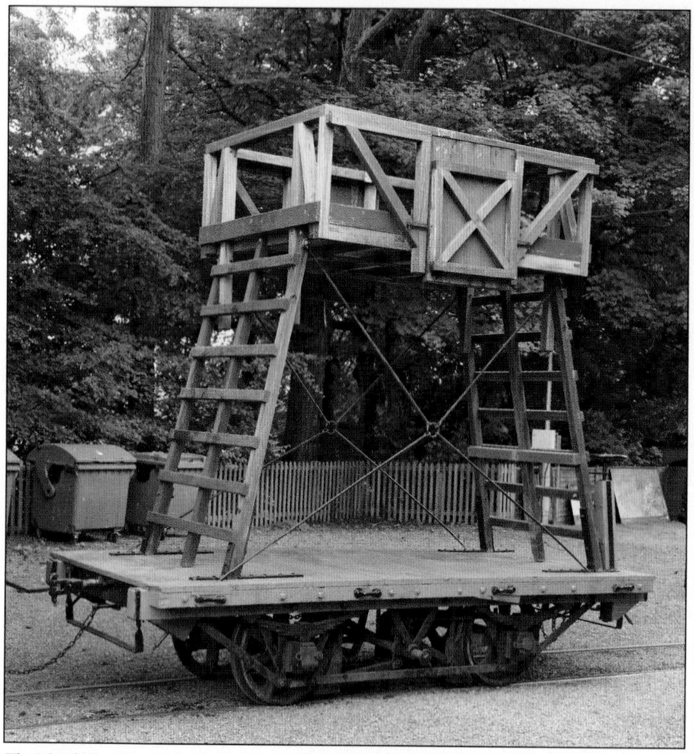

The Isle of Man Electric Railway has a small number of non-passenger vehicles, these are mainly for engineering work, such as this tower wagon, converted from a flat. This is used by the lines power supply department to reach the overhead power line for repair or overhaul. The wagon is unbraked and would be powered by one of the electric trams to near a work site and then man-handle to the site of work. **CJM**

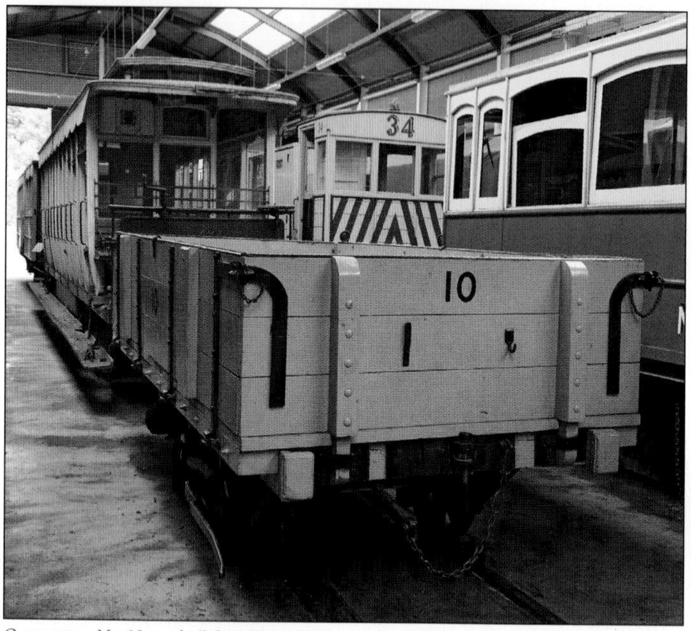

Open wagon No. 10 was built by Milnes of Birkenhead in 1897, apart from freight demonstration purposes the wagon is no longer used on work sites, it is shown stored out of harms way at Laxey, along with 'loco' No. 34 and 'Winter Saloon' No. 21. **CJM**

Snaefell Mountain Railway

Power Cars

No.	Type	Builder / Year	Notes
1	Vestibuled saloon	G F Milnes / 1895	
2	Vestibuled saloon	G F Milnes / 1895	
4	Vestibuled saloon	G F Milnes / 1895	
5	Vestibuled saloon	H D Kinnin / 1971	Original car destroyed in fire August 1970
6	Vestibuled saloon	G F Milnes / 1895	New body 2021-2022

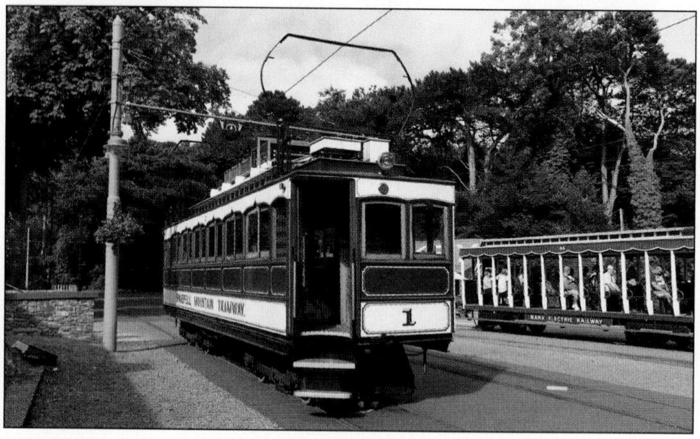

A fleet of five Snaefell Mountain Railway trams are in use, based at a small depot in Laxey, the vehicles are confined by gauge to the Snaefell Mountain route. No. 1 painted in white and blue Snaefell Mountain Tramway livery is seen at Laxey station in August 2021. **CJM**

Non Passenger Stock

No.	Type	Builder / Year	Notes
-	Flat wagon	MER / 1981	
-	Flat wagon	P Keefe	
-	Flat with tipper	Allens / 1940	
-	Tower wagon	MER / 1998	
4	Wickham (11730)	Wickham / 1991	
-	Flat wagon	MER / 2019	Fitted with Fell brake

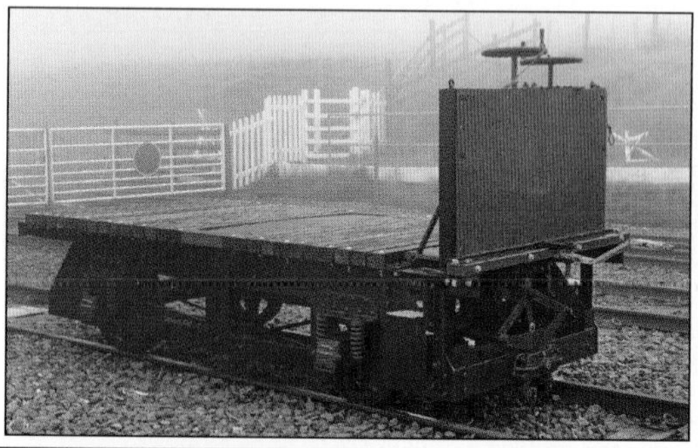

This 'modern' Fell-Brake' fitted freight wagon was built at Laxey depot in 2019 and can be used to move light engineering equipment on the mountain line, it would be hauled by a tram car. It is seen stabled at Bungalow. **CJM**

Isle of Man Works Locomotive

No.	Name	Type	Builder / Year	Notes
LM344	*Pig*	60SL 4-wheel	Simplex / 1980	Works No. 60SL751, ex-Bord na Mona Peat Railway, Ireland as No. LM344.

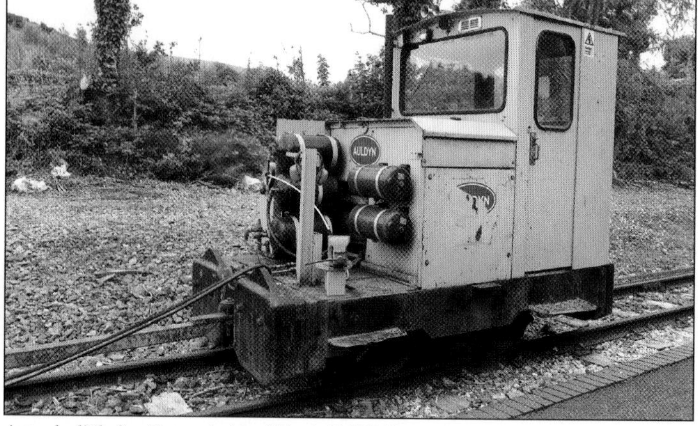

A popular little diesel loco on he Isle of Man is LM233 Pig, now owned and operated by engineering company Auldyn. From the Bord na Mona Peat Railway in Ireland, the loco can be found on both steam and electric railway. It is seen in this view at Santon. **CJM**

Douglas Bay Horse Tram

Passenger Cars

No.	Type	Builder / Year	Notes
1	Single-ended saloon	Milnes Voss / 1913	
11	Toastrack saloon	Starbuck / 1886	At Jurby Transport Museum
12	Toastrack saloon	G F Milnes / 1888	
14	Double-deck car	Metro C&W / 1883	At Manx Museum, Douglas
18	Double-deck car	Metro C&W / 1883	
21	Toastrack saloon	G F Milnes / 1890	
22	Toastrack saloon	G F Milnes / 1890	At Jurby Transport Museum
27	Single-deck saloon	G F Milnes / 1892	
29	Single-deck saloon	G F Milnes / 1892	
32	Toastrack saloon	G F Milnes / 1896	
35	Toastrack saloon	G F Milnes / 1896	Home of Rest for Old Horses, Douglas
36	Toastrack saloon	G F Milnes / 1896	
38	Toastrack saloon	G F Milnes / 1902	
42	Toastrack saloon	G F Milnes / 1905	
43	Toastrack saloon	United Elec / 1907	
44	Toastrack saloon	United Elec / 1907	Royal Car
45	Toastrack saloon	Milnes Voss / 1908	
47	Toastrack saloon	Milnes Voss / 1911	At Jurby Transport Museum

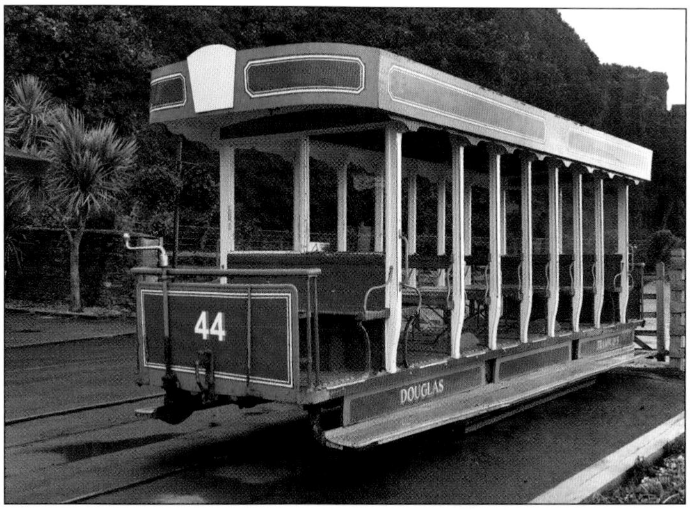

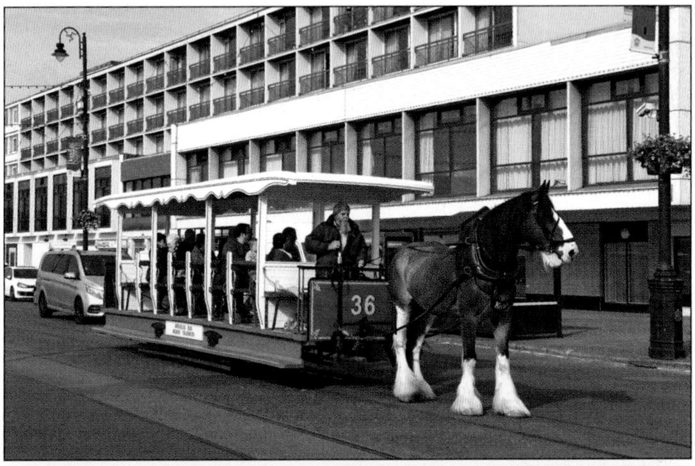

For the 2021-2022 seasons, the historic Douglas Bay Horse Tramway did not operate, this was due to Covid-19 restrictions and major rebuilding of the main promenade at Douglas, seeing a diversion of the tramway from the middle to the side of the road for part of its route. It is hoped that the line will re-open for the 2023 season. In the above view 'Toastrack' saloon No. 44, built in 1907 is seen at Derby Castle. The view left, shows one of the lines horses Keith, powering 1896-built 'Toastrack' saloon No. 36 passing The Palace Hotel and Casino. Both: **CJM**

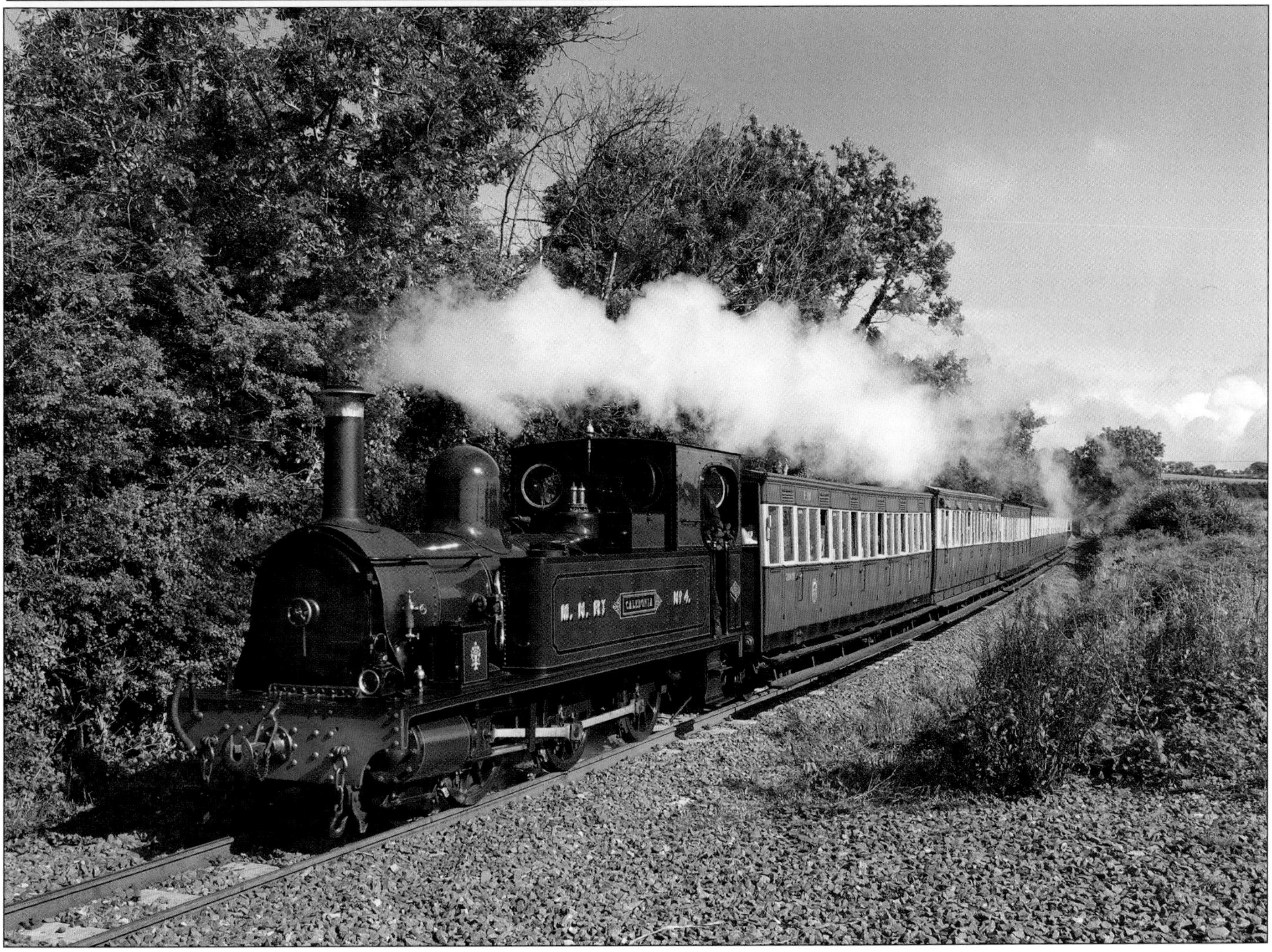

The Isle of Man Steam Railway is a very photogenic line with hundreds of possible photo viewpoints. On 12 August 2021, No. 4 Caledonia *passes Mearyveg near Santon with the first southbound train of the day, the 09.50 from Douglas to Port Erin.* **CJM**

Preserved Steam Locomotives

No.	Name	Group	Class	Wheel Arrangement	Location	Notes
GNR 1		NER	Stirling	4-2-2	National Railway Museum	
3	*Coppernob*	LMS	FR	0-4-0	National Railway Museum	
5	*Cecil Raikes*	LMS		0-6-4T	Liverpool Museum	
FR20		LMS		0-4-0	Ribble Valley Steam Railway	
W24	*Calbourne*	Southern	O2	0-4-4T	Isle of Wight Steam Railway	
FR25		LMS		0-4-0ST	Furness Railway trust, Ribble Valley Railway	
49	*Columbine*	LMS		2-2-2	Science Museum	
54	*Waddon*	Southern	A1X	0-6-0T	Canadian Railway Museum, Saint-Constant, Quebec	
57	*Lion*	LMS	L&M	0-4-2	Liverpool Museum	
66	*Aerolite*	NER	X1	2-2-4T	National Railway Museum	
103		LMS		4-6-0	Riverside Museum, Glasgow	
B110		Southern	E1	0-6-0T	East Somerset Railway	
123		LMS		4-2-2	Riverside Museum, Glasgow	
158A		LMS		2-4-0	National Railway Museum Shildon	
214	*Gladstone*	Southern	B	0-4-0	National Railway Museum York	
251		NER	C1	4-4-2	Danum Gallery & Museum, Doncaster (Part of National Collection)	
419		LMS		0-4-4T	Bo'ness and Kinneil	
426		GWR		0-6-2T	Keighley & Worth Valley Railway	
450		GWR		0-6-2T	NRM at Gwili Railway	
563		Southern	T3	4-4-0	Flower Mill / Swanage	
600	*Gordon*	WD	WD	2-10-0	Severn Valley Railway	
670		-	LNWR	2-2-2	Tyseley Locomotive Works	Replica New Build
673		LMS	Spinner	4-2-2	National Railway Museum	
790	*Hardwicke*	LMS	LNWR	2-4-0	National Railway Museum York	
813		GWR		0-6-0ST	Telford Steam Railway	
828		LMS	812	0-6-0	Strathspey Railway at Spa Valley Rilway for 2022	
910	*Fletcher*	NER		2-4-0	NRM at Kirkby Stephen East	
990	*Henry Oakley*	NER	C2	4-4-2	National Railway Museum York	
1000		LMS	MC	4-4-0	NRM at Barrow Hill	
1014	*County of Glamorgan*	-	1000	4-6-0	Discot Railway Centre	Replica New Build
1275		NER	1001	0-6-0	National Railway Museum	
1310		NER	Y7	0-4-0T	Middleton Railway	
1338		GWR		0-6-0ST	Didcot Railway Centre	
1340	*Trojan*	GWR		0-6-0ST	Didcot Railway Centre	
1363		GWR	1361	0-6-0ST	Didcot Railway Centre	
1369		GWR	1366	0-6-0PT	South Devon Railway	
1420		GWR	1400	0-4-2T	South Devon Railway	
1439		LMS		0-4-0ST	NRM at Ribble Steam Railway	
1442		GWR	1400	0-4-2T	Tiverton Museum	
1450		GWR	1400	0-4-2T	Severn Valley Railway	
1463	*Tennant*	NER	E5	2-4-0	NRM at Darlington	
1466		GWR	1400	0-4-2T	Dean Forest Railway	
1501		GWR	1500	0-6-0PT	Severn Valley Railway	
1621		NER	D17	4-4-0	National Railway Museum	
1638		GWR	1600	0-6-0PT	Kent & East Sussex Railway	
1719	*Lady Nan*	LMS		0-4-0ST	East Somerset Railway	
1759		-	G5	0-4-4T	Shildon	Replica New Build
2007	*Prince of Wales*	-	P2	2-8-2	Darlington Locomotive Works	Replica New Build
2271		LMS		0-6-2T	National Railway Museum at Foxfield	Also No. NSR 2
2516		GWR	Dean Goods	0-6-0	Swindon Museum, Swindon	
2807		GWR	2800	2-8-0	Gloucestershire Warwickshire Railway	
2818		GWR	2800	2-8-0	Steam, Swindon	
2857		GWR	2800	2-8-0	Severn Valley Railway	
2859		GWR	2800	2-8-0	Private in Congleton	
2861		GWR	2800	2-8-0	Barry	
2873		GWR	2800	2-8-0	South Devon Railway	Parts for 3803
2874		GWR	2800	2-8-0	Gloucestershire Warwickshire Railway	
2885		GWR	2800	2-8-0	Tyseley	

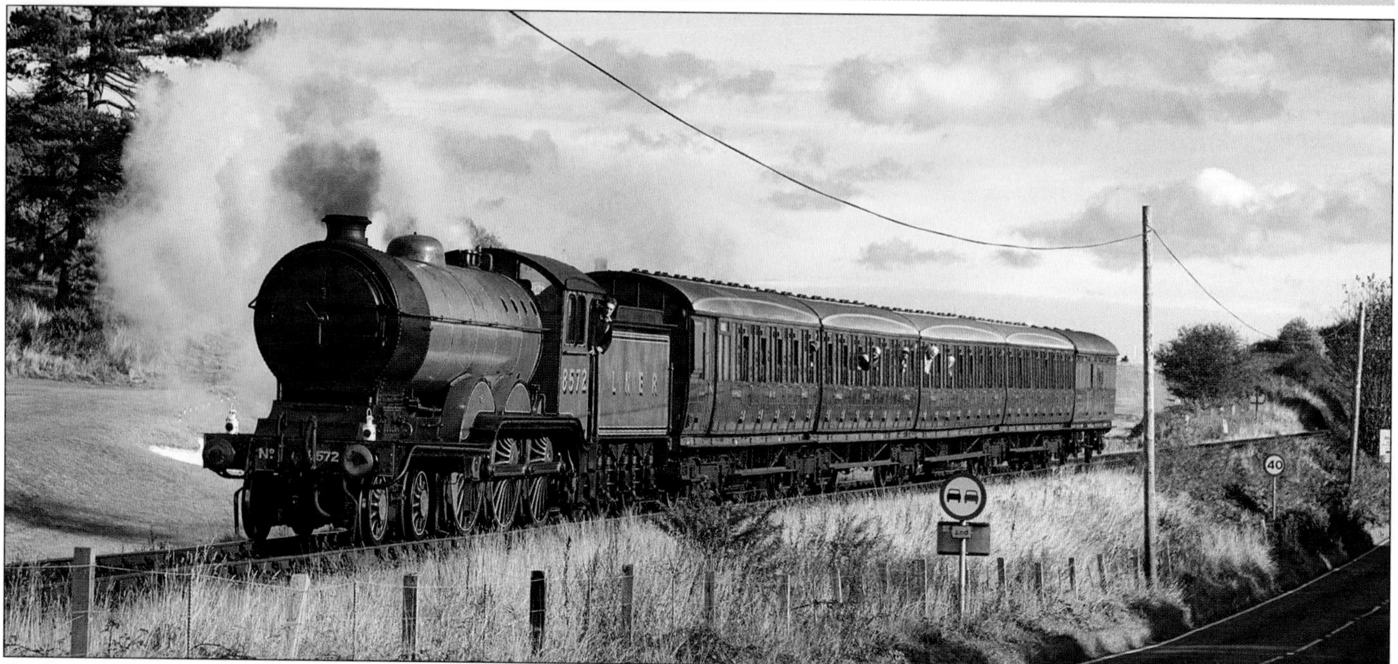

Superbly restored B12 No. 8572 is seen on the North Norfolk Railway on 30 October 2021 passing Sheringham Golf Course bound for Hold. This loco was withdrawn from service at the end of 2021 for an overhaul. **Ian Williams**

2999	*Lady of Legend*	GWR	2900	4-6-0	Didcot Railway Centre	Replica New Build
3020	*Cornwall*	LMS	LNWR	2-2-2	NRM at Buckingham Railway	
3205		GWR	2251	0-6-0	South Devon Railway	
3440	*City of Truro*	GWR	City	4-4-0	Steam Museum, Swindon	
3650		GWR	5700	0-6-0PT	Didcot Railway Centre	
3738		GWR	5700	0-6-0PT	Didcot Railway Centre	
3802		GWR	2800	2-8-0	Llangollen Railway	
3803		GWR	2800	2-8-0	Dartmouth Steam Railway	
3814		GWR	2800	2-8-0	Northern Steam Engineering, Stockton	
3822		GWR	2800	2-8-0	Gloucestershire Warwickshire Railway	
3840		-	3800	4-4-0	Tyseley Loco Works	Replica New Build
3845		GWR	2800	2-8-0	West Somerset Railway	
3850		GWR	2800	2-8-0	Gloucestershire Warwickshire Railway	
3855		GWR	2800	2-8-0	East Lancashire Railway	
3862		GWR	2800	2-8-0	Northampton & Lamport	
4003	*Lode Star*	GWR	Star	4-6-0	National Railway Museum York	
4073	*Caerphilly Castle*	GWR	Castle	4-6-0	Steam Museum, Swindon	
4079	*Pendennis Castle*	GWR	Castle	4-6-0	Didcot Railway Centre	
4110		GWR	5101	2-6-2T	East Somerset Railway	
4115		GWR	5101	2-6-2T	Didcot Railway Centre	
4121		GWR	5101	2-6-2T	Tyseley Museum	
4141		GWR	5101	2-6-2T	Epping and Ongar Railway	
4144		GWR	5101	2-6-2T	Didcot Railway Centre, on loan to Kent & East Sussex Rly	
4150		GWR	5101	2-6-2T	Severn Valley Railway	
4160		GWR	5101	2-6-2T	South Devon Railway	
4247		GWR	4200	2-8-0T	Dartmouth Steam Railway	
4248		GWR	4200	2-8-0T	Steam Museum, Swindon	
4253		GWR	4200	2-8-0T	Kent & East Sussex Railway	
4270		GWR	4200	2-8-0T	Gloucestershire Warwickshire Railway	
4277		GWR	4200	2-8-0T	Dartmouth Steam Railway	
4555	*Warrior*	GWR	4500	2-6-2T	Dartmouth Steam Railway	
4561		GWR	4500	2-6-2T	West Somerset Railway	
4566		GWR	4500	2-6-2T	Severn Valley Railway	
4588		GWR	4500	2-6-2T	Tyseley Museum	
4612		GWR	5700	0-6-0PT	Bodmin & Wenford Railway	
4709		-	4700	2-8-0	Tyseley Loco Works	Replica New Build
4920	*Dumbleton Hall*	GWR	Hall	4-6-0	Exported to Japan, at Harry Potter Museum, Warner Bros Studio, Toshimean	
4930	*Hagley Hall*	GWR	Hall	4-6-0	Severn Valley Railway	
4936	*Kinlet Hall*	GWR	Hall	4-6-0	Tyseley Museum	
4953	*Pitchford Hall*	GWR	Hall	4-6-0	Epping and Ongar Railway	
4965	*Rood Ashton Hall*	GWR	Hall	4-6-0	Tyseley Museum	
4979	*Wootton Hall*	GWR	Hall	4-6-0	Ribble Steam Railway	
5029	*Nunney Castle*	GWR	Castle	4-6-0	Didcot Railway Centre	
5043	*Earl of Mt Edgecumbe*	GWR	Castle	4-6-0	Tyseley Museum	
5051	*Earl Bathurst*	GWR	Castle	4-6-0	Didcot Railway Centre	
5080	*Defiant*	GWR	Castle	4-6-0	Tyseley Museum	
5164		GWR	5101	2-6-2T	Barrow Hill	
5193		GWR	5101	2-6-2T	West Somerset Railway	Rebuilt as Mogul 9351
5199		GWR	5101	2-6-2T	West Somerset Railway (until Dec-22)	
5224		GWR	5205	2-8-0T	West Somerset Railway	
5227		GWR	5205	2-8-0T	Barry	
5239	*Goliath*	GWR	5205	2-8-0T	Dartmouth Steam Railway	
5322		GWR	4300	2-8-0T	Didcot Railway Centre	
5521		GWR	4500	2-6-2T	Epping and Ongar Railway (loan) as L150	
5526		GWR	4500	2-6-2T	Swanage Railway	
5532		GWR	4500	2-6-2T	Llangollen Railway	
5538		GWR	4500	2-6-2T	Flower Mill	
5539		GWR	4500	2-6-2T	Barry Railway	
5541		GWR	4500	2-6-2T	Dean Forest Railway	
5542		GWR	4500	2-6-2T	South Devon Railway	
5552		GWR	4500	2-6-2T	Bodmin & Wenford Railway	
5553		GWR	4500	2-6-2T	Peak Rail	
5572		GWR	4500	2-6-2T	Didcot Railway Centre	
5619		GWR	5600	0-6-2T	Epping and Ongar Railway (on loan)	
5637		GWR	5600	0-6-2T	Swindon & Cricklade Railway	
5643		GWR	5600	0-6-2T	East Lancashire Railway (loan)	
5668		GWR	5600	0-6-2T	Kent & East Sussex Railway	
5764		GWR	5700	0-6-0PT	Severn Valley Railway	
5775		GWR	5700	0-6-0PT	Keighley & Worth Valley Railway	
5786		GWR	5700	0-6-0PT	South Devon Railway as L92	
5900	*Hinderton Hall*	GWR	Hall	4-6-0	Didcot Railway Centre	
5952	*Cogan Hall*	GWR	Hall	4-6-0	Tyseley Railway Centre	
5967	*Bickmarsh Hall*	GWR	Hall	4-6-0	Northampton & Lamport	
5972	*Olton Hall*	GWR	Hall	4-6-0	Warner bros, Harry Potter Museum, Leavesden, Watford	
6000	*King George V*	GWR	King	4-6-0	Swindon Museum, Swindon	
6023	*King Edward II*	GWR	King	4-6-0	Didcot Railway Centre	
6024	*King Edward I*	GWR	King	4-6-0	West Somerset Railway (GWS)	
6106		GWR	6100	2-6-2T	Didcot Railway Centre	
6412		GWR	6400	0-6-0PT	South Devon Railway	
6430		GWR	6400	0-6-0PT	South Devon Railway	
6435		GWR	6400	0-6-0PT	Bodmin & Wenford	
6619		GWR	5600	0-6-2T	Kent & East Sussex Railway	
6634		GWR	5600	0-6-2T	Peak Rail	
6686		GWR	5600	0-6-2T	Barry	
6695		GWR	5600	0-6-2T	Swindon & Cricklade Railway	
6697		GWR	5600	0-6-2T	Didcot Railway Centre	
6880	*Betton Grange*	-	Grange	4-6-0	Llangollen Raileway	Replica New Build
6960	*Raveningham Hall*	GWR	Mod Hall	4-6-0	1:1 Museum, Margate	
6984	*Owsden Hall*	GWR	Mod Hall	4-6-0	Buckingham Railway Centre	
6989	*Wightwick Hall*	GWR	Mod Hall	4-6-0	Quainton Railway	
6990	*Witherslack Hall*	GWR	Mod Hall	4-6-0	Great Central Railway	
6998	*Burton Agnes Hall*	GWR	Mod Hall	4-6-0	Didcot Railway Centre	
7027	*Thornbury Castle*	GWR	Castle	4-6-0	Private at Great Central Railway	
7029	*Clun Castle*	GWR	Castle	4-6-0	Tyseley Museum	
7200		GWR	7200	2-8-2T	The Buckinghamshire Railway Centre, Quainton	
7202		GWR	7200	2-8-2T	Didcot Railway Centre	
7229		GWR	7200	2-8-2T	East Lancashire Railway	
7325		GWR	4300	2-6-0	Severn Valley Railway	

7714		GWR	5700	0-6-0PT	Severn Valley Railway	
7715		GWR	5700	0-6-0PT	The Buckinghamshire Railway Centre, Quainton as L99	
7752		GWR	5700	0-6-0PT	Tyseley Museum	
7754		GWR	5700	0-6-0PT	Llangollen Railway	
7760		GWR	5700	0-6-0PT	Tyseley Museum	
7802	*Bradley Manor*	GWR	Manor	4-6-0	Severn Valley Railway	
7808	*Cookham Manor*	GWR	Manor	4-6-0	Didcot Railway Centre	
7812	*Erlestoke Manor*	GWR	Manor	4-6-0	Tyseley Museum	
7819	*Hinton Manor*	GWR	Manor	4-6-0	Severn Valley Railway	
7820	*Dinmore Manor*	GWR	Manor	4-6-0	Gloucestershire Warwickshire Railway	
7821	*Ditcheat Manor*	GWR	Manor	4-6-0	Retail Park, Swindon	
7822	*Foxcote Manor*	GWR	Manor	4-6-0	West Somerset Railway	
7827	*Lydham Manor*	GWR	Manor	4-6-0	Dartmouth Steam Railway	
7828	*Odney Manor*	GWR	Manor	4-6-0	West Somerset Railway	
7903	*Foremarke Hall*	GWR	Mod Hall	4-6-0	Gloucestershire Warwickshire Railway	
7927	*Willington Hall*	GWR	Mod Hall	4-6-0	Llangollen Railway	
9017	*Earl of Berkeley*	GWR	Dukedog	4-4-0	Bluebell Railway	
9351		GWR		2-6-0	West Somerset Railway	Replica New Build
9400		GWR	9400	0-6-0PT	Steam Museum, Swindon	
9466		GWR	9400	0-6-0PT	West Somerset Railway	
9600		GWR	5700	0-6-0PT	Tyseley Museum	
9629		GWR	5700	0-6-0PT	Pontypool & Blaenavon	
9642		GWR	5700	0-6-0PT	Gloucestershire Warwickshire Railway	
9681		GWR	5700	0-6-0PT	Dean Forest Railway	
9682		GWR	5700	0-6-0PT	Dean Forest Railway	
11243		LMS		0-4-0ST	Ribble Steam Railway	
11456		LMS		0-6-0ST	Keighley & Worth Valley Railway	Also No. 752
16379		LMS	GSWR	0-6-0T	Glasgow Museum	
30053		Southern	M7	0-4-4T	Swanage Railway	
30064		Southern	USA	0-6-0T	Bluebell Railway	
30065		Southern	USA	0-6-0T	Kent & East Sussex Railway	
30070		Southern	USA	0-6-0T	Kent & East Sussex Railway	Also No. DS238
30072		Southern	USA	0-6-0T	Keighley & Worth Valley Railway	
30075		Southern	USA	0-6-0T	Mid-Hants Railway	Yugoslav loco
30076		Southern	USA	0-6-0T	Mid-Hants Railway	Yugoslav loco
30096	*Normandy*	Southern	B4	0-4-0T	Bluebell Railway	
30102	*Granville*	Southern	B4	0-4-0T	Bressingham	
30120		Southern	T9	4-4-0	Swanage Railway, part of National Collection	
30245		Southern	M7	0-4-4T	National Railway Museum	
30499		Southern	S15	4-6-0	Mid Hants Railway	
30506		Southern	S15	4-6-0	Mid-Hants Railway	
30541		Southern	Q	0-6-0	Bluebell Railway	
30583		Southern	0415	4-4-2T	Bluebell Railway	
30585		Southern	0298	2-4-0WT	Buckingham Railway Centre	
30587		Southern	0298	2-4-0WT	National Railway Museum Shildon	
30777	*Sir Lamiel*	Southern	N15	4-6-0	Great Central Railway	
30825		Southern	S15	4-6-0	North Yorkshire Moors Railway	
30828		Southern	S15	4-6-0	Mid-Hants Railway	
30830		Southern	S15	4-6-0	North Yorkshire Moors Railway	
30847		Southern	S15	4-6-0	Bluebell Railway	
30850	*Lord Nelson*	Southern	LN	4-6-0	Mid-Hants Railway	
30925	*Cheltenham*	Southern	V	4-4-0	Mid-Hants Railway	
30926	*Repton*	Southern	V	4-4-0	North Yorkshire Moors Railway	
30928	*Stowe*	Southern	V	4-4-0	Bluebell Railway	
31027		Southern	P	0-6-0T	Bluebell Railway	
31065		Southern	O1	0-6-0	Bluebell Railway	Also No. 65
31178		Southern	P1	0-6-0T	Bluebell Railway	
31263		Southern	H	0-4-4T	Bluebell Railway	
31323		Southern	P	0-6-0T	Bluebell Railway	Also No. 323
31556		Southern	P	0-6-0T	Kent & East Sussex Railway Southern	
31592		Southern	C	0-6-0	Bluebell Railway	
31618		Southern	U	2-6-0	Bluebell Railway	
31625		Southern	U	2-6-0	Swanage Railway	
31638		Southern	U	2-6-0	Bluebell Railway	
31737		Southern	D	4-4-0	National Railway Museum York	
31806		Southern	U	2-6-0	Swanage Railway	
31874		Southern	N	2-6-0	Swanage Railway	
32110	*Cannock Wood*	Southern	E1	0-6-0T	Isle of Wight Steam Railway	
32424	*Beachy Head*	-	H2	4-4-2	Bluebell Railway	Replica New Build
32473	*Birch Grove*	Southern	E4	0-6-2T	Bluebell Railway	
32636	*Fenchurch*	Southern	A1X	0-6-0T	Bluebell Railway	
32640	*Newport*	Southern	A1X	0-6-0T	Isle of Wight Steam Railway	Also No. W11
32646	*Freshwater*	Southern	A1X	0-6-0T	Isle of Wight Steam Railway	
32650	*Whitechapel*	Southern	A1X	0-6-0T	Spa Valley Railway	
32655	*Stepney*	Southern	A1X	0-6-0T	Bluebell Railway	
32662	*Martello*	Southern	A1X	0-6-0T	Bressingham	
32670	*Poplar*	Southern	A1X	0-6-0T	Kent & East Sussex Railway	
32672	*Fenchurch*	Southern	A1X	0-6-0T	Statfold Barn Railway	
32678	*Knowle*	Southern	A1X	0-6-0T	Kent & East Sussex Railway	
32682	*Boxhill*	Southern	A1X	0-6-0T	National Railway Museum	
33001		Southern	Q1	0-6-0	National Railway Museum	
34007	*Wadebridge*	Southern	WC	4-6-2	Mid-Hants Railway	
34010	*Sidmouth*	Southern	WC	4-6-2	Hope Farm, Sellinge, Kent	
34016	*Bodmin*	Southern	WC	4-6-2	WCRC Carnforth	
34023	*Blackmore Vale*	Southern	WC	4-6-2	Bluebell Railway	
34027	*Taw Valley*	Southern	WC	4-6-2	Severn Valley Railway	
34028	*Eddystone*	Southern	WC	4-6-2	Swanage Railway	
34039	*Boscastle*	Southern	WC	4-6-2	Great Central Railway	
34046	*Braunton*	Southern	WC	4-6-2	Southall	
34051	*Winston Churchill*	Southern	BB	4-6-2	National Railway Museum, York	
34053	*Sir Keith Park*	Southern	BB	4-6-2	Spa Valley Railway	
34058	*Sir Frederick Pile*	Southern	BB	4-6-2	Midland Railway Centre	
34059	*Sir Archibald Sinclair*	Southern	BB	4-6-2	Bluebell Railway	
34067	*Tangmere*	Southern	BB	4-6-2	WCRC Carnforth	
34070	*Manston*	Southern	BB	4-6-2	Swanage Railway	
34072	*257 Squadron*	Southern	BB	4-6-2	Swanage Railway	
34073	*249 Squadron*	Southern	BB	4-6-2	East Lancashire Railway	
34081	*92 Squadron*	Southern	BB	4-6-2	Nene Valley Railway	

Great Western Railway 'Star' 4-6-0 No. 4003 Lode Star, *is a part of the National Collection an is available for inspection at the National Railway Museum, York. This view shows the loco stabled next to Great Western 'Railbus' No. 4.* **CJM**

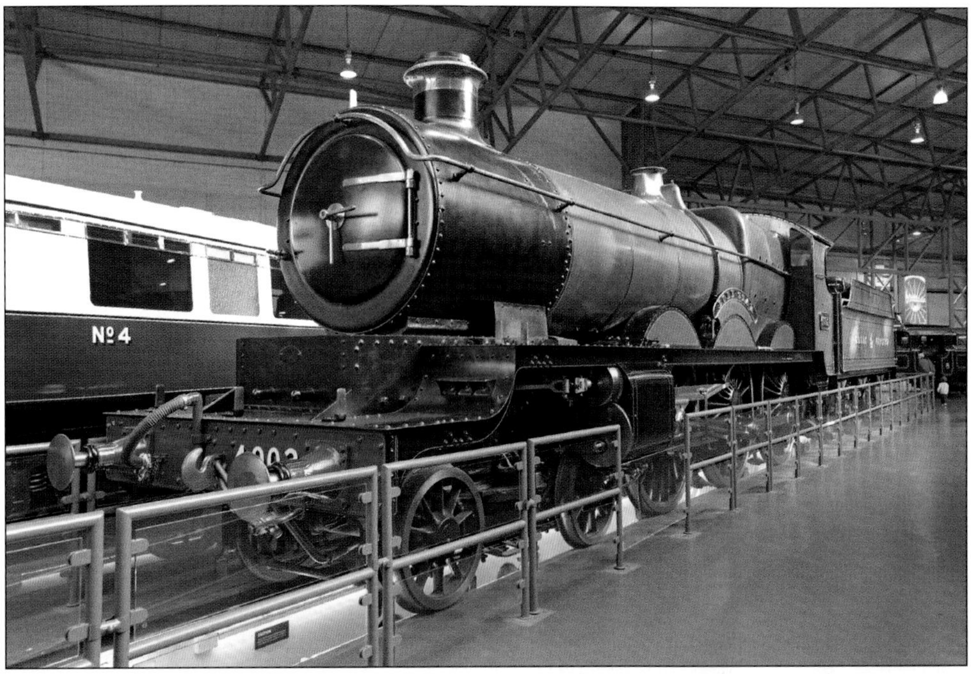

34092	*City of Wells*	Southern	WC	4-6-2	East Lancashire Railway	
34101	*Hartland*	Southern	WC	4-6-2	North Yorkshire Moors Railway	
34105	*Swanage*	Southern	WC	4-6-2	Mid-Hants Railway	
35005	*Canadian Pacific*	Southern	MN	4-6-2	Mid-Hants Railway	
35006	*Peninsular & Oriental S. N Co*	Southern	MN	4-6-2	Gloucestershire Warwickshire Railway	
35009	*Shaw Savill*	Southern	MN	4-6-2	Riley & Son, Heywood	
35010	*Blue Star*	Southern	MN	4-6-2	Colne Valley Railway	
35011	*General Steam Navigation*	Southern	MN	4-6-2	Sellinge (restoration)	
35018	*British India Line*	Southern	MN	4-6-2	WCRC Carnforth	
35022	*Holland America Line*	Southern	MN	4-6-2	Private at Bury	
35025	*Brocklebamk Line*	Southern	MN	4-6-2	Private at Sellindge	
35027	*Port Line*	Southern	MN	4-6-2	Private in Bury	
35028	*Clan Line*	Southern	MN	4-6-2	Stewarts Lane	
35029	*Ellerman Lines*	Southern	MN	4-6-2	National Railway Museum, York	
41241		LMS	Class 2	2-6-2T	Keighley & Worth Valley Railway	
41298		LMS	Class 2	2-6-2T	Isle of Wight Steam Railway	
41312		LMS	Class 2	2-6-2T	Mid-Hants Railway	
41313		LMS	Class 2	2-6-2T	Isle of Wight Steam Railway	
41708		LMS	1F	0-6-0T	Barrow Hill	
41966	*Thundersley*	LMS		4-4-2T	Bressingham	
42073		LMS		2-6-4T	Lakeside and Haverthwaite Railway	
42085		LMS		2-6-4T	Lakeside and Haverthwaite Railway	
42500		LMS		2-6-4T	National Railway Museum York	
42700		LMS	Crab	2-6-0	National Railway Museum York	
42765		LMS	Crab	2-6-0	East Lancashire Railway	
42859		LMS	Crab	2-6-0	RAF Binbrook	
42968		LMS	Crab	2-6-0	Severn Valley Railway	
43106		LMS	4MT	2-6-0	Severn Valley Railway	
43924		LMS	4F	0-6-0	Keighley & Worth Valley Railway	
44027		LMS	4F	0-6-0	Vale of Berkeley Railway	
44123		LMS	4F	0-6-0	Avon Valley Railway	
44422		LMS	4F	0-6-0	Churnet Valley Railway	
44767	*George Stephenson*	LMS	Black 5	4-6-0	WCRC Carnforth	
44806	*Kenneth Aldcroft*	LMS	Black 5	4-6-0	North Yorkshire Moors Railway	
44871	*Sovereign*	LMS	Black 5	4-6-0	East Lancashire Railway	
44901		LMS	Black 5	4-6-0	Vale of Berkeley Railway	
44932		LMS	Black 5	4-6-0	WCRC Carnforth	
45000		LMS	Black 5	4-6-0	National Railway Museum, Shildon	
45025		LMS	Black 5	4-6-0	Strathspey Railway as 5025	
45110	*RAF Biggin Hill*	LMS	Black 5	4-6-0	Severn Valley Railway	
45163		LMS	Black 5	4-6-0	Churnet Valley Railway	
45212		LMS	Black 5	4-6-0	Keighley & Worth Valley Railway	
45231	*The Sherwood Forester*	LMS	Black 5	4-6-0	Crewe LSL	
45293		LMS	Black 5	4-6-0	Churnet Valley Railway	
45305		LMS	Black 5	4-6-0	Great Central Railway	
45337		LMS	Black 5	4-6-0	East Lancashire Railway	
45379		LMS	Black 5	4-6-0	One:One Railway Museum, Margate	
45407	*Lancashire Fusilier*	LMS	Black 5	4-6-0	East Lancashire Railway	
45428	*Eric Treacy*	LMS	Black 5	4-6-0	North Yorkshire Moors Railway	
45491		LMS	Black 5	4-6-0	Great Central Railway	
45551	*The Unknown Warrior*	-	6P	4-6-0	Midland Railway Centre	Replica New Build
45593	*Kolhapur*	LMS	Jubilee	4-6-0	Tyseley Museum	
45596	*Bahamas*	LMS	Jubilee	4-6-0	Tyseley Museum	
45690	*Leander*	LMS	Jubilee	4-6-0	WCRC Carnforth	
45699	*Galatea*	LMS	Jubilee	4-6-0	WCRC Carnforth	
46100	*Royal Scot*	LMS	Royal Scot	4-6-0	WCRC Southall	
46115	*Scots Guardsman*	LMS	Royal Scot	4-6-0	WCRC Carnforth	
46201	*Princess Elizabeth*	LMS	Princess	4-6-2	WCRC Carnforth	
46203	*Princess Margaret Rose*	LMS	Princess	4-6-2	Midland Railway Centre	
46229	*Duchess of Hamilton*	LMS	Coronation	4-6-2	National Railway Museum	
46233	*Duchess of Sutherland*	LMS	Coronation	4-6-2	Midland Railway Centre	
46235	*City of Birmingham*	LMS	Coronation	4-6-2	Millenium Point, Birmingham	
46428		LMS	2MT	2-6-0	East Lancashire Railway	
46441		LMS	2MT	2-6-0	Lakeside & Haverthwaite Railway	

46443		LMS	2MT	2-6-0	Severn Valley Railway	
46447		LMS	2MT	2-6-0	East Somerset Railway	
46464		LMS	2MT	2-6-0	Strathspey Railway	
46512		LMS	2MT	2-6-0	Strathspey Railway	
46521		LMS	2MT	2-6-0	Great Central Railway	
47279		LMS	Jinty	0-6-0T	Keighley & Worth Valley Railway	
47298		LMS	Jinty	0-6-0T	East Lancashire Railway	
47324		LMS	Jinty	0-6-0T	East Lancashire Railway	
47327		LMS	Jinty	0-6-0T	Midland Railway Centre	
47357		LMS	Jinty	0-6-0T	Midland Railway Centre	
47383		LMS	Jinty	0-6-0T	Severn Valley Railway	
47406		LMS	Jinty	0-6-0T	Mountsorrel & Rothley Heritage Centre	
47445		LMS	Jinty	0-6-0T	Midland Railway Centre	
47493		LMS	Jinty	0-6-0T	Spa Valley Railway	
47564		LMS	Jinty	0-6-0T	Midland Railway Centre	
48151		LMS	8F	2-8-0	WCRC Carnforth	
48173		LMS	8F	2-8-0	Churnet Valley Railway	
48274		LMS	8F	2-8-0	Great Central Railway-Nottingham	Ex-Turkey
48305		LMS	8F	2-8-0	Great Central Railway	
48431		LMS	8F	2-8-0	Keighley & Worth Valley Railway	
48624		LMS	8F	2-8-0	Great Central Railway	
48773		LMS	8F	2-8-0	Severn Valley Railway	
49395		LMS	7F	0-8-0	National Railway Museum	
50621		LMS	LYR	2-4-2T	National Railway Museum	
51218		LMS	LYR	0-4-0ST	Keighley & Worth Valley Railway	
52044		LMS	LYR	0-6-0	Keighley & Worth Valley Railway	
52322		LMS	LYR	0-6-0	East Lancashire Railway	
53808		LMS	7F	2-8-0	Mid Hants Railway	Also No. 88
53809		LMS	7F	2-8-0	Midland Railway, Butterley	
55189		LMS		0-4-4T	Scottish Railway Pres Society	
57566		LMS		0-6-0	Strathspey Railway	
58850		LMS		0-6-0T	Barrow Hill	
58926		LMS		0-6-2T	Keighley & Worth Valley Railway	
60007	*Sir Nigel Gresley*	NER	A4	4-6-2	Loco Services Ltd, Crewe	
60008	*Dwight D Eisenhower*	NER	A4	4-6-2	Green Bay, Wisconsin, USA	
60009	*Union of South Africa*	NER	A4	4-6-2	Bury Transport Museum	
60010	*Dominion of Canada*	NER	A4	4-6-2	Canadian Railway Museum	
60019	*Bittern*	NER	A4	4-6-2	One:One Railway Museum, Margate	
60022	*Mallard*	NER	A4	4-6-2	National Railway Museum	
60103	*Flying Scotsman*	NER	A3	4-6-2	National Railway Museum	
60163	*Tornado*	-	A1	4-6-2	Great Central Railway	Replica New Build
60532	*Blue Peter*	NER	A2	4-6-2	LNWR Crewe	
60800	*Green Arrow*	NER	V2	2-6-2	Danum Gallery & Museum, Doncaster (part of National Collection) (as 4771)	
61264		NER	B1	4-6-0	North Yorkshire Moors Railway	
61306	*Mayflower*	NER	B1	4-6-0	LSL Southall	
61572		NER	B12	4-6-0	North Norfolk Railway	
61994	*Great Marquess*	NER	K4	2-6-0	Severn Valley Railway	
62005		NER	K1	2-6-0	West Coast Railway, Carnforth	
62277	*Gordon Highlander*	NER	D40	4-4-0	Glasgow Transport Museum	
62469	*Glen Douglas*	NER	D34	4-4-0	Scottish Railway Pres Society	
62660	*Butler Henderson*	NER	D11	4-4-0	NRM at Great Central Railway	
62712	*Morayshire*	NER	D49	4-4-0	Scottish Railway Pres Society	
62785		NER	E4	2-4-0	Bressingham	
63395		NER	Q6	0-8-0	North Yorkshire Moors Railway	
63460		NER	Q7	0-8-0	NRM at Darlington Museum	
63601		NER	O4	2-8-0	Great Central Railway	
65033		NER	J21	0-6-0	Loco Services, Loughborough	
65243	*Maude*	NER	J36	0-6-0	Scottish Railway Pres Society	
65462		NER	J15	0-6-0	North Norfolk Railway	
65567		NER	J17	0-6-0	NRM at Barrow Hill	
65894		NER	J27	0-6-0	North Yorkshire Moors Railway	
68011		NER	J94	0-6-0ST	In Belgium	
68030		NER	J94	0-6-0ST	Churnet Valley Railway	
68077		NER	J94	0-6-0ST	Spa Valley Railway	
68088		NER	Y7	0-4-0T	Great Central Railway	
68095		NER	Y9	0-4-0ST	Scottish Railway Pres Society	
68153		NER	Y1/2	4w	Middleton Railway	

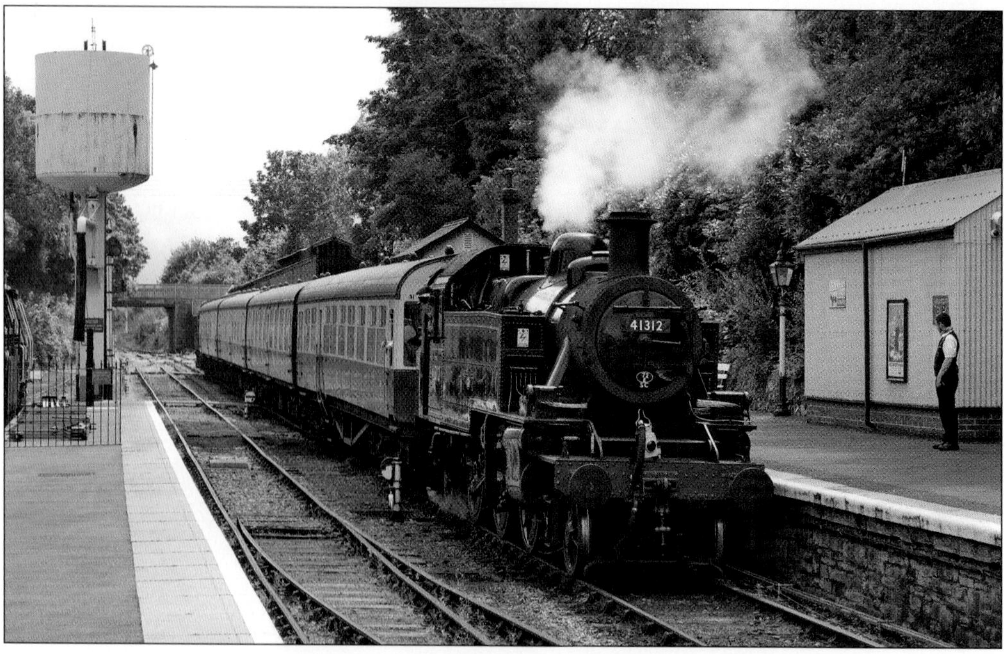

Although of LMS Ivatt design, Class 2 2-6-2T No. 41312, built in 1952 was a Southern Region loco all its life. It is now preserved on the Mid-Hants Railway. It is seen when visiting the Bodmin & Wenford Railway at Bodmin General in August 2021. **Antony Christie**

68633		NER	J69	0-6-0T	National Railway Museum	
68846		NER	J52	0-6-0ST	NRM at Great Central Railway	
69023		NER	J72	0-6-0T	Wensleydale Railway	
69523		NER	N2	0-6-2T	North Norfolk Railway	
69621		NER	N7	0-6-2T	East Anglian Railway Museum	
70000	*Britannia*	BR	Class 7	4-6-2	Crewe LSL	
70013	*Oliver Cromwell*	BR	Class 7	4-6-2	Great Central Railway	
71000	*Duke of Gloucester*	BR	Class 8	4-6-2	Tyseley Museum	
72010	*Hengist*	-	Class 6	4-6-2	CTL, Sheffield	Replica New Build
73050	*City of Peterborough*	BR	Class 5	4-6-0	Nene Valley Railway	
73082	*Camelot*	BR	Class 5	4-6-0	Bluebell Railway	
73096	*Merlin*	BR	Class 5	4-6-0	Mid-Hants Railway	
73129		BR	Class 5	4-6-0	Midland Railway Centre	
73156		BR	Class 5	4-6-0	Great Central Railway	
75014		BR	Class 4	4-6-0	Dartmouth Steam Railway	
75027		BR	Class 4	4-6-0	Bluebell Railway	
75029	*The Green Knight*	BR	Class 4	4-6-0	North Yorkshire Moors Railway	
75069		BR	Class 4	4-6-0	Severn Valley Railway	
75078		BR	Class 4	4-6-0	Keighley & Worth Valley Railway	
75079		BR	Class 4	4-6-0	Mid-Hants Railway	
76017		BR	Class 4	2-6-0	Mid-Hants Railway	
76077		BR	Class 4	2-6-0	Gloucestershire Warwickshire Railway	
76079		BR	Class 4	2-6-0	North Yorkshire Moors Railway	
76084		BR	Class 4	2-6-0	North Norfolk Railway	
78018		BR	Class 2	2-6-0	Great Central Railway	
78019		BR	Class 2	2-6-0	Great Central Railway	
78022		BR	Class 2	2-6-0	Keighley & Worth Valley Railway	
80002		BR	Class 4	2-6-4T	Keighley & Worth Valley Railway	
80064		BR	Class 4	2-6-4T	Bluebell Railway	
80072		BR	Class 4	2-6-4T	Llangollen Railway	
80078		BR	Class 4	2-6-4T	Mangapps Farm	
80079		BR	Class 4	2-6-4T	Severn Valley Railway	
80080		BR	Class 4	2-6-4T	Ecclesbourne Valley Railway	
80097		BR	Class 4	2-6-4T	East Lancashire Railway	
80098		BR	Class 4	2-6-4T	Midland Railway Centre	
80100		BR	Class 4	2-6-4T	Bluebell Railway	
80104		BR	Class 4	2-6-4T	Tyseley Works	
80105		BR	Class 4	2-6-4T	Scottish Railway Pres Society	
80135		BR	Class 4	2-6-4T	North Yorkshire Moors Railway	
80136		BR	Class 4	2-6-4T	North Yorkshire Moors Railway	
80150		BR	Class 4	2-6-4T	Mid-Hants Railway	
80151		BR	Class 4	2-6-4T	Bluebell Railway	
82045		-	Class 3	2-6-2T	Severn Valley Railway	Replica New Build
84030		-	Class 2	2-6-2T	Bluebell Railway	Replica New Built
90733		WD	WD	2-10-0	Keighley & Worth Valley Railway	
90775		WD	WD	2-10-0	North Norfolk Railway	Ex-Greece
92134		BR	9F	2-10-0	North Yorkshire Moors Railway	
92203	*Black Prince*	BR	9F	2-10-0	North Norfolk Railway	
92207		BR	9F	2-10-0	Shillingstone Station	
92212		BR	9F	2-10-0	Midland Railway Centre	
92214	*Lieicester City*	BR	9F	2-10-0	Great Central Railway	
92219		BR	9F	2-10-0	Private site near Tebay	
92220	*Evening Star*	BR	9F	2-10-0	National Railway Museum	
92240		BR	9F	2-10-0	Bluebell Railway	
92245		BR	9F	2-10-0	Barry Island Railway	

US Army Transportation Corps

No.		Type	Former Railway	Preservation Site
1631		S160	Hungarian Railways 411.388	Nottingham Transport Heritage Centre
2138		S160	Hungarian Railways 411.009	Nottingham Transport Heritage Centre
2253	*Omaha*	S160	Polish Railways Tr203.288	Dartmouth Steam Railway
2364		S160	Hungarian Railways 411.377	Nottingham Transport Heritage Centre (Frame only)
3278	*Franklin D. Roosevelt*	S160	Italian Railways 736.073	Churnet Valley Railway
5197		S160	Chinese Railways KD6-463	Churnet Valley Railway
5820		S160	Polish Railways Tr203.474	Keighley & Worth Valley Railway
6046		S160	Hungarian Railway 411.144	Churnet Valley Railway

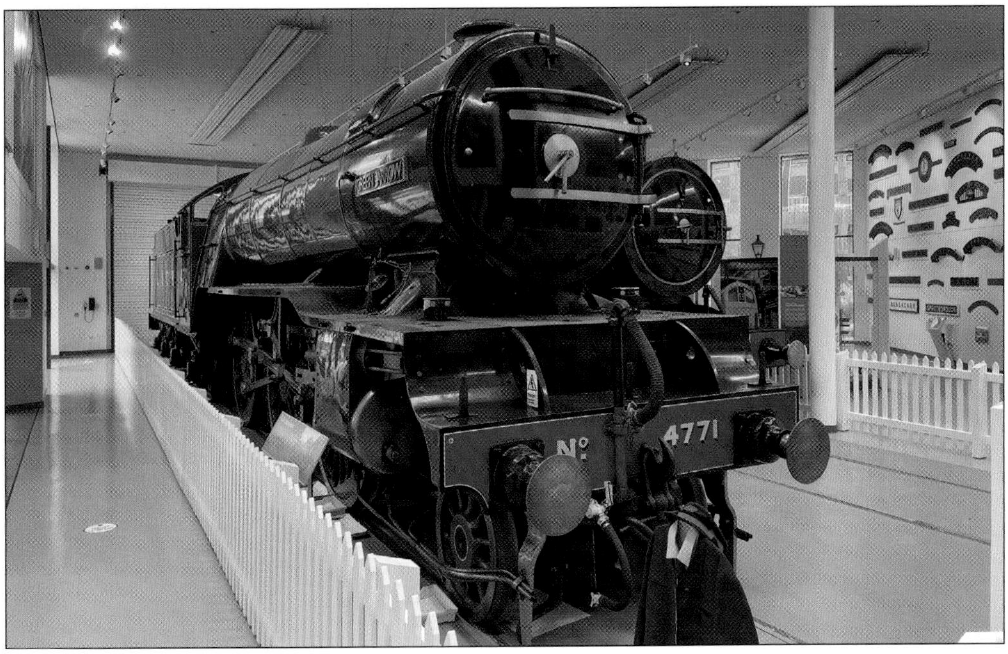

A new location for preserved steam locomotives is the Danum Gallery & Museum in the town centre of Doncaster, which is free to visit with the small railway collection on the lower floor. Locos 4771 Green Arrow *and North Eastern Railway No. 251 are seen on display on October 2021.* **CJM**

Replica Heritage Locomotives

Name	Type	Former Railway	Preserbation Site
Locomotion	0-4-0	Stockton & Darlington Railway	NRM, Shildon
Rocket	0-2-2	Liverpool & Manchester Railway	NRM, York (two locos)
Sans Pareil	0-4-0	Liverpool & Manchester Railway	NRM, Shildon
Planet	2-2-0	Liverpool & Manchester Railway	Science & Industry Museum, Manchester
Novelty	0-2-2WT	Braithwaite & Ericosson	Science & Industry Museum, Manchester
North Star	2-2-2	Great Western Railway	Steam Mueum, Swindon
Fire Fly	2-2-2	Great Western Railway	Didcot Railway Centre
Iron Duke	4-2-2	Great Western Railway	Didcot Railway Centre

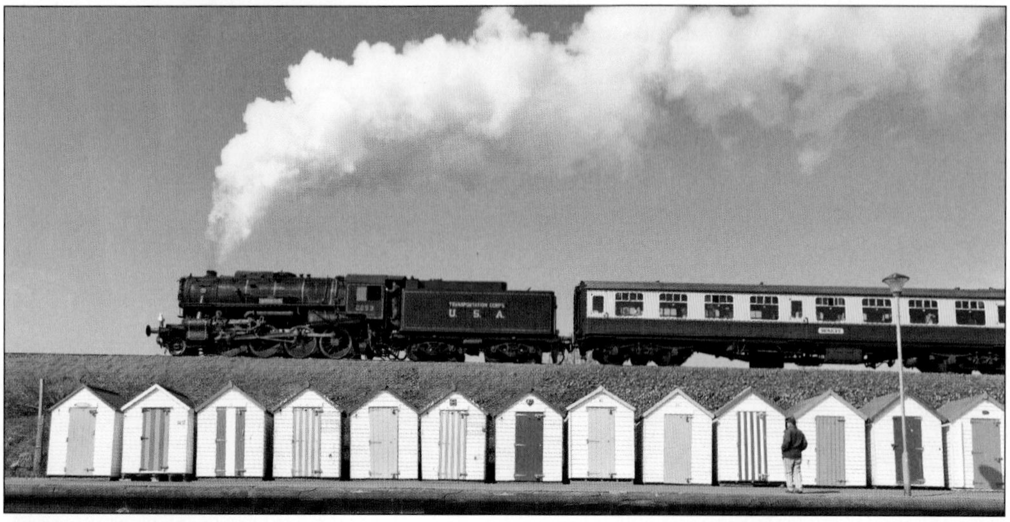

US Army Transportation Corps 2-8-0 No. 2253 Omaha, *a S160 loco is currently operating on the Dartmouth Steam Railway. This loco operated with Polish Railways as No. Tr203.288 before being moved to the UK for restoration. Eight examples of the S160 design are in the UK, but not all are operational. No. 2253 is seen climbing the bank between Goodrington and Churston on 27 April 2021.* **CJM**

Preserved Irish Locos (Standard Gauge)
Steam

Great Southern & Western Railway

No.	Name	Class	Arrangement	Location
36	-	23	2-2-2	Cork station
90	-	J30	0-6-0T	Sownpatrick & County Down Rly
184		J15	0-6-0	RPSI, Whitehead
186	-	J15	0-6-0	RPSI, Whitehead

Doublin & South Eastern Railway

15	-	K2	2-6-0	RPSI, Whitehead

Great Southern Railway

800	*Maedhbh*	B1a	4-6-0	NI Transport Museum, Cultra

LMS (Northern Counties Committee)

4	-	WT	2-6-4T	RPSI, Whitehead
74	*Dunluce Castle*	U2	4-4-0	NI Transport Museum, Cultra

Belfast & County Down Railway

30	-	1	4-4-2T	NI Transport Museum, Cultra

Sligo, Leitrim & Northern Counties Railway

27	*Lough Erne*	Z	0-6-4T	RPSI, Whitehead

GBR(I) & GNRB

85	*Merlin*	V	4-4-0	RPSI, Whitehead
93	*Sutton*	JT	2-4-2T	NI Transport Museum, Cultra
131	*Uranus*	Q	4-4-0	RPSI, Whitehead
171	*Slieve Gullion*	S	4-4-0	RPSI, Whitehead

Diesel

CIE / Irish Rail

No.		Class	Arrangement	Location
A3	003	A 001	A1A-A1A	West Clare Railway
A15	015	A 001	A1A-A1A	West Clare Railway
A39	039	A 001	A1A-A1A	Downpatric & County Down Railway
A55	055	A 001	A1A-A1A	Hell's Kitchen Museum, Castlerea
B103		B 101	A1A-A1A	Irish Traction Group, Carrick-on-Suir
B113	1100	C2a 113	Bo-Bo	NI Transport Museum, Cultra
C226	B226/226	C 201	Bo-Bo	Irish Traction Group, Carrick-on-Suir
C227	B227/106/202	C 201	Bo-Bo	Don Butler Ltd, Skeard
C231	B231/231	C 201	Bo-Bo	Downpatric & County Down Railway
E421	421	E 421	C	Downpatric & County Down Railway
E428	428	E 421	C	Dunsandle Station, Co Galway
E432	432	E 421	C	Downpatric & County Down Railway
G601		G 601	B	Irish Traction Group, Carrick-on-Suir
G611		G 611	B	Downpatric & County Down Railway
G613		G 611	B	Downpatric & County Down Railway
G616		G 611	B	Irish Traction Group, Carrick-on-Suir
G617		G 611	B	Downpatric & County Down Railway
B124	124	121	Bo-Bo	Irish Traction Group, West Clare Railway
B134	134	121	Bo-Bo	RPSI at Inchicore Works
B141	141	141	Bo-Bo	RPSI, Connolly Depot, Dublin
B142	142	141	Bo-Bo	RPSI, Whitehead
B146	146	141	Bo-Bo	Downpatric & County Down Railway
B152	152	141	Bo-Bo	Irish Traction Group, West Clare Railway
B175	175	141	Bo-Bo	RPSI, Connolly Depot, Dublin
B190	190	181	Bo-Bo	Irish Traction Group, West Clare Railway

Northern Ireland Railways

No.	Name	Class	Arrangement	Location
1, 5	-	1	0-6-0	Beaver Power, Merthyr Tydfil, Wales
102	*Falcon*	101	Bo-Bo	NI Transport Museum, Cultra

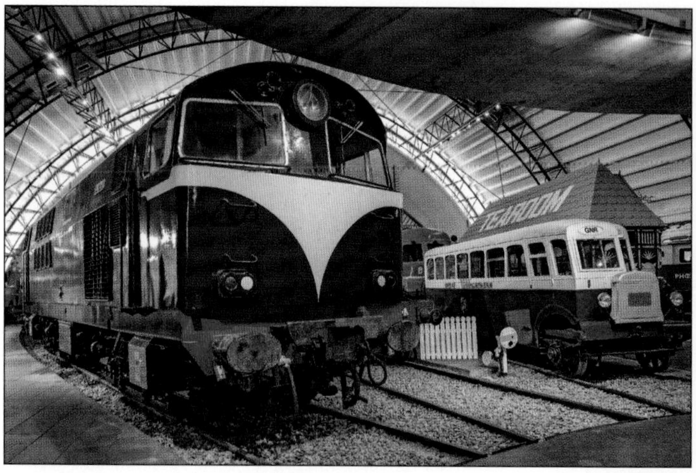

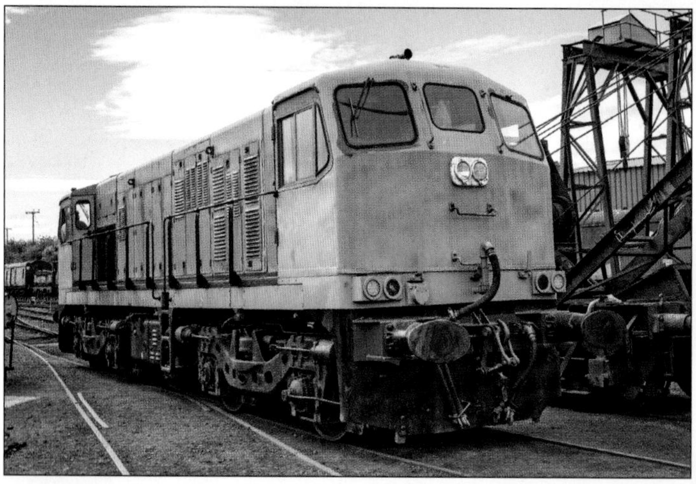

In the right upper image, the preserved Hunslet/BREL-Doncaster 1970s built 'Enterprise' Northern Ireland Railways diesel-electric loco No. 102 Falcon *is illustrated inside the main railway hall at the Northern Ireland Transport Museum at Cultra on 28 May 2022. This museum holds the vast majority of preserved Irish historic locos and trains and is well worth a visit.* **CJM**

On the right, Railway Preservation Society of Ireland General Motors Class 141 Bo-Bo No. 142 is seen at the groups Whitehead depot and workshop on 28 May 2022. The loco is currently receiving cosmetic attention, but is fully operational. The RPSI site at Whitehead is open to the public on selected days, check website for details. **CJM**

Preserved Railways and Museums

Aln Valley Railway	Aln Valley Railway Trust, Lionheart Railway Station, Lionheart Enterprose Park, Alnwick, Northumberland. NE66 6EZ
Appleby Frodingham Railway	Appleby Frodingham Railway, British Steel, Gate E, Brigg Road, Scunthorpe, Lincolnshire. DN16 1XA
Avon Valley Railway	Bitton Station, Bath Road, Bristol, South Gloucestershire. BS30 6HD
Barrow Hill Roundhouse	Barrow Hill Roundhouse, Campbell Drive, Barrow Hill, Chesterfield, Derbyshire. S43 2PR
Battlefield Line	Shackerstone Railway Society Ltd, Shackerstone Station, Shackerstone, Leicestershire. CV13 6NW
Beamish Museum & Railway Centre	Beamish Museum, Beamish, County Durham. DH9 0RG
Bideford Railway Heritage Centre	Bideford Railway Centre, Bideford Station, Bideford, Devon. EX39 4BB
Bluebell Railway	The Bluebell Railway, Sheffield Park Station, East Sussex. TN22 3QL
Bodmin & Wenford Railway	Bodmin & Wenford Railway, Bodmin General Station, Bodmin, Cornwall. PL31 1AQ
Bo'ness & Kinneil Railway	Bo'ness & Kinneil Railway, Bo'ness Station, Union St, Bo'ness. EH51 9AQ
Bressingham Steam & Gardens	Bressingham Steam & Gardens, Low Road, Bressingham, Diss, Norfolk. IP22 2AA
Bristol Harbour Railway	Bristol Harbour Railway, Wapping Road, Bristol. BS1 4RN
Buckinghamshire Railway Centre	Quainton Road Station, Station Road, Quainton, Aylesbury. HP22 4BY
Caledonian Railway	Caledonian Railway, The Station, Park Road, Brechin, Angus. DD9 7AF
Chasewater Railway	Chasewater Country Park, Brownhills West Station, Pool Lane, Burntwood, Staffordshire. WS8 7NL
Chinnor & Princes Risborough Railway	Chinnor & Princes Risborough Railway, Station Road, Chinnor, Oxfordshire. OX39 4ER
Churnet Valley Railway	Churnet Valley Railway, Consall Station, Consall, Leek, Staffordshire. ST13 7EE
Colne Valley Railway	Colne Valley Railway, Castle Hedingham, Halstead. CO9 3DZ
Crewe Heritage Centre	(The Railway Age) The Railway Age, Vernon Way, Crewe. CW1 2DB
Cultra Northern Ireland Museum	Cultra, Holywood, Northern Ireland. BT18 0EU
Dean Forest Railway	Dean Forest Railway, Forest Road, Lydney, Gloucestershire. GL15 4ET
Derwent Valley Light Railway	Derwent Valley Light Railway, Murton Park, Murton Lane, Murton, York. YO19 5UF
Didcot Railway Centre	Didcot Parkway railway station, Didcot, Oxfordshire. OX11 7NJ
East Anglian Railway Museum	East Anglian Railway Museum, Chappel Station, Colchester, Essex. CO6 2DS
East Kent Railway	East Kent Railway, Station Road, Shepherdswell, Dover. CT15 7PD
East Lancashire Railway	East Lancashire Railway, Bury Bolton Street Station, Bolton Street, Bury, Lancashire. BL9 0EY
East Somerset Railway	East Somerset Railway, Cranmore Railway Station, Cranmore, Shepton Mallet, Somerset. BA4 4QP
Ecclesbourne Valley Railway	Ecclesbourne Valley Railway, Wirksworth Station, Coldwell Street, Wirksworth, Derbyshire. DE4 4FB
Eden Valley Railway	Eden Valley Railway, Warcop Station, Warcop, Appleby, Cumbria. CA16 6PR
Elsecar Heritage Railway	Elsecar Heritage Railway, The Railway Office, Wath Road, Elsecar, Barnsley. S74 8HJ
Embsay and Bolton Abbey Steam Railway	Embsay Railway, Embsay Station, Embsay, Skipton, North Yorkshire. BD23 6QX
Epping Ongar Railway	Epping Ongar Railway, Ongar Station, Station Approach, Ongar, Essex. CM5 9BN
Foxfield Railway	Foxfield Railway, Foxfield Station, Caverswall Road, Blythe Bridge, Stoke-on-Trent. ST11 9BG
Glasgow Museum of Transport	(Riverside Museum) Riverside Museum, Pointhouse Place, Glasgow. G3 8RS
Gloucestershire Warwickshire Railway	Gloucestershire Warwickshire Railway, Railway Station, Toddington, Gloucestershire. GL54 5DT
Great Central Railway	Great Central Railway PLC, Loughborough Central Station, Great Central Road, Loughborough, Leicestershire. LE11 1RW
Great Central Railway (Nottingham)	Great Central Railway - Nottingham, Mere Way, Ruddington, Nottinghamshire. NG11 6JS
Gwili Railway	Gwili Railway, Bronwydd Arms Station, Carmarthen. SA33 6HT
Head of Steam, Darlington	Head of Steam - Darlington Railway Museum, Station Road, Darlington. DL3 6ST
Helston Railway	Helston Railway, Trevarno Farm, Prospidnick, Helston. TR13 0RY
Isle of Wight Steam Railway	Isle of Wight Steam Railway, The Railway Station, Havenstreet, Isle of Wight. PO33 4DS
Kent & East Sussex Railway	Kent & East Sussex Railway, Tenterden Town Station, Station Road, Tenterden, Kent. TN30 6HE
Keith & Dufftown Railway	Keith & Dufftown Railway, Dufftown Station, Dufftown, Banffshire. AB55 4BA
Keighley & Worth Valley Railway	Keighley & Worth Valley Railway, The Railway Station, Haworth, West Yorkshire. BD22 8NJ
Llangollen Railway	Llangollen Railway, The Station, Abbey Road, Llangollen, Denbighshire. LL20 8SN
Llanelli & Mynydd Mawr Railway	Llanelli & Mynydd Mawr Railway, Cynheidre, Llanelli, Carmarthenshire. SA15 5YF
Lavender Line	Lavender Line, Isfield Station, Isfield, Near Uckfield, East Sussex. TN22 5XB
Lakeside & Haverthwaite Railway	Lakeside & Haverthwaite Railway, Haverthwaite Station, Near Ulverston, Cumbria. LA12 8AL
Lincolnshire Wolds Railway	Lincolnshire Wolds Railway, Ludborough Station, Station Road, Ludborough, Lincolnshire. DN36 5SQ
Locomotion, Shildon	(National Railway Museum) Locomotion - NRM Dale Road Industrial Estate, Dale Road, Shildon, County Durham. DL4 2RE
London Transport Museum	Covent Garden Piazza, London. WC2E 7BB
London Transport Museum Depot	118-120 Gunnersbury Lane, Acton Town, London, W3 9BQ
Mangapps Railway Museum	Mangapps Railway Museum, Southminster Road, Burnham-on-Crouch, Essex. CM0 8QG
Middleton Railway	Middleton Railway Trust Ltd, The Station, Moor Road, Hunslet, Leeds. LS10 2JQ
Midland Railway Centre	Midland Railway, Butterley Station, Ripley, Derbyshire. DE5 3QZ
Mid Hants Railway	Mid Hants Railway, The Railway Station, Alresford, Hampshire. SO24 9JG
Mid-Norfolk Railway	Mid-Norfolk Railway, Dereham Station, Station Road, Norfolk. NR19 1DF
Mid Suffolk Light Railway	Mid-Suffolk Light Railway, Brockford Station, Wetheringsett, Stowmarket, Suffolk. IP14 5PW
Monkwearmouth Station Museum	Monkwearmouth Station Museum , North Bridge Street, Sunderland. SR5 1AP
National Railway Museum	National Railway Museum, Leeman Road, York. YO26 4XJ
Nene Valley Railway	Nene Valley Railway, Wansford Station, Stibbington, Peterborough. PE8 6LR
North Dorset Railway	Shillingstone Station, Station Road, Shillingstone, Blandford Forum, Dorset. DT11 0SA
North Norfolk Railway	North Norfolk Railway, Sheringham Station, Station Approach, Sheringham, Norfolk. NR26 8RA
North Tyneside Steam Railway	Stephenson Railway Museum, Middle Engine Lane, North Shields, Tyne and Wear. NE29 8DX
North Yorkshire Moors Railway	North Yorkshire Moors Railway, Pickering Station, Pickering, North Yorkshire. YO18 7AJ
Northampton & Lamport Railway	Northampton & Lamport Railway, Pitsford & Brampton Station, Pitsford Road, Chapel Brampton. NN6 8BA
Dartmouth Steam Railway	Dartmouth Steam Railway, Queens Park Station, Torbay Road, Paignton, Devon. TQ4 6AF
Peak Rail	Peak Rail, Matlock Station, Matlock, Derbyshire. DE4 3NA
Plym Valley Railway	Plym Valley Railway, Coypool Road, Plympton, Plymouth. PL7 4NW
Pontypool & Blaenavon Railway	Pontypool & Blaenavon Railway, Railway Station, Furnace sidings, Garn Yr Erw, Blaenavon. NP4 9SF
Railway Preservation Society Ireland	RPSI Whitehead Railway Museum, Castleview Road, Whitehead, Co. Antrim. BT38 9NA
Ribble Steam Railway	Ribble Steam Railway, Chain Caul Road, Preston, Lancashire. PR2 2PD
Rocks by Rail	(Rutland Railway Museum) Rocks by Rail, Ashwell Road, Cottesmore, Oakham, Leicestershire. LE15 7FF
Royal Deeside Railway	The Royal Deeside Railway, Milton of Crathes, Banchory, Aberdeenshire. AB31 5QH
Rushden Transport Museum	Rushden Transport Museum, Rushden Station, Station Approach, Rushden, Northamptonshire. NN10 0AW
Severn Valley Railway	Severn Valley Railway, Kidderminster Station, Kidderminster. DY10 1QR
Somerset & Dorset Railway	Somerset & Dorset Railway Heritage Trust, Midsomer Norton Station, Silver Street, Midsomer Norton. BA3 2EY
South Devon Railway	South Devon Railway, Buckfastleigh Station, Dartbridge Road, Buckfastleigh, Devon. TQ11 0DZ
Spa Valley Railway	Spa Valley Railway, Tunbridge Wells West Station, Royal Tunbridge Wells, Kent. TN2 5QY
Stainmore Railway	Stainmore Railway, Station Road, Kirkby Stephen, Cumbria. CA17 4LA
Steam – Museum of the GWR	Steam, Fire Fly Avenue, Swindon. SN2 2EY
Strathspey Railway	Strathspey Railway, Aviemore Station, Dalfaber Road, Aviemore, Invernessshire. PH22 1PY
Swanage Railway	Swanage Railway, Station House, Swanage, Dorset. BH19 1HB
Swindon & Cricklade Railway	Swindon & Cricklade Railway, Blunsdon Station, Tadpole Lane, Swindon. SN25 2DA
Tanfield Railway	Tanfield Railway, Marley Hill, Engine Shed, Old Marley Hill, Gateshead. NE16 5ET
Telford Steam Railway	Telford Steam Railway, The Old Loco Shed, Bridge Road, Horsehay, Telford, Shropshire. TF4 3UH
Tyseley Railway Centre	Vintage Trains, 670 Warwick Road, Tyseley, Birmingham. B11 2HL
Vale of Berkeley Railway Museum	Vale of Berkeley Railway, The Old Engine House, Dock Road, Sharpness, Gloucestershire. GL13 9UD
Weardale Railway	Weardale Railway, Stanhope Station, County Durham. DL13 2YS
Wensleydale Railway	(Auckland Project) Wensleydale Railway, Leases Road, Leeming Bar, North Yorkshire. DL7 9AR
West Somerset Railway	West Somerset Railway, The Railway Station, Minehead, Somerset. TA24 5BG
Yeovil Railway Centre	Yeovil Railway Centre, Yeovil Junction Station, Stoford, Yeovil, Somerset. BA22 9UU

Railway Operators (Passenger)

Avanti West Coast

Business:	National Rail Contract to 3/31
Owning Company:	First Group (70%), Trenitalia (30%)
Managing Director:	Phil Whittingham
Address:	North Wing Offices, Euston Station London. NW1 2HS
Phone:	0845 000 8000
E-mail:	Customer.Resolutions@avantiwestcoast.co.uk
Rolling Stock:	Class 221, 390

c2c

Business:	National Rail Contract to 11/29
Owning Company:	Trenitalia
Managing Director:	Rob Mullen
Address:	2nd Floor, Cutlers Court, 115 Houndsditch - London. EC3A 7BR
Phone:	03457 444422
E-mail:	contact@c2crail.co.uk
Rolling Stock:	Class 357, 387, 720

Caledonian Sleeper

Business:	Emergency Recovery Measures Agreements / franchise to 3/30
Owning Company:	Serco
Managing Director:	Kathryn Darbandi
Address:	1 Union Street, Inverness. IV1 1PP
Phone:	03300 600500
E-mail:	enquiry@sleeper.scot
Rolling Stock:	Mk5 stock

Chiltern Railways

Business:	National Rail Contract to 2027
Owning Company:	Arriva
Managing Director:	Richard Allan
Address:	Banbury ICC, Merton Street, Banbury. OX16 4RN
Phone:	03456 005165
E-mail:	customer.service@chilternrailways.co.uk
Rolling Stock:	Class 68, 165, 168, Mk3 stock

CrossCountry Trains

Business:	National Rail Contract to 10/23
Owning Company:	Arriva
Managing Director:	Tom Joyner
Address:	Cannon House, 18 The Priory Queensway, Birmingham. B4 6BS
Phone:	03447 369123
E-mail:	customer.relations@crosscountrytrains.co.uk
Rolling Stock:	Class 43, 170, 220, 221, Mk3 HST stock

East Midlands Railway

Business:	National Rail Contract to 3/22
Owning Company:	Abellio
Managing Director:	Will Rogers
Address:	Prospect House, 1 Prospect Place, Millennium Way, Pride Park, Derby. DE24 8HG
Phone:	03457 125678
E-mail:	contact@eastmidlandsrailway.co.uk
Rolling Stock:	Class 08, 156, 158, 180, 222, 360

Eurostar

Business:	Private Company
Owning Company:	Eurostar
CEO:	Jacques Damas
Address:	Times House, Bravingtons Walk, London. N1 9AW
Phone:	01777 777879
E-mail:	traveller.care@eurostar.com
Rolling Stock:	Class 08, 373, 374

Govia Thameslink Railway

Business:	National Rail Contract to 4/25
Owning Company:	Govia
CEO:	Angie Doll
Address:	Hertford House, 1 Cranwood Street, London. EC1V 9QS
Phone:	03451 272920
E-mail:	comments@southernrailway.com, customerservices@greatnorthernrail.com customerservices@thameslinkrailway.com
Rolling Stock:	Class 73, 171, 313, 377, 387, 700, 717

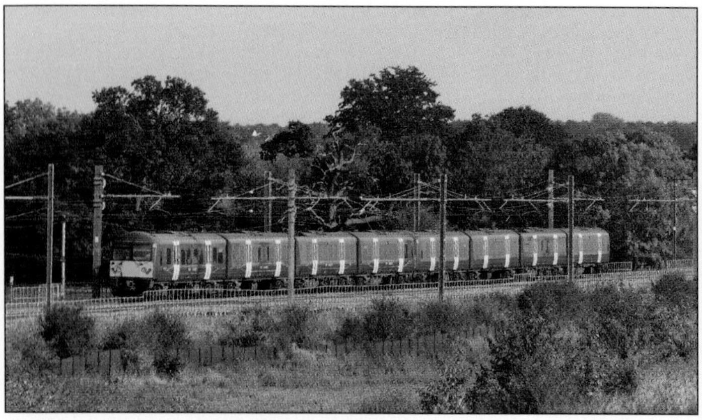

The Siemens 'Desiro' Class 360/1 fleet, introduced for use on Anglia outer-suburban routes have now transferred to East Midland Railway, following introduction of Class 720 stock on the Greater Anglia route. EMR deploy the sets on the EMR Connect route between ST Pancras International and Corby. Set No. 360110 passes Great Oakley near Corby on 11 October 2021 with the 10.15 St Pancras International to Corby. **CJM**

Grand Central

Business:	Open Access Operator, until December 2026
Owning Company:	Arriva
Managing Director:	Richard McClean
Address:	3rd Floor, Northern House, Rougier Street, York. YO1 6HZ
Phone:	03456 034852
E-mail:	customer.services@grandcentralrail.com
Rolling Stock:	Class 180

Great Western Railway

Business:	National Rail Contract to 3/23
Owning Company:	First Group
Managing Director:	Mark Hopwood
Address:	Milford House, 1 Milford Street, Swindon. SN1 1HL
Phone:	03457 000125
E-mail:	GWR.feedback@GWR.com
Rolling Stock:	Class 08, 43, 57, 150, 158, 165, 166, 387, 769, 800, 802, Mk3 stock

Greater Anglia

Business:	National Rail Contract to 10/25
Owning Company:	Abellio (60%), Mitsui (40%)
Managing Director:	Jamie Burles
Address:	The Hub, Colchester North Station, North Station Road, Colchester, Essex. C01 1JS
Phone:	03456 007245
E-mail:	contactcentre@greateranglia.co.uk
Rolling Stock:	Class 317, 321, 322, 720, 745, 755

Heathrow Express

Business:	Private company, operated by Great Western
Owning Company:	Heathrow
Managing Director:	Sophie Chapman
Address:	Compass Centre, Nelson Road, Hounslow. TW6 2GW
Phone:	03456 001515
E-mail:	queries@heathrowexpress.com
Rolling Stock:	Provided by GWR, Class 387

Hull Trains

Business:	Open Access Operator, until 12/29
Owning Company:	First Group
Managing Director:	Louise Cheeseman
Address:	4th Floor, Europa House, 184 Ferensway, Hull. HU1 3UT
Phone:	03450710222
E-mail:	customerservices.hull@firstgroup.com
Rolling Stock:	Class 802

London North Eastern Railway (LNER)

Business:	Operated by DfT (operator of last resort) 6/25
Owning Company:	DfT, UK Government
Managing Director:	David Horne
Address:	East Coast House, 25 Skeldergate, York, Y01 6DH
Phone:	03457 225333
E-mail:	customers@LNER.co.uk
Rolling Stock:	Class 91, 800, 801, Mk4 stock

London Overground

Business: Concession, operated by Arriva
Owning Company: Transport for London
Managing Director: Will Rogers
Address: 125 Finchley Road, Swiss Cottage, London. NW3 6HY
Phone: 03432 221234
E-mail: overgroundinfo@tfl.gov.uk

Rolling Stock: Class 09, 378, 710

Lumo

Business: Open Access Operator
Owning Company: First Group
Managing Director: Temp-Phil Cameron
Address: 4th Floor, Central Square South, Orchard Street, Newcastle-upon-Tyne. NE1 3PG
Phone: 0345 528 0409
E-mail: lumo.co.uk

Rolling Stock: Class 803

Merseyrail

Business: Local concession, due to end 19/7/28
Owning Company: Serco (50%), Abellio (50%)
Managing Director: Jan Chaudhry
Address: 9th Floor Rail House, Lord Nelson Street, Liverpool, L1 1JF
Phone: 0151 702 2534
E-mail: comment@merseyrail.org

Rolling Stock: Class 507, 508, 777

Northern

Business: Operated by DfT (operator of last resort 06/25)
Owning Company: DfT, UK Government
Managing Director: Nick Donovan
Address: Northern House, 9 Rougier Street, York. YO1 6HZ
Phone: 08002 006060
E-mail: enquiries@northernrailway.co.uk

Rolling Stock: Class 150, 155, 156, 158, 170, 195, 319, 323, 331, 333, (399), 769

ScotRail

Business: Operated by Scottish Government (Scottish Rail Holdings)
Owning Company: Scottish Government
Managing Director: Alex Haynes
Address: Atrium Court, 50 Waterloo Street, Glasgow. G2 6HQ
Phone: 03448 110141
E-mail: customer.relations@scotrail.co.uk

Rolling Stock: Class 43, 153, 156, 158, 170, 318, 320, 334, 380, 385, Mk3 stock

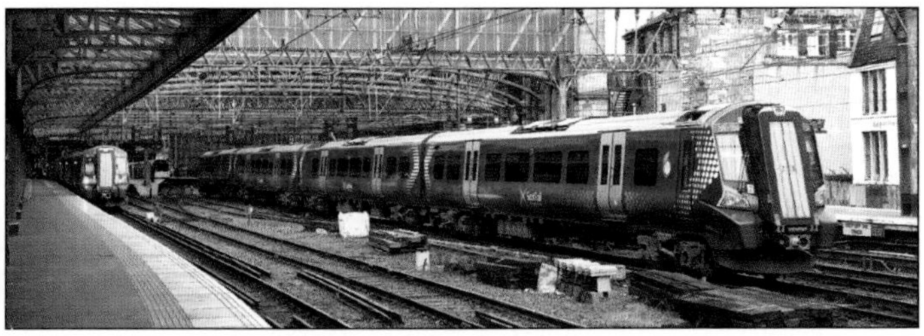

Four-car Class 380/1 No. 380108, one of a fleet of 38 main line Siemens 'Desiro' units operated by Scottish Railways is shown arriving at Glasgow Central in November 2021. **CJM**

South Eastern Trains

Business: Operated by DfT (operator of last resort)
Owning Company: DfT, UK Governmentt
Managing Director: Steve White
Address: Friars Bridge Court, 41-45 Blackfriars Road, London. SE1 8NZ
Phone: 03453 227021
E-mail: info@southeasterntrains.co.uk

Rolling Stock: Class 375, 376, 377, 395, 465, 466, 707

South Western Railway

Business: National Rail Contract to 4/23
Owning Company: First Group (70%), MTR (30%)
Managing Director: Claire Mann
Address: 4th Floor, South Bank Central, 30 Stamford Street, London SE1 9LQ
Phone: 03456 000650
E-mail: customerrelations@swrailway.com

Rolling Stock: Class 158, 159, 444, 450, 455, 458, 484, 701, 707

Transport for London (Elizabeth Line)

Business: Concession, operated by MTR Corporation
Owning Company: TfL
Managing Director: Nigel Holness
Address: 4th Floor, 14 Pier Walk, London. SE10 0ES
Phone: 03432 221234
E-mail: helpdesk@crossrail.co.uk

Rolling Stock: Class 345

Transport for Wales

Business: Welsh Government, Transport for Wales (operator of last resort)
Owning Company: Welsh Government
Managing Director: Kevin Thomas
Address: St Mary's House, 47 Penarth Road, Cardiff. CF10 5DJ
Phone: 03333 211202
E-mail: Via website - https://tfwrail.wales/contact-us

Rolling Stock: Class 67, 150, 153, 158, 170, 175, 230, 231, 756, 769, Mk 4 stock

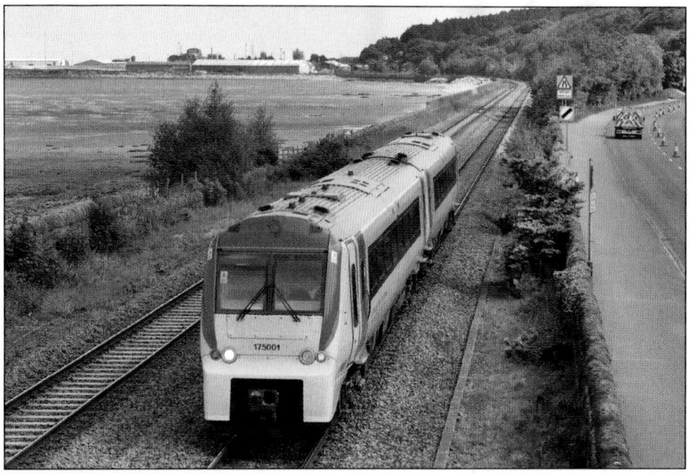

Currently Transport for Wales, operates a fleet of refurbished Class 175s on longer distance services, based at the Alstom-operated depot at Chester. Two-car set No. 175001 is seen on North Wales coast near Mostyn on 1 June 2021 with the 13.27 Shrewsbury to Holyhead service. **CJM**

TransPennine Express

Business: Direct Award Contract to mid 2031
Owning Company: First Group
Managing Director: Matthew Golton
Address: 7th Floor, Bridgewater House, 60 Whitworth Street, Manchester, M1 6LT
Phone: 03456 001671
E-mail: tpecustomer.relations@firstgroup.com

Rolling Stock: Class 68, 185, 397, 802, Mk5a stock

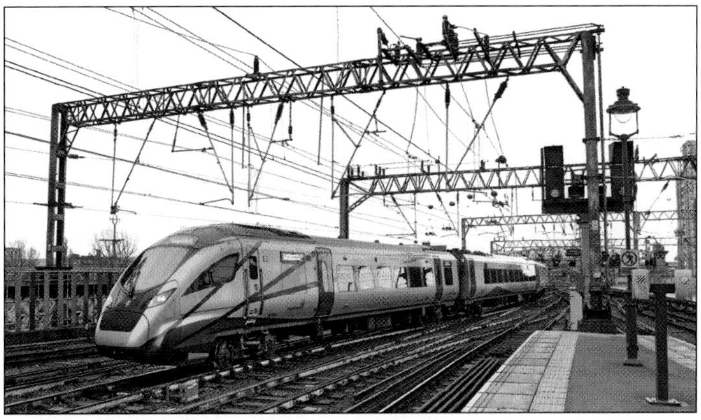

The streamlined CAF-built five-car Class 397 sets operated by TransPennine Express are usually deployed on West Coast Services to and from Glasgow and Edinburgh. The sets display the standard TPE livery without a yellow front end. Set No. 397004 is shown arriving at Glasgow Central on 11 November 2021. **CJM**

West Midlands Railway

Business: National Rail Contract to 3/26
Owning Company: Abellio (70%), East Japan Railway (15%), Mitsui (15%)
Managing Director: Ian McConnell
Address: 134 Edmund Street, Birmingham, West Midlands. B3 2ES
Phone: 03333 110039
E-mail: comments@westmidlandsrailway.co.uk

Rolling Stock: Class 08, 139, 170, 172, 196, 230, 323, 350

Railway Operators (Freight / Specialist)

Colas Rail Freight

Owning Company:	Colas
Managing Director:	Iain Anderson
Address:	25 Victoria Street, London, SW1H 0EX
Phone:	020 7593 5353
E-mail:	marketing@colasrail.com
Rolling Stock:	Class 37, 56, 66, 70, Hauled stock, Track Machines

DB-Cargo

Owning Company:	DB
Managing Director:	Andrea Rossi
Address:	Lakeside Business Park, Caroline Way, Doncaster. DN4 5PN
Phone:	0870 140 5000
E-mail:	info@dbcargo.com
Rolling Stock:	Class 58, 60, 66, 67, 90, 92, Hauled stock

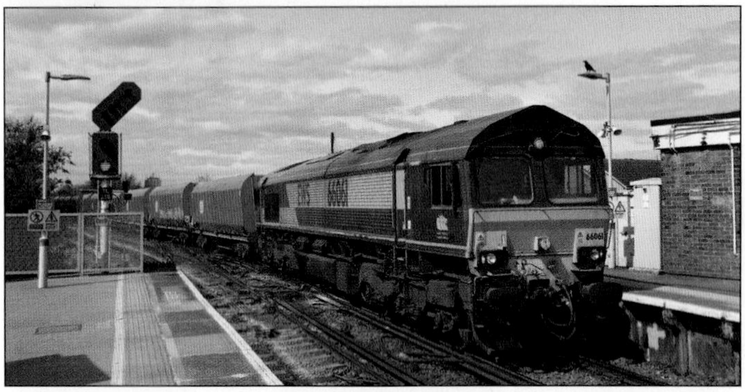

The DB Class 66/0 fleet currently carry a mix of EWS maroon and gold and the recent DB red livery. Still without DB branding on 8 April 2021, No. 66061 passes Lewisham with an aggregate train from. Paddington to Hither Green. CJM

Direct Rail Services (DRS)

Owning Company:	Nuclear Decommissioning Authority
Managing Director:	Chris Connelly
Address:	Kingmoor Depot, Etterby Road, Carlisle, Cumbria. CA3 9NZ
Phone:	01228 406600
E-mail:	info@directrailservices.com
Rolling Stock:	Class 37, 57, 66, 68, 88, Hauled stock

GB Railfreight (GBRf)

Owning Company:	GB Railfreight
Managing Director:	John Smith
Address:	15-25 Artillery Lane, London. E1 7HA
Phone:	0207 983 5177
E-mail:	gbrfinfo@gbrailfreight.com
Rolling Stock:	Class 08, 09, 18, 47, 50, 56, 59, 60, 66, 67, 69, 73, 92, Di8, Industrial

Freightliner

Owning Company:	Genesee & Wyoming Inc
CEO UK/Europe:	Eddie Austin
Address:	G&W UK, 3rd Floor, 90 Whitfield Street, London. W1T 4EZ
Phone:	03330 169545
E-mail:	press.office@freightliner.com
Rolling Stock:	Class 08, 47, 59, 66, 70, (86), 90, Industrial

Devon Cornwall Rail (DCR)

Owning Company:	Cappagh Group
Managing Director:	David Fletcher
Address:	DCRail, Days Space Business Centre, Litchurch Lane, Derby. DE24 8AA
Phone:	01332 977 008
E-mail:	dfletcher@cappagh.co.uk
Rolling Stock:	Class 56, 60

Loco Services Ltd (LSL)

Managing Director:	Tony Bush
Address:	Crewe Diesel Depot, off Nantwich Road, Crewe. CW2 6GT
Phone:	01270 256088
E-mail:	customerservices@lsltoc.co.uk
Rolling Stock:	Class 08, 20, 37, 40, 43, 47, 55, 60, 73, 86, 87, 89, 90, Hauled stock

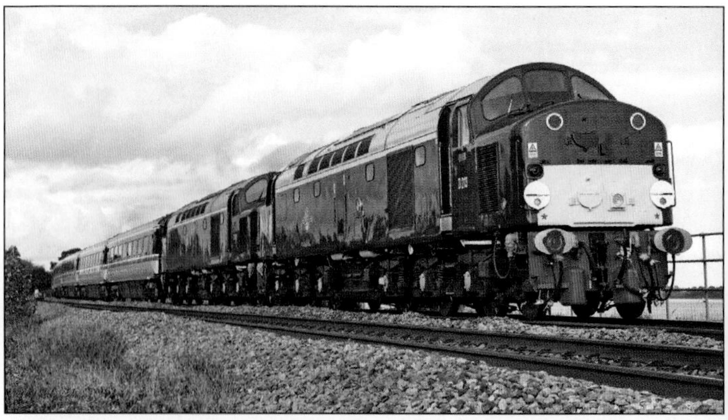

Loco Services Ltd, based at Crewe operate a well presented fleet of locos for charter and hire use. Green-liveried Class 40 No. D213 heads through Devon at Cockwood on 30 October 2021 with a charter from Preston to Plymouth, Class 40 Preservation Society No. D345 is coupled behind. CJM

Rail Operations Group (ROG)

Managing Director:	Karl Watts / David Burley
Address:	Wyvern House, Railway Terrace, Derby. DE1 2RU
Phone:	01332 343295
E-mail:	inforailopsgroup.co.uk
Rolling Stock:	Class 37, 43, 91, 319, 360, 769, Hauled stock

Riviera Trains

Address:	116 Ladbroke Grove, London, W10 5NE
Phone:	0207 727 4036
E-mail:	enquiries@riviera-trains.co.uk
Rolling Stock:	Hauled stock

Loram UK Ltd

Address:	Kelvin House, RTC Business Park, London Road, Derby. DE24 8UP
Phone:	01332 293035
E-mail:	commercial@loram.co.uk
Rolling Stock:	Class 20, 950, Hauled stock, Track machines

Network Rail

Chief Executive:	Andrew Haines OBE
Address:	1 Eversholt Street, London NW1 2DN
Phone:	0207 557 8000
Website:	www.networkrail.co.uk

Network Rail operate a sizable fleet of locos and ex passenger vehicles forming test trains. The Overhead Line Inspection Coach, No. 975091 is shown. This ex-BCK was previously known as test car Mentor - Mobile Electronic Network Testing & Observation Recorder. CJM

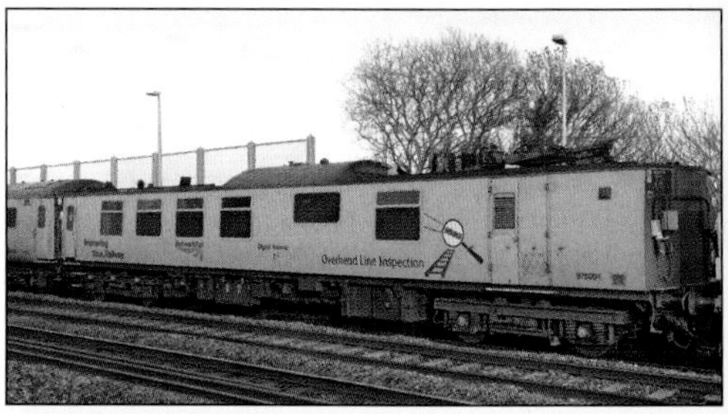

Irish Rail

Chief Executive:	Jim Meade
Address:	Iarnród Éireann HQ, Connolly Station, Amien Street, Dublin 1, D01 V6V6
Phone:	00 353 1 836 6222
Website:	www.irishrail.ie

Northern Ireland Railways

General Manager:	Richard Knox
Address:	Translink Contact Centre, Falcon Road, Belfast, BT126PU
Phone:	02890 666630
E-mail:	feedback@translink.co.uk

Isle of Man Railways

Address:	Transport Headquarters, Banks Circus, Douglas, Isle of Man. IM1 5PT
Website:	www.rail.im
E-mail:	publictransport@gov.im

Railway Operators (Light Rail)

London Underground

Managing Director: Andy Lord
Address: Floor 11, Windsor House, 50 Victoria Street, London. SW1H 0TL
Phone: 08456 044141
E-mail: customerservice@tfl.gov.uk

Rolling Stock: Tube and Surface vehicles

Docklands Light Railway

Managing Director: Gareth Powell
Address: 4th Floor, 14 Pier Walk, London. SE10 0ES
Phone: 034322 21234
E-mail: customerservice@tfl.gov.uk

Rolling Stock: DLR fleet

Croydon Tramlink

Operator: First Group
Managing Director: John Rymer
Address: 4th Floor, 14 Pier Walk, London. SE10 0ES
Phone: 03432 221234
E-mail: customerservice@tfl.gov.uk

Rolling Stock: Tramlink fleet

Edinburgh Tramway

Operator: Transport for Edinburgh
Managing Director: Lea Harrison
Address: Customer Relations, 1 Myreton Drive, Edinburgh. EH12 9GF
Phone: 0131 338 5780
E-mail: customer@edinburghtrams.com

Rolling Stock: Edinburgh Tram fleet

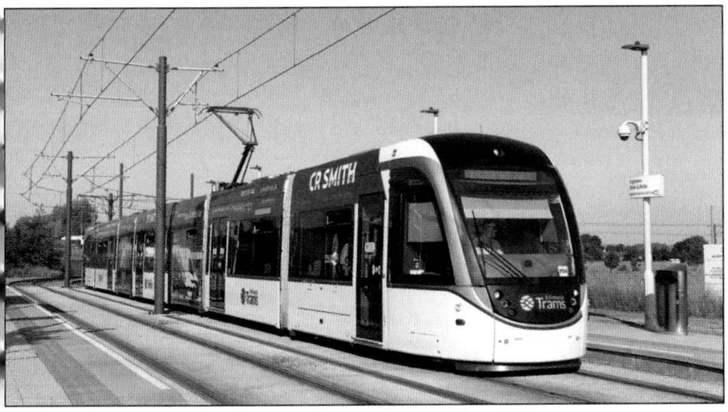

The Edinburgh Tramway system which currently operates between Edinburgh Airport and Edinburgh City Centre, has quickly become a norm for local travel. The system will soon be extended. CAF Urbos-3 7-section tram No. 259 is seen arriving at Ingliston Park & Ride. **CJM**

Blackpool Trams

Operator: Blackpool Council
Managing Director: Jane Cole
Address: Rigby Road, Blackpool, Lancashire. FY1 5DD
Phone: 01253 473001
E-mail: enquiries@blackpooltransport.com

Rolling Stock: Blackpool Tram fleet

Glasgow Subway

Operator: Strathclyde Passenger Transport
Managing Director: Antony Smith
Address: Consort House, 12 West George Street, Glasgow. G2 1HN
Phone: 0141 332 6811
E-mail: enquiry@spt.co.uk

Rolling Stock: Glasgow Underground fleets

Manchester Metrolink

Operator: Keolis/Amey
Managing Director: Danny Vaughan
Address: Trafford Depot, Warwick Road South, Stretford, Manchester. M16 0GZ
Phone: 0161 205 2000
E-mail: customerservices@metrolink.co.uk

Rolling Stock: Manchester Tram fleet

West Midlands Metro

Operator: Transport for West Midlands
Managing Director: Laura Shoaf
Address: Potters Lane, Wednesbury. WS10 0AR
Phone: 0345 835 8181
E-mail: customerservices@westmidlandsmetro.com

Rolling Stock: West Midlands Tram fleet

The expanding West Midlands Metro system operates a fleet of CAF-Urbos 3 five-section trams. No. 21 is seen arriving at The Hawthorns with a service from Wolverhampton to central Birmingham. **CJM**

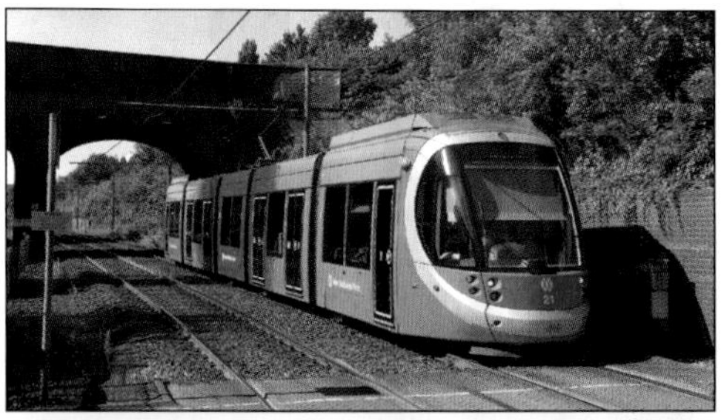

Nottingham Express Transit

Operator: Tramlink Nottingham Ltd
Managing Director: Paul Robinson
Address: Queens Chambers, King Street, Nottingham. NG1 2BH
Phone: 0115 824 6060
E-mail: info@thetram.net

Rolling Stock: Nottingham Tram fleets

South Yorkshire Super Tram

Operator: Stagecoach
Managing Director: Tim Bilby
Address: Nunnery Depot, Woodburn Road, Sheffield. S9 3LS
Phone: 0114 272 8282
E-mail: enquiries@supertram.com

Rolling Stock: Sheffield Tram fleet and Class 399

Tyne & Wear Metro

Operator: Tyne and Wear Passenger Transport Executive
Managing Director: Martin Kearney
Address: Station Road, Gosforth, Newcastle upon Tyne
Phone: 0191 20 20 747
E-mail: contactmetro@nexus.org.uk

Rolling Stock: Tyne & Wear Tram fleet

Great Orme Tramway

Operator: Conwy County Borough Council
Address: Victoria Station, Church Walks, Llandudno, North Wales, LL30 2NB
Phone: 01492 577877
E-mail: tramwayenquiries@conwy.gov.uk

Rolling Stock: Great Orme Tram fleets

Hythe Pier Tramway

Operator: Blue Funnel Ferries Ltd
Address: The Pier, Prospect Place, Hythe, Southampton. SO45 6AU
Phone: 02380 840722
E-mail: ticketoffice@hytheferry.co.uk

Rolling Stock: Hythe Pier Stock

Southend Pier Tramway

Operator: Southend Council
Address: Western Esplanade, Southend-on-Sea. SS1 2EL
Phone: 01702 611214
E-mail: council@southend.gov.uk

Rolling Stock: Southend Pier Stock

Volks Electric Railway

Operator: City of Brighton and Hove
Address: 285 Madeira Drive, Brighton. BN2 1EN
Phone: 01273 292718
E-mail: via website - www.volkselectricrailway.co.uk

Rolling Stock: Volks Electric Fleet

Livery Codes

ADV	Advertising/promotional livery
AFG	Arlington Fleet Group, green
AGI	Aggregate Industries green/silver/blue
ALS	Alstom
ANG	Anglia turquoise
ASB	Abellio Scottish Railways with pictograms branding
ASR	Abellio Scottish Railways blue
ATC	Arriva Train Care turquoise
ATT	Arriva Trains Wales unbranded turquoise
ATW	Arriva Trains Wales turquoise
AWC	Avanti West Coast white/branded Avanti West Coast, green cab sides
AWW	White, de-branded Virgin West Coast, Avanti
AWF	Anglia white with Freightliner brand
AWT	Anglia white, Greater Anglia branding
AXC	Arriva CrossCountry silver/dark crimson
BLG	BR blue/grey
BLK	Black
BLL	Blue Large Logo
BLP	Blue (Midland) Pullman Nankin blue
BLU	Blue
BOM	Bombardier Transportation
CAL	Caledonian Sleeper
CAR	Carmine and cream
C2C	c2c Railway, white with blue doors
CHC	Chocolate and cream
COL	Colas Rail Freight yellow/orange/black
COR	Corus Steel silver
COT	Cotswold Rail silver
CRG	Chiltern Railways two tone grey
CRW	Chiltern Railways white/blue
DBC	Deutsche Bahn red/grey
DBS	Deutsche Bahn Schenker red/grey
DCR	Devon Cornwall Railway grey
DRA	Direct Rail Services mid blue with simplified branding
DRC	Direct Rail Services blue with compass branding
DRS	Direct Rail Services blue
ELZ	Elizabeth Line CrossRail white/mauve
EMI	East Midlands Railway white/aubergine
EMR	East Midlands Railway blue
EMP	East Midlands Railway all over aubergine
EPG	European Passenger Services grey
EPX	Europhoenix grey/silver/red
EUB	Eurostar, blue/grey
EUS	Eurostar white/yellow
EWD	As EWS with DRS branding
EWE	Silver with DB branding
EWS	Maroon and gold
FEC	First East Coast blue
FER	Fertis Rail. grey
FGB	First Group blue, with pink doors
FHT	First Hull Trains blue, pictogram branding
FLP	Freightliner Powerhaul green/yellow
FLR	Freightliner green/yellow
FNA	First blue, Greater Anglia branding
FNO	First blue, no branding
FSL	Fastline Freight grey
FSR	First ScotRail
FTN	First Trans Pennine silver, blue and mauve
GAR	Greater Anglia white with red doors
GAT	Gatwick Express red
GAZ	Greater Anglia Retanus white/grey/red
GBC	GB Railfreight/Trainload Construction
GBB	GB Railfreight blue
GBN	GB Railfreight blue, revised cab sides
GBR	GB Railfreight blue/orange
GBS	GB Railfreight with speed whiskers
GEM	Gemini Rail Blue/white
GNH	GBRf with National Health Service branding
GOV	Govia, white with green doors
GRN	Green
GRY	Grey
GSW	Great Scottish & Western maroon/gold
GTO	Grand Central black/orange
GWF	Genesee & Wyoming Freightliner orange/black
GWG	Great Western Railway green
GWR	Great Western Railway green historic colours
HAN	Hanson Aggregate blue
HEC	Heathrow Connect
HEL	Heathrow Connect Link
HEX	Heathrow Express/GW grey
HNR	Harry Needle Railroad yellow
HRA	Hanson & Hall / RailAdventure
HS1	High Speed 1 blue, South Eastern
HSB	HSBC blue/cream
HUN	Hunslet blue/orange
ICS	InterCity Swallow
LEM	As LNE with East Midland Railway branding
LHL	Loadhaul black/orange
LMI	London Midland green/grey
LMT	Ex Thameslink white with WMR branding
LNE	LNER red/white
LNN	LNER red with Network Rail badge
LNR	LNER red, white
LNW	London Northwestern Railway, grey, two-tone green
LOG	London Overground white/blue
LON	London Overground revised black/grey/blue
LOM	Loram grey
LUL	London Transport/Underground maroon or white
MAR	Maroon
MEN	Mendip Rail blue
MEY	Merseyrail grey/yellow
MEZ	Merseyrail black/yellow, Class 777
MGR	Meridian-Generic Rail blue
MIM	Maritime Freight blue, DB branding
MSC	Mediterranean Shipping Co with GBRf branding
NBL	Northern Belle blue/cream
NNE	Northern Rail white/blue EMR decals
NNR	Northern Rail white/blue
NOR	Northern Railways blue, unbranded
NRL	Network Rail yellow
NSE	Network SouthEast blue/grey/red/white
NXU	Ex National Express white/grey, Greater Anglia
ONE	ONE pink, grey with Freightliner branding
ORI	Rail Operations Group Orion blue
PIT	Pitstop black
PTR	Porterbrook white/mauve
PUL	Pullman umber/cream
RCG	Rail Charter Services green/white
RCS	Rail Charter Services white/grey

By far the most supportive rail company in terms of rail enthusiasts and photographers is GB Railfreight, who, so far, have applied a different livery to each of the delivered Class 69s. In February 2022 No. 69004 emerged from the paint shop at Arlington Fleet Services at Eastleigh, displaying a version of BR Research blue and red livery, with a large bodyside GBRf badge, a BR double arrow logo, GB Railfreight branding and the legend on the bodyside reading 'GBRf NR Research Department Rail Innovation and Development Centre Old Dalby' The loco is captured at Tonbridge yard on 22 February 2022, before entering service. **Spencer Conquest**

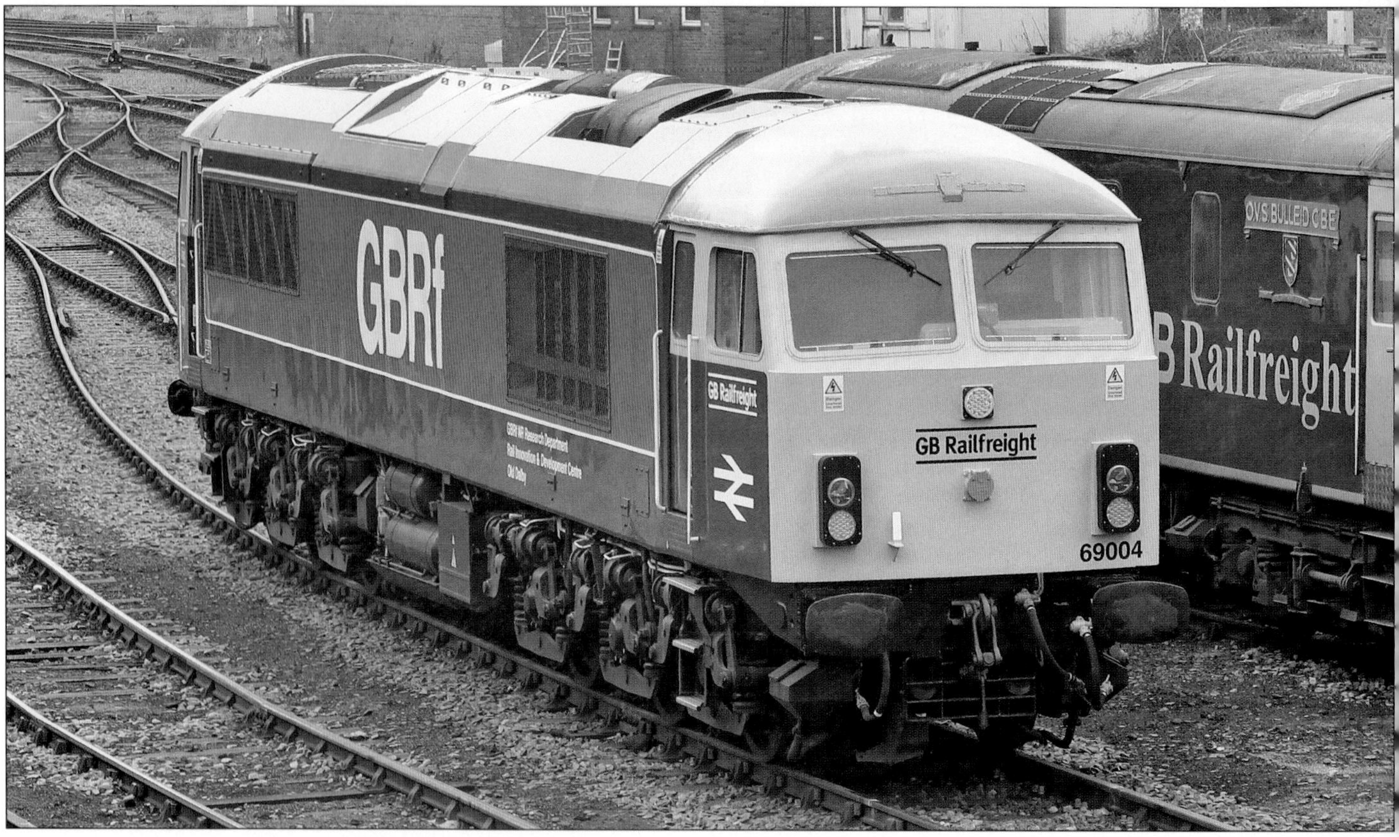

RED	Unbranded ex DB red
REG	Regional Railways blue/grey
RES	Rail express systems red/grey
RFE	Railfreight grey with EWS branding
RFD	Railfreight Distribution grey
RIV	Riviera blue
RMR	Royal Mail red
RMS	RMS Locotech Blue/grey
ROG	Rail Operations Group blue
ROJ	Royal Jubilee silver
ROS	Royal Scotsman/GBRf maroon & gold
ROY	Royal Train claret, DB branding
RSS	Railway Supply Services dark grey
RTC	Railway Technical Centre red/blue
S7C	Scotrail Inter7City grey/blue
SEB	South Eastern blue
SET	South Eastern white/grey/blue
SCE	Stagecoach blue/red with EMR brand
SCI	ScotRail grey/white, blue band
SCR	ScotRail/Scottish Railways blue/white
SCS	Scottish Caledonian Sleeper teal green
SOU	Southern white/green
SPL	Special livery scheme
SRB	ScotRail blue
SST	Sheffield Super Tram blue
SWI	South West Railway Island Line
SWS	South Western Railway red, swirl ends
SWR	SWR dark blue, grey, lemon ends
SWN	South Western Railway white/swirl ends
SWO	South Western Railway blue, swirl ends
TAT	Tata Steel silver
TFG	Trainload Freight grey
TFW	Transport for Wales white/red
TMK	Thameslink, grey/white light blue doors
VIR	Virgin Trains red
VIV	Vivarail white with branding
WAB	Wabtec black
WCE	West Coast Railway maroon
WMG	West Midlands Railway green/white
WMR	West Midlands Railway mauve/gold
WMT	West Midland Railway white/gold
YEL	Yellow

Owner Codes

AFG	Arlington Fleet Group
AGT	Agility Trains
AKI	Akiem Rail
ANG	Angel Trains Leasing
ATR	Arriva Trains (DB)
BAA	British Airports Authority
BEL	Belmond Pullman
BEA	Beacon Rail
BRO	Brodie Engineering
BRE	Boden Rail Engineering
BR8	BR Class 8 Steam Loco Trust
C2L	Class 20 Locomotives
CAL	Caledonian Rail Leasing
CAP	Cappaga Group
CBR	CB Rail
CLT	Cross London Trains
COL	Colas Rail Freight
COR	Corlink Rail
CRS	Continental Railway Services
D05	D05 Preservation Group
DAS	Data Acquisition and Testing Services
DBC	Deutsche Bahn Cargo UK
DCR	Devon Cornwall Railway
DRS	Direct Rail Services
EEP	English Electric Preservation
EMD	Electro-Motive Diesels
EMR	East Midlands Railway
EMS	Ed Murray & Sons
ERS	Eastern Rail Services
EPX	Europhoenix
EUS	Eurostar UK
EVL	Eversholt Leasing
FGP	First Group
FLR	Freightliner (Genesee & Wyoming)
GBR	GB Railfreight (GBRf)
GSW	Great Scottish & Western Railway
HAN	Hanson
HNR	Harry Needle Railroad Co
HRA	Hanson & Hall / RailAdventure
LIV	Liverpool Authority
LOG	London Overground
LOM	Lombard Finance
LSL	Locomotive Services Limited
MGR	Meridian-Generic Rail
MRC	Midland Railway Centre
MON	Michael Owen
NEM	Nemesis Rail
NRL	Network Rail Ltd
NYM	North Yorkshire Moors Railway
PMO	Pre Metro Operations
PRI	Private
PRO	Progress Rail
PTR	Porterbrook Leasing
QWR	QW Rail Leasing
RAM	Rampart Engineering
RFL	Rail for London
ROG	Rail Operations Group
ROK	Rock Rail
RIV	Riviera Trains
RML	Royal Mail Ltd
RMS	Rail Management Services/Locotec
S4G	Stratford 47 Group
SMB	SMB/Equitix Leasing
SNF	SNCF French Railways
SRP	Scottish Rail Preservation
SST	Sheffield Super Tram
TFL	Train Fleet (2019) Ltd [DfT]
TFW	Transport for Wales
TTS	Transmart Trains
URL	UK Rail Leasing
VIN	Vintage Trains
VIV	Vivarail
WCR	West Coast Railway Co
WMR	West Midlands Railway
189	Class 20189 Ltd
37G	Scottish 37 Group
3RL	345 Rail Leasing
50A	Class 50 Alliance
56G	Class 56 Group
71A	71A Locomotives Ltd

Operator Codes

50A	Class 50 Alliance
ABC	ABC Electrification
AFS	Arlington Fleet Services
ASR	Abellio Scottish Railways
AWC	Avanti West Coast
AXC	Arriva Cross Country
BAB	Babcock Rail
BAL	Balfour Beatty
BEL	Belmond Pullman
BOD	Boden Rail
BRO	Brodie Rail Engineering
C2C	c2c Railway
COL	Colas Rail Freight
CRW	Chiltern Railways
DAS	Data Acquisition and Testing Services
DBC	Deutsche Bahn Cargo
DB-F	Deutsche Bahn in France
DB-P	Deutsche Bahn in Poland
DCR	Devon Cornwall Railways
DRS	Direct Rail Services
ELZ	Elizabeth Line
EMR	East Midland Railway
EPX	Europhoenix
ERS	Eastern Rail Services
EUR	Eurotunnel
EUS	Eurostar
FHT	First Hull Trains
FLR	Freightliner
GAR	Greater Anglia Railway
GBR	GB Railfreight
GTL	Grand Central Railway
GTR	Govia Thameslink Railway
GWR	Great Western Railway
HAN	Hanson
HER	Hersco Rail Technology
HNR	Harry Needle Railroad Co
HRA	Hanson & Hall / RailAdventure
LNE	London North Eastern Railway
LOG	London Overground
LOR	Loram Rail
LSL	Loco Services Ltd
MER	Merseyrail
MGR	Meridian-Generic Rail
NOR	Northern Rail
NRL	Network Rail
NYM	North Yorkshire Moors Railway
OLS	Off lease
RAC	Rail Vac
RIV	Riviera Trains
RMS	Rail Management Services/Locotec
ROG	Rail Operations Group
S4G	Stratford 47 Group
SBR	Swietelsky Baugesellschaft/Babcock
SCS	Caledonian Sleepers
SET	South Eastern Trains
SH	Spot Hire
SRP	Scottish Rail Preservation
SST	Sheffield Super Tram
SWR	South Western Railway
TFW	Transport for Wales
TPE	TransPennine Express
URL	UK Rail Leasing
VIV	Vivarail
VRL	Volker Rail Ltd
VTN	Vintage Trains
WAB	Wabtec
WCR	West Coast Railway Co
WMR	West Midland Railways
(S)	Stored

Pool Codes

AWCA	West Coast Railway locos operational
AWCX	West Coast Railway locos stored
CFOL	Class 50 locos operational
COFS	Colas Rail Class 56
COLO	Colas Rail Class 66 and Class 70
COTS	Colas Rail Class 37 and Class 67
DCRO	Devon Cornwall Rail Class 56
DCRS	Devon Cornwall Rail Class 60
DFGI	Freightliner Class 70
DFHG	Freightliner Class 59
DFHH	Freightliner Class 66/6
DFIM	Freightliner Class 66/5
DFIN	Freightliner Class 66 low emission
DFLC	Freightliner Class 90
DFLH	Freightliner Class 47
DFLS	Freightliner Class 08
DHLT	Freightliner locos not in traffic
EFOO	Great Western Class 57
EFPC	Great Western Class 43
EFSH	Great Western Class 08
EJLO	West Midlands Railway Class 08
EMPC	East Midlands Railway Class 43
EMSL	East Midland Railway Class 08
EPEX	Europhoenix traction for export
EPUK	Europhoenix locos operational
ERSL	Eastern Rail Services Locomotives
EROG	DATS/Rail Operations Group testing
GBBT	GB Railfreight Class 66 extended tanks
GBCS	GB Railfreight Class 73/9 Caledonian Sleeper
GBCT	GB Railfreight Class 92 Channel Tunnel use
GBDF	GB Railfreight Class 47
GBEB	GB Railfreight Class 66 ex-Europe large tanks
GBED	GB Railfreight Class 73
GBEL	GB Railfreight Class 66 reduced fuel capacity

GBFM	GB Railfreight Class 66 fitted with RETB
GBGD	GB Railfreight Class 56 operational
GBGS	GB Railfreight Class 56 stored
GBHH	GB Railfreight Class 66 low gear 65mph
GBKP	GB Railfreight Class 67
GBLT	GB Railfreight Class 66 reduced fuel capacity
GBNB	GB Railfreight Class 66
GBNR	GB Railfreight Class 73/9 Network Rail
GBOB	GB Railfreight Class 66 ex DB-C with combination couplers
GBRT	GB Railfreight locos with restricted use
GBSD	GB Railfreight stored locos
GBSL	GB Railfreight Class 92 Caledonian Sleeper
GBTG	GB Railfreight Class 60
GBWM	GB Railfreight Class 08 and Class 09
GBYH	GB Railfreight Class 59
GPSS	Eurostar UK Class 08
GBST	GB Railfreight Class 92 Caledonian Sleeper & Channel Tunnel
GROG	Rail Operations Group, active locos
HAPC	Abellio ScotRail Class 43
HHPC	Hanson & Hall Class 43
HNRL	Harry Needle Railroad hire locos
HNRS	Harry Needle Railroad stored locos
HTLX	Hanson & Hall Rail Services
HVAC	Hanson & Hall Class 50
HYWD	South Western Railway Class 73
IECA	London North Eastern Railway Class 91
LSLO	Locomotive Services Ltd operational locos
LSLS	Locomotive Services Ltd stored locos
MBDL	Privately owned diesel locos
MBED	Privately owned electro-diesel locos
MBEL	Privately owned electric locos
MOLO	Class 20189 Locos owned traction
QADD	Network Rail owned locomotives
QCAR	Network Rail Class 43s
QETS	Network Rail Class 97 (37)
RAJV	Scottish Railway Preservation Society Class 37
RTLO	Privately owned Shunting locos
SAXL	Eversholt Rail stored locos
SBXL	Porterbrook Leasing stored locos
SROG	Rail Operations Group stored locos
TPEX	TransPennine Express Class 68
UKRL	UK Rail Leasing operational locos
UKRS	UK Rail Leasing stored locos
WAAC	DB Cargo Class 67
WABC	DB Cargo Class 67 fitted with RETB
WAWC	DB Cargo Class 67 on hire to TFW
WBAE	DB Cargo Class 66 fitted with auto-start
WBAR	DB Cargo Class 66 fitted with remote monitoring
WBAT	DB Cargo Class 66
WBBE	DB Cargo Class 66 with RETB and auto-start
WBBT	DB Cargo Class 66 with RETB
WBEN	DB Cargo Class 66 working in France
WBEP	DB Cargo Class 66 working in Poland
WBLE	DB Cargo Class 66 with Lickey incline mods
WCAT	DB Cargo Class 60
WCBT	DB Cargo Class 60 with extended fuel capacity
WEAC	DB Cargo Class 90
WEDC	DB Cargo Class 90 with Mk4 passenger stock mods
WFBC	DB Cargo Class 92 fitted with TVM430 for HS1 use
WQAA	DB-Cargo stored locos - short term
WQAB	DB-Cargo stored locos
WQBA	DB-Cargo stored locos - not operational
WQCA	DB-Cargo stored locos - not operational
XHAC	Direct Rail Services Class 37/4 and Class 57/3
XHCE	Direct Rail Services with Chiltern Railways modifications
XHIM	Direct Rail Services locos for Intermodal traffic
XHSO	Direct Rail Services Operational
XHTP	Direct Rail Services locos for TransPennine use
XHVE	Direct Rail Services Class 68 and Class 88
XHVT	Direct Rail Services Class 57/3 for use on Avanti West Coast
XWSS	Direct Rail Services Stored

Multiple Unit Coach Types

BDMSO	Battery Driving Motor Standard Open
DM	Driving Motor
DMC	Driving Motor Composite
DMCL	Driving Motor Composite Lavatory
DMCO	Driving Motor Composite Open
DMF	Driving Motor First
DMRFO	Driving Motor Restaurant First Open
DMS	Driving Motor Standard
DMSO	Driving Motor Standard Open
DMSL	Driving Motor Standard Lavatory
DTC	Driving Trailer Composite
DTCO	Driving Trailer Composite Open
DTLO	Driving Trailer Luggage Open
DTPMV	Driving Trailer Parcels Mail Van
DTRF	Driving Trailer Restaurant First
DTS	Driving Trailer Standard
DTSO	Driver Trailer Standard Open
MBS	Motor Brake Standard
MC	Motor Composite
MF	Motor First
MLO	Motor Luggage Open
MPMV	Motor Parcels Mail Van
MS	Motor Standard
MSO	Motor Standard Open
MSL	Motor Standard Lavatory
MSRB	Motor Standard Restaurant Buffet
MSRMB	Motor Standard Restaurant Miniature Buffet
PDTF	Pantograph Driver Trailer First
PDTRF	Pantograph Driving Trailer Restaurant First
PDTS	Pantograph Driving Trailer Standard
PMS	Pantograph Motor Standard
PP	Power Pack
PTRMB	Pantograph Trailer Restaurant Miniature Buffet
PTF	Pantograph Trailer First
PTS	Pantograph Trailer Standard
PTSO	Pantograph Trailer Standard Open
PTSOL	Pantograph Trailer Standard Open Lavatory
PTSW	Pantograph Trailer Standard Wheelchair
TBK	Trailer Buffet Kitchen
TBF	Trailer Brake First
TC	Trailer Composite
TF	Trailer First
TLO	Trailer Luggage Open
TPMV	Trailer Parcels Mail Van
TS	Trailer Standard
TSO	Trailer Standard Open
TSOL	Trailer Standard Open Lavatory

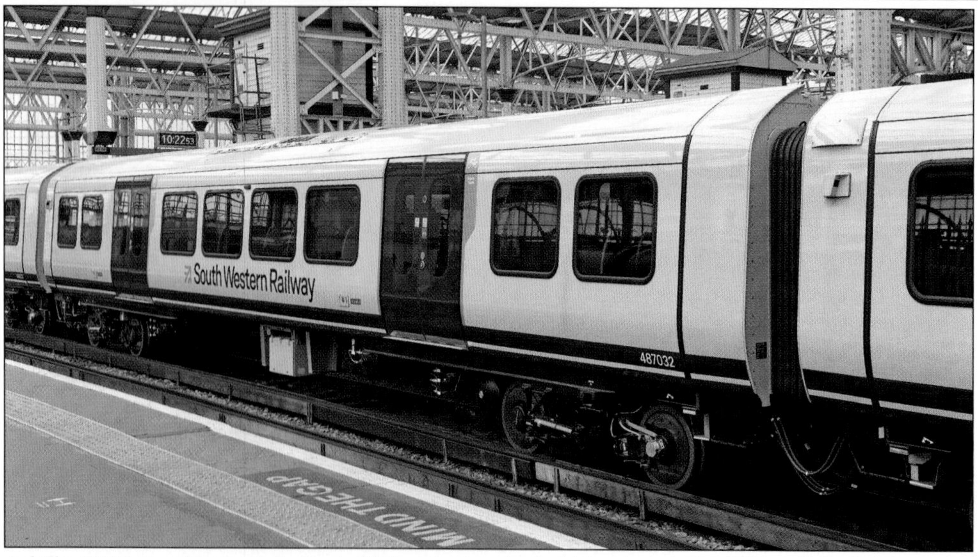

Each Class 701 10-car set have two Trailer Standard (TS) coaches, formed as the third coach from each end of the train. On five-car sets, one TS coach is formed in the middle of the consist. In full South Western Railway grey and blue livery, TS No. 487032 from set 701032 is seen at Waterloo in September 2021. **CJM**

Coupling Types

A. BSI Coupling. 1: Emergency air connection, 2: Main coupling with gathering horn, 3: Electrical connection box, 4: Main reservoir air connection.

B. Tightlock Coupling. 1: Emergency air connection, 2: Manual release handle, 3: Semi rotary electric/pneumatic cover, 4: Physical Tightlock coupling.

C. Dellner Coupling. 1: Emergency air connection, 2: Dellner coupling face, 3: Pneumatic (main reservoir) connection, 4: Roller cover to protect electrical connections, 5: Emergency air supply line.
All: **CJM**

Front End Equipment

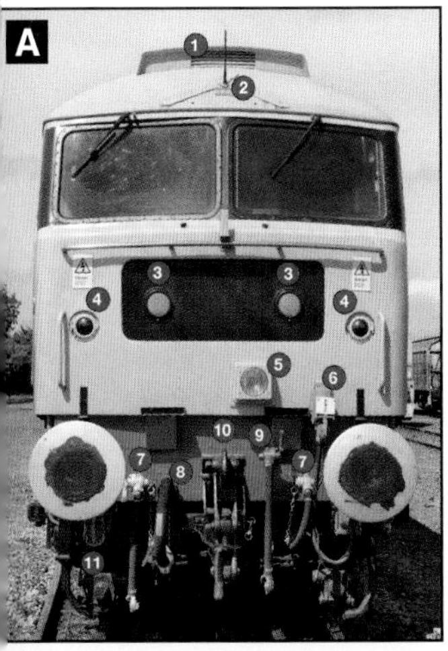

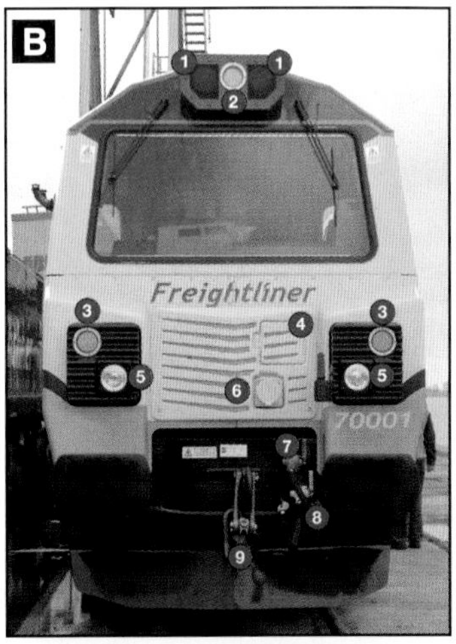

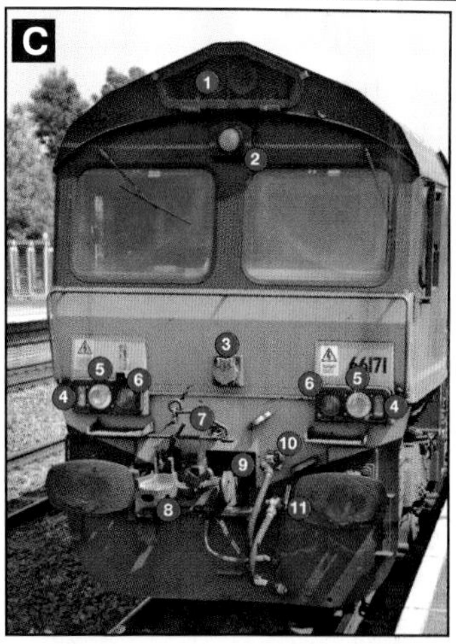

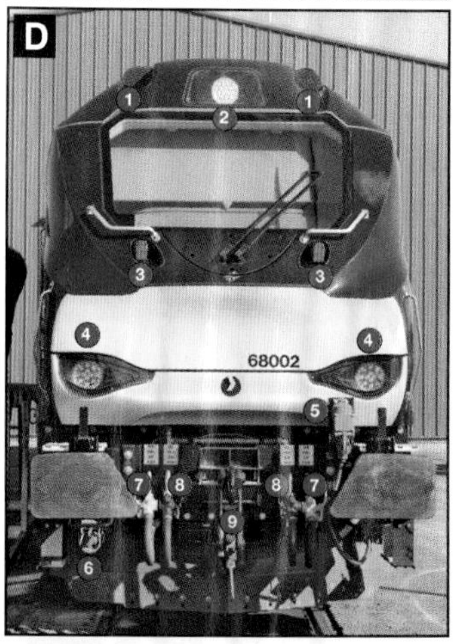

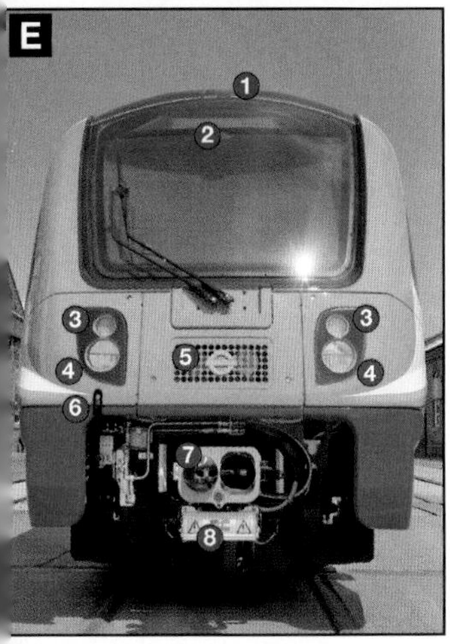

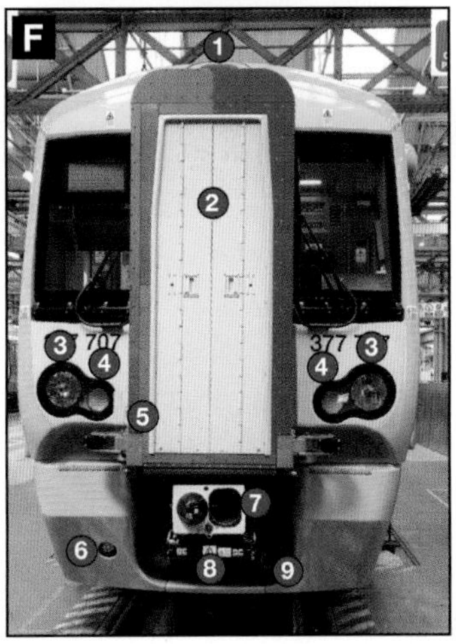

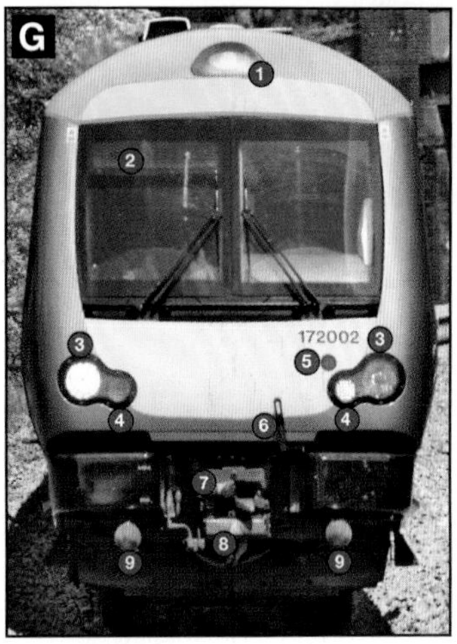

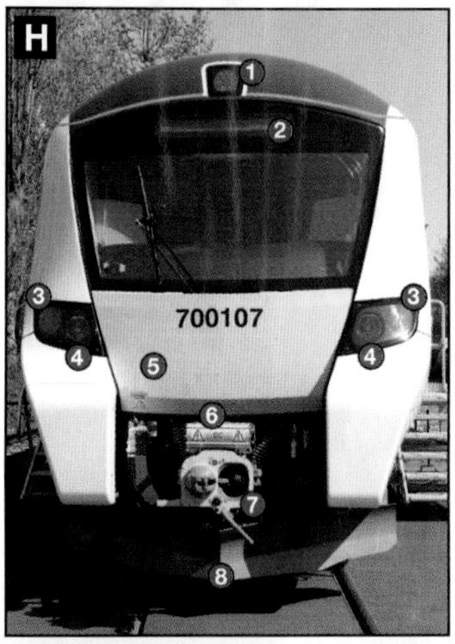

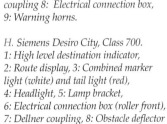

Throughout *Rail123*, we see and discuss the wide number of different front end designs in respect of equipment carried and how it is positioned. Standard design is something the rail industry just does not have. Here we show nine different designs, to try and assist readers to understand the equipment fitted. A trains front end has three main functions, to provide a safe location for the driver with a good clear view of the track ahead, a method of attachment to another train and provide a warning of either the trains front or rear end using lights.

A. A traditional main line diesel, Class 47. 1: Warning horn grille, 2: Radio aerial, 3: Marker lights (white), 4: Tail lights (red), 5: Headlight, 6: Electric train supply jumper cable, 7: Main reservoir pipe, 8: Vacuum brake pipe, 9: Air brake pipe, 10: Coupling hook and shackle, 11: Electric train supply jumper socket.

B. Class 70. 1: Warning horns behind grilles, 2: High level marker light, 3: Combined marker (white) and tail light (red), 4: Windscreen washer filler port, 5: Headlight, 6: AAR type multiple control jumper socket (cable stowed in cab cross-walk). 7: Air brake pipe, 8: Main reservoir pipe, 9: Coupling hook and shackle.

C. Class 66. 1: Warning horns behind grille, 2: High level marker light, 3: AAR type multiple control jumper socket (cable stowed in engine compartment), 4: Marker light (white), 5: Headlight, 6: Tail light (red), 7: Combination coupler release mechanism, 8: Combination swing head coupling, 9: Coupling hook (shackle stowed in engine compartment), 10: Air brake pipe, 11: Main reservoir pipe.

D. Class 68 (also applicable to Class 88). 1: Warning horn, 2: High level marker light, 3: Multiple working jumper cable sockets (cable stowed in engine compartment), 4: Joint head, marker and tail light, 5: Electric train supply jumper cable, 6: Electric train supply jumper socket, 7: Main reservoir pipe, 8: Air brake pipe, 9: Coupling hook and shackle.

E. Class 710 (Bombardier Aventra EMU). 1: Cant rail height marker light, 2: Destination display, 3: Combined white marker and red tail light (LED type), 4: Headlight, 5: Warning horns behind grille, 6: Emergency lamp bracket, 7: Dellner coupling, 8: Electrical connection box with roller cover.

F. Class 377, also applicable to Class 375 and 385. 1: High level marker light, 2: Gangway doors, 3: Headlight, 4: Combined white marker / red tail light, 5: Lamp bracket, 6: Track light, 7: Dellner coupling, 8: Electrical connection box, 9: Warning horns, located within coupling pocket.

G. Modern 'Turbostar' DMU, Class 172. 1: High level marker light, 2: Destination indicator, 3: Headlight, 4: Combined marker light (white) and tail light (red), 5: forward facing camera, 6: fold away lamp bracket, 7: BSI coupling 8: Electrical connection box, 9: Warning horns.

H. Siemens Desiro City, Class 700. 1: High level destination indicator, 2: Route display, 3: Combined marker light (white) and tail light (red), 4: Headlight, 5: Lamp bracket, 6: Electrical connection box (roller front), 7: Dellner coupling, 8: Obstacle deflector

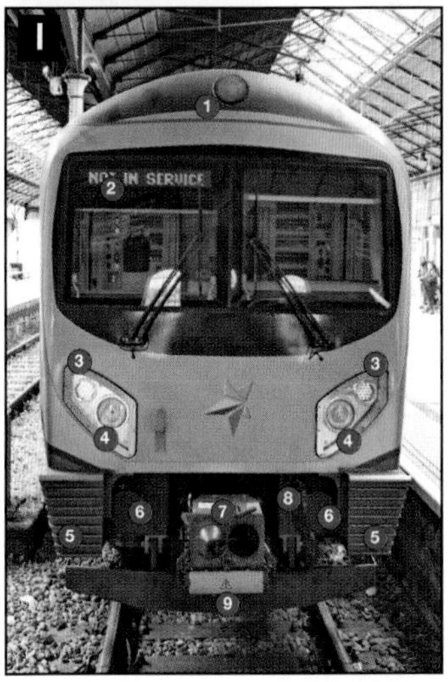

plate (snowplough).

I. Class 185. 1: High level marker light, 2: Destination indicator, 3: Combined marker light (white) and tail light (red), 4: Headlight, 5: Anti-climber blocks, 6: Warning horns, 7: Dellner 12 coupling, 8: Coupling air supply, 9: Electrical connection box (roller front).
CJM / Antony Christie

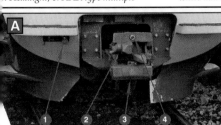

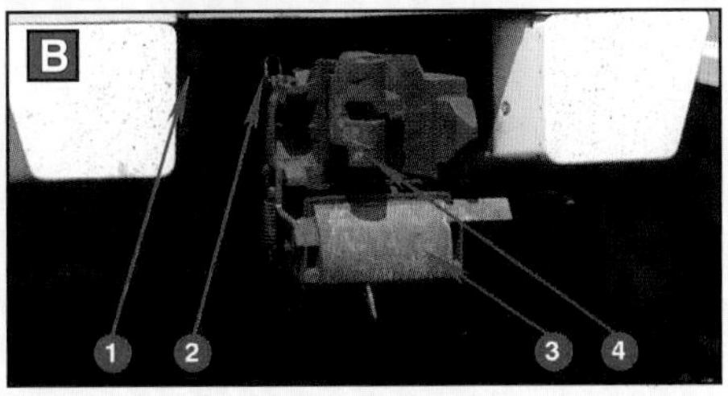

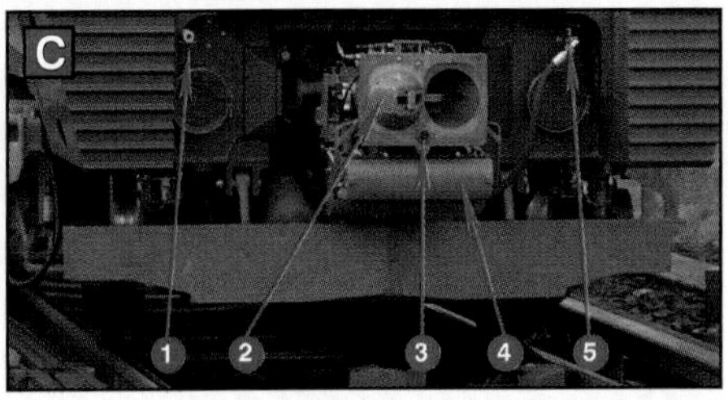

Loco and Multiple Unit Depots and Servicing Facilities

National Network

AD	Ashford
AK	Ardwick
AL	Aylesbury
AN	Allerton
AZ	Alizay, France
BD	Birkenhead North
BF	Bedford
BH	Barrow Hill
BI	Brighton
BM	Bournemouth
BN	Bounds Green
BO	Bo'ness
BQ	Bury ELR
BU	Burton
BY	Bletchley
CB	Crewe Basford Hall
CD	Castle Donnington
CE	Crewe Electric
CF	Cardiff Canton
CH	Chester
CK	Corkerhill
CL	Crewe LSL
CN	Castle Donnington
CQ	Coquilles
CR	Crewe Gresty Bridge
CS	Carnforth WCRC
CV	Cardiff Canton (TFW)
CY	Crewe CS
CZ	Central Rivers
DN	Doncaster IET
DR	Doncaster
DY	Derby
EC	Edinburgh Craigentinny
EL	Ely
EH	Eastleigh
EM	East Ham
EX	Exeter
FL	Freightliner - various
GA	Gascogne Wood
GW	Glasgow Shields Road
HA	Haymarket
HC	Hope cement plant
HE	Hornsey
HJ	Hoo Junction
HN	Hamilton, Assenta Rail
HQ	Headquarters
HT	Heaton
IL	Ilford
IS	Inverness
KK	Kirkdale
KM	Carlisle Kingmoor
KR	Kidderminster, SVR
LA	Laira
LD	Leeds Midland Road
LE	Landore
LN	Longtown
LM	Long Marston
LR	Leicester
LT	Longport
LY	La Landy
MA	Manchester International
MB	Mod Bicester
MD	Merehead
MN	Machynlleth
NC	Norwich Crown Point
NG	New Cross Gate
NH	Newton Heath
NL	Neville Hill
NM	Nottingham Eastcroft
NN	Northampton
NR	North Norfolk Railway
NP	North Pole
NT	Northampton
NY	North Yorkshire Moors Railway
OC	Old Oak Common

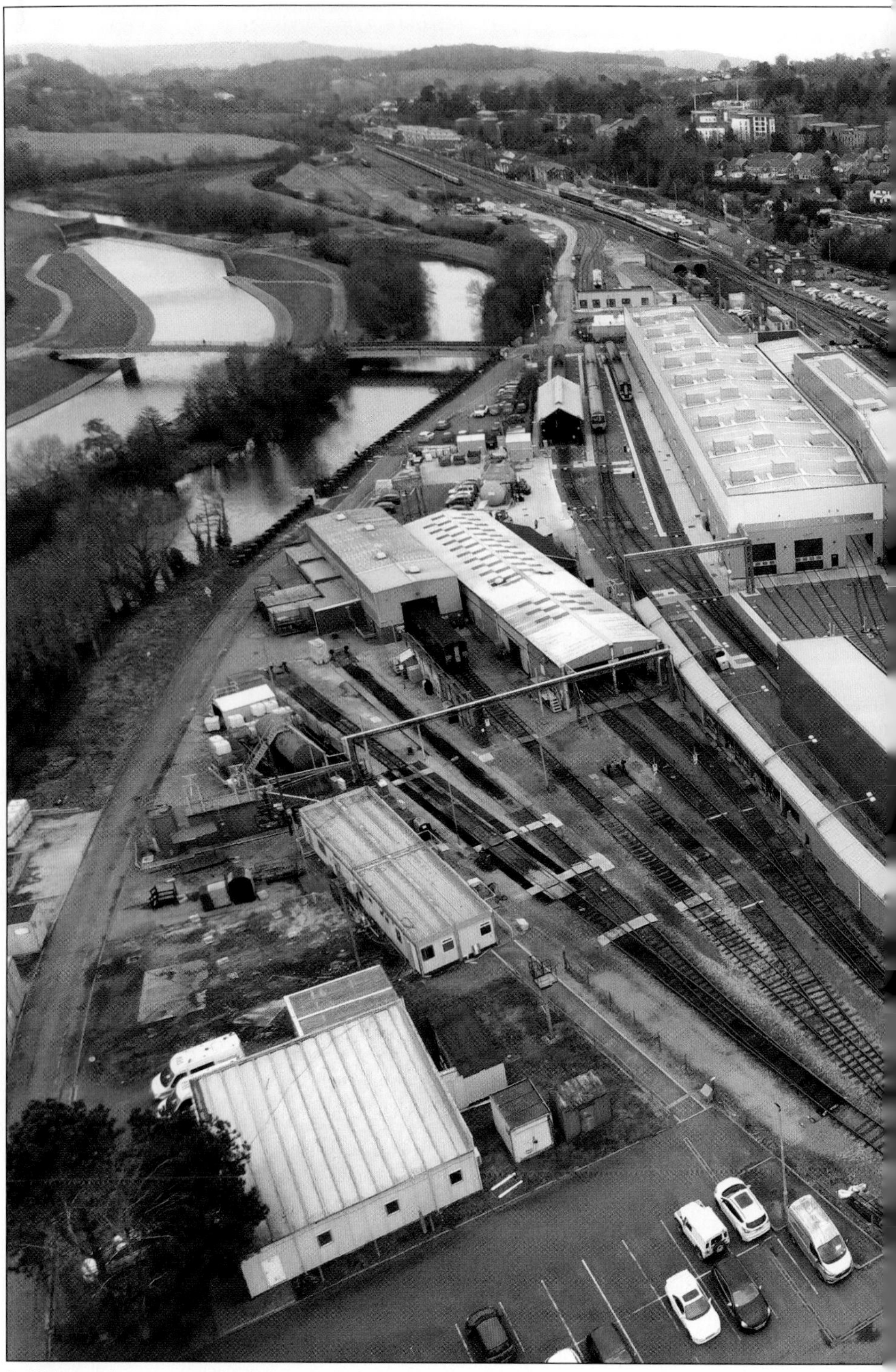

In 2021 a new depot was opened at Exeter to look after the West fleet of GW Class 150, 158 and 166 units operating in the Devon and Cornwall area. Located adjacent to Exeter St Davids station, a large admin building houses the local staff accommodation. The depot is also equipped to handle 2+4 HST 'Castle' sets and IETs if needed. This aerial view of the depot was captured in February 2022 and shows examples of Class 150, 158 and 166 stock 'on shed', while 'Voyager' IET and 150 sets are seen in St Davids station. **Mark Gibbs**

A sizable Scottish Railways depot is located in the triangle of lines next to Inverness station, which handles Class 158 and 170 DMU stock as well as HST stock operated on the Scottish I7C services. This is one of the few depots which still maintains the use of a Class 08 pilot loco. No. 08523 with power cars 43032 and 43168 are seen on shed on 17 October 2018. **Antony Christie**

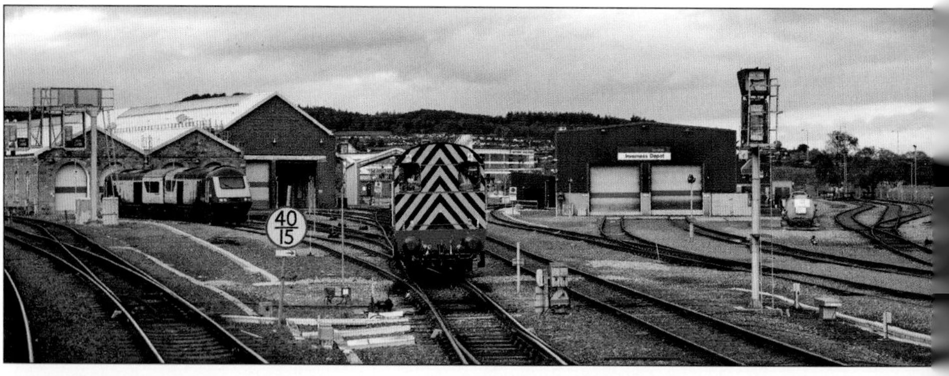

OD	Old Dalby
OY	Oxley
PM	St Philips Marsh
PN	Poznan, Poland
PO	Polmadie
PZ	Penzance
RG	Reading
RJ	Rectory Junction
RM	Ramsgate
RR	Roberts Road
RU	Rugby
RY	Ryde
SA	Salisbury
SC	Scunthorpe Steelworks
SE	St Leonard's
SG	Slade Green
SH	Southall
SI	Soho
SK	Swanick Junction
SL	Stewart's Lane
SP	Springs Branch
SU	Selhurst
SW	Swanage SR
TB	Three Bridges
TI	Temple Mills
TM	Tyseley Loco Works
TN	Tonbridge
TO	Toton
TS	Tyseley
WB	Wembley
WD	Wimbledon
WN	Willesden
WO	Wolsingham
WS	Worksop
YM	Yarmouth
ZA	Derby RTC
ZB	Doncaster Works
ZG	Eastleigh Works
ZH	Springburn Works
ZM	Brodie, Kilmarnock
ZN	Wolverton Works
ZR	York Holgate

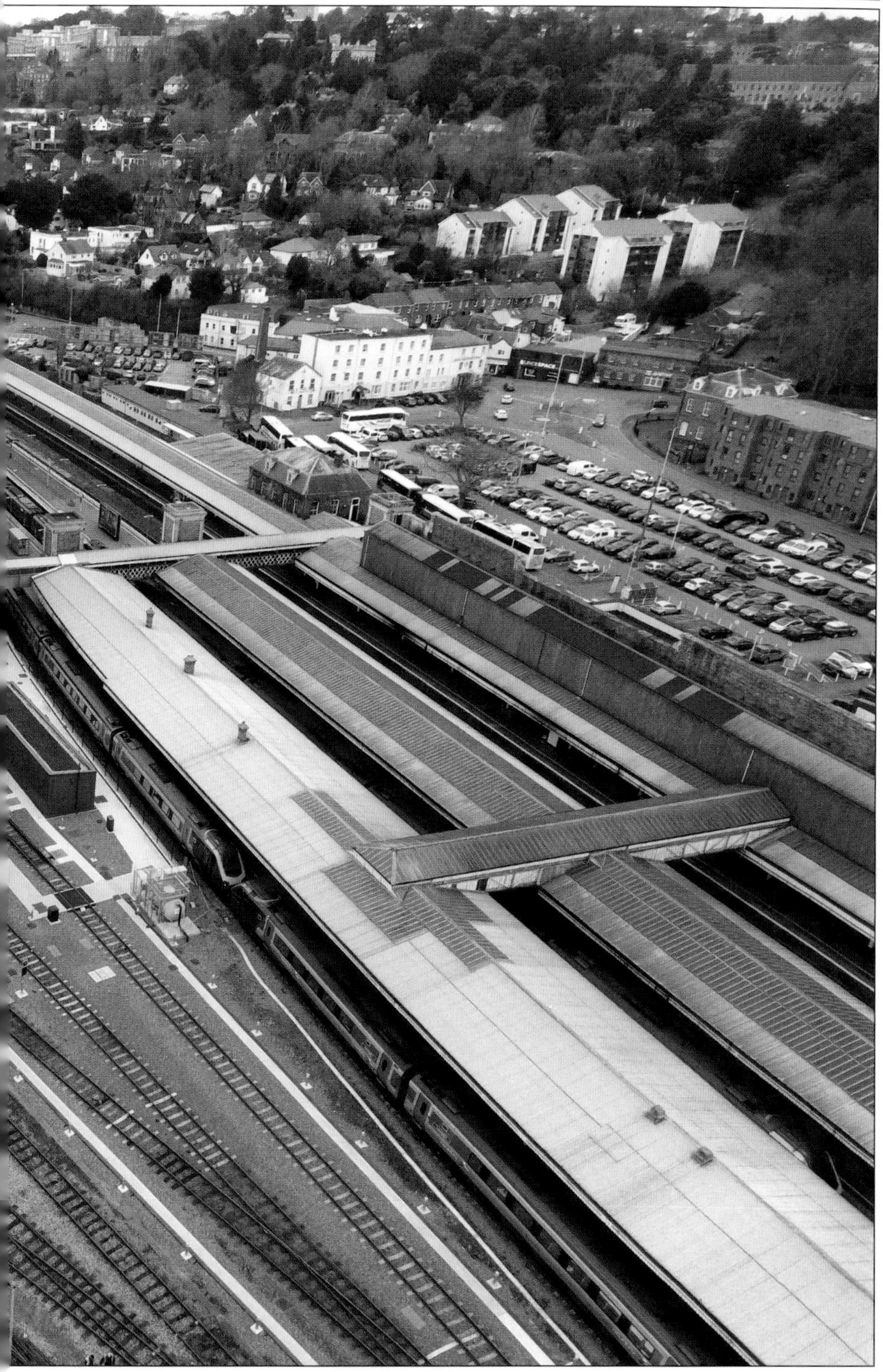

London Transport

Cockfosters (Piccadilly)
Golders Green (Northern)
Ealing Common (Circle/H&C)
Hainault (Central)
Morden (Northern)
Neasden (Metropolitan)
Northfields (Piccadilly)
Northumberland Park (Victoria)
Ruislip (Central)
Stonebridge Park (Northern)
Stratford Market (Jubilee)
Upminster (Circle H&C)
Waterloo (Waterloo & City)

Most of the London Underground lines concentrate fleet maintenance on one or two main depots, with stabling and overnight cleaning done at major turn round points. This is a view of the large Piccadilly Line depot at Northfields, which is responsible along with Cockfosters depot for the upkeep of the 516 cars of 1972 stock. **Antony Christie**

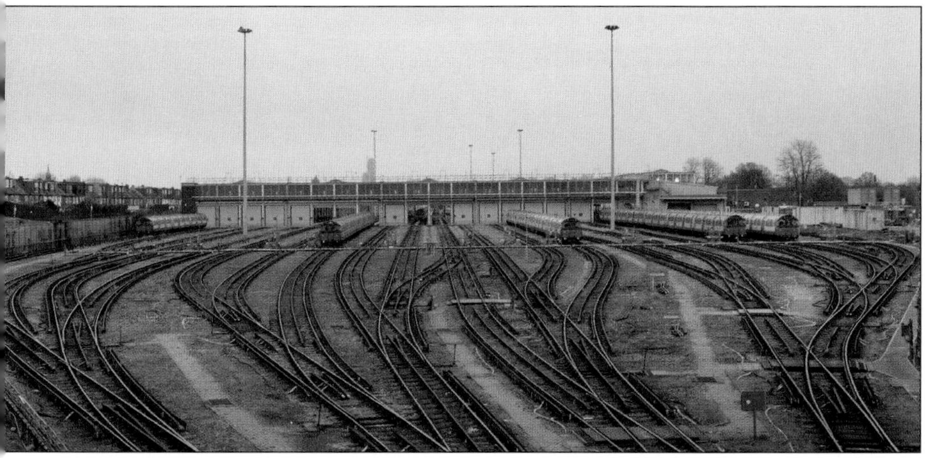

Light Rail

Coydon Tramlink	Therapia Lane
Docklands Light Rail	Beckton, Poplar
Edinburgh Tramway	Gogar
Blackpool	Star Gate
Blackpool Heritage	Rigby Road
Manchester Metrolink	Queens Road, Trafford
West Midlands Metro	Wednesbury
Nottingham Tramway	Wilkinson Street
South Yorkshire Super Tram	Nunnery
Tyne & Wear Metro	Gosforth, Howdon
Glasgow Subway	Broomloan

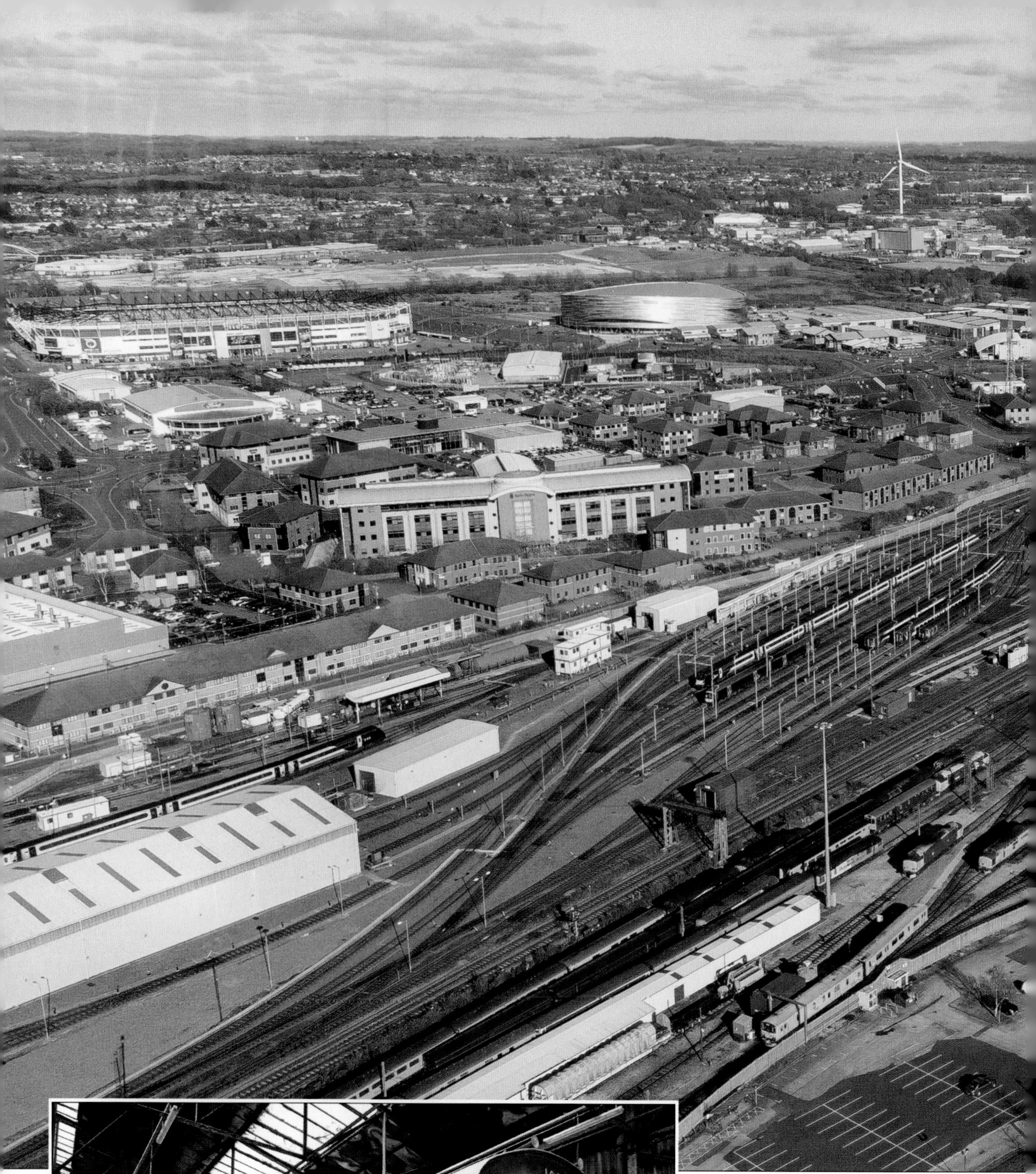

One of the most important sites and facilities in the UK is the Railway Technical Centre, located in Derby. For many years this has been the headquarters of the CM&EE and BR Research. Today, it is operated as a multi-function site, including Network Rail, Loram UK Ltd and many other engineering-based businesses. The facilities and yard, full of Network Rail rolling stock is seen in this 27 March 2022 view. The main Derby-Trent Junction line runs adjacent to the site and beyond is the ever expanding East Midlands Railway Derby Etches Park facility, with workshops to the left and right and stabling sidings towards the centre. On the far right, are the sidings of Alstom Derby Litchurch Lane. **Steve Donald**

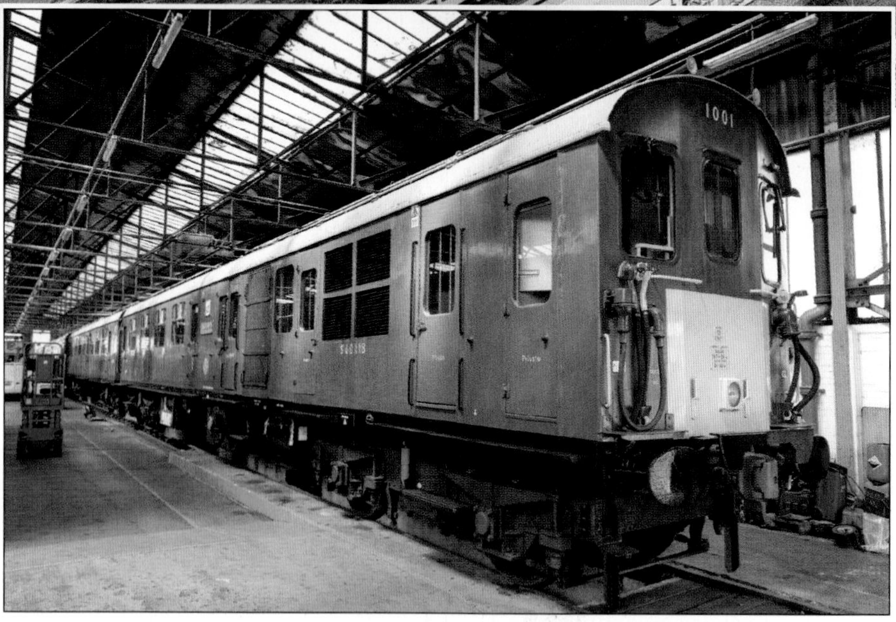

The former DEMU 'Hastings' depot at St Leonards, Hastings is now operated by Hastings Diesels Ltd and is the home base and restoration site for the 'Hastings' fleet and some Class 205 vehicles. St Leonards also does contract work for TOC and FOCs, including GTR-Southern and GB Railfreight. Set No. 1001 in immaculate condition is seen inside the shed on 17 May 2022. **CJM**

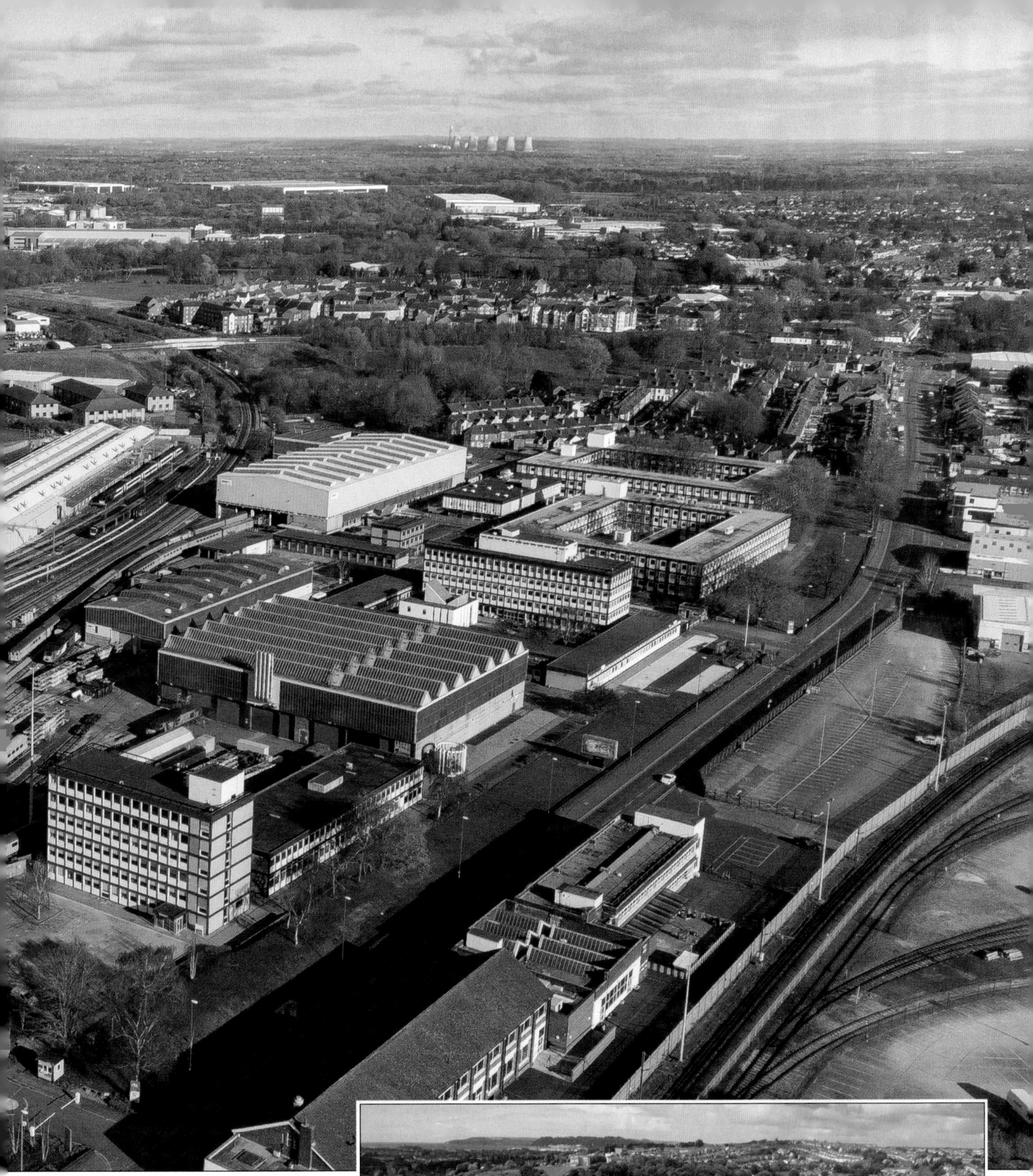

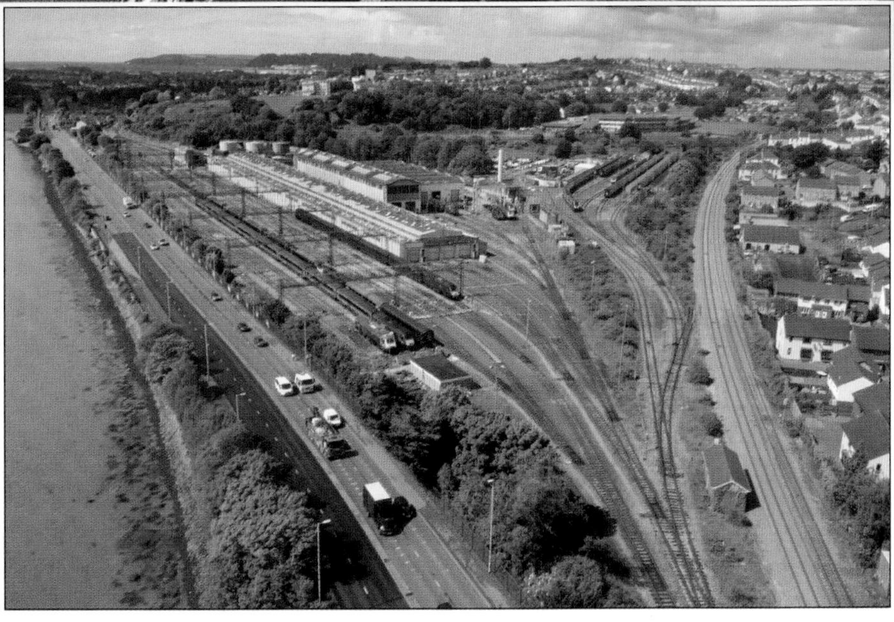

Great Western Railway operate a sizable facility at Plymouth Laira, once the home of GW steam locos and later the 'Warship', 'Western' and D6300 hydraulic fleets. After the demise of the hydraulic classes, the depot maintained the Class 50s and HST fleet. Today, Laira is the base for the 2+4 GWR 'Castle' sets, the CrossCountry HST fleet as well as performing maintenance and stabling of InterCity IET and 'Voyager' stock. This overall view of the depot recorded in May 2022 shows from left to right the stabling roads to the left, the 4-track HST/stock shed, the two road heavy repair bays, the four track maintenance shed, with further stabling sidings on the right. The two track GW main line to/from Plymouth is on the far right. **Eddie Holden**

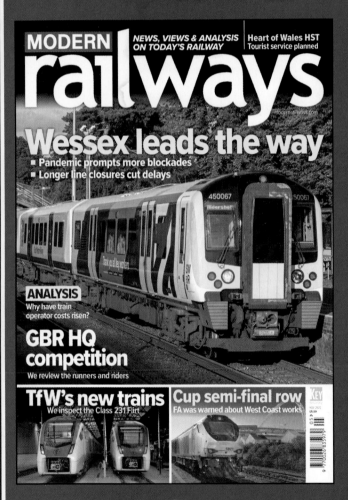

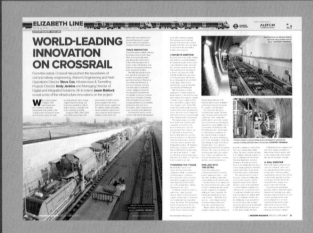